Pharmaceutical Dosage Forms

Capsules

Pharmaceutical Dosage Forms

Capsules

Edited by
Larry L. Augsburger
Stephen W. Hoag

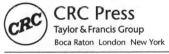

CRC Press
Taylor & Francis Group
Boca Raton London New York

CRC Press is an imprint of the
Taylor & Francis Group, an **informa** business

CRC Press
Taylor & Francis Group
6000 Broken Sound Parkway NW, Suite 300
Boca Raton, FL 33487-2742

First issued in paperback 2022

ISBN-13: 978-1-841-84976-8 (hbk)
ISBN-13: 978-1-03-233942-9 (pbk)
DOI: 10.1201/9781315111896

Library of Congress Cataloging-in-Publication Data

Names: Augsburger, Larry L., editor. | Hoag, Stephen W., editor.
Title: Pharmaceutical dosage forms. Capsules / [edited by] Larry L. Augsburger and Stephen W. Hoag.
Other titles: Capsules
Description: Boca Raton : CRC Press, [2017] | Includes bibliographical references and index.
Identifiers: LCCN 2017014862| ISBN 9781841849768 (hardback : alk. paper) | ISBN 9781315111896 (ebook)
Subjects: | MESH: Capsules--pharmacology | Drug Compounding
Classification: LCC RS200 | NLM QV 786.5.C3 | DDC 615.1/9--dc23
LC record available at https://lccn.loc.gov/2017014862

Visit the Taylor & Francis Web site at
http://www.taylorandfrancis.com

and the CRC Press Web site at
http://www.crcpress.com

We dedicate this book to Dr. Fridrun Podczeck whose untimely death prevented her from seeing its publication after having worked so hard on her chapters. Fridrun's long and valiant battle with her illness, as well as her strength of character as she dealt with its challenges, was simply amazing. An internationally recognized researcher in pharmaceutics and process engineering, Dr. Podczeck was one of the most productive pharmaceutical scientists of our time who made outstanding contributions to the underlying material and physicochemical science of solids and solid dosage forms, especially capsules. Her research significantly promoted systematic formulation development, rather than old-school pharmaceutical art and empiricism.

We also dedicate this book to our wives, Jeanette and Cathy, and our families whose loving forbearance makes all things we do possible, including editing and writing books. Thank you for all your love and support.

Contents

Preface

Invented more than 160 years ago, the capsule today is second only to the compressed tablet among solid dosage in frequency of utilization for drug delivery, and its utilization is growing. According to one estimate,* approximately 10–15% of FDA-approved drugs in 2014 were capsule formulations, about double that in 2007. Originally intended to mask the unpleasant taste of certain medications, today there are many other advantageous reasons and drivers for selecting the capsule for drug delivery, as discussed in the various chapters of this book. Despite the growing utilization of the capsule and the important roles it plays as a dosage form, the capsule has been relatively under-served in the literature. To our knowledge, there have been only two prior published edited texts[†,‡] devoted entirely to capsules, the most recent of which was published about 12 years ago. These books were intended to fulfill the need to provide in one place a concise summary of the making and filling of capsules, and of developing formulations for capsules. We are honored to have the opportunity to join the efforts of these prior editors in providing an updated discussion and description of capsule formulation and filling technology and the role of capsules in drug delivery. We are especially honored that Fridrun Podczeck, Brian E. Jones, and J. Michael Newton, editors and/or authors of chapters of those earlier books, have also contributed to this book.

---

* Seuffert K. HPMC capsules gain credibility as alternative to gelatin. *Tablets & Capsules* 2016; 14: 41–45.
† Ridgway K, ed., *Hard Capsules, Development & Technology*, London, The Pharmaceutical Press 1987.
‡ Podczeck F, Jones BE, eds., *Pharmaceutical Capsules*, 2nd edition, London, The Pharmaceutical Press 2004.

Editors

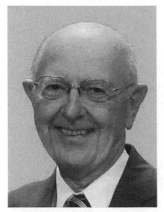

Larry L. Augsburger is an emeritus professor at the University of Maryland School of Pharmacy. He previously served as the Shangraw Professor of Industrial Pharmacy and Pharmaceutics, chair of the Department of Pharmaceutics, and director of Pharmaceutics Graduate Programs. A founding member of UPM Pharmaceuticals, Inc., he served for 5 years as UPM's VP of Pharmaceutical Development and Manufacture, and later as a senior scientific advisor. He was a senior research scientist for Johnson & Johnson before joining the Maryland faculty. His research has focused on the design and has optimization of immediate- and extended-release oral solid dosage forms for both their drug delivery performance and manufacturability, excipient functionality, and in later years, the quality and performance of botanical dietary supplement products. He was a principal investigator for and directed the research programs of the UM/FDA (US Food and Drug Administration) Collaborative Agreements that supported science-based FDA policies codified in "SUPAC" publications and guidance documents. His research has been disseminated through over 500 publications, abstracts, and presentations. He is an elected Fellow and former president of the American Association of Pharmaceutical Scientists (AAPS). Among others, his awards include FIP's Industrial Pharmacy Medal, FDA Commissioner's Special Citation, AAPS Outstanding Educator Award, AAPS Dale E. Wurster Research Award in Pharmaceutics, and the first Dr. Patricia Sokolove Outstanding Mentor Award from the UM Graduate School.

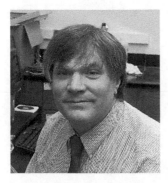

Stephen W. Hoag, PhD, is a professor of pharmaceutical sciences at the University of Maryland, Baltimore; he earned a PhD in pharmaceutics at the University of Minnesota–Twin Cities and a BS in biochemistry at the University of Wisconsin–Madison. Dr. Hoag has been a visiting professor at 3M Pharmaceuticals and Abbott Laboratories. His primary research interests are in the area of tablet and capsule formulation, excipient functionality testing, QbD, tablet coating, coating polymer formulation, tablet press instrumentation, and compaction modeling. His research has included studies in formulation and process development of tablets and capsules, formulation of folic acid in multivitamin and mineral supplements, controlled-release formulation, polymer science, pigment stability in coating polymers and thermal analysis of polymers, powder flow, and formulation stability. Hoag has studied the application of near-infrared spectroscopy to the analysis of excipient identification, tablet and capsule quality, and production monitoring for process analytical technology applications. He is also the director of the UMB GMP facility, and he has extensive experience using capsules to make clinical supplies for research studies. Dr. Hoag is a member of NIPTE (National Institute of Pharmaceutical Technology and Education) Executive Committee, he has been elected to the USP Counsel of Experts, he serves on the FDA compounding advisory committee, and he is an AAPS fellow. In addition, he serves on the International Steering Committee for the *Handbook of Pharmaceutical Excipients* and he serves on the editorial board of the *Journal of Pharmaceutical Development Technology*.

Contributors

Amusa Adebayo
Roosevelt University
Schaumburg, Illinois

Moji Christianah Adeyeye
Roosevelt University
Schaumburg, Illinois

Vikas Agarwal
TARIS Biomedical LLC
Lexington, Massachusetts

Larry L. Augsburger
University of Maryland
Baltimore, Maryland

Lawrence H. Block
Duquesne University
Pittsburgh, Pennsylvania

Stuart L. Cantor
Ei Solution Works
Kannapolis, North Carolina

Asish K. Dutta
Notre Dame of Maryland University
Baltimore, Maryland

Reza Fassihi
Temple University
Philadelphia, Pennsylvania

Pavan Heda
Johnson & Johnson
Medical Devices R&D
New Brunswick, New Jersey

Stephen W. Hoag
University of Maryland
Baltimore, Maryland

Brian E. Jones
Cardiff University
Cardiff, UK

Mansoor Khan
US Food and Drug Administration
Silver Spring, Maryland

Ammar Khawam
Boehringer Ingelheim Roxane Inc.
Columbus, Ohio

Michael Levin
Measurement Control Corporation
East Hanover, New Jersey

Donald K. Lightfoot
Independent Consultant
Tucson, Arizona

Paul Lukas
Technophar Equipment and Services
Tecumseh, Ontario, Canada

Vikas Moolchandani
Nutrilite
Buena Park, California

and

US Food and Drug Administration
Silver Spring, Maryland

Dennis Murachanian
Independent Consultant
Brick, New Jersey

J. Michael Newton
University College London
London, UK

Fridrun Podczeck*
University College London
London, UK

Shailesh K. Singh
Assembly Biosciences, Inc.
Carmel, Indiana

*Deceased

Sven Stegemann
Graz University of Technology
Graz, Austria

and

Capsugel
Bornem, Belgium

Huiquan Wu
US Food and Drug Administration
Silver Spring, Maryland

Lin Xie
Merck & Co. Inc.
Kenilworth, New Jersey

1 Advances in Capsule Formulation Development and Technology

Larry L. Augsburger and Stephen W. Hoag

CONTENTS

Among solid dosage forms, the capsule is second only to the compressed tablet in frequency of utilization for drug delivery, and the hard shell capsule continues to be the more frequently used form. Because hard shell capsules are often perceived as "simpler" than other oral dosage forms, they are frequently the first dosage form administered to humans and sometimes the final marketed dosage form. Even when the marketed product is to be a tablet, firms may sometimes make a tablet formulation and initially fill it in hard shell capsules to facilitate clinical testing. During the past 15 years or so, there have been several interesting and important advances in capsule formulation science and technology, including (1) alternative (to gelatin) shell compositions and enhanced shell function such as enteric capsules, (2) unique drug delivery systems, (3) using capsules to manage poorly soluble drugs, (4) filling small doses of drugs into capsules without excipients, (5) capsule filling machine simulation, and (6) application of artificial intelligence and other modeling methods in support of formulation development and Quality by Design (QbD).

ALTERNATIVE SHELL COMPOSITIONS

Capsules made from gelatin continue to predominate; however, recent years have seen an increased interest in and utilization of hard and soft non-gelatin capsules. Such alternative shell compositions may be preferred to satisfy religious, cultural, or vegetarian needs to avoid animal sources and because they may offer some important technological advantages. In Chapter 4, Brian Jones, Fridrun Podczeck, and Paul Lukas discuss the manufacture of hard and soft capsule shells formed from both gelatin and alternative shell compositions. They also address the historical development of capsule making and such topics as capsule sorting, printing, storage and quality. In Chapter 5, Sven Stegemann addresses non-gelatin-based capsules specifically, focusing particularly on such topics as hypromellose capsules, pullulan capsules, thermogelation, and capsule performance.

The improved capsule performance includes new developments in delayed release capsules designed to avoid the stomach and deliver their contents to the small intestine and colon.

UNIQUE DRUG DELIVERY SYSTEMS

Modern filling technology enables the filling into hard shell capsules of various combinations of diverse systems, for example, beads/granules, tablets, liquid/semisolids, small soft gelatin capsules, or smaller hard shell capsules. This ability to produce multicomponent capsules offers formulators many options in dosage form design.[1] Incompatibilities can be overcome by separating problem ingredients within the same capsule; for example, one component could be filled as a coated pellet. Novel modified or controlled drug delivery systems can be created by combining modified-release beads or granules and immediate-release formulations in the same capsule. In some configurations, drugs with pharmacokinetic properties that require different modified-release profiles can be filled into the same capsule as different species of beads. These modern capsule and formulation approaches are discussed in detail in Chapter 6, where Donald Lightfoot reviews capsule filling machines and how various components can be filled into capsules, and in Chapter 12, where Reza Fassihi discusses modified-release delivery systems and strategies for formulating controlled-release capsules. In addition to being a unique delivery system, capsules can come in a wide range of colors and can have unique logos printed on them. The ability to create a unique appearance is very advantageous to the marketing of capsule products. For example, most US consumers have probably seen an ad for the purple pill and this unique color really helps to create a product brand identity. Dennis Murachanian in Chapter 2 discusses these latter issues.

Capsules have always played an important role in early development stages. The PIC (powder in capsule) direct filling of small doses of drugs into capsules without excipients is another unique delivery system that has gained much attention in recent years and increases this important role. PIC direct filling of actives potentially offers a number of advantages, such as reduced time of getting candidates into Phase I clinical trials, reduced waste of API early on when only limited amount is available, fewer technical problems, and no formulation development. In their chapter on hard shell capsules in clinical trials (Chapter 3), Moji Adeyeye and Amusa Adebayo discuss PIC filling, including equipment and methods, potential advantages, and limitations.

LIQUID AND SEMISOLID CAPSULE FILLING

Historically the domain of soft gelatin capsules, which are inherently hermetically sealed as they formed and filled, modern technology has made possible the practical filling of liquids or semisolid matrices into both soft and hard shell capsules. Filling liquids into hard shell capsules was once popular up until the 1900s, but fell into disuse due to leakage problems.[2] The development of self-locking capsules, sealing techniques such as banding and liquid sealing, and high resting-state viscosity fills have now made liquid/semisolid filled hard shell capsules a feasible dosage form.[3] Brian Jones, Fridrun Podczeck, and Paul Lukas discuss in Chapter 4 the manufacture of both hard and soft capsules. In Chapter 6, Donald Lightfoot discusses the liquid filling and sealing equipment for hard shell capsules. The rheological aspects of hard and soft shell capsule filling are discussed by Lawrence Block in Chapter 14.

Capsules may be filled with a single liquid, a combination of miscible liquids, a solution of a drug in a liquid, or a suspension of a drug in a liquid, provided the liquid does not have an adverse effect on the shell walls.[4] In general, semisolid matrices consist of high proportions of solid material dispersed in a liquid phase. Often active ingredients are dissolved or suspended in a thermosoftening base, that is, waxy or fatty substances requiring that the formulation be filled into the capsule as a melt. Suitable thermosoftening excipients are liquid at filling temperatures up to ~70°C and solid or semisolid in the capsule at room temperature. These include such materials as hydrogenated vegetable oils, carnauba wax, cocoa butter, fatty derivatives (e.g., Gelucires), and certain molecular weight grades of polyethylene glycol.

In other semisolid matrices, the liquid formulation containing the active ingredient may be thickened by the addition of an excipient such as colloidal silicon dioxide to form a thixotropic gel.[5] Thixotropic gels undergo shear thinning when agitated and thus are pumpable: when agitation stops, the system rapidly reestablishes a gel structure.

Liquid/semisolid filled capsules offer numerous advantages in both technology and drug delivery.[6–11] In liquid/semisolid filled capsules, the drug is a liquid or a solid dissolved, solubilized or suspended in a liquid vehicle. The liquid fill is metered into individual capsules via high-precision pumps, thereby achieving a much higher degree of reproducibility than is possible with the powder or granule flow and feed required for the manufacture of dry filled capsules. Furthermore, a far higher degree of homogeneity is possible in liquid systems than can be achieved in typical dry powder blends. Volatile drugs and drugs subject to atmospheric oxidation often may also be formulated satisfactorily in sealed liquid/semisolid filled capsules.[12]

The liquid/semisolid matrix capsule platform also provides formulators with an important tool for addressing poor drug aqueous solubility, which can lead to variable and poor bioavailability. Formulating the drug substance in solution or solubilized form essentially eliminates dissolution of the solid as a rate-limiting step. When the drug cannot be solubilized, it can be delivered as a dispersion of micronized or nanometer-sized particles in a suitable vehicle that promotes rapid dispersion of capsule contents and dissolution. A Vitamin E solid dispersion in Gelucire 44/14 melt filled in hard gelatin capsules was reported to exhibit increased bioavailability.[13] In an early study, Hom and Miskal[14,15] found more rapid *in vitro* dissolution rates of 20 drugs from soft gelatin capsules compared to tablets. In the soft shell capsules, the drugs were either dissolved in polyethylene glycol 400 or suspended in polyols or non-ionic surfactants. Single dose studies in man comparing the sedative temazepam as a powder-filled hard gelatin capsule and as a polyethylene glycol solution filled in soft-gelatin capsules revealed earlier and higher peak plasma levels from the polyethylene glycol formulation, although there was no significant difference in their total availabilities.[16] In still another example, digoxin dissolved in a polyethylene glycol 400, ethanol, propylene glycol, and water vehicle and filled in soft gelatin capsules elicited higher mean plasma levels in man during the first 7 h after administration than an aqueous solution or commercial tablets.[17] The AUCs (areas under the 14-h plasma concentration curves) were also greater for the soft shell capsule.

The liquid/semisolid matrix platform can also provide a practical solution to the problems of formulating with low-melting point and hygroscopic substances, as well as materials that are liquid at room temperatures. Smith et al. reported that ibuprofen, a low-melting point, thermostable drug, could be successfully filled into hard gelatin capsules as a melt using 10% or less of such excipients as AcDiSol, maize starch, arachis oil, stearic acid, beeswax, and others.[18] In another example, Doelker et al. demonstrated the successful filling of four liquid or deliquescent drugs (benzonatate, nicotinic acid, chloral hydrate, and paramethadione) in hard gelatin capsules using Gelucire excipients (glycerides and other fatty acid esters available with different hydrophilic–lipophilic balance [HLB] values) as the vehicle or matrix.[19] The drugs were first incorporated in the melted vehicle before pouring into the capsules. A successful stable semisolid matrix hard gelatin capsule product of the highly hygroscopic antibiotic vancomycin HCl by incorporating the drug in polyethlene glycol 6000 was reported by Bowtle et al.[20] This was the product Vancocin, originally developed by Eli Lilly and later licensed to Viro Pharma in 2004.

USING CAPSULES TO MANAGE POORLY SOLUBLE DRUGS

Currently, much interest is being focused on hard and soft shell capsules as vehicles for lipid-based drug delivery systems designed to improve the dissolution and bioavailability of poorly soluble, hydrophobic drug substances.[21,22] That lipids can enhance oral bioavailability has been well recognized and arises from observations that the bioavailability of some drugs increases when administered with food.

Lipid drug delivery systems may be solid/semisolid or liquid at room temperature. The drug is delivered essentially dissolved or solubilized in a lipid phase. Improved bioavailability from these systems is still under study, but is believed to involve at least solubilization and dispersal in physiological fluids with transfer to the bile salt mixed micellar phase from which absorption across the intestinal epithelium may readily occur.[23,24]

Lipid-based drug delivery systems can be complex compositions of three main classes of components: lipids, surfactants, and, possibly, cosolvents.[25,26] The lipid may be a single lipid or a blend of fatty materials. The most important lipids are fatty acids or their derivatives (e.g., mono-, di-, and triglycerides, and propylene glycol esters). They are either solid or liquid at room temperature, depending on their chain length and degree of unsaturation of the fatty acid chains. The presence of the surfactant (emulsifier) assists in the breakup and dispersion of the capsule content in gastrointestinal fluids. Typically, these are the non-ionic type (e.g., polyoxyl 40 stearate, polysorbate 80, and sorbitan monopalmitate) of varying HLB values. Cosolvents (e.g., alcohol, polyethylene glycol 400, and propylene glycol) may be included to help solubilize the drug substance.

Hard shell capsules liquid-filled with poorly soluble etodolac dispersed in a carrier consisting of Gelucire 44/14 and/or TPGS (D-α-tocopheryl polyethylene glycol 100 succinate) exhibited more rapid *in vitro* dissolution than the pure drug, owing possibly to increased wetting and micellization.[27] Stability studies (ICH guidelines) of the filled capsules revealed etodolac to be chemically stable under tested conditions, but changes in dissolution behavior that occurred after storage at high humidity and temperature were thought possibly related to formation of etodolac microcrystals and water absorption by the carrier during aging. A rapid vehicle screening method was proposed for developing suitable lipid-based formulations of low solubility compounds for hard gelatin capsules.[28]

Self-emulsifying lipid-based systems are unique compositions of these components with solubilized drug molecules, that is, physically stable isotropic mixtures that emulsify spontaneously in the presence of water with only gentle agitation, as may occur when delivered to the aqueous content of gastrointestinal tract where the gentle agitation is provided by digestive motility.[24] Emulsions (particle size greater than about 0.15 μm) may be formed if the ratio of surfactant to lipid is <1 or microemulsions (particle size less than about 0.15 μm) may be formed if the ratio is >1.[29] Nanoemulsions (<50 nm) may also be formed. The efficiency of "self-emulsification" appears to correlate strongly with the HLB of the surfactant, with values of 12–15 generally considered to have good efficiency.[29] Various acronyms have been used to describe these self-emulsifying systems, for example, SEDDS (self-nano-emulsifying drug delivery system), SMEDDS (self-emulsifying microemulsion drug delivery system), and SNEDDS (self-emulsifying nanoemulsion drug delivery system). The composition of drug, lipid(s), surfactant(s), and cosolvent is sometimes referred to as a "preconcentrate."[30] Initial interest in this dosage form may be attributable to the successful commercialization of Neoral, which consists of cyclosporine in a SMEDDS preconcentrate and which exhibited improved and more reliable bioavailability independent of food intake over the original Sandimmune.[31,32]

Such systems are usually studied and developed through the construction of pseudo-ternary phase diagrams, as illustrated in Figure 1.1, to identify the regions of interest. An excellent example of the use of such a diagram is a case study on the development of a SMEDDS delivery system for atorvastatin.[33] The lipid formulation was filled into capsules and the oral bioavailability of atorvastatin in dogs was increased nearly 150% over that of the conventional tablet formulation.

The broader adoption of SEDDS may in part be impeded by the limited solubility of some hydrophobic drugs in preconcentrates. Based on research with simvastatin SNEDDS, it has been suggested that supersaturation of the preconcentrate may be a feasible approach to increase drug loads and bioavailability.[34] Supersaturated preconcentrates containing up to 200% simvastatin (compared to 75% conventional loading) were formed by subjecting the preconcentrates to heating and cooling

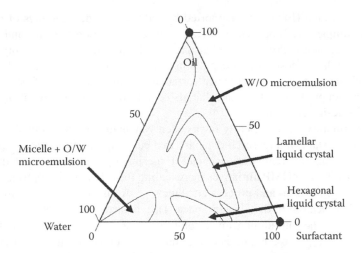

FIGURE 1.1 Diagrammatic ternary phase diagram for studying the relationship between oil, water and surfactant for self-emulsifying lipid-based drug delivery systems. (Adapted from JB Cannon, MA Long. Emulsions, microemulsions, and lipid-based drug delivery systems for drug solubilization and delivery— Part II: Oral applications. In: R. Liu, ed., *Water-Insoluble Drug Formulation*, 2nd edition, CRC Press, Boca Raton, FL, 2008, Chapter 11, pp. 227–254.)

cycles. In beagle dogs, the 200% super SNEDDS exhibited markedly greater bioavailability than the same dose in multiple units of the conventional SNEDDS.

The broader adoption of SEDDS in capsules may also be impeded by lack of stability on aging and possible adverse interactions of some preconcentrates with soft or hard shells. To remedy this problem, solid SEDDSs have been proposed, formed by such processes as spray drying or freeze drying the preconcentrate, and physical adsorption onto silica and silicate-based carriers.[35,36] The resultant powdery formulations, mixed as needed with suitable excipients, may be encapsulated or tableted.

SYSTEMATIC APPROACHES FOR UNDERSTANDING HARD SHELL CAPSULE FORMULATION AND FILLING

MODELING OF PLUG FORMATION

That most powder formulations are filled on machines that form powder plugs by compression and eject the plugs into capsules has stimulated interest in exploring filling machine operating characteristics and low-force compression physics. Advanced through the instrumentation of capsule filling machines and laboratory simulation of plug formation, discussed in Chapter 7, this research has revealed that several powder compression models (e.g., Heckel, Shaxby–Evans, and Kawakita) can be used to parameterize the low-force compression profiles related to capsule filling, as discussed by Podczeck in Chapter 9. Based in part on understandings developed through such research, a theoretical model was developed by Khawam, discussed in Chapter 10, that may prove to be useful as an *in silico* analysis tool for developing formulations for dosator machines that can be used in conjunction with other development tools, for example, experimental design/ response surface analysis.

MODELING IN SUPPORT OF FORMULATION DEVELOPMENT

More than ever before, pharmaceutical scientists are adopting systematic approaches to the design, formulation, and optimization of dosage forms. Driven in part by the QbD initiative of the US Food and Drug Administration (FDA) and supported by enhanced understandings of biopharmaceutic principles, for example, the Biopharmaceutical Drug Classification System, and software-driven optimization and decision-making tools, pharmaceutical scientists have the ability to make logical and deliberate formulation design decisions. Using such tools to model the interplay of formulation and process variables not only can enhance formulators' understanding of how formulation and process factors affect product performance but also can lead to an optimized drug delivery system with respect to its design criteria.

The current regulatory climate clearly favors such systematic development approaches. Systematic approaches can establish a research database that can help justify SUPAC (scale-up and post-approval changes) changes to regulatory agencies. Experimental design and modeling also supports FDA's QbD and risk-based cGMP initiatives by revealing the relationships between product quality attributes and critical material and process attributes.[37,38] An understanding of these relationships can lead to the identification of the Design Space (DS), a particularly useful QbD tool. The DS is formally defined as "The multidimensional combination and interaction of input variables (e.g., material attributes) and process parameters that have been demonstrated to provide assurance of quality."[39] Thus, these operational ranges determine the DS space within which movement is not considered a change for regulatory purposes.

Among the tools being employed by today's formulation scientists are multivariate analysis and response surface methodology[40,41] and artificial intelligence.[42-44] A discussion of the mathematical principles and statistical bases for these tools is beyond the scope of this discussion. For these, the interested reader is referred to Fridrun Podczeck's chapter entitled "Aims and Objectives of Experimental Design and Optimization in Formulation and Process Development"[45] and the Peng and Augsburger chapter on "Knowledge-Based Systems and Other AI Applications for Tableting,"[46] both of which appear in *Pharmaceutical Dosage Forms: Tablets*. However, several interesting examples of applications to hard shell formulation development have been selected for discussion here.

Multivariate Analysis and Response Surface Methodology

One example of response surface analysis applied to capsules examines the critical formulation variables for a piroxicam capsule formulation.[41] This example is particularly interesting because it links *in vitro* outcomes with *in vivo* outcomes in human subjects. Piroxicam is a BCS Class II drug (low solubility and high permeability) drug. Thirty-two batches of 20-mg piroxicam capsules were manufactured according to a *resolution V* central composite (face-centered) experimental design. Five formulation (independent) variables were studied at each of three levels (see Table 1.1 and

---

TABLE 1.1

Variables and Levels of the Piroxicam Capsule Study

Formulation or Process Variable	Level Studied		
	Low	Medium	High
Surfactant: sodium lauryl sulfate	0%	0.5%	1.0%
Lubricant: magnesium stearate	0.5%	1.0%	1.5%
Lubricant blend time	2 min	10 min	18 min
Filler (expressed as % lactose in binary mixtures with microcrystalline cellulose)	0%	50%	100%
Drug particle size (expressed as % milled [4.91 M^2/g] piroxicam in binary mixtures with unmilled [1.79 M^2/g] piroxicam)	0%	50%	100%

Source: DA Piscitelli, S Bigora, C Propst, S Goskonda, P Schwartz, L Lesko, LL Augsburger, D Young. The impact of formulation and process changes on in vitro dissolution and bioequivalence of piroxicam capsules. *Pharm Devel Tech* 1998; 3(4): 443–452.

additional comments in Chapter 15). Colloidal silica (glidant) and sodium starch glycolate (disintegrant) were fixed at 0.1% and 5%, respectively, in all batches. Because it is a BCS II drug, the effect of piroxicam particle size on drug dissolution was of particular importance. This aspect was evaluated by comparing the piroxicam powder as received (termed *unmilled* in the study) with the same lot of piroxicam that was remilled (termed *milled* in the study). The remilling of piroxicam substantially reduced its particle size, as reflected in a nearly threefold increase in its specific surface area from 1.79 to 4.91 m^2/g. The capsules were filled with a consistent plug compression force using an instrumented Zanasi LZ-64 automatic capsule filling machine. USP monograph dissolution profiles (% piroxicam dissolved vs. time) were obtained for the batches. Statistical analysis revealed a number of interesting insights. For example, the percent lactose, and an interaction between piroxicam particle size and sodium lauryl sulfate level were the most important variables affecting the percentage of piroxicam dissolved at 10 min. However, the most important variable affecting the percent dissolved in 45 min was the wetting agent, sodium lauryl sulfate, followed closely by piroxicam particle size. When the piroxicam is milled, the sodium lauryl sulfate level has comparatively little effect on dissolution (see Figure 1.2), presumably because the milled drug is more rapidly dissolving because of its larger specific surface area. The apparent reduced significance of the level of lactose at 45 min may be attributed to its complete dissolution by that time. Overall, the magnesium stearate level and its blending time were either not significant or among the least significant factors affecting piroxicam dissolution in these formulations. This observation may be largely explained by the ability of sodium lauryl sulfate to overcome the hydrophobicity of magnesium stearate. The water solubility of lactose and the presence of the disintegrant, sodium starch glycolate, may also help overcome hydrophobic lubricant effects.

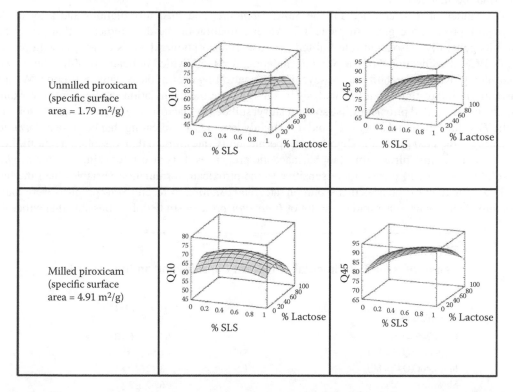

FIGURE 1.2 Effect of piroxicam-specific surface area, sodium lauryl sulfate (SLS), and lactose on dissolution. (Plotted from University of Maryland–FDA data [Food and Drug Administration, RFP 223-91-3401].) Q10 = percent dissolved in 10 min; Q45 = percent dissolved in 45 min; % SLS = percent sodium lauryl sulfate; % lactose = percentage of lactose in a binary filler consisting of a blend of lactose and microcrystalline cellulose.

Three formulations from this study having *Fast*, *Moderate*, and *Slow* dissolution were chosen for comparison to a lot of the innovator's product in a human bioavailability study.[41] The resulting pharmacokinetic data provided still another opportunity to examine the effects of formulation variables. Using the following previously developed deconvolution-based model (Equation 1.1),[47] Polli developed an *in vitro–in vivo* relationship (*IVIVR*) that pointed up the role of formulation in overcoming piroxicam's low solubility/high permeability properties.[48]

$$F_a = \frac{1}{f_a}\left(1 - \frac{\alpha}{\alpha-1}(1-F_d) + \frac{1}{\alpha-1}(1-F_d)^\alpha\right)$$
(1.1)

F_d is the fraction of the dose dissolved in time t, F_a is the fraction of the dose of the drug absorbed in time t, f_a is the fraction of the total amount of drug absorbed at $t = \infty$, and α is the ratio of the apparent first-order permeation rate constant, k_p^1, to the first-order dissolution rate constant, k_d. The model makes the following simplifying assumptions: apparent first-order permeability, first-order dissolution under sink conditions, drug is stable in the gastrointestinal lumen or at the gastrointestinal wall, *in vitro* and *in vivo* dissolution profiles are identical, and the absence of a lag time for permeation or dissolution. The term α is of particular interest to this discussion. If an analysis reveals $\alpha \gg 1$, the permeation rate constant is much greater than the dissolution rate constant and drug absorption is expected to be dissolution rate-limited. If $\alpha \ll 1$, then the permeation rate constant is much less than the dissolution rate constant, signifying that the rate-limiting step to absorption is intestinal permeation.

The values of α determined for the *Slow*, *Moderate*, and *Fast* formulations and a lot of the *Innovator* product are given in Table 1.2. An examination of the data indicates that piroxicam exhibits generally dissolution rate-limited (i.e., $\alpha > 1$) absorption, which is consistent with piroxicam's BCS classification. For the *Slow* formulation, $\alpha = 6.50$, which indicates that dissolution was dominating over permeability about sevenfold in controlling overall piroxicam absorption. What is particularly interesting about the analysis in Table 1.2 are the formulation implications. For example, the use of milled piroxicam, 1% sodium lauryl sulfate, and lactose filler so promoted dissolution in the *Fast* formulation that $k_d \cong k_p^1$ and α is slightly less than 1, indicating that because of *formulation design*, the *Fast* product is slightly more permeability rate-limited than dissolution rate-limited, thereby overcoming piroxicam's biopharmaceutic properties. It is also interesting that the *in vitro* dissolution test (USP) proved more sensitive to the piroxicam formulation variables than the biodata. Despite their differences in dissolution rate, the *Fast*, *Moderate*, and *Slow* products were found bioequivalent to each other and to the lot of *Innovator* product studied. It is possible that either the

TABLE 1.2
Values of α for Experimental Piroxicam Capsules and an Innovator Lot

Formulation	$\alpha = \dfrac{k_p^1}{k_d}, \pm SE$
Fast (Q45 = 95)	0.896 ± 0.138
Moderate (Q45 = 87)	1.54 ± 0.24
Innovator (Q45 = 80)	3.42 ± 0.84
Slow (Q45 = 65)	6.50 ± 2.17

Source: JE Polli. Analysis of in vitro–in vivo data. In: GL Amidon, JR Robinson, RL Williams, eds. *Scientific Foundations for Regulating Drug Products*. Arlington, VA, AAPS Press, 1997, pp. 335–351.

Note: Q45 = percent labeled content dissolved in 45 min; SE = standard error.

formulation variables studied did not affect *in vivo* dissolution or the differences were not discernible because of the long biological half-life of piroxicam.[49]

Statistical methods have also been applied to the formulation development of dry powder inhalation (DPI) capsules. Nearly half of marketed DPIs are single-dose delivery systems consisting of a powder formulation in a hard shell gelatin capsule. In practice, the capsule is punctured in a specially designed inhalation device and the powder is inhaled by the patient. In one example, Faulhammer et al.[50] undertook a study aimed at development of a predictive model for the filling of the typically low fill-weight capsule inhalation products with a dosator nozzle. Based on an assessment of the effects of the critical process parameters (CPPs) and critical material attributes (CMAs) on fill weight and weight variability, they developed and validated a predictive model for fill weight variation for two groups of powders: those that flow well and those that are cohesive. The model provided a "good approximation" of fill weight variability for each powder group and permitted the establishment of a DS for different types of inhalation grade lactose in low-fill weight capsule filling.

In another study of low-fill weight capsule filling, Faulhammer et al.[51] examined the effect of CMAs on the critical quality attributes (CQAs) of capsules filled on a dosator machine using six different grades of microcrystalline cellulose representing a wide range in physical properties. An experimental design was developed using four filling machine process parameters as controllable variables: dosator size, dosing chamber length (sometimes referred to as the *piston height* setting), powder layer height (often also called *powder bed height*), and filling speed. The data were analyzed by multivariate analysis with partial least squares regression (PLA). The Faulhammer group also used experimental design to evaluate the effect of these dosator machine process parameters on the capsules with various forms of lactose.[52] A partial least square (PLS) method was used to examine the correlations between the material properties and process parameters and capsule fill weight and weight variability.

Expert Systems

An expert system is a computer program that is constructed to emulate the decision making of human experts in a particular domain. Perhaps most commonly, an attempt is made to represent the knowledge of experts as a set of rules that express the relationship between various pieces of information in the form of conditional statements, represented mainly as if–then rules.[46] Bateman et al.[53] described a customized expert system for capsule formulations that incorporates the practices and policies of the Sanofi Research Center. Developed using Logica's PFES shell, knowledge acquired through a series of meetings with formulators was incorporated by encoding an appropriate set of rules that reproduce the formulation experts' decision making. Another component of the system important to making formulation decisions is an excipients database. Based on formulation experts' input, the most important properties to consider, for example, particle size, bulk density, acid–base reactivity, amine reactivity, aqueous solubility, hygroscopicity, and others were determined. Since information on these properties found in the literature is based on different analytical methods and couldn't be correlated, these measurements were made in-house. Preliminarily, the system was challenged by three chemical entities and the formulations generated were judged by experienced formulators to be acceptable for manufacture and initial stability evaluation.

Capsugel's CAPEX expert system for the formulation of powders in hard gelatin capsules was developed as a centralized system that incorporates broad, worldwide industrial experience.[54] Development of the system was begun at the University of London under the sponsorship of Capsugel, a division of Pfizer, Inc. at the time. The expert system consists of three databases: (1) "past knowledge" collected from the published literature, including information on excipients used in many marketed formulations in Europe and the United States, (2) experiential and non-proprietary information acquired from industrial experts through the use of classical knowledge engineering techniques, and (3) information generated by conducting statistically designed laboratory studies intended to fill knowledge gaps and provide quantitative information. The decision trees and production rules used to construct the expert system were developed based on these databases. The expert system was programmed in Microsoft C and the core system was linked to a dBase-driven database. The system has since been converted to a Microsoft Windows-based platform. The program was further enhanced by the efforts of the University of Kyoto and the University of Maryland through additional laboratory research and a series of panel meetings in Europe, Japan, and the United States with industrial, regulatory, and academic experts.

Neuro-Nets (NNs)

NNs are computer programs that attempt to simulate certain brain functions, such as learning, generalizing, and abstracting from experience. They can discern relationships or patterns in response to exposure to facts ("learning").[46] The nonlinear processing ability of NNs makes them particularly attractive as a way to manage and solve pharmaceutical problems because the relationships that exist between formulation and process variables and desired outcomes are complex and typically nonlinear. The goals of applying NNs to pharmaceutical problems primarily are optimization and prediction. The predominant NN model in these areas is the feed forward/back propagation network, which is often referred to simply as the backpropagation network. Most reported applications in pharmaceutical formulation and technology involve immediate- and modified-release tablet formulation and many of these have been previously summarized.[46] However, one reported study involves capsule formulations and thus deserves discussion here. Under the sponsorship of Capsugel, the University of Maryland conducted a feasibility study aimed at linking an expert system for capsule formulation support with a neural net.[55,56] The intent was to create a hybrid intelligent system capable of generating capsule formulations that would meet specific drug dissolution criteria for BCS Class II drugs, that is, drugs expected to exhibit dissolution rate-limited absorption. Based on prior experience with this drug, the Maryland group selected piroxicam as its model Class II drug with which to demonstrate feasibility. A simplified expert system patterned after the Capsugel system was developed, which provided an opportunity to build certain additional features into the decision process and to use a more effective and more flexible programming language package. Unlike the original Capsugel system, this modified expert system was constructed as a rule-based system and encoded in Prolog. This structure was chosen because it offers certain technical advantages over the original Capsugel system and is more suited to managing complex formulation problems than a decision tree because it can represent more-complicated decision logic and more abstract situations.

The expert system is linked to a neural network to form the hybrid system in the form of modules. The "decision module" is the expert system that generates a proposed formula based on data and requirements input by the user. The "prediction module" is the NN. Trained by a backpropagation algorithm, the NN predicts the dissolution performance of the proposed formulation. The optimization process, controlled by a third module, the "control module," is driven by the difference that might exist between the desired dissolution rate and the predicted dissolution rate of the proposed formulation. The control module thus inputs the formulation proposed by the decision module to the prediction module to compute the predicted dissolution rate. The control module then asks for the user's acceptance of the currently recommended formulation based on that predicted dissolution rate. If the formulation is acceptable, the control module will terminate the formulation process. If it is not acceptable, the control module will then present a set of options to the user for parameter adjustments (e.g., excipient levels) for improving the dissolution rate. This prototype exhibited good predictability for the model compound, piroxicam. A more generalized version of this system was developed by Wilson et al.,[57] which included parameters to address wettability, and the intrinsic dissolution characteristics of the drugs was found to show good predictability for several BCS II drugs having broad differences in solubilities. Following up on this work, Wilson et al. found that a Bayesian network could successfully model the cause–effect relationships between the variables used in the generalized expert network.[58]

Product development is a complex multifactorial problem requiring specialized knowledge and often years of experience. The need to both accelerate the development process and modernize manufacture and control will continue to drive researchers in academia and industry to develop a more fundamental understanding of products and processes that will enable them to identify and measure critical formulation and process attributes that relate to product quality and to model the relationships between product quality attributes and measures of critical material and process attributes.

REFERENCES

1. See, for example, http://www.innercap.com/index.cfm?fuseaction=site.multiphase
2. BE Jones. History of the medicinal capsule. In: F Podczek, BE Jones, eds., *Pharmaceutical Capsules*, 2nd edition, Pharmaceutical Press, 2004, London, pp. 1–20.
3. D Francois, BE Jones. Making the hard capsule with the soft center. *Manuf Chem Aerosol News* 1979; 50(3): 37, 38, 41.
4. BE Jones. Liquid-filled capsules: The New frontier. Brochure. Shionogi Qualicaps, S.A., Madrid, Spain.
5. SE Walker, JA Ganley, K Bedford, T Eaves. The filling of molten and thixotropic formulations into hard gelatin capsules. *J Pharm Pharmacol* 1980; 32: 389–393.
6. IR Berry. Improving bioavailability with soft gelatin capsules. *Drug Cos Ind* 1983; 133(3): 32, 33, 102, 105–108.
7. H Seager. Soft gelatin capsules: A solution to many tableting problems. *Pharm Technol* 1985; 9(9): 84–104.
8. ET Cole. Liquid-filled hard-gelatin capsules. *Pharm Technol* 1989; 13(9): 124–140.
9. M Richardson, S Stegemann. Capsule filling. *Tablets & Capsules* 2007; 5(1): 12–18.
10. F Nink. Liquid-filled capsules. *Tablets & Capsules* 2007; 5(6): 44–49.
11. ET Cole, D Cade, H Benameur. Challenges and opportunities in the encapsulation of liquid and semi-solid formulations for oral administration. *Advanced Drug Del Rev* 2008; 60(6): 747–756.
12. FS Hom, SA Veresh, WR Ebert. Soft gelatin capsules II. Oxygen permeability study of capsule shells. *J Pharm Sci* 1975; 64: 851–857.
13. SA Barker, SP Yap, KH Yuen, CP McCoy, JR Murphy, DQ Craig. An investigation into the structure and bioavailability of alpha-tocopherol dispersions in gelucire. *J Control Rel* 2003; 91: 477–488.
14. FS Hom, JJ Miskel. Oral dosage form design and its influence on dissolution rates for a series of drugs. *J Pharm Sci* 1970; 59: 827–830.
15. FS Hom, JJ Miskel. Enhanced drug dissolution rates for a series of drugs as a function of dosage form design. *Lex et Scientia* 1971; 8(1): 18–26.
16. LJ Fuccella, G Bolcioni, V Tamassia, L Ferario, G Tognoni. Human pharmacokinetics and bioavailability of temazepam administered in soft gelatin capsules. *Europ J Clin Pharmacol* 1977; 12: 383–386.
17. BF Johnson, C Bye, G Jones, GA Sabey. A completely absorbed oral preparation of digoxin. *Clin Pharmacol Therap* 1976; 19: 746–757.
18. A Smith, JF Lampard, KM Carruthers, P Regan. The filling of molten ibuprofen into hard gelatin capsules. *Int J Pharm* 1990; 59: 115–119.
19. C Doelker, E Doelker, P Buri, L Waginaire. The incorporation and in vitro release profiles of liquid, deliquescent or unstable drugs with fusible excipients in hard gelatin capsules. *Drug Devel Ind Pharm* 1986; 12(10): 1553–1565.
20. WJ Bowtle, NJ Barker, J Wodhams. A new approach to vancomycin formulation using filling technology for semisolid matrix capsules. *Pharm Technol* 1988; 12(6): 86–97.
21. CH Dubin. Liquid-filled and multiphase capsules: Overcoming solubility, reducing costs % improving commercial viability. *Drug Development & Delivery* 2011; 11(4): 48–51.
22. R Savla, J Browne, V Plassat. Bringing poorly soluble molecules to market with bioavailability enhancement technologies. *Amer Pharm Rev* 2016; 19(4): 10–12.
23. DJ Hauss. Lipid-based systems for oral drug delivery: Bioavailability of poorly water soluble drugs. *Am Pharm Rev* 2002; 5(4): 88–93.
24. HD Williams, NL Trevaskos, YY Yeap, MU Anby, CW Pouton, CJH Porter. Lipid-based formulations and drug supersaturation: Harnessing the unique benefits of the lipid digestion/absorption pathway. *Pharm Res* 2013; 30: 2976–2992.
25. DG Fatouros, DM Karpf, FS Nielson, A. Mullertz. Clinical studies with oral lipid based formulations of poorly soluble compounds. *Therapeutics and Clinical Risk Management* 2007; 3(4): 591–604.

26. JB Cannon, MA Long. Emulsions, microemulsions, and lipid-based drug delivery systems for drug Solubilization and delivery—Part II: Oral applications. In: R. Liu, ed., *Water-Insoluble Drug Formulation*, 2nd edition, CRC Press, Boca Raton, FL, 2008, Chapter 11, pp. 227–254.
27. NS Barakat. Etodolac-liquid-filled dispersion into hard gelatin capsules: An approach to improve dissolution and stability of etodolac formulation. *Drug Devel Ind Pharm* 2006; 32: 865–876.
28. A Kheur, A Kane, M Aleem, M McLaughlin. A rapid vehicle-screening approach for formulating a low-solubility compound into liquid-filled capsules. *Tablets & Capsules* 2014; 12(1): 10–15.
29. P Gao, M Charton, W Morozowich. Speeding development of poorly soluble/poorly permeable drugs by SEDDS/S-SEDDS formulations and prodrugs (Part II). *Pharm Rev* 2006; 9(4): 16, 18, 19–23.
30. TM Serajuddin, P Li, TF Haefele. Development of lipid-based drug delivery systems for poorly water-soluble drugs as viable oral dosage systems—Present status and future prospects. *Am Pharm Rev* 2008; 11(3): 34–42.
31. JM Kovarik, EA Mueller, JB van Bree, W Tetzloff, K Kutz. Reduced inter- and intraindividual variability in cyclosporine pharmacokinetics from a microemulsion formulation. *J Pharm Sci* 1994; 83(3): 444–446.
32. EA Muller, JM Kovarik, JB van Bree, J Grevel, PW Lücker, K Kutz. Influence of a fat-rich meal on the pharmacokinetics of a new oral formulation of cyclosporine in a crossover comparison with the market formulation. *Pharm Res* 1994; 11(1): 151–155.
33. H Shen, M Zhong. Preparation and evaluation of self-microemulsifying drug delivery systems (SMEDDS) containing atorvastatin. *J Pharm Pharmacol* 2006; 58: 1183–1191.
34. N Thomas, R Holm, M Garmer, JJ Karlsson, A Müllertz, T Rades. Supersaturated self-nanoemulsifying drug delivery systems (Super-SNEDDS) enhance bioavailability of the poorly water-soluble drug simvastatin. *The APAPS J* 2012; 15(1): 219–227.
35. TJ Dening, S Rao, N Thomas, CA Prestidge. Novel nanostructured solid materials for modulating oral drug delivery from solid-state lipid-based drug delivery systems. *The AAPOS J* 2016; 18(1): 23–40.
36. DH Truong, TH Tran, T Ramasamy, JY Choi, HH Lee, C Moon, H-G Choi, JO Kim. Development of solid self-emulsifying formulation for improving the oral bioavailability of erlotiib. *AAPS Pharm Sci Tech* 2016; 17(2): 466–473.
37. RA Lionberger, SL Lee, L Lee et al. Quality by design: Concepts for ANDAs. *The AAPS J* 2008; 10(2): 268–276.
38. PD Lunney, RP Cogdill, JK Drennen III. Innovation in pharmaceutical experimentation. Part I: Review of experimental designs used in industrial pharmaceutics research and introduction to Bayesian D-optimal experimental design. *J Pharm Innov* 2008; 3: 188–203.
39. E Korkakianiti, D Rekkas. Statistical thinking and knowledge management for quality driven design and manufacturing in pharmaceuticals. *Pharm Res* 2011; 28: 1465–1479.
40. J Hogan, P-I Shue, F Podczeck, JM Newton. Investigations into the relationship between drug properties, filling, and the release of drugs from hard gelatin capsules using multivariate statistical analysis. *Pharm Res* 1996; 13: 944–949.
41. DA Piscitelli, S Bigora, C Propst, S Goskonda, P Schwartz, L Lesko, LL Augsburger, D Young. The impact of formulation and process changes on in vitro dissolution and bioequivalence of piroxicam capsules. *Pharm Devel Tech* 1998; 3(4): 443–452.
42. AS Hussain, X Yu, RD Johnson. Application of neural computing to pharmaceutical product development. *Pharm Res* 1991; 8: 1248–1252.
43. J Bourquin, H Schmidli, P van Hoogevest, H Leuenberger. Application of artificial neural networks (ANN) in the development of solid dosage forms. *Pharm Devel Tech* 1997; 2(2): 111–121.
44. B Aksu, A Paradkar, M de Matas, Ö Özer, T Güneri, P York. Quality by design approach: Application of artificial intelligence techniques to tablets manufactured by direct compression. *AAPS PharmSciTech* 2012; 13(4): 1138–1146.
45. F Podczeck. Aims and objectives of experimental design and optimization in formulation and process development In: LL Augsburger, SW Hoag, eds. *Pharmaceutical Dosage Forms: Tablets*, 3rd edition, Volume 2, Chapter 3, Taylor & Francis: New York, 2008, pp. 105–135.
46. Y Peng, LL Augsburger. Expert systems and other AI applications. In: LL Augsburger, SW Hoag, eds. *Pharmaceutical Dosage Forms: Tablets*, 3rd edition, Volume 2, Chapter 4, Taylor & Francis: New York, 2008, pp. 137–172.
47. JE Polli, JR Crison, GL Amidon. Novel approach to the analysis of an in vitro–in vivo relationships. *J Pharm Sci* 1996; 85: 753–760.
48. JE Polli. Analysis of in vitro–in vivo data. In: GL Amidon, JR Robinson, RL Williams, eds. *Scientific Foundations for Regulating Drug Products*. Arlington, VA, AAPS Press, 1997, pp. 335–351.

49. TA Hicks, B Patel, LL Augsburger, R Shangraw, L Lesko, V Shah, D Young. The effect of the relative magnitudes of absorption and elimination half-lives on the decision of C_{max}-based bioequivalence (abstr). American Association of Pharmaceutical Scientists, 8th annual meeting, Orlando, FL, Nov. 1993.

50. E Faulhammer, M Llusa, PR Wahl, A Paudel, S Lawrence, S Biserni, V Calzolari, JG Khinast. Development of a design space and predictive statistical model for capsule filling of low-fill-weight inhalation products. *Drug Dev Ind Pharm* 2016; 42(2): 221–230.

51. E Faulhammer, M Llusa, C Radeke, O Scheibelhofer, S Lawrence, S Biserni, V Calzolari, JG The effects of material attributes on capsule fill weight and weight variability in dosator nozzle machines. *Int J Pharm* 2014; 471: 332–338.

52. E Faulhammer, M Fink, M Llusa, SM Lawrence, S Biserni, V Calzolari, JG Khinast. Low-dose capsule filling of inhalation products: Critical material attributes and process parameters. *Int J Pharm* 2014; 473: 617–626.

53. SD Bateman, J Verlin, M Russo, M Guillot, SM Laughlin. The development of a capsule formulation knowledge-based system. *Pharm Technol* 1996; 20(3): 174, 178, 180, 182, 184.

54. S Lai, F Podczeck, JM Newton, R Daumesnil. An expert system to aid the development of capsule formulations. *Pharm Technol Eur* 1996; 8(Oct.): 60–65.

55. M Guo, G Kalra, W Wilson, Y Peng, LL Augsburger. A prototype intelligent hybrid system for hard gelatin capsule formulation development. *Pharm Technol* 2002; 26(9): 44–60.

56. G Kalra, Y Peng, M Guo, LL Augsburger. A hybrid intelligent system for formulation of BCS Class II drugs in hard gelatin capsules. Proceedings, International Conference on Neural Information Processing, Singapore, November 2002.

57. W Wilson, Y Peng, LL Augsburger. Generalization of a prototype intelligent hybrid system for hard gelatin capsule formulation development. *AAPS PharmSciTech* 2005; 6(3): E449–E457.

58. W Wilson, Y Peng, LL Augsburger. Comparison of statistical analysis and Bayesian networks in the evaluation of dissolution performance of BCS Class II model drugs. *J Pharm Sci* 2005; 94: 2764–2776.

2 An Introduction to Two-Piece Hard Capsules and Their Marketing Benefits

Dennis Murachanian

CONTENTS

INTRODUCTION

Two-piece hard capsules are a well-established dosage form that provides solutions to many of today's drug delivery and nutraceutical formulation challenges.[1] Widely used in the pharmaceutical and nutritional industry for more than a century, two-piece capsules are still a recognized and trusted dosage form.[2] When viewed as an empty container, they are highly flexible and amenable to many fill material types including powders, granulations, pellets, minitablets, semisolids, and liquids.[3] Uses for two-piece capsules are equally flexible, including immediate release, sustained release, enteric release, clinical blinding, inhalation therapy, and vaccines.[4,5] While the majority of hard capsules are composed of gelatin, hydroxypropylmethyl cellulose (HPMC) has emerged as a naturally sourced, lower water content alternative offering further flexibility to the formulator.

Modern drug discovery has yielded insoluble and complex molecules that challenge the pharmaceutical formulator to develop an orally available dosage form while meeting aggressive timelines. Likewise, the nutraceutical formulator is under even more aggressive development timelines and is usually constrained by the inability to use traditional formulation aids such as binders, flow aids, and disintegrants. For both formulators, the hard capsule typically offers a quicker and simpler developmental path than tablets, resulting in a faster time to market and considerable cost advantages.

Hard capsules are available in a wide range of sizes to meet most requirements. Colorants and printing options improve product identification and product branding, aid in anti-counterfeiting, and help improve patient compliance. For patients, hard capsules are frequently a preferred dosage form for their visual appeal, ease of swallowing, and taste and odor masking.

Market Growth of Two-Piece Hard Capsules

The pharmaceutical and nutraceutical industries are undergoing significant changes globally, and many of these changes are expected to increase usage of two-piece hard capsules. The global empty capsule market is forecast to grow at a compound annual growth rate of 7% per year from 2014 to 2019. Market growth in both the pharmaceutical and nutraceutical industries will be driven by many factors including growth in the aging population, increased availability of information on personal health, increased intake of nutraceuticals as preventative therapy, an increasing number of prescription medicines becoming available without a prescription, and government programs that subsidize the cost of prescription medications.

In the pharmaceutical segment, growth continues to be driven largely by an aging population in the developed world, leading to an overall increase in the consumption of medications. A growing demand for innovative drug delivery formulations has positively affected the growth of the hard capsule market. For example, there has been an increasing trend toward the use of multiple fill formulations as a tool to achieve multiple release rates or drug combinations. Multiple fill formulations usually consist of combinations of pellets, powders, tablets, or minitablets, and are discussed later in the chapter. Minitablets in particular have been increasingly used as a formulation tool owing to their ease of development and manufacture as compared to pellets. Additionally, minitablets may be employed to either strengthen a patent or circumvent an existing one. In all of these cases, two-piece hard capsules are an indispensable tool to support innovative drug development.

Nutraceuticals are an important and growing driver of hard capsule consumption. According to Euromonitor International, the dietary supplement market has grown 23%, to $51 billion, in the past 5 years. Increasingly, consumers of natural products are demanding that all of the ingredients in the product be all natural, including the capsule shell. Traditionally, capsules have been produced using gelatin, an animal-derived material. All of the major capsule suppliers now produce capsules composed of HPMC, a naturally derived material from plants. The growing demand for all natural gelatin alternative capsules such as HPMC is driving the usage of two-piece capsules. Additionally, the increased consumption of dietary supplements on a daily basis is expected to drive the demand for empty capsules in the coming years.

Improvements in capsule filling machines are also helping drive capsule usage. Significant advances have been made by the leading manufacturers of high-speed capsule filling machines that make the process faster and more precise.[2] An important advancement has been the implementation of onboard weight control systems. Modern control systems are capable of dynamically measuring empty and filled capsule weights during the filling operation at speeds up to 200,000 capsules per hour.[6] These systems continuously monitor the filling operation and adjust fill weights when necessary. Such controls help meet the regulatory requirements for process control and are an integral component of process analytical technology and continuous manufacturing. These advances help drive the market for capsule usage by making their use more efficient and thus more acceptable to manufacturing operations.

HISTORICAL DEVELOPMENT OF THE CAPSULE DOSAGE FORM

Capsules are one of the oldest known dosage forms dating back to the ancient Egyptians. One of the oldest and longest papyri is the Ebers Papyrus dating to approximately 1500 BC. The document mentions more than 800 mixtures to be administered in various dosage forms including capsules. Further specifics on how they defined a capsule or its design are not provided in the papyri.[7] The first modern reference to capsules in literature is in 1730 by the Viennese pharmacist de Pauli. His invention described oval-shaped capsules designed to mask the unpleasant taste of turpentine, which he prescribed for patients afflicted with gout. More than a century would pass before gelatin capsules would again appear. In 1834, the first patent was granted in Paris to pharmacist Joseph Gérard Dublanc and pharmacy student François Achille Barnabé Mothès for the invention and manufacture of gelatin capsules. These first capsules were "bladders made of gelatin" produced by immersing a small leather bag filled with mercury in a gelatin solution. As soon as the gelatin film dried, the mercury was emptied from the leather bag, and the firm gelatin capsule was stripped off. The capsules were used for liquid medications, which were introduced by pipette, following which the capsule was sealed with a drop of gelatin. Mothès ended his collaboration with Dublanc in 1837 and continued to work on developing the gelatin capsule and taking out additional patents for their manufacture and use.

The invention was widely recognized as addressing an important medicinal need, and by the following year, capsules were being produced in many parts of the world. Eventually, other inventors began applying for patents for gelatin capsules for among other reasons to circumvent patents held by Mothès. One such inventor, Jules César Lehuby, was credited with the invention of the two-piece gelatin capsule and, on October 20, 1846, was granted a French patent for his "medicine coverings." Lehuby was the first to describe two-piece capsules, which were produced by dipping silver-coated metal pins into a gelatin solution and then drying them.[7] Lehuby described his capsules as "cylindrical in the shape of a silk-worm cocoon and consisting of two parts which fit into each other to form a box." Although Lehuby's principles for manufacturing two-piece capsules established the method still used today, technical difficulties in manufacturing the separate bodies and caps limited their manufacture mainly to pharmacists who also filled them.

In 1888, John B. Russell patented a process for making gelatin coatings that was first made use of by Parke, Davis & Co. The manufacturing process was improved, and in 1895, Arthur Colton patented, on behalf of the company, a machine with an hourly output of 6000–10,000 capsules. In 1924, Arthur Colton Company, again on behalf of Parke, Davis & Co., designed an improved capsule manufacturing machine. Patented in 1931, this machine was the first to simultaneously make both caps and bodies on the same machine, which enabled two-color capsules to be made.[7] This machine still represents the basic design of machinery used today (see Chapter 6). Numerous improvements have been made over the years to include locking mechanisms, printing for product identification, and improved tolerances to meet the demands of high-speed filling machines.[1] Additionally, capsule designs have been developed for specific applications such as clinical blinding and liquid formulations. With advances made in hard capsule technology, the use and importance of capsules as a delivery system have steadily increased, and the market has enjoyed continuous growth. In the past, capsules were filled either manually by a very labor-intensive process or by slower filling machines. Today, automatic encapsulation machines can fill as many as 200,000 capsules per hour. Modern capsule filling machines are fully automated and instrumented to monitor and adjust fill weights to stay within target specifications, making for an efficient and modern manufacturing process.

CAPSULE SHELL MANUFACTURING PROCESS

The manufacturing process for two-piece hard capsules is still quite similar to the process first proposed and patented by Colton in 1931 (see Chapter 6). In the ensuing years, the process has been refined and modernized to become highly efficient and capable of producing capsules at high speeds, yielding capsules of consistent quality, with tightly controlled dimensional tolerances. The following description of the capsule manufacturing process is by far not exhaustive but designed to provide the reader with a general idea of how capsules are produced.

GELATIN SOLUTION PREPARATION

While two-piece capsules may be composed of various materials, the vast majority are still made using high-quality gelatin prepared from collagen. Collagen is a fibrillary protein that contains 18 different amino acids. The collagen of bones and hides is subject to a maceration and purification process employing acids and alkalis that split the collagen hydrolytically into an almost unbranched amino acid chain of variable length; this end product is known as gelatin. Gelatin used in hard capsule manufacture must meet the requirements of all major pharmacopeias.

A gelatin solution is prepared by dissolving the gelatin in demineralized water, which has been heated to 60–70°C in jacketed stainless steel tanks. This solution contains 30–40% w/w of gelatin and is highly viscous, which causes bubbles as a result of air entrapment. The presence of these bubbles in the final solution would yield capsules of inconsistent weight and would also become problematic during capsule filling and upon storage. To remove the air bubbles, a vacuum is applied to the solution; the duration of this process varies with batch size.

Following the above steps, colorants and pigments are added to attain the desired final capsule appearance.[8] At this stage, other processing aids may be added, such as sodium lauryl sulfate, to reduce surface tension. The solution viscosity is measured and adjusted as needed with hot demineralized water to achieve the target specification. The viscosity of the gelatin solution is a critical parameter as it affects the downstream manufacturing process and plays a major role in capsule shell wall thickness. After physical, chemical, and microbiological testing, the gelatin is released for capsule production. The gelatin solution is then transferred to temperature-controlled tanks on the dipping machine where it is fed continuously into the dipping dishes.

CAPSULE SHELL PRODUCTION

Capsules are manufactured under strict climatic conditions by a dipping process on high capacity machines. Standardized steel pins arranged in rows on metal bars are dipped into a temperature-controlled solution to a precisely regulated depth. The rows of pins are arranged so that caps are formed on one side of the machine while bodies are simultaneously formed on the opposite side of the machine. After dipping, the bars are rotated to evenly distribute the solution around the pins, correct gelatin distribution being critical to uniform and precise capsule wall thickness and dome strength. The pins are then passed through several drying stages to achieve the target moisture content. Once dried, the capsule halves are stripped from the pins and cut to the correct length, and the cap and body are joined to the pre-closed position. Figure 2.1 depicts steel pins immediately after dipping into a gelatin solution. Figure 2.2 shows dried capsules just before removal from mold pins.

After formation, the capsule shells can be printed to improve identification. Printing can be achieved using one or two colors, containing information such as the following:

Product name or code number
Manufacturer's name or logo
Dosage details

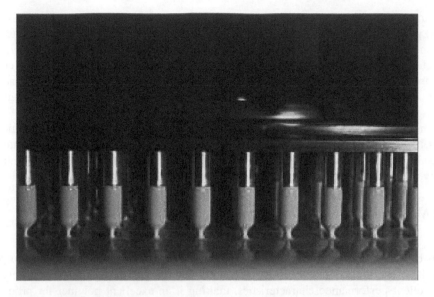

FIGURE 2.1 Capsule shells being formed on mold pins.

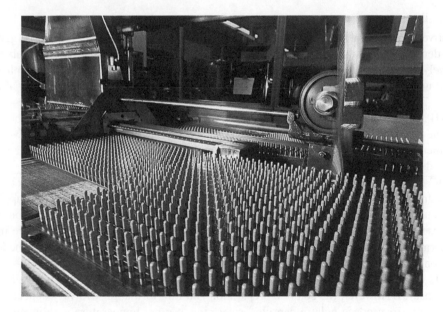

FIGURE 2.2 Dried capsule shells on mold pins just before removal.

Printing reduces the risk of product confusion by the numerous handlers and users of the product including manufacturers, pharmacists, nurses, doctors, caregivers, and patients. Capsule printing will be further covered in a later section.

QUALITY CONTROL

The capsule manufacturing process is carried out according to Good Manufacturing Practices during all phases of production from gelatin preparation through printing and packaging. A large number of quality control tests are conducted at each stage to ensure that the finished product meets all specifications.

In the raw material stage, gelatin is tested for Bloom strength (gelling properties), viscosity, solubility, pH value, chemical purity, heavy metals, and microbial count. Water is tested for electrolyte content, pH value, and microbial count. Coloring agents are tested for identity, solubility, heavy metals, and microbial count. The final gelatin solution is tested for viscosity, temperature, color composition, and color shade. Finished capsules are tested for capsule characteristics including water content, shell wall thickness, cap and body length, open and closed shell length, ovality, separation force, color shade, and print quality/defects.

Modern capsule manufacturing processes yield capsules with highly consistent critical quality attributes including weight, length, and shell wall thickness. Studies have demonstrated that the hard capsule is a suitable excipient for QbD drug development and manufacturing with acceptable variability within a consistent and narrow range, and is well defined by its specifications.

CAPSULE MATERIALS

Gelatin

Gelatin is by far the most common and most well-known material used to produce two-piece hard capsules. Its origin has been previously described.[9] Gelatin has a long history of safety and possesses excellent performance characteristics, making it an excellent polymer for producing capsules. It is nontoxic, widely used in foods, acceptable for use worldwide, and recognized in all pharmaceutical pharmacopeia.

Hypromellose

Alternatives have been investigated to gelatin either for reasons of stability or objections to animal-derived materials.[10,11] The most common gelatin alternative is HPMC, which has been extensively studied and successfully developed into two-piece capsules for use in the pharmaceutical and nutritional industries. Important benefits of HPMC include a water content of approximately 4–7% as compared to gelatin capsules, which are typically in the range of 13–16%. This makes HPMC capsules an excellent container for water-sensitive drugs; as a result, they are also less prone to brittleness owing to drying. However, capsules made with HPMC have a higher gas permeation rate than those from gelatin, which may be a consideration for oxygen-sensitive compounds.

HPMC is a cellulose ether of vegetable origin and therefore answers the need for religious, cultural, and dietary restrictions. HPMC capsules are available from most capsule suppliers, but unlike gelatin capsules, HPMC capsules may differ somewhat among suppliers. Consequently, these capsules may not be readily interchangeable between suppliers and it is therefore important for the formulator to fully understand the composition of the capsule being procured. The following description will lead to a fuller understanding of this issue.

HPMC capsules are molded according to a steel pin dipping process as described above for gelatin capsules. However, the solution preparation and film formation will vary depending on the manufacturer. To produce gelatin capsules, steel pins at room temperature are dipped into a hot gelatin solution. This approach may also be used for HPMC capsules; however, doing so requires the addition of a gelling aid. Common gelling agents include gellan gum and various types of carrageenan. Each of these gelling agents imparts unique performance characteristics that may affect capsule dissolution.

An alternative approach is to dip hot steel pins into a room temperature solution of HPMC solution, thus eliminating the need for a gelling agent. The value of this approach is a reported improvement in capsule dissolution. Each approach, hot steel pin or gelling agent, has its advantages and disadvantages that may affect the rate of dissolution as well as capsule dimensions. It then becomes clear that supplier interchangeability is not as simple as for gelatin capsules. Switching among suppliers will likely require additional manufacturing trials and stability studies and may affect any regulatory documents.

CAPSULE SHELL FEATURES (CAPSULE DESIGN)

Hard capsules are designed not only to contain pharmaceutical and nutritional formulations but also to withstand the rigors of handling on high-speed filling machines, packaging, and shipping. The filling machine process involves feeding of capsules into the machine, rectification, separation of cap and body, filling, closing of cap and body, and ejection. These steps may occur at rates in excess of 200,000 capsules per hour, making the design and integrity of the capsule of paramount importance. Figure 2.3 shows the operational steps of a capsule filling machine.

Capsule designs are often patented by their respective manufacturers, the net result being a capsule sufficiently robust for all phases of handling. Figure 2.4 shows a capsule design containing a prelocking feature, a locking mechanism, air venting, and an alignment feature on the body. The following will discuss each of these features to fully understand their function.[2,12]

Capsules were originally produced as simple caps and bodies with no additional locking features or design elements to support filling at commercial scale. However, with the advent of high-speed filling machines, it quickly became apparent that this design was inadequate to meet the needs of the industry. One common problem was the ease with which cap and body would separate after filling and during shipping. After some study, it was discovered that this was often attributed to air entrapment in the capsule during the filling process, thus creating sufficient internal pressure to cause separation of the cap and body. To remedy this problem, matching lock-rings were introduced onto the cap and body to assure a tight closure. There are multiple methods for achieving this, and these vary by manufacturer, but all perform the same function of locking the cap and body together. As capsule filling became ever more efficient and faster, the lock-rings alone were often not sufficient to withstand internal forces. To further improve the capsule design, air vents were introduced

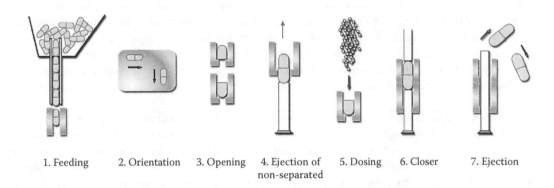

| 1. Feeding | 2. Orientation | 3. Opening | 4. Ejection of non-separated | 5. Dosing | 6. Closer | 7. Ejection |

FIGURE 2.3   The basic operational steps of all capsule filling machines.

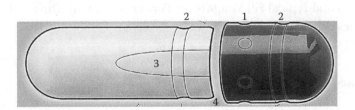

FIGURE 2.4   Capsugel Coni-Snap® Capsule: (1) dimples maintain body and cap in pre-joined position; (2) rings lock cap and body together after closing; (3) vents allow air to escape during closing; (4) tapered rim provides additional closing tolerance.

onto the body. These allow air to escape at the closing station and thus eliminate a common cause of cap–body separation.

As described earlier, after the molding step, the cap and body are joined together for packaging and shipping. The separation of caps and bodies during shipping and handling was initially a common occurrence. Unfortunately, shipping capsules in the fully closed or locked position is not feasible as this requires excessive separation force on the filling machine, which results in capsule damage. To address this challenge, indentations are molded into the cap that provides a firmer fit known as the prelock force. The placement, depth, and number of indentations are optimized to assure that the cap and body are sufficiently held in place during shipping and handling but not so much so that separation on the filling machine is difficult. As with the other capsule features, the various manufacturers offer different approaches to address this challenge.

An alignment feature on the body was another productivity enhancement made to the original capsule design. Similar to the other design features, an alignment feature was introduced in response to the demands of high-speed filling machines. Previously, even slight variances in lateral cap–body alignment would cause improper closing, resulting in split and deformed capsules. The alignment feature provides for additional tolerance during this operational step. Unique approaches have been taken by various manufacturers to enhance closing variance. These include tapered body rims that increase variance or circular grooves indented into the body near the end to maintain circularity. Of course, proper filling machine setup is still critical to ensure an efficient and smooth filling operation.

CAPSULE SIZES

Capsule sizes are designated numerically from sizes 000 to 5, with 000 being the largest size and 5 being the smallest. Table 2.1 lists commonly available capsule sizes and their respective fill capacities based on tapped density.[12] Determination of the optimal capsule size for a given product is straightforward. First, determine the density of the formulation using tapped density for powders and bulk density for pellets, minitablets, and granules. Refer to a capsule volume chart such as Table 2.1; this type of information is available from the capsule supplier.[12] The appropriate capsule size may then be calculated using the measured density of the formulation, the target fill weight, and capsule volume.

Specialized capsule sizes have also been developed to overencapsulate dosages for blinding in clinical trial administration.[13] Two important requirements for blinded clinical trial materials are that the patient not being able to see the contents of the capsule and that it would be difficult for the patient to open the capsule and thus break the blind. A unique capsule design was developed to support these requirements with a cap that covers most of the body, creating a double layer of shell

TABLE 2.1
Capsule Volumes and Typical Fill Weights for Formulations with Different Tapped Densities

Size	000	00el	00	0el	0	1 el	1	2el	2	3	4	5
Capsule volume (mL)	1.37	1.02	0.91	0.78	0.68	0.54	0.50	0.41	0.37	0.30	0.21	0.13
Powder tapped density					Capsule capacity (mg)							
0.6 g/mL	822	612	546	468	408	324	300	246	222	180	126	78
0.8 g/mL	1096	816	728	624	544	432	400	308	296	240	168	104
1.0 g/mL	1370	1020	910	780	680	540	500	410	370	300	210	130
1.2 g/mL	1644	1224	1092	936	816	648	600	492	444	360	252	156

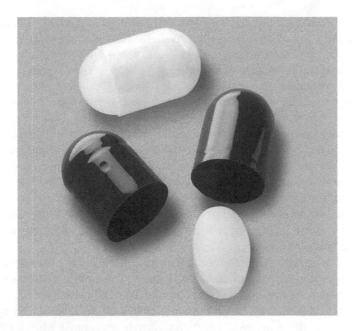

FIGURE 2.5   Capsule for clinical blinding.

so that only the rounded end is visible, as shown in Figure 2.5. This dual layer not only ensures the opacity of capsule contents but also makes it extremely difficult to open, maintaining the integrity of the blind. As the size and cost of clinical studies increase, the need to maintain study integrity becomes ever more critical. The two-piece capsule can be an invaluable tool in preventing patient bias by making it difficult for the patient to break the blind, thus assuring study integrity. Another unique capsule was developed specifically to contain liquids using special design and locking features. Such capsules are typically sealed after filling either by applying a band across the seam or by a hydroalcoholic seal.[14,15]

CAPSULE COLORANTS AND PRINTING

Capsule colorants are an important means of creating a strong brand identity and for avoiding product confusion, especially for elderly patients taking multiple medications.[16–18] Capsule printing is an additional means of product identification and is required by most regulatory agencies for pharmaceutical capsules, though typically not for nutritional products. Capsule colorants must satisfy three key requirements:

1. Regulatory approval in the countries intended for distribution
2. Brand image and marketing
3. Patient acceptance

First, the color must meet the regulatory requirements of those countries where the product will be sold.[13] Since color regulations vary from country to country, this is an important consideration when developing a capsule for a new product. Each country or region has a list of acceptable colorants along with their allowable levels. The leading capsule suppliers can usually assist with this regulatory information. Additionally, the full composition of colorant, by weight is available on the capsule supplier's specification sheet. This information is used to ensure that the patient's daily intake does not exceed approved limits. The daily intake of each colorant is calculated by assuming the highest daily dosage (highest number of capsules) times the weight of colorant in each capsule.

The term *globally acceptable* generally refers to the regions of the United States, the European Union, and Japan. For a global presentation, the available palette of colorants is vastly reduced and mainly consists of the iron oxides, titanium dioxide, and blue #2. It is important to note that blue #2 is a light-sensitive dye that is prone to fading; therefore, light protective packaging should be used to avoid capsule discoloration. Iron oxides present a special challenge as they contain elemental iron, which can be toxic at elevated levels. This is an especially important consideration since the iron oxides are one of the few classes of globally acceptable coloring agents. For reasons of patient safety, guidelines have been established for the daily intake of iron oxides and elemental iron. For example, the World Health Organization has established a limit of 0.5 mg/day/kg of iron oxide, while the US Code of Federal Regulations has an established limit of 5 mg/day of elemental iron. It is therefore incumbent on the formulator to be aware of the levels of iron oxide in their capsule color formulation. This information enables the back calculation of elemental iron levels per capsule; the maximum theoretical intake of elemental iron can be calculated based on the number of capsules to be dosed daily. A reputable capsule supplier can provide assistance in this matter and reformulate to lower iron oxide levels if necessary.

Capsule printing is usually required by regulatory authorities for pharmaceutical products to comply with product identification requirements. Printing is typically not required for nutritional supplements. The print must contain some form of product identification such as the product name, strength, or code number. Colorants for printing inks follow the same regulatory approach as those for capsules. Printing is often a means of improving capsule appearance when a global presentation results in an otherwise dull-looking capsule.

Legibility is the most important consideration when creating a capsule print design. Ink selection and design type must be optimized to ensure that the print is applied evenly and does not smear during the printing and drying process. Very fine or crowded print, as well as exotic logos, can be problematic when printing at commercial scale. An experienced print department can assist in developing a print design that meets the requirements for product identification while ensuring that the print will be legible when applied at high speeds.

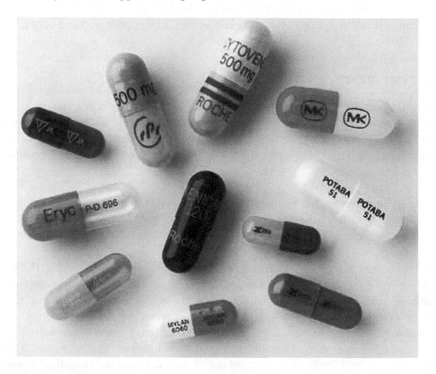

FIGURE 2.6   Examples of capsule shells printed along the axis and around the radius.

Capsules may be printed either lengthwise along the axis (axial printing) or around the circumference (radial printing). The benefit of radial printing is the ability to cover a greater surface area than with axial printing. Of the 360° of the circumference, approximately 270° are available for printing when allowance has been made for good legibility. This means that the print area is five times greater than for axial printing. Because of the larger area available for printing, identification characteristics of both the product and the manufacturer can be clearly printed. Thus, product identification is greatly increased and product confusion is greatly reduced.

In addition to product identifiers such as product name or strength, capsules may also be printed with a company logo or other identifiers to further enhance the capsule image. Figure 2.6 shows examples of capsules printed along the axis and around the radius. The wide array of printing options provides greater possibilities in brand protection and identification. Novel colors and printing also help deter counterfeiting by making capsules more difficult to copy.

BRAND IMAGE AND MARKETING

A single globally acceptable capsule color will eliminate the need for multiple capsule presentations and thus reduce stability testing and inventory requirements. The use of globally acceptable colorants can be applied to both commercial and clinical supplies. In the case of clinical supplies, this approach allows for maintenance of a readily available inventory of capsules when clinical materials are needed on short notice regardless of the clinical site. To avoid introducing bias into a clinical trial where blinding by overencapsulation is required, it is important to choose a colorant that is sufficiently opaque to fully hide the contents of the capsule.

Colorants play an important role in product identification and enhancing brand image. Capsule suppliers can produce customized color combinations and may offer exclusivity on color combinations. For clinical supplies, the use of a standardized color reduces possible confusion and product mix-ups at the clinical site and acts as an additional means of reassurance to the clinician.

PATIENT ACCEPTANCE

Patient acceptance is the third key consideration in color choice.[16] With distinct colors, patients can more easily identify their medications, which aids in improved patient compliance and safety. In various studies, it has been consistently demonstrated that the color of the dosage form is the attribute most readily recognizable by patients, followed by other key attributes including product name, dosage form, shape, and size. Patients are often immediately aware when their medication or brand is switched based on a new color.

The psychology of color selection based on therapeutic indication has been studied and applied for many years.[16] Broadly defined rules exist for associating colors with certain indications; studies have also demonstrated the psychological influence of capsule colors on the therapeutic effect of a drug. For example, a capsule designed for anxiety or sedation would probably be viewed as more effective by the patient if a soft color such as light blue were used as opposed to a stimulating, bright color such as orange.

MOISTURE CONTENT AND STORAGE

Two-piece hard gelatin capsules normally contain an equilibrium moisture content of 13–16%. This moisture is critical to the physical properties of the shells; at lower moisture contents, shells become brittle, while higher moisture contents result in capsule softening and deformation. Gelatin capsule water content can vary greatly based on packaging and storage conditions. Gelatin capsules should be stored in tightly sealed containers with typical storage conditions of 15–25°C and 35–55% relative humidity. Capsule water content can also affect product stability, and potential drug–water interactions should be considered during early formulation screening. For example, moisture-sensitive drugs may degrade in the presence of capsule moisture. It is also good practice to ensure that all fill materials are compatible with the hard gelatin capsule as some excipients may be hygroscopic and cause the capsule shell to become brittle.

Gelatin cross-linking is another important consideration. This is a phenomenon wherein amino acids from adjacent protein strands or within a protein strand bind together resulting in gelatin cross-linking.[19–21] Cross-linking causes the formation of a swollen, rubbery, water-insoluble membrane (pellicle) during dissolution testing in distilled water. The insoluble film acts as a barrier to drug release and may result in out-of-specification dissolution results. Common causes of gelatin cross-linking include aldehydes (in the active or excipients), high heat and humidity, and rayon coilers.

HPMC capsules offer the advantage of having a lower water content than gelatin capsules, typically in the range of 4–7% depending on the supplier. Since water is not a plasticizer for HPMC capsules, they do not become brittle when dried to water contents of 1% or less. Additionally, HPMC capsules are not protein based and thus do not cross-link under stress conditions. As a result, they are a useful alternative to gelatin capsules for moisture-sensitive and hygroscopic formulations or where cross-linking is a concern.

Capsule Fill Materials

Two-piece capsules offer flexibility and speed of development, and are an excellent tool for containing many different types of fill materials including those that are difficult to compress into tablets. Importantly, capsule formulations typically require less excipient than tablet formulations and are easier to formulate. This being the case, capsule formulations are by far the most common dosage form used for early phase clinical studies where speed to clinic and early proof of safety and efficacy studies are required. Examples exist on the market where a capsule was chosen as the commercial dosage form over a tablet purely for reasons of competitive environment and speed to market.

Some of the more common fill materials for capsules are discussed below and shown in Figure 2.7.

Powders

The most common fill materials for two-piece capsules are immediate-release powders. Powder formulations require fewer processing steps, reduce excipient requirement, and offer overall time savings as compared to tablet development. It is often possible to go directly from a dry powder blend to the capsule filling machine with no intermediate steps.

Granules

Granules are useful in cases where a powder formulation exhibits poor flow or inadequate content uniformity. Granules may be coated with gastric-resistant polymers in cases where the drug is destroyed by stomach acids. Other polymer applications can be used to yield a delayed release

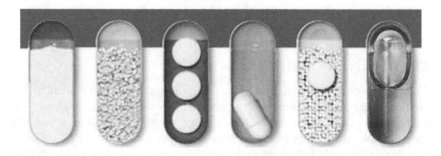

FIGURE 2.7 Examples of possible fill materials that can be filled into capsule shells.

profile and to improve drug stability. Granules are often denser than comparable powder formulations; this enables higher fill weights and thus a smaller capsule size.

Pellets

Pellets are an excellent tool for numerous applications. Pellets can be coated with sustained-release and enteric film coatings to achieve unique release profiles, or multiple release rates in a single dosage unit by mixing pellets having different film coatings. Pellets also offer the ability to mix multiple active ingredients or incompatible active ingredients.

Minitablets

Minitablets offer many of the advantages of pellets but with reduced processing steps. Minitablets are nearly round in shape with a typical diameter of 2.0–3.0 mm and are produced by conventional tableting methods. Minitablets are compressed using specially designed multiple headed punches; this eliminates many of the processing steps associated with pellet manufacture. Additionally, they often yield higher drug loads owing to inclusion of active ingredients directly into the tablet core. Coating of minitablets provides for a variety of release rates, and they can be mixed to yield combination products as well as a combination of release rates. Modern encapsulation machines have been designed to precisely dose minitablets into capsules at commercial-scale speeds.

Tablets

The filling of tablets alone or in combination with powders, granules, or pellets is a common formulation approach. The use of tablets allows for combination products and combination release rates. Another common application is the overencapsulation of tablets for clinical blinding.

Liquid and Semisolids

As drug discovery continues to yield poorly water-soluble molecules, there is an increasing need for formulation techniques that can improve drug solubility. One such approach is the use of liquid-based formulations containing lipids, solvents, or surfactants, usually in combination, to improve drug solubility and bioavailability. The final formulation may be filled as a room temperature liquid, or as a molten semisolid. Two-piece hard capsules, either gelatin or HPMC, are a useful dosage form for such formulations.

Dosing of Pure API

Capsules can be filled directly with pure active ingredient as a means of achieving speed to clinic without the time requirement for preformulation, formulation, or stability studies. This approach is becoming increasingly popular as developers face escalating demands to reduce costs and determine proof of concept more quickly. Filling machines are available, designed specifically for this application and can dose accurately to weights as low as 100 µg.

Dry Powder Inhalers

Two-piece hard capsules, especially those composed of hypromellose, are used in conjunction with specially designed inhalation devices for pulmonary delivery of dry powders.[4] The benefit of this approach is an inexpensive and portable delivery system that does not require propellants. Dry powder inhalation also has the benefit of bypassing the hurdles of oral delivery for peptide molecules. Inhaled insulin is one such example that uses this approach.

BENEFITS OF MARKETING TWO-PIECE CAPSULES

Two-piece capsules continue to play a vital role in today's cost-constrained medical environment. As the population of octogenarians, nonagenarians, and even centenarians grows, issues related to medication management will become ever more critical. Patient compliance and safety are a primary focus for improved therapeutic outcomes with the goal of fewer hospital admissions and an overall reduction in healthcare costs. Product identification is greatly enhanced when capsules are marketed using unique identifiers such as color combinations and print designs. Improved product identification results in fewer product mix-ups at all levels of the healthcare system, improved patient compliance, and patient safety.[17,18]

Medication swallowing is another important consideration in patient compliance and safety. Studies have demonstrated that patients often prefer taking capsules instead of tablets as their oblong shape and smooth surface make them easier to swallow.[16,22] Evidence of this is the use of gelatin-coated oblong tablets for consumer pharmaceuticals, especially for therapies requiring chronic administration such as analgesics. There is often confusion among formulators as to why gelatin coatings are applied to tablets with the assumption that the coating must impart a functional effect such as delayed or enteric release. However, the presence of such coatings is purely to improve swallowing, an issue that is a challenge for many patients, especially for larger dosage forms. Additionally, capsules improve medication compliance by masking objectionable tastes and odors.

Two-piece capsules also support marketing strategies for over-the-counter medications. The image of efficacy associated with prescription capsule medications is often used by marketers to promote nonprescription capsule products. The association being that the over-the-counter product is as strong and effective as a prescription medicine and will be worth the price. Additionally, capsule colors play a significant role in developing a brand image in television, internet, and print advertising. The power of brand image cannot be underestimated since, unlike prescription medications, the consumer will make the purchase decision.

The two-piece capsule remains a relevant and modern tool for today's pharmaceutical products. As a product container, it offers excellent versatility, especially with the enhanced selection of polymers now available. Combination products, incompatible medications, and multiple release rates can all be accommodated by the capsule dosage form. Capsules support the QbD requirements of the regulatory authorities through sophisticated and well-controlled manufacturing techniques. QbD is also supported through high-speed filling machines capable of dynamic weight measurement and adjustment (filling machines will be discussed in a later chapter). Color selection and print design make product recognition easier, aiding in improved patient compliance and safety. A broad array of color and print options also support marketing efforts to build brand image and patient loyalty for both prescription and nonprescription products.

REFERENCES

1. Stegemann S. 2002. Hard gelatin capsules today and tomorrow.
2. Capsugel Library 1997. All About the Hard Gelatin Capsules.
3. Keerthi ML, Kiran RS, Rao VUM, Sannapu A, Dutt AG, Krishna KS. 2014. Pharmaceutical mini-tablets, its advantages, formulation possibilities and general evaluation aspects: A review. *Int. J. Pharm. Sci. Rev. Res.,* 28(1):214–21.
4. Plourde R. Performance of hypromellose (V-Caps®) capsules for unit dose dry powder inhalation. *Proc. Devices Respiratory Drug Delivery Europe, Libson, Portugal, 2009.*
5. Edwards D. 2010. Applications of capsule dosing techniques for use in dry powder inhalers. *Therapeutic Delivery* 1:195–201.
6. Augsburger LL. 1996. Hard and soft shell capsules. In *Modern Pharmaceutics,* eds. GS Banker, CT Rhodes. New York: Marcel Dekker, pp. 395–440.
7. Jones B. 2004. The history of the medicinal capsule. In *Pharmaceutical Capsules,* eds. F Podczek, B Jones. London: Pharmaceutical Press, pp. 1–22.
8. Nyamweya N, Hoag SW. 2007. Influence of pigments in the properties of polymeric coating systems. In *Aqueous Polymeric Coatings for Pharmaceutical Dosage Forms,* eds. L Felton, J McGinity. New York: Informa Healthcare.
9. Jones BE, Turner TS. 1975. Century of commercial hard gelatin capsules. *Pharmaceutical Journal (England)* 213:614–17.

10. Ku MS, Lu Q, Li W, Chen Y. 2011. Performance qualification of a new hypromellose capsule: Part II. Disintegration and dissolution comparison between two types of hypromellose capsules. *International Journal of Pharmaceutics* 416:16–24.
11. Sherry Ku M, Li W, Dulin W, Donahue F, Cade D et al. 2010. Performance qualification of a new hypromellose capsule: Part I. Comparative evaluation of physical, mechanical and processability quality attributes of Vcaps Plus®, Quali-V® and gelatin capsules. *International Journal of Pharmaceutics* 386:30–41.
12. Capsugel Library 2008. Technical Reference File Hard Gelatin Capsules.
13. Capsugel Library 2009. DBcaps Daily Intakes for Colorants.
14. Cole ET. 2000. Liquid filled and sealed hard gelatin capsules.
15. Cole ET, Cadé D, Benameur H. 2008. Challenges and opportunities in the encapsulation of liquid and semi-solid formulations into capsules for oral administration. *Advanced Drug Delivery Reviews* 60:747–56.
16. Buckalew LW, Coffield KE. 1982. An investigation of drug expectancy as a function of capsule color and size and preparation form. *Journal of Clinical Psychopharmacology* 2:245–8.
17. Col N, Fanale JE, Kronholm P. 1990. The role of medication noncompliance and adverse drug reactions in hospitalizations of the elderly. *Archives of Internal Medicine* 150:841–5.
18. Schwartz D, Wang M, Zeitz L, Goss ME. 1962. Medication errors made by elderly, chronically ill patients. *American Journal of Public Health and the Nation's Health* 52:2018–29.
19. Digenis GA, Gold TB, Shah VP. 1994. Cross-linking of gelatin capsules and its relevance to their in vitro-in vivo performance. *Journal of Pharmaceutical Sciences* 83:915–21.
20. Brown J, Madit N, Cole ET, Wilding IR, Cadé D. 1998. The effect of cross-linking on the in vivo disintegration of hard gelatin capsules. *Pharmaceutical Research* 15:1026–30.
21. Meyer MC, Straughn AB, Mhatre RM, Hussain A, Shah VP et al. 2000. The effect of gelatin cross-linking on the bioequivalence of hard and soft gelatin acetaminophen capsules. *Pharmaceutical Research* 17:962–6.
22. Overgaard ABA, Moller-Sonnergaard J, Christrup LL, Hojsted J, Hansen R. 2001. Patients' evaluation of shape, size and colour of solid dosage forms. *Pharmacy World & Science* 23:185–8.

3 Hard Shell Capsules in Clinical Trials

Moji Christianah Adeyeye and Amusa Adebayo

CONTENTS

INTRODUCTION

The choice and use of capsule shell type in formulation and development for clinical trials are generally based on the drug delivery goals (gastrointestinal site-specific delivery), acceptable dietary norms and patient preferences, and ease of blinding in clinical trials. Another important reason for choice is the need for use of small amount of actives in the early phase.

PRECLINICAL PHASE

In early stage development (including discovery and preclinical stages), formulations are evaluated in animals via different routes such as oral and intravenous in order to generate activity, efficacy, pharmacokinetics, and toxicity data. With the realization that nearly 40% of all compounds discovered have aqueous solubility and poor bioavailability limitations [1], it becomes a challenge for the development scientist to develop formulations that are simple to deliver via a route that could provide useful data.

Several *in silico* software and methods could be used to determine the solubility at the initial stage. These include the C log$P$ [2] and Lipinsky "Rule of 5" that states that compounds that possess the following properties could have oral absorption and permeability problems: molecular weight ≥ 500; log$P \geq 5$; H-bond donor ≥ 5, and H-bond acceptors ≥ 10 [3]. Having established the low water solubility, there are many approaches to improving it using different delivery systems. These include use of cosolvents, cyclodextrins, microemulsions, self-emulsifying delivery systems (SMEDDS), nanosuspensions, and solid dispersions. The products can then be used as such or filled into hard shell capsules for the early phase studies. The oral route is the common dosing route in animals where solutions, suspensions, and capsules can be used. Oftentimes, hard gelatin capsules are used in bigger animal models such as dogs.

Hard shell capsules made for preclinical trials (PCcaps) can be used in animals for oral dosing of formulations or drugs alone with or without excipients or incorporation of solvents [4]. The advantages of PCcaps include assurance of delivering consistent dosage levels, avoidance of regurgitation and upper gastrointestinal tract (GIT) irritation, taste and odor masking, and ease of dosing. PCcaps can be used for encapsulating powders and granules, semisolids, and nonaqueous liquids.

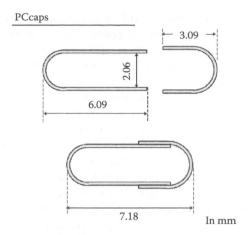

FIGURE 3.1 PCcaps overall length and dimensions showing locking ring. (Courtesy of Capsugel.)

The capsules can also be enterically coated for controlled-release studies. The capacity of PCcaps is 21.8 µL, the average weight of the capsule is 0.01 g, and the overall closed length is 7.2 mm, as shown in Figure 3.1. The capsules are available in a kit that includes the two boxes of 50 PCcaps, dosing syringe, funnel stand, and tamper.

Shen and Zhong [5] studied the bioavailability of atorvastatin in beagle dogs using SMEDDS consisting excipients such as Labrafil and Cremophor RH40. The SMEDDS formulation was encapsulated in hard gelatin capsules. The authors compared the bioavailability (BA) data in comparison to the conventional tablet equivalent.

They reported higher BA in the encapsulated formulation. In an earlier study, Serajuddin et al. [6] investigated the dissolution and bioavailability of a poorly water-soluble drug (REV-5901) in different polyethylene glycols and in Gelucire 44/14 filled in hard gelatin capsule. Sherif et al. [7] also used hard gelatin capsules to contain a coprecipitate of danazol–hydroxypropyl-β-cyclodextrin for the purpose of studying the bioavailability of the poorly water-soluble danazol in beagle dogs. The oral absorption was reported to be rapid in the dogs and comparable to oral dosing in rats.

Clinical Phase

The use of hard shell capsules for developing "first" clinical batch formulation has increased within the last 15 years owing to the timelines that have to be met in the process of clinical batch manufacturing [8]. In addition, encapsulation as a technology is relatively simple and cost-effective in blinding investigators and clinical subjects compared to other dosage forms that could be used such as tablets, pellets, semisolids, liquids, and parenterals. The goal during early phase (Phase 0 or Phase I) is to assess safety of the molecule and proof of concept for the intended therapy. Limited quantity of active pharmaceutical ingredient (API) is available and the decision is often skewed toward use of capsule dosage form. The clinical supply capsule units can range from several hundreds to several thousands.

Realizing that more than 90% of drugs at the drug discovery and development stage do not make it to the market, it behooves the early preformulation stage scientist to use appropriate dosage form for the safety and effectiveness assessment. Despite the fact that the physicochemical properties (e.g., dissociation constant, partition coefficient, solution-state stability, solubility, polymorphism, thermal events) of a potential drug candidate might have been identified, there is no assurance that including excipients at this stage with the drug in tablet dosage form will result in a promising formulation; therefore, a provisional formulation, such as hard gelatin capsules containing only the drug, is often used at this early phase [9]. Several types of shells made of different materials are now being used for early phase clinical trials. As will be discussed in more detail later in the chapter, these include materials such as hard gelatin, soft gelatin, hydroxypropyl methylcellulose (hypromellose) or HPMC [10] starch [11], calcium pectinate [12], chitosan [13], and various polymer-coated capsules intended for delivery in the lower part of the intestine and the colon [14,15].

Based on the preclinical and clinical trial phase considerations in early phase development, capsule engineering has evolved to accommodate different types of capsule fabrications and technologies, and this will be discussed in the chapter. The manufacturing of hard shells for clinical trials will also be considered for the different capsule technologies such as miniaturization, over-encapsulation, and liquid- or semisolid-filled hard shells. In particular, the manufacturing variables that could affect the delivery of the drug in preclinical and clinical trials will be discussed. The challenges associated with choice are usually related to manufacturability, cost–benefit ratio, and therapeutic outcomes. The chapter will underscore the uniqueness of hard shells in polyherbal formulation in clinical trials and in commercially available products. The functionality of hard shells in targeted oral delivery of small molecules and peptides/proteins in chronotherapy for drugs that follow circadian rhythm is emphasized. References will be made to drugs that otherwise could not be delivered orally because of the poor water solubility and which are delivered in lipid-based formulations using hard shells.

Irrespective of the capsule type, clinical development goal, and targeted delivery outcomes, the hard shell formulation development and subsequent use in preclinical or clinical trial should be approached from the quality of the product attributes or design of the formulation (i.e., quality-by-design [QbD] approach). This will eventually determine the quality of *in vivo* performance. Thus, QbD, relative to hard shells and clinical trials will be examined. Knowing the inevitability of regulatory oversight in product development, approval, and registration, perspectives of *in vitro* dissolution and respective *in vivo* performance and regulatory concerns regarding the choice of hard shell in the oral delivery of drugs over tablets will be discussed.

MINIATURIZATION TECHNOLOGY

Miniaturization is a new concept in pharmaceutical technology of solid dosage forms that involves the use of smaller quantities of new chemical entities (NCEs). This is to allow for essential information at the preformulation stage that would expedite the potential formulation development to be gathered. Formulations could be delivered earlier using smaller, and more readily available APIs and all clinical studies can be supported with more realistic and representative dosage forms [16]. Aside from this, a go–or–no-go decision could be made earlier regarding the formulation process, thus saving precious development time and improving efficiency. This is unlike the traditional formulation method where relatively large amount of API is typically needed and which may not be available until late Phase I or early Phase II. Knowing that the NCE is available only for clinical demands, the development team can become very creative in using precision dosing technologies available as part of miniaturization.

XCELODOSE TECHNOLOGY

It incorporates the miniaturization concept, and one of these technologies is Meridica's non-excipient filling Xcelodose. It allows for the use of very little drug (100 μg to 100 mg) filled into a hard gelatin capsule for early preformulation or formulation studies in early clinical trials. It is also called powder in capsule (PIC), API in capsule, or chemical in capsule. It has been reported that 9 out of the top 10 pharmaceutical companies use Xcelodose [17], and it reduces time to Phase I significantly [18]. The technology makes go–no-go decisions earlier without too much overhead that usually comes with the conventional program. This is because technical problems or delays that otherwise could arise as a result of preformulation studies, such as drug-excipient compatibility, and formulation and analytical development are avoided. It allows the API to be screened according to the Critical Path Initiative strategy of the US Food and Drug Administration (FDA) that allows a drug to fail quickly without incurring too much costs and time [19]. Xcelodose is particularly suited for oral and inhalation delivery. The goal of this pharmaceutical technology should be to produce safe and quality formulations that can be achieved by built-in robust science via design of experiment (DOE).

Knowing that 0.02% of NCEs will reach the market, typically 10–15 years after discovery, and that it costs at least $500 million to successfully develop an approved molecule, the concept of miniaturization becomes very logical. It will expedite rapid selection of drug candidates and development of lead compounds [20]. As companies strive to accelerate time to market, the paradigm increases the chances of taking a market advantage, period of market exclusivity, and greater yield of revenues [16].

One of the challenges of miniaturization is use of machines (capsule filling machines) that can provide adequate information with the use of not more than 10 g. The machines should be capable of producing capsules that are equivalent to those produced by large-scale machines. The machines used in miniaturization technology need not be based on geometric similarity; however, the instrumentation should be such that equivalent products will be produced. The equipment will be discussed in "Clinical Batch Manufacturing or Fabrication of Hard Gelatin Capsules" section. Other disadvantages of the Xcelodose technology include the following: poorly water-soluble drugs (Classes II and IV Biopharmaceutics Classification System [BCS] drugs) will not be suited for the technology [21]; high-dose and low-bulk density drugs will not be suitable for the filling into capsules [22]; APIs that are micronized and susceptible to electrostatic charge, agglomeration, and moisture may also create a problem during filling; the technology may be limited to only Phase I clinical trials; and API incompatible with hard gelatin will be excluded.

It is inevitable that the technology will be well used as a twenty-first century-adopted formulation development approach especially considering the genomic-driven revolution in drug discovery that calls for elucidation of 4000 new drug targets within the next 10 years. As reported by the author, miniaturization will need to be combined with high-throughput screening and combinatorial chemistry in order to achieve rational lead information [16].

CAPSULE DESIGN AND SPECIALTY SHELLS

HARD GELATIN CAPSULES PCCAPS

The fabrication of PCcaps is based on easy oral dosing in preclinical trials. The capsules have locked rings for improved closure (Figure 3.2), and it is available in a kit that contains a stainless steel tamper for filling powder with poor flow properties (Figure 3.3). The volume as stated earlier is 21.8 μL or 0.02 mL. The capacity in weight, which varies from 12 to 24 mg, depends on the bulk density of the powder that also varies from 0.6 to 1.2, respectively.

CONI-SNAP HARD GELATIN CAPSULES

The standard Coni-Snap hard gelatin capsules are widely used for clinical trials or for overencapsulation of double-blind clinical trials. In these cases, size 0 and size 00 capsules are often used, and in some instances, the larger size 000 capsules are used. However, the Coni-Snap capsules might not always provide the features that are needed for the broad variety of clinical trial goals and for comparison to other solid dosage forms. To overcome these limitations for certain trials, specific double-blind capsules (DBcaps) are now available.

HARD GELATIN DBCAPS

DBcaps are two-piece hard gelatin capsules designed for double-blind clinical trials in which the capsule body is completely covered by the elongated design of the cap. The design is such that it is virtually

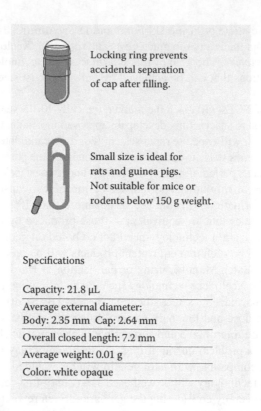

Locking ring prevents accidental separation of cap after filling.

Small size is ideal for rats and guinea pigs. Not suitable for mice or rodents below 150 g weight.

Specifications

Capacity: 21.8 µL	
Average external diameter: Body: 2.35 mm Cap: 2.64 mm	
Overall closed length: 7.2 mm	
Average weight: 0.01 g	
Color: white opaque	

FIGURE 3.2   PCcaps with locking rings. (Courtesy of Capsugel.)

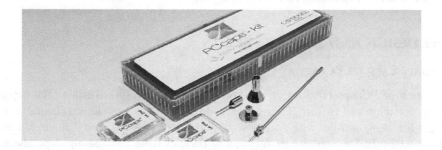

FIGURE 3.3   **(See color insert.)** PCcaps for a preclinical trial study. (Courtesy of Capsugel.)

impossible to open the capsule without causing clearly visible damage, thus alerting investigators of blind breaking and bias. The importance of blinding is underscored in clinical trials involving antipsychotic drugs where patients may not want to participate in placebo-controlled clinical trials [23]. The refusal can be attributed to fear of deterioration of disease state if a placebo is given. Therefore, use of a capsule such as DBcaps provides the added security of blinding that cannot be easily broken.

There are eight different sizes of DBcaps—AAA, AAel, AA, A, B, C, D, and E (Table 3.1). The wider diameter of DBcaps offers an advantage of relative ease of containment of several shapes and sizes of tablets, while the shorter length facilitates ease of swallowing. More than 90% of most commonly tableted drugs can be overencapsulated using DBcaps. The sizing guide of DBcaps for overencapsulation of Coni-Snap capsules, tablets, and caplets of different shapes are shown in the table.

DBcaps allow direct filling of whole tablets of various shapes without a need for breaking or grinding of tablets, thus eliminating the concern for inaccurate dosage or modification of intended

TABLE 3.1
DBcap Clinical Trials Overencapsulation Sizing Guide Information Clinical Trial

For capsules
If you need to overencapsulate a capsule, use the sizing guide below.

Coni-Snap® capsule size	5	4	3	2	1
Use DBcaps capsule size	B*, AA	A	A*, AAeL	AAeL	AAeL*

*May be suitable, depending on specific filling machine used.

For round or diametric shaped tablets
Measure the diameter (d) of your comparator product and compare it to the size ranges below.[1]

	Diameter					
Millimeters	≤5.49	5.50–6.05	6.06–6.73	6.74–7.56	7.57–8.82	8.83–11.00
Inches	≤.216	.217–.238	.239–.265	.266–.297	.298–.347	.348–.433
Use DBcaps capsule size	E	D	C	B	AA	AAA

As marketed comparator products may be manufactured in multiple global locations, there can be subtle country-to-country differences in actual tablet dimensions.

For oblong shaped tablets and caplets
Measure the height (h) and width (w) of your comparator product and compare it to the size ranges below.[1]

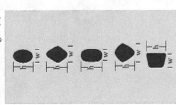

		Width					
Millimeters		≤5.49	5.50–6.05	6.06–6.73	6.74–7.56	7.57–8.82	8.83–11.00
Inches		≤.216	.217–.238	.239–.265	.266–.297	.298–.347	.348–.433
Height ≤8.74	≤.344	E	D	C	B	AA	AAA
8.75–9.64	.345–.379	D	D	C	B	AA	AAA
9.65–10.34	.380–.407	C	C	C	B	AA	AAA
10.35–10.54	.408–.415	B	B	B	B	AA	AAA
10.55–13.06	.416–.514	A/AA	A/AA	A/AA	A/AA	AA	AAA
13.07–14.44	.515–.568	A	A	A	A	AA	AAA
14.45–15.76	.569–.620	AAel/AAA	AAel/AAA	AAel/AAA	AAel/AAA	AAel/AAA	AAA
15.77–18.39	.621–.724	AAel	AAel	AAel	AAel	AAel	–

This chart assumes that the shape of the comparator allows it to drop fully to the base of the body section of the DBcaps capsule. To confirm this assumption, use the outline drawings of the DBcaps capsule bodies shown on the reverse side. [1]All tables include a conservative adjustment factor of –.2 mm or –.008″ versus the minimum range of DBcaps dimensional specifications.

DBcaps®

Source: Courtesy of Capsugel.

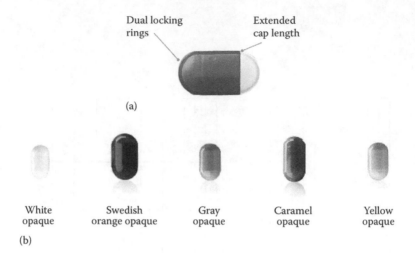

FIGURE 3.4 **(See color insert.)** DBcaps showing dual locking rings and extended cap length. (a) Extended cap length of DBcaps capsules that completely covers the sidewall of the capsule body. This makes it virtually impossible to open the capsule without causing visible damage. A dual locking ring design provides a full-circumference, leak-free closure. (b) DBcaps capsules formulated in a wide array of colors. The five standard color formulations were developed based on globally accepted colorants and on sufficient opacity to ensure blinding. (Courtesy of Capsugel.)

performance of drug (Figure 3.4). When the standard two-piece hard gelatin capsules (Coni-Snap) are used for blinding tablets for clinical trials, the smaller diameter (compared to DBcaps) limits the size of the tablet that can be filled into the capsule.

Hypromellose (HPMC) Capsules

The use of HPMC capsules commonly called VCaps has gained attention in recent years in over-the-counter formulations, especially in the encapsulation of herbs and dietary supplements (Figure 3.5).

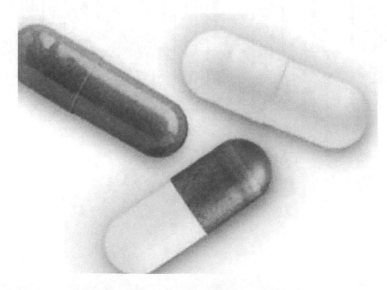

FIGURE 3.5 Hypromellose capsules (VCaps). (Courtesy of Capsugel.)

The reason is that it is preferred over bovine-derived material like gelatin to rule out the possibility of transmission of bovine spongiform encephalopathy and spongiform encephalopathy.

Preference for HPMC has also been attributed to the lack of cross-linking potential and drug–shell interaction that the gelatin capsule has shown [24]. Because of its vegetable origin, some cultural and religious preferences have become part of the reasons for the increased use of HPMC. However, because HPMC is bioadhesive, esophageal sticking tendency exists. This has been widely reported in literature.

Perkins et al. [25] reported this observation in a study involving elderly healthy subjects and use of radiolabeled capsules and tablets for comparison. Longer residence time (20.9 s) was observed in the HPMC capsule compared to tablet dosage form with a residence time of 4.3 s. Other investigators such as Cole et al. [26], McCargar et al. [27], and Osmanoglou et al. [28] also made similar observations. Hypromellose capsules are available in physical dimensions and shell weights similar to hard gelatin capsules, although the latter have wider size ranges.

HPMC capsules have been recommended for use in unit dose inhalers over hard gelatin capsules because of the higher moisture content of the latter (13–16%) compared to HPMC capsules with 4–6% moisture content. The higher moisture content of the gelatin capsules can cause interaction with the powdered material, resulting in the adherence of the powder to the capsule wall, inadequate discharge of powder, and possible dose failing [24]. Being a bioadhesive material, HPMC capsules are expected to stick to the esophagus compared to gelatin capsules, slowing down the transit time. As referred to earlier, Perkins et al. studied the esophageal transit time of HPMC capsules versus gelatin capsules [25]. The authors observed that the HPMC detached more easily compared to gelatin. Based on the nature of the two materials, it has been recommended that at least 150–200 mL of water be used when taking either capsule with the patient in an upright position that is maintained for several minutes [29]. An earlier study had indicated that there was tendency for HPMC capsules to stick to isolated porcine esophagus. However, it has been shown by gamma scintigraphy that the esophageal transit in the porcine model does not correlate with the human model [27].

In another study by Honkanen et al. [30], where six human subjects were used, the disintegration of two prolonged-release, radiolabeled formulations containing different grades of HPMC (K100 and K4M) in size 0 capsules was monitored. The disintegration time was measured at the midpoint of the time interval between the last image of the capsule with clear outlines and visually detectable spreading of the radioactivity plus the time of first detection of spreading radiation. It was observed that 4 out of the 12 capsules were lodged in the esophagus for 22–43 min. The initial disintegration

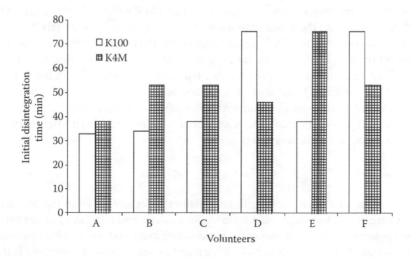

FIGURE 3.6 *In vivo* initial disintegration time (minutes) for the HPMC capsules in six healthy volunteers filled with two different prolonged formulations containing different viscosity grades of HPMC powder (HPMC K100 and HPMC K4M). (From www.oclc.org.)

time range was from 33 to 75 min, with very little difference between the two polymers at the 5% level. The profiles are shown in Figure 3.6.

Tuleu et al. [31] also compared the *in vivo* disintegration of uncoated 4-aminosalicylic acid Na (550 mg) HPMC capsules (that included carrageenan as gelling agent) with hard gelatin capsules in fasting eight healthy male volunteers. The two capsules were radiolabeled with indium 111 and technetium-99m and filled with a plug of lactose formulation. The capsule was administered to the subjects with 180 mL of water. The disintegration time was recorded when the scintigraphic image first shows the spread of radioactivity from the "core" of the capsule. It was observed that the disintegration times for both capsules are not significantly different.

Comparison of HPMC and Hard Gelatin Encapsulation and Performance

Unlike hard gelatin capsules, there was low correlation between the *in vitro* dissolution/disintegration and *in vivo* performance of HPMC capsules. Cole et al. [26] reported this in their investigation where ibuprofen-filled formulations in hard gelatin and HPMC capsules (containing gellan gum for gelling [HPMC$_{gell}$]) were used. The study was a crossover experiment involving 11 subjects in fasted and fed states. Scintigraphic and pharmacokinetics parameters were used to evaluate the disintegration and extent of drug distribution (AUC).

The authors reported significant differences in the time before absorption was detected (T_{lag}) for the two capsules whether in fasted or fed state due to the delayed initial disintegration. However, the study revealed longer *in vivo* opening of the HPMC$_{gell}$ capsules compared to hard gelatin capsules. This was attributed to the gelling agent such as carrageenan and gellan gum that are usually used in HPMC capsule formulation. The cations such as potassium used in the gelling system of HPMC capsule and which are present in the *in vivo* media interacted with the HPMC, causing persistent gelling of the capsule shells. *In vivo* disintegration/dissolution of HPMC$_{gell}$ capsules has been reported to also decrease in acidic medium [24]. Avoiding the gelling agent may reduce the delay in disintegration/dissolution.

In addition, unlike hard gelatin capsules, the disintegration/dissolution of HPMC decreases with an increase in temperature; therefore, it has been suggested that hard gelatin capsules should be administered with a warm drink (>30°C), while HPMC capsules, which is soluble below 30°C, could be taken with cold water. The disintegration/dissolution and machinability of HPMC capsules have been their major drawbacks, while their main advantage is the preference based on cultural or religious reasons. Manufacturing of HPMC is more expensive compared to hard gelatin because of needed modification in the processing and accommodation of the gelling system that will need to be added. Other advantages of HPMC capsules are the better compatibility with hygroscopic materials based on its lower moisture content and the non-cross-linking tendency compared to hard gelatin capsules [24].

In a recent report by Cade [32], a newer type of HPMC capsules was developed (VCaps Plus) without the gelling agent using a proprietary thermal gelling process. The impact of the mold pin temperature and the conditions to achieve optimal capsule drying were assessed. The author reported that capsules that had no delay in dissolution/disintegration were produced because of the absence of cations in the gelling system that otherwise would have interacted with the *in vivo* media and slowed down the dissolution/disintegration.

Plantcaps

It is a plant-based capsule made from pullulan—naturally fermented from tapioca. Its vegetable-origin, preservative-free, gluten-free, starch-free, allergen-free, and non-GMO identity makes it very attractive for customers who want purely organic supplement and those with discerning healthy lifestyle. The capsule has GRAS (generally recognized as safe) status, Kosher and Halal certifications, and approval by the Vegetarian Society [33]. Its vegetable origin makes it suitable for Asian regulatory agencies especially for use in Japan. Pullulan offers the best oxygen barrier of all available plant-based products and is therefore suitable for encapsulation of vitamin C known to produce "spotting" associated with encapsulation using gelatin capsule. It is also suitable for masking pungent tastes and odors and will find suitability in encapsulation of pungent herbal or polyherbal products. Plantcaps can be easily manufactured using the regular capsule filling machines.

STARCH CAPSULES

Starch capsules may be an alternative to hard gelatin or HPMC capsules if there is a need for such choice. The capsule is made from potato starch using injection molding. For filling and sealing, modification of the existing capsule manufacturing process is needed because the body and cap are manufactured separately. A benchtop, a semiautomatic, and an automatic machine can be used for the filling and sealing of starch capsules [11]. The capsules are manufactured in different sizes—0, 1, 2, 3, and 4. An advantage of starch capsules over other hard shells is the fact that the same size cap is made to fit all the different sizes. The cap fits evenly in place over the body, resulting in a good surface finish unlike the "lipped" seal on gelatin capsules.

The moisture content of starch capsules is comparable to that of hard gelatin capsules, although the moisture may be more tightly bound to the starch, thus reducing migration of moisture to the product. In an unpublished data, West Pharmaceuticals studied the stability of acetaminophen starch capsules in blister packages and reported acceptable stability after storage for 18 months. It would have been more informative if the blister packaging was compared to bulk packaging in a bottle.

SPECIALTY SHELLS DESIGN FOR TARGETED DRUG DELIVERY

PIC TECHNOLOGY

As referred to in "Miniaturization Technology" section, the Xcelodose miniaturization technology has gained a lot of attention in recent years for the filling of small amounts of drugs (usually without excipients) into capsule (PIC) for Phase I clinical trials. Some advantages and disadvantages of the technology have been highlighted in the section earlier. The emphases that could further be made of PIC are the contradictions of the technology. Although PIC could expedite Phase I clinical trials (3–6 months faster) compared to the conventional method, it could add to overall clinical and development cost since development work usually goes beyond Phase I trials. Therefore, the needed development work that should go into Phase II clinical trials is essentially postponed, thus slowing down New Drug Application (NDA) filing, approval, and overall development time and cost [21,22]. Pharmacokinetic data gathered using PIC technology for poorly soluble drugs could also be misleading, causing manufacturers to immaturely terminate the development without robust consideration of other means of improving the dissolution and absorption characteristics [21]. Another issue with PIC technology is the absence of the QbD requirements in the FDA guidance. More on this will be discussed in "Elements of QbD in Development of Capsules for Clinical Trial" section.

IMPERMEABLE OR COATED HARD GELATIN ENCAPSULATION AND PULSATILE DELIVERY

The use of impermeable or coated hard gelatin capsules has increased in recent years as investigators develop oral dosage forms that can deliver new drugs and new vaccines or target the colon specifically during preclinical and clinical phases.

A comparison of the coated hard gelatin and HPMC capsules was made by Dvorakova et al. [15], where they used different levels of Eudragit L and S 12.5, respectively, to target the intestine and ileum. Bhat et al. [34] devised a hard gelatin in which the capsule body was rendered impermeable without the cap or the plug by cross-linking via exposure to formaldehyde plus potassium permanganate (to facilitate generation of formalin vapor). The cross-linking was processed in a dessicator. The meltable erodible plug was made in a mold using several polymers such as Xanthan gum, Karaya gum, and Veegum, and processed by direct compression. The plug was placed by hand on the content inside the capsule body followed by the replacement of the cap. The whole capsule assembly was then dip-coated using 5% ethanolic solution of ethyl cellulose. The goal was to achieve a pulsatile drug delivery that can be used for nocturnal asthma. The authors reported that the drug release was dependent on the polymer level and the lag time before pulsatile release was determined by the properties of the plug. They also observed programmable pulsatile delivery that varied between 2 and 36 h as expected with chronopharmaceutical drug delivery. More of the release mechanism will be discussed later in the chapter.

Capsular systems are more independent of the capsule content and more dependent on the capsule device. Pulsincap system, as an example, is an osmotic system that has an impermeable or insoluble capsule body and a swellable plug [35,36]. The impermeable capsule half is filled with the drug formulation while the capsule half (the cap) is closed at the open end with a swellable hydrogel plug. The drug is released rapidly once the plug swells and is ejected when in contact with dissolution media or gastrointestinal fluids [37,38].

Fused and Banded Hard Gelatin Capsules

In an invention reported by Samantaray et al. [39], fused hard gelatin capsule was designed to deliver a liquid formulation of paricalcitol (synthesized form of calcitriol, an active metabolite of vitamin D) for the prevention and treatment of hyperparathyroidism in chronic kidney disease. The formulation contains solubilizers such as Cremophor ELP and other pharmaceutically acceptable excipients. The capsules are filled and then sealed by spraying a water–ethanol mixture at the cap and body interface, followed by warming to fuse the cap and body together. Banding is done by rectifying the capsules and passing over a serrated revolving wheel that revolves in a gelatin bath. The gelatin that is picked up by the wheel is applied to the cap and body interface. A two-way crossover single-dose comparative bioavailability study of the liquid-filled fused capsules and commercially available tablets (Zemplar) of the drug showed similar pharmacokinetic profiles.

Acid-Resistant HPMC Capsules

Acid-resistant DRCaps have been developed to meet the challenges often encountered in manufacturing [40]. The goal is targeted delivery of drugs to the intestine. Acid-sensitive drugs and drugs/excipients that may be prone to acid-reflux will qualify for encapsulation using DRCaps. Because of its low moisture content, DRCaps will be useful for moisture-sensitive drugs and excipients. Unlike enteric-coated HPMC capsules, DRCaps development does not include a laborious coating process that may include solvents and heat that could compromise the stability of the drugs and excipients. The capsule is fully compatible with Capsugel's Xcelodose S precision powder microdosing system.

Gastro-Resistant (Enteric-Coated) HPMC Capsules

Enteric-coated capsules have been used in a double-blind, placebo-controlled clinical trial in children (5–16 years) with Crohn's disease [41]. In the study, one group received 5-aminosalicylic acid (5-ASA) + ω-3 fatty acids as triglycerides in gastroresistant capsules and 3 g/day Triolip capsule containing 400 mg eicosapentaenoic acid and 200 mg docosahexaenoic acid. The other group received 5-ASA + olive placebo capsules. The authors reported that the enteric-coated 5-ASA capsules in addition to the ω-3 fatty acids delayed the relapse of the disease even if it could not prevent it compared to the 5-ASA alone. The capsule material was not mentioned.

In a publication by Kadri and Greene, enteric-coated HPMC was developed using cellulose acetate phthalate (Aquacoat CPD) and polyvinyl acetate phthalate (Sureteric). The authors reported that the Aquacoat CPD-coated capsules were weaker at the cap/body junction than the Sureteric-coated capsules that remained rigid after 1 h. The testing was done in simulated gastric fluid although both provided similar gastric media protection at comparable coating levels [42]. If the coating is intended for colonic delivery, the pH solubility has to be chosen to accommodate the physiological condition. The pH solubilities for enteric delivery and colonic delivery are pH 5.5 and pH 7, respectively.

Examples of other polymers include cellulose trimellitiate, hydroxypropylmethyl cellulose phthalate, polyvinyl acetate phthalate, shellac copolymer of methacrylic acid and methylmethacrylate, azopolymers, disulfide polymers, and amylase [15]. Direct pan coating of HPMC capsule has been reported to be much easier than coating of gelatin when Eudragit L and S 12.5 were used because of insufficient surface adhesion to the smoother surface of gelatin and its relative brittleness [43].

Coated Hypromellose Capsules

Hydroxypropyl methylcellulose capsules containing 4-aminosalicylic acid was coated with amylose-ethylcellulose film coat by a dip coating process in an investigation. The coated capsules, monitored by scintigraphic imaging, remained intact throughout transit in the upper GIT before arrival in the colon. Plasma and urine concentrations of N-acetyl-4-aminosalicylic acid (a metabolite of 4-aminosalicylic acid) were used as primary endpoints in in-vivo evaluation monitoring of drug release in the healthy adults. Amylose/ethylcellulose coating film is called COLAL and prednisolone sodium metasulfobenzoate integrated into this system is designated COLAL-PRED [44,45].

In another related study, COLAL-PRED oral capsules were used in multicentered Phase III clinical trials involving 796 participants for the treatment of moderate acute ulcerative colitis. The 8-week randomized parallel study involved once-daily dosing of 40-, 60-, and 80-mg COLAL-PRED oral capsules, with prednisolone tablets as the active comparator. Colitis activity index and cortisol level were used as the endpoints of this safety and efficacy study. Although there were no differences in efficacy, the authors suggested that the safety profile of the test product was better than that of the comparator [46] COLAL-PRED has the potential to become the first bacteria-aided biomaterials and pH-sensitive polymeric film (BPSF)-coated delivery system approved for use in humans. Guar gum/Eudragit RS PO/S100 blend was used in coating hypromellose theophylline capsules using triethyl citrate as plasticizer and the dip coating method in another study [47]. The intent of the study was colon-delivery but there was no justification made in the report for colonic delivery of theophylline [14].

Enteric-Coated Starch Capsules

For drugs that may be destroyed by acidic medium in the gastric region or may cause gastric irritation or nausea, or targeted delivery, especially to the colon (for ulcerative colitis or Crohn's disease therapy), starch capsules have been coated for delayed release for these purposes. The coating was reported in an unpublished report not to be problematic owing to the smoothness of the cap/body seal and the higher bulk density of the capsules. In a different study, Vilivalam et al. [48] evaluated the stability of 5-ASA starch capsules by monitoring the dissolution and disintegration indices at 25°C and 55% relative humidity (RH), and at 40°C and 75% RH. They reported that the to be 5-ASA release remains unchanged at the temperature and RH conditions.

Watts and Illum [49] studied the development of coated starch capsules for colon-targeted delivery and reported delayed release to meet the objective. To follow the transit characteristics of dosage forms through the GIT, scintigraphic study has been used in healthy human volunteers [50]. Doll et al. studied the release characteristics (capsule opening) and transit times of coated starch capsules and hard gelatin capsules though the GIT [51]. The GIT transit data were compared to plasma concentrations of the drug amoxicillin. In the study, coated starch or gelatin capsule containing 250 mg of the drug and a radiolabel was administered to the volunteers under fasted conditions. Analysis of the data showed no significant differences between the plasma concentrations and the transit time for both capsules.

In another study, Wilding et al. [52] studied the gastro-resistance of starch capsules enteric-coated using Aquateric coating. The authors observed capsule integrity in the stomach following administration after either an overnight fast or a medium breakfast, confirming the gastro-resistance of the capsules. Effect of food on the gastro-resistance was studied in another investigation [53] and the authors reported that the capsules remained intact for more than 2 h in 0.1 N hydrochloric acid but disintegrated within 20 min after the acid medium was exchanged for pH 6.8 phosphate buffer (simulated intestinal fluid pH). Gamma scintigraphy confirmed the gastro-resistance of the capsules in the stomach until disintegration occurred in the small intestine at 68 ± 28 and 95 ± 3.3 min following fasted and fed administrations, respectively, after leaving the stomach.

Targit Technology

It is an enteric-coated starch capsule designed for targeted delivery to different sites within the colonic region. Eudragit L and S were used for the coating to provide timed dissolving of the capsule as it enters the small intestine after leaving the stomach [54]. The coating is designed such that the capsule disintegrates at a predetermined region such as the terminal ileum and the ascending, the transverse, and the descending colon (Figure 3.7). Therefore, drug release from the Targit system is pH- and time-dependent, which is preferred or fail-safe compared to a system that is only dependent on pH change in the environment.

Osmotic Capsules

Waterman et al. [55] developed osmotic capsule technology for the purpose of controlling the delivery of the drug based on the water permeability of the capsule shell and the ratio of the combination polymers used to compose the capsule. The osmotic capsule was made with the combination of a water-insoluble polymer (cellulose acetate) and a water-soluble polymer (polyethylene glycol 3350).

The intent of the capsule device was to rapidly develop a delivery system in the early development phase that could facilitate the understanding of the drug release profiles using needed additives but with minimal formulation optimization. The ultimate goal is to shorten the time to market. The osmotic capsule features include drug-independent drug release profiles, easily varied drug

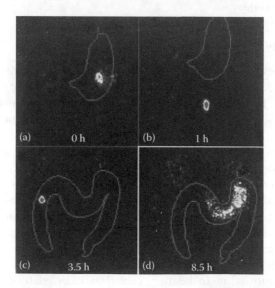

FIGURE 3.7 **(See color insert.)** Scintigraphic images of a radiolabeled TARGIT capsule in a human after oral administration. At 0 h, the capsule is in the stomach (a); 1 h, small intestine (b); 3.5 h, ascending colon (c); and 8.5 h, dispersed in transverse and descending colon (d). (Courtesy of Taylor & Francis.)

loading and simple fabrication without specialized equipment, simple formulation, and good *in vitro–in vivo* correlation. The device is made of a capsule body (which has a laser-drilled hole through the closed end), an active tablet, a push tablet, and a capsule cap.

Other osmotic capsular systems have been reported by several authors to provide a sustained drug release throughout the large bowel after a silent phase that coincides with the time necessary for their activation. In an investigation by Crison et al., osmotic excipients were added to the formulation in the capsule body to expedite the plug ejection at the end of the lag phase. In a capsule-like delivery system, an erodible plug made using the injection-molding technology was positioned at each open end of an impermeable shell cylinder that has the drug in the core [56]. The system can also be made such that an insoluble plug was matched with a semipermeable capsule body containing the active ingredient along with an osmotic charge (programmable oral release technology [PORT]) [57]. Upon inflow of aqueous fluid, hydrostatic pressure that develops inside the capsule pushes the plug out. The mechanism was used to create lag phases that could be suitable for time-dependent colonic delivery.

The osmotic pump mechanism was also exploited to achieve lag phases potentially suitable for time-based colonic delivery [58]. As stated in "Capsule Design and Specialty Shells" section, Zhang et al. reported a similar system in an earlier investigation [35].

CLINICAL BATCH MANUFACTURING OR FABRICATION OF HARD GELATIN CAPSULES

MINIATURIZATION TECHNOLOGY ENCAPSULATION

The miniaturization technology used in the Xcelodose system is a precision micro-dose automated encapsulator (Figure 3.8). It allows for direct filling of minute quantities of drug (100 µg to 100 mg) into hard gelatin capsules (PIC) without excipients at a rate of several hundred capsules per hour. This is particularly suited in clinical batch manufacturing or production of formulations for clinical trials.

The Xcelolab dispenser or encapsulator is used for Xcelodose technology [59]. The Xcelodose 120S system can be used to manually fill capsules and small vials, tubes, and cassettes. The programmable dispensing of dose weight through the weighing balance assembly ensures dose accuracy. It has a closed-loop dispensing mechanism into the capsules and for powder characterization, preparation, and stability setup. The encapsulation can be done in a regular laboratory, under a laminar flow setting containment enclosure. It uses a tapping mechanism that involves a building a

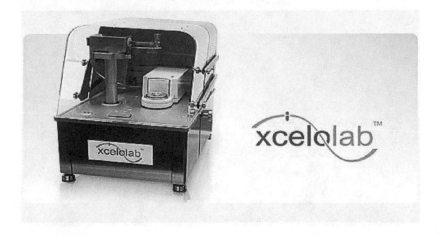

FIGURE 3.8 Xcelolab encapsulator. (Courtesy of Capsugel.)

micro-bridge (Figure 3.9) that upon impact breaks down and rebuild [60]. The technology ensures that the drug is not compacted and the stability is not compromised as a result of compaction. The technology is suitable for free-flowing actives, including cohesive substances and micronized or inhalation powders. The filling occurs without segregation, and for moisture-sensitive actives, operation can be done under humidity-controlled environment, for example, <5% RH.

The capacity for Xcelolab to fill drug alone makes analysis and stability testing easier and the development time faster. It also reduces waste of actives especially at the early development phase when limited amount of active is available.

Xcelodose 600 is an automated programmable 21 CFR Part 11 compliant machine (Figure 3.10) that is used for precise metering of API or simply blending of formulations (100 µg to 300 mg) into capsules of varied sizes (00 to 4) [61]. The powder is dispensed through dispensing heads (a and b) through dispensing fingers (c) for cohesive materials (Figure 3.11).

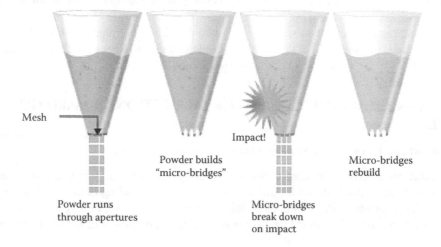

FIGURE 3.9   Xcelolab tapping and micro-bridging powder encapsulation. (Courtesy of Capsugel.)

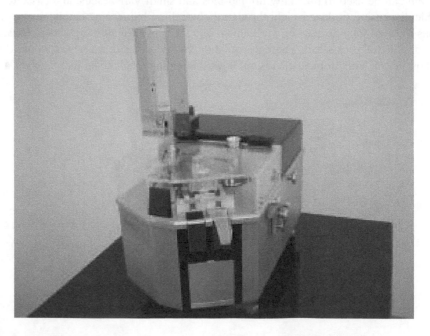

FIGURE 3.10   Xcelodose 600 micro filling system. (Marketed by Capsugel BVBA.)

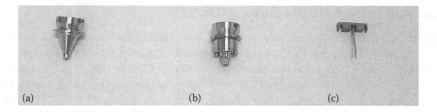

FIGURE 3.11 **(See color insert.)** Xcelodose 600 micro filling system dispensing heads (a and b) and fingers (c). (Courtesy of Capsugel.)

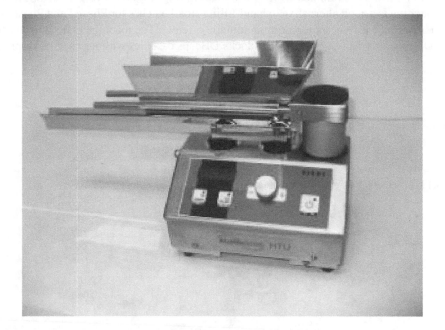

FIGURE 3.12 Xcelience automatic feeding high-throughput unit (HTU). (Courtesy of Capsugel.)

Clinical trial (Phase I) supplies up to several thousand capsules can be manufactured using the automatic feeding high-throughput unit (HTU) (Figure 3.12) attached to Xcelodose.

LIQUID OR SEMISOLID FILLED HARD GELATIN CAPSULES

Hard gelatin capsules are used to contain liquids and semisolids during the early stages of drug development. This is applicable where the drug is poorly water-soluble or there is a problem of recrystallization if the formulation is developed as a solution form. At this stage, there is limited supply of the active. Therefore, producing small batches of formulations for clinical trials becomes critical. Manual filling can be done in the laboratory using a pipette or a semiautomatic machine. An example of a simple machine used for such clinical batch manufacturing is CFS 1200 that was developed by Capsugel. The machine can fill up to 1200 capsules/h with hot melt liquid or cold thixotropic semisolid/liquid materials. Liquid filling and sealing technologies for hard shell capsules provide the formulator with the flexibility of in-house development of formulations from a small scale, as required for Phase I studies, up to production [62]. If hard gelatin capsules cannot be used because of any formulation, preference, or cultural reason in early stage development, alternative materials such as polymer-based shells or hypromellose may be used.

Overencapsulation Hard Gelatin Capsules (DBcaps)

Overencapsulation is a process that hides a dosage form (tablets and capsules) in another capsule shell for the purpose of blinding in clinical trials. The DBcaps are available in eight different sizes to accommodate various sizes of comparator tablet, caplet, or capsule shapes in clinical trials blinding (Figure 3.13). Because there is no need for modification of comparator dosage forms, the process of blinding becomes easier and the errors that could be associated with the bioequivalence data become reduced.

The capsules can be filled manually (Profiller 3700), as shown in Figure 3.14, and with most semiautomatic and automatic capsule filling machines such as the ProFiller 3800 DB machine, CFS 1200, and Ultra 8 II combined with TFR 8 loading ring (Figures 3.15 and 3.16). The ProFiller 3800 DB machine is a good alternative to hand-filling small batches for Phase I and Phase II double-blind studies because it comes with a semiautomatic orienter. The machine is designed specifically for filling DBcaps. It orients, separates, and locks DBcaps capsules without vacuum or pneumatics.

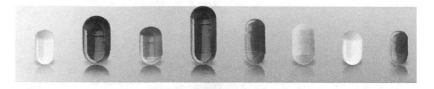

FIGURE 3.13 **(See color insert.)** Different DBcaps sizes. (Courtesy of Capsugel.)

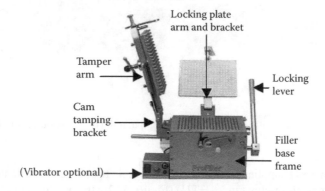

FIGURE 3.14 ProFiller 3700 and 3800 stainless steel upgrade series. (Courtesy of Capsugel.)

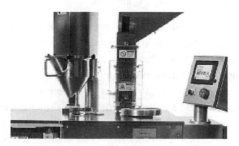

Ultra™ III semiautomatic capsule filling machine

FIGURE 3.15 Ultra III semiautomatic capsule. (Courtesy of Capsugel.)

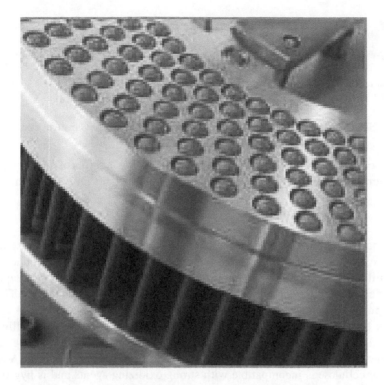

FIGURE 3.16 TFR 8 tablet filling ring filling machine. (Courtesy of Capsugel.)

It can double blind 1000 to 1500 doses of caplets, tablets, or capsules per hour. A separate attachment is used for different capsule sizes.

Manufacturing Considerations of DBcaps and Clinical Trials

The intent to use DBcaps in clinical trials should be based on several factors such as capsule size, target population, the cultural acceptance of the capsule color, the influence of backfill on capsule filling, the capsule filling machine and change parts, and ordering of clinical supplies.

Target Population

Geriatric and pediatric populations cannot swallow bigger size capsules easily; therefore, in clinical trials, this factor has to be taken into consideration. When a smaller capsule size is needed for overencapsulation, the regular Coni-Snap sizes 1, 2, or 3 may be used for blinding.

Choice of Capsule Color

The choice of color is crucial in clinical trials, and DBcaps has the advantage of availability in many colors, which can be chosen to completely hide the encapsulated or enclosed unit (Figure 3.17). Examples of colors are shown below.

The DBcaps should not reveal any shadow or air pockets resulting from the backfill or any printing or monogram on the encapsulated unit [63]. The choice of color dyes and pigments may sometimes be based on cultural acceptance. Regulatory agencies such as the World Health Organization, the US Code of Federal Regulations, and the Japanese Pharmaceutical Excipients Directory have set guidelines on ingestion of iron oxide and elemental iron. The reason is that iron oxides are commonly used in pharmaceutical grade colorants in DBcaps. Although several colors are accepted globally, many countries have restrictions on some colors. This must be confirmed before clinical

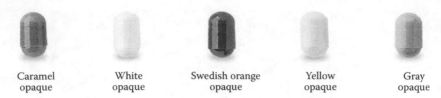

| Caramel | White | Swedish orange | Yellow | Gray |
| opaque | opaque | opaque | opaque | opaque |

FIGURE 3.17 (**See color insert.**) DBcaps in different colors. (Courtesy of Capsugel.)

investigation in order to dialogue with capsule vendor according in terms of ordering of the capsules in the right colors. A good lead time of 2–3 months should be built into the planning for ordering the capsules.

Backfill

The choice of backfill (excipient that can be added to the encapsulated unit) is sometimes determined by the excipients that are used for the formulation of the comparator product [64]. It is best to choose a similar excipient but it is not required. This is to avoid problems of excipient–excipient interaction that could result in compromise of disintegration or dissolution results. The information regarding excipients used in the comparator product is usually listed in the package insert or in Physician Desk Reference. The most commonly used excipients are microcrystalline cellulose or lactose monohydrate.

The preference for the two excipients is attributed to their hydrophilicity and water solubility. Microcrystalline cellulose is incompatible with strong oxidizing agents and is hygroscopic; it also has disintegrating properties depending on the amount in the formulation. Lactose monohydrate is incompatible with primary and some secondary amine drugs such as aminophylline and amphetamines due to browning that results from the Maillard reaction. Therefore, lactose should be avoided in lactose-intolerant populations especially if a larger amount is needed in the backfill.

Faust [64] studied the effect of variations in the excipients on disintegration and dissolution. Lactose anhydrous, which is sometimes used as backfill, may contain 5-(hydroxymethyl)-2 furfuraldehyde as an impurity that could cause cross-linking. Examples of other excipients that may form aldehyde upon autooxidation are starch, polysorbate 80, and polyethylene glycol. Therefore, drug or excipients should not contain aldehydes that could cross-link with the gelatin. It was reported that backfill with a high amount of microcrystalline cellulose pulled more water from the shell, thus causing faster disintegration of the shells compared to backfill made up of lactose monohydrate. However, mounding (coning of excipients under the dissolution paddle) occurred in the microcrystalline backfill that resulted in slower dissolution of the comparator product compared to lactose monohydrate. The author then concluded that a 50:50 blend of both excipients would counterbalance the effect of each and provide the expected outcomes in disintegration and dissolution of the comparator product. The blend also met the SUPAC-IR guidance for sameness/equivalence as compared to the comparator product.

Huynh-Ba and Aubry [65] reported that the dissolution profiles of two encapsulated forms of the same tablet with different overfill or backfill excipient gave significantly different results in dissolution (Figure 3.18). The difference could be attributed to the excipients, which the authors did not include in the report.

Use of DBcaps can significantly reduce the amount of backfill or overfill that will be used during manufacturing. Thus, the potential for drug–excipient or excipient–excipient interaction is reduced. For example, using a size C DBcaps instead of size 0 of the regular Coni-Snap reduces the volume for overfilling by 40% (Figure 3.19). The manufacturing considerations highlighted above and other formulation and process attributes can be used to design a formulation in a systematic manner in order to ensure quality and reduce risk in early phase development using the QbD approach that will be discussed later in the chapter.

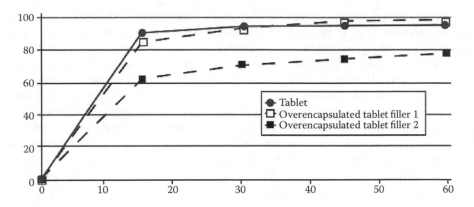

FIGURE 3.18 Comparison of dissolution profiles of innovator's tablet and two overencapsulated formulations. (From Huynh-Ba K, Aubry AF. Analytical development strategies for comparator products. *American Pharmaceutical Review* 2003; 6(2): 92–97.)

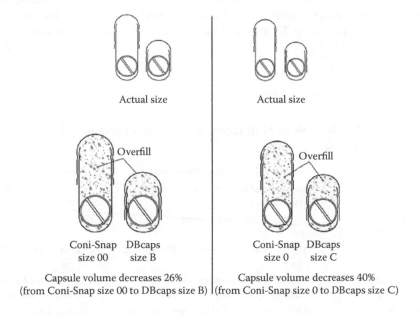

FIGURE 3.19 Size comparison of DBcaps capsules versus standard capsules. (From Huynh-Ba K, Aubry AF. Analytical development strategies for comparator products. *American Pharmaceutical Review* 2003; 6(2): 92–97.)

Dissolution of DBcaps Capsules

The dissolution of drug from an overencapsulated product is dependent on the drug BCS, the characteristics of the product (e.g., tablets, capsules, mini-tablets, pellets, etc.), and the nature of the backfill. It has been reported that the profiles of overencapsulated and un-encapsulated products are comparable enough not to affect the dissolution endpoint; however, there could be a lag time of 5–10 min as a result of the capsule opening.

Esseku et al. [8] studied the dissolution of DBcaps overencapsulated tablets of drugs that belonged to different BCS groups—propranolol, a highly soluble, highly permeable BCS class I, and rofecoxib, a low-solubility and high-permeability BCS class II drug that is susceptible to oxidation and photolysis [8]. The influence of moisture on the disintegration and dissolution of the encapsulated tablets has not been studied for either class of drugs. Two blocks of $2 \times 2 \times 2$ randomized full factorial design were used to determine the effect of three independent parameters. Two levels, that is, two drug types (propranolol and rofecoxib), two capsule types (DBcaps and Coni-Snap), and two filler levels (microcrystalline cellulose/lactose 1:1 mixture and no filler), were used in the design. They reported that the disintegration time (D-time) for rofecoxib was slightly higher than the D-time for propranolol, possibly because of the lower solubility of the former. D-times for the capsule and filler effects were similar, ranging from 3.67 to 3.85 min, respectively, an indication that the variables had no effect on the D-times and were not statistically significant ($P > 0.05$).

To compare the dissolution profiles, the similarity factor F_2 was used. For propranolol tablets, the F_2 between CS and DBcaps was 60.67, indicating that the dissolution profiles of the two were similar. The similarity factor between rofecoxib tablets encapsulated in standard and DBcaps was 62.48. This was also indicative of similarity in dissolution profiles.

ENCAPSULATED POLYHERBAL FORMULATIONS AND CLINICAL TRIALS

Hard shell capsules have found great utility in nutraceuticals and polyherbals. HPMC capsules have particularly drawn interest from manufacturers of herbal formulations and nutraceuticals because of the non-bovine origin. Encapsulation using different hard shells in general is also preferred because of convenience of manufacturing. Examples of the products in the market that have sufficient information are shown in Table 3.2.

TABLE 3.2

Some Examples of Polyherbals or Nutraceuticals Products Formulated in HPMC Capsules and Their Manufacturers

Product	Nature of the Formulation	Manufacturing Company
Damiana Herb 300 mg	Pure powdered herbs (*Damiana turnera aphrodisiaca*)	Bio-Health Ltd., UK
Thera Veda's Ajay-Allergy Support Formula	Vegetable extracts and powders	Organix South, USA
Natren Life Start 2	Bacteria, vitamin C, potato powders and whole goat milk	NATREN, Inc., USA
Coloclear (in VegiCap)	Flax seeds, slippery elm and other herbs	Higher Nature Ltd., USA
Jarro-Dophilus EPS	8 probiotic species and ascorbic acid	Jarrow Formulas, USA
Culturelle HS Capsules	80 mg *lactobacillus GG* (*L. rhamnosus GG*) Vegetarian formula	Kirkman Labs, USA
Align Daily Probiotic Supplement Capsules	*Bifidobacterium infantis*	Procter & Gamble, USA
Sportlegs Supplement	Vitamin D, calcium and magnesium	Sportlegs, USA
Planetary Herbals Cinnamon Extract	Cinnamomum aromacticum 300 mg, bark extract 10:1 yielding 8% flavonoids, cinnamomum aromaticum bark 100 mg	Planetary Herbals, USA
Ex-Tox II	Folic acid, cilantro powder (leaf), ethylenediamine tetra-acetic acid, N-acetyl L-cysteine, fulvic (humic) acid, R-lipoic acid (K-RALA), L-methionine	Progressive Labs, USA

Source: Al-Tabakha MM, HPMC capsules: Current status and future prospects. *J Pharm Pharm Sci* 2010; 13 (3): 428–442. Permission granted by the Canadian Society of Pharmaceutical Sciences.

Establishment of safety and efficacy of polyherbals has had some pitfalls in the past because of lack of adequate evaluation. Therefore, to overcome this, encapsulation has been used for the formulation and evaluation of polyherbals; Khan et al. [66] evaluated the physicochemical parameters including the preformulation characteristics of four anti-stress plants, namely, *Withania somnifera*, *Tinospora cordifolia*, *Emblica officinalis*, and *Eugenia caryophyllus*. Each plant was prepared after drying and milling by wet granulation in readiness for encapsulation into size 00 hard gelatin capsules. Among other tests conducted, high-performance thin-layer chromatography and differential scanning calorimetry indicated that the plants contain withanolide, berberine, gallic acid, and eugenol markers, respectively. Disintegration test of the capsules was performed using a digital microprocessor disintegration apparatus. The authors reported that the disintegration was 8 min 28 s.

Another pitfall in herbal product evaluation is lack of assessment of the effectiveness of the blind. Lack of blinding may lead to bias in performance assessment and in the choice of analytical strategies and methods. Based on this premise, Zick et al. [67] conducted a randomized placebo-controlled clinical trial to assess blinding with ginger (*Zingiber officinale*) using healthy individuals. The goal of the study is to establish whether the participants can determine accurately if they receive a ginger or placebo capsule in blister pack and a bottle filled with ginger or placebo capsules. The authors reported that volunteers couldn't determine which type of individual capsule they receive but could distinguish a bottle with ginger capsules. This outcome of the research is that use of ginger capsules in blister packs enhanced blinding. They recommended that, for studies that include powdered standardized ginger root, one should place the ginger capsules in blister packs where the participants receive individual capsules and where the distinctive ginger aroma that otherwise is present in bulk packing of many capsules in a bottle is absent. The authors also recommended that, in general, clinical trials of herbal products include blinding procedures for the above-stated reasons.

Hard shell capsules were used in another clinical study where a comparative clinical evaluation of a polyherbal formulation with multivitamin formulation was undertaken for learning and memory enhancement [68]. In the randomized, placebo-controlled, double-blind study, the authors used 47 human volunteers (18–24 years) that were given either a capsule of the placebo or two capsules of the polyherbal formulation (500 mg) at night or one capsule of the multivitamin formulation (500 mg) two times a day for a period of 3 months. The subjects were monitored for neuropsychological tests such as short-term memory and IQ scores. They reported an increase in short-term memory and IQ scores in the polyherbal- and multivitamin-treated group, suggesting that both formulations improved learning and memory compared to the placebo in young healthy subjects. The polyherbal appeared more effective than the multivitamin formulation.

A clinical evaluation of herbal formulation was also reported by Tasawar et al. [69] where *Nigella sativa* was studied for the lowering of body total lipid concentration and prevention of atherosclerosis. The authors used 80 subjects (in fasted state) that were divided into two groups—an interventional group (given capsules of *N. sativa* and statin) and a non-interventional group that received statin capsule only. The study, which lasted 6 months, showed that there was a significant decrease in cholesterol, LDL, VLDL, and triglycerides and a significant increase in HDL in the interventional group compared to the non-interventional group that received only statin. This is an indication that *N. sativa* has the therapeutic effectiveness to reduce lipid profile in patients with coronary artery disease.

The pharmacokinetics and bioavailability of soy extract capsules were studied and compared with a soy beverage in a randomized two-phase crossover design. The two products have isoflavones—daidzein and genistein—but in different ratios. The results revealed that the normalized bioavailability of daidzein, following a single oral administration of soy beverage, was slightly (but significantly) less than that of soy extract capsules, whereas the bioavailability of genistein from both soy preparations was comparable. The other pharmacokinetic parameters of daidzein and genistein, including C_{max} adjusted for the dose, T_{max}, and $t_{1/2}$, were similar for both soy preparations.

HARD SHELL CAPSULES AND TARGETED ORAL DRUG DELIVERY

As oral delivery remains the most common route of administration because of its flexibility and convenience, the differences in the GIT physiology makes the delivery of drug to the different sites more challenging. Therefore, the need to tailor the dosage form device to a specific site is heightened. The use of hard shell capsules in oral targeted delivery will be brought to focus in this section although the targeted delivery was referred to earlier in different sections of the chapter. The advances in capsule technology and in coating processes make it necessary to capture the importance of the hard shell as a utility vehicle to deliver drugs to different segments of the GIT to maximize therapeutic effectiveness.

STOMACH

It is easier to study the *in vivo* performance of dosage forms such as mini-tablets or pellets designed with a purpose and contained in hard gelatin capsules than the tablets because, in the latter, the manufacturing variables—excipients, granulation methods, and compression process variables—could modify the *in vivo* dissolution and bioavailability. Sawicki [70] studied the *in vivo* performance of verapamil and norverapamil from controlled-release floating pellets in humans. The pellets were contained in hard gelatin capsules. The authors found out that for verapamil (40 mg), pharmacokinetic parameters such as C_{max}, T_{max}, and area under the curve (AUC) for the pellets were more favorable compared to the reference tablets. This was because the pellets, which were found to float for 6 h during *in vitro* studies, maintained the dissolution attributes as a result of the containment in hard gelatin capsules before their release.

Dhaliwal et al. [71] reported the use of hard gelatin capsules in the delivery of mucoadhesive acyclovir microspheres to the stomach. The microspheres were prepared using chitosan, carbopol, and methylcellulose polymers and emulsion and chemical cross-linking techniques. The capsule delivered the multiunits to the stomach, and because of the mucoadhesive property, the multiunits were retained in the stomach and released the drug for over a period of 12 h. In an earlier study, Sakr [72] reported the use of a programmable, controlled-release drug delivery oral non-digestible capsule containing levonorgestrel designed as a floating device and made up of different grades of HPMC. The device has a built-in triggering ballooning system with predetermined erosion rates to control retention times, which, after the release of the drug, becomes flattened and returns to normal size to enable elimination.

INTESTINE

Hard gelatin capsules have also been used to deliver drugs farther down into the intestinal region. Schellekens et al. [73] coated the capsule with a pH-responsive polymer (Eudragit S) and related the responsiveness to the swelling index of the disintegrant, particularly croscarmellose. Studies in humans showed that the coat was able to resist the acidic gastric conditions in the stomach and duodenum, delaying the delivery of the drug until the distal segments of the intestine was reached. A more sophisticated targeted drug delivery system using capsules was reported earlier by Hinderling et al. [74] in which the drug Fasudil was delivered at different GI sites using the InteliSite capsule. The authors achieved the delivery by remote control following activation by a magnetic signal.

COLON

The colon has become a drug delivery target site especially for therapy of diseases localized in the colon. The site will become more popular as investigators (Ishibashi et al. [75] and Pinto [76]) assess the technology for delivery of many drugs including proteins and peptides. Ishibashi et al. referred to the capsular system (coated with Eudragit E as a colon-targeted delivery capsule). In different instances, Ishibashi and other authors had reported that the erosion of a functional Eudragit E coating was induced by the delayed dissolution and ionization of an organic acid enclosed within the capsule core [77,78]. The obvious advantages are improvement in patient compliance and treatment efficacy. Abdul and Bloor [79] underscored this importance and the challenges that the drug faces at the different segments of the GIT en route to the delivery site. Based on this, pharmaceutical technological approaches have been implored to target colonic delivery. The approaches are either drug-specific or formulation-specific. In the latter, coated hard shell capsules or other delivery units are used. The targeting mechanisms are pH-dependent, time-dependent, pressure-dependent, or bacteria-dependent. There are many researchers that have documented colon-targeted delivery using gastric-resistant or coated hard shell. Some of these mechanisms will be discussed next.

Tuleu et al. [31] compared amylose-ethylcellulose-coated HPMC capsule (size 0) with uncoated capsules for the delivery of 4-aminosalicylic acid Na (550 mg) to the colon. The goal for the use of ethylcellulose in preclinical studies is to control the drug release and target the lower part of the intestine. Drug release is dependent on the disintegration lag time that can be determined by the thickness of the water-insoluble membrane (ethylcellulose), and the tolerability and the amount of the swellable excipients. In the study, seven healthy volunteers were used and pharmacokinetic parameters were monitored using a scintigraphic method. The authors reported that based on the T_{max} (29 ± 9 min), percent absolute bioavailability, and AUC (118 ± 41), capsule content was released and absorbed completely and rapidly from the uncoated capsules.

In another study, a time-delayed oral drug delivery using insoluble (coated) gelatin capsule was reported by McConville et al. [80]. The delivery device contained an erodible tablet sealing the mouth of an insoluble capsule that controls the lag time for the delayed release. Erosion rates and drug release profiles were investigated using different excipients—calcium sulfate dihydrate, dicalcium phosphate, HPMC, and silicified microcrystalline cellulose. The authors reported that ethylcellulose coating on the capsule controlled the drug release and lag time.

Colon-coated capsules were used in the treatment of ulcerative colitis in a double-blinded randomized clinical trial in which Fufangkushen colon-coated (FCC) capsules were compared with mesalazine [81]. The FCC capsules contained extracts of Chinese herbal medicines Radix Sophorae Flavescentis (Kushen), Radix Sanguisorbae (Diyu), Indigo Naturalis (Qingdai), Bletilla hyacinthina reichb (Baiji), and Radix Glycyrrhizae (Gancao). All the extracts were contained in a coated capsule that ensures that the medicine is released in the colon. The type of capsule and the coating was not mentioned in the report. The use of FCC was based on the Chinese medicine pattern of damp-heat accumulation interior. A total of 240 patients were treated with capsules of FCC plus mesalazine (HD) placebo treatment, and 80 were treated with HD plus FCC placebo. The drugs and their corresponding placebos were administrated at advised dosages for 8 weeks. The primary endpoint was a positive clinical response at week 8, and Mayo scoring system (0–12) was employed for assessment of ulcerative colitis activity where higher scores (6–12) indicated more severe disease activity. On the 8th week, 72.50% of patients in the FCC group (170 of 234) and 65.00% of patients in the HD group (52 of 80) had achieved a clinical response. There was no statistically significance between the two groups ($P > 0.05$). Sometimes, the delivery system may be designed to deliver the drug through the GIT.

Amidon and Leesman [82] developed controlled-release propranolol beads (units) that can be filled into capsules and that could deliver the drug in a pulsed manner. Each unit has a core containing the drug and it is surrounded by two polymer membranes chosen to protect the drug until a preprogrammed time when the drug is released based on the pH of the environment. Each unit is expected to deliver the drug content in respective pulses through the GIT and into the portal vein in a pattern similar to an immediate release dosage form administered at predetermined time intervals. The intent is to avoid the first-pass effect. The formulation contained citric acid that can cause drastic pH change upon pulsed release of the drug and will make tracking of the pH by the Heidelberg capsule (designed for monitoring and clinical diagnosis) easier. The dosage form was administered to dogs and pH in the GIT was monitored using the Heidelberg capsule. Based on the variable pH in the small intestine and the possibility of its affecting the pulsing, the authors developed an osmotic system for the same purpose.

PEPTIDE/PROTEIN COLONIC DELIVERY IN HARD SHELLS

Recent investigations into the delivery of peptides and proteins have resulted in potential orally delivered hard shell colon-targeted systems. The proximal colon has been viewed as a potential release site for insulin and other peptide or protein drugs. However, absorption from the colon is hindered by the presence of proteases and lack of permeability. Therefore, protease inhibitors and permeation enhancers are generally co-administered with oral peptide/protein drug candidates. The proximal colon has significantly reduced proteolytic activities when compared with the small intestine; it is more responsive to absorption enhancers, and the lengthy transit may improve the extent of absorption, while the viscosity of the contents is not as high as in the descending and sigmoid branches, thus allowing for better absorption. The release of the drug from oral colonic delivery systems of small molecules or peptides, like insulin, can be dependent on colonic factors such as microflora, pH, or time. Consequently, capsular systems intended for colonic delivery are designed based on any of the factors.

In the report of Saffran et al., insulin was delivered to the colon using hard gelatin capsules coated with an azoaromatic polymer [83]. 5-Methoxysalicylic acid was added to the insulin as an absorption enhancer, and sodium bicarbonate was also included in the insulin formulation to react with the acid, to form carbon dioxide that could aid in the release of the insulin. The system is time-dependent. Pancreatectomized dogs were used to avoid proteases that could breakdown the insulin. The insulin was preserved through the intestine because of the resection of the pancreas and the subsequent absence of proteases, although the animal diet was supplemented with digestive enzymes until the day before the experiment. The endpoints that the authors used were portal insulin, arterial glucose production, portal blood flow, and glucagon-like immunoactivity. Azoaromatic hydrogel (that can be degraded by colonic bacteria) was also used and reported by Bronsted and Kopecek [84].

The coating of hard shell with deacetylated chitosan was reported by Tozaki et al. [85] and Yamamoto et al. [86]. The capsular system was used in the investigations as carrier for bovine insulin to the distal colon. The enteric-coated capsules contained protease inhibitors such as aprotinin, bacitracin, and absorption enhancers (e.g., sodium glycocholate and sodium oleate). The delivery system was administered intragastrically to rats, and plasma insulin and glucose concentrations were used as endpoints. The chitosan capsular container was reported to cause increased insulin absorption compared to gelatin capsule formulation.

Eudragit S and Eudragit NE at a 3:7 ratio was reportedly used by several authors [87–89] to coat formaldehyde-treated hard gelatin capsules filled with a gelled insulin microemulsion. The system was pH-dependent based on the composition of the coat. Cellulose acetate phthalate was used to provide gastro-resistance. The colon-targeted capsules, administered to dogs, showed significantly greater pharmacological availability in comparison with a non-encapsulated liquid insulin microemulsion and an insulin-free colon-targeted capsule. The potential for utilization of the delivery system is high for oral delivery of peptides and proteins.

HARD GELATIN CAPSULES AND CHRONOTHERAPY

The delivery of drug may sometimes need to be modified or adapted to meet drug needs to circadian rhythms of body functions or diseases. Such diseases include asthma, arthritis, duodenal ulcer, cancer, cardiovascular diseases, diabetes, hypercholesterolemia, neurological disorders, and so on. Many investigations have been documented in literature where capsular systems (coated hard shells) were used to create a lag time for the drug to be delivered in a pulsatile manner to match the circadian rhythm. The PORT system is a capsular system of hypromellose capsule that provides programmed drug release using the osmotic device as stated earlier in "Coated Hypromellose Capsules" section and reported by other authors [90].

Bhat et al. [34] reported a design of hard gelatin capsule that has an impermeable capsule body filled with the formulation (theophylline pellets) and sealed with erodible polymer plug placed in the opening of the capsule body. The investigators' goal was to develop a pulsatile drug delivery system of theophylline for nocturnal asthma. In pulsatile delivery, the drug is released rapidly within a short window or period after a predetermined lag time when little or no drug is released. The result is better absorption and more effective plasma concentration–time profiles.

A capsular system containing one or more propranolol/verapamil HCL particles (e.g., beads, pellets, granules, etc.) was also used and reported by Mandal et al. Each bead is preprogrammed to deliver the drug in a rapid or sustained-release manner with or without lag time. The technology is based on chronopharmaceutical drug delivery—DIFFUCAPS—and the rationale is to treat hypertension because blood pressure measurements have shown a significant circadian variation to characterize blood pressure [91].

Barzegar-Jalali et al. [92] developed an osmotic capsule for the treatment of pain. Pain in disease states such as arthritis has been reported to exhibit circadian rhythm based on the plasma concentration of pro-inflammatory markers such as C-reactive protein and interleukin-6 in patients with arthritis. The authors used hard gelatin capsules filled with acetaminophen, with sorbitol as osmotic agent and sodium dodecyl sulfate as release promoter. The capsule was coated with semipermeable cellulose acetate containing castor oil as hydrophobic plasticizer and sealed with white beeswax. The drug was released when the system came in contact with the water and the semipermeable membrane permitted water into the system. Upon dissolving the osmotic agent, increase in the osmotic pressure inside the shell resulted in expulsion of the plug and the release of the drug.

ENCAPSULATED LIPID-BASED FORMULATIONS AND CLINICAL TRIAL RELEVANCE

Hard gelatin capsules are now used in filling liquids and semisolids of drugs with low melting point, low dose, and some critical stability that may make other solid oral dosage form development challenging [93]. For example, drugs with low melting points may liquefy at room temperature and may need a significant amount of other excipients to make the solids flow during manufacturing. If the drug is used in high dose, then the bulkiness of the formulation may not be suitable for a single dose. Moreover, low-melting point solids may become unsuitable to compress because the compaction process introduces added heat that could melt the solid drug. In addition, a low-dose drug, such as hormones and anticancer agents, may be too low in a formulation to be formulated as a solid. Moreover, the dust-free processing of such drugs reduces chances of exposure to production staff. A disadvantage of hard gelatin liquid-filled capsules is improper sealing and leaking that could occur. However, new technological advances have significantly solved the closure problem; it involves spraying the capsule body/cap joint with ethanolic solution [94].

There are many reports in literature on clinical investigations involving use of hard gelatin filled with liquids and semisolids. Seta et al. [95,96] compared the extent of absorption or AUC of captopril semisolid formulation filled into hard gelatin capsules with a tablet formulation. They reported that the semisolid filled capsules had higher AUC than the tablet and ascribed this to the longer transit time, adhesion of the hard gelatin formulation to the mucosa, and protection of the drug against degradation by food particles. The captopril formulation has been translated into a commercial formulation.

As mentioned in "Introduction" section, Shen and Zhong [5] studied the bioavailability of atorvastatin, a poorly soluble drug. The drug was formulated as a self-(micro)emulsifying drug delivery system (SEDDS [or SMEDDS]) (to improve the solubility) that contained Labrafil, polyethylene glycol, and Cremophor RH40. The formulation was filled into capsules and administered to six beagle dogs. The authors reported that the bioavailability was increased in the SMEDDS-filled capsule formulation compared to the conventional tablet.

DRUG RELEASE MECHANISMS AND HARD SHELL ENCAPSULATION

The utilization of hard shells in oral drug delivery is a technologically simpler method when compared to tablet dosage form. However, the intent of use to targeted sites in the GIT or to release drug at predetermined times as a modified-release dosage form underscores the importance of understanding the release mechanisms. As discussed earlier in the chapter, hard shells can be designed for different drug delivery outcomes; the shell can be made impermeable until it reaches a particular site in the GIT.

It can also be made to deliver the drug based on osmotic pressure within the dosage form; the intent can be to protect the drug from enzymes in the GI or it can be as an overencapsulated product that contains an immediate release or modified release tablet, capsule, or multiunits (immediate release or modified release) in the capsule.

Aside from the uniqueness of the capsular system, the drug or excipient or the coating material can greatly influence the drug release pattern. Qiu and Zhang emphasized the release mechanisms of modified-release dosage forms in their review [97]. They underscored the importance of the need for the application of a holistic approach in rational dosage form development. This encompasses multidisciplinary knowledge of the drug, excipients, delivery technology mentioned above, basic unit operations, and interactions between the formulation and process variables. Four different delivery systems—matrix, reservoir, osmotic, and pulsatile capsular systems—will be considered in this section.

MATRIX CAPSULAR SYSTEMS

These are dosage forms in which the drug is dispersed into the unit containing the excipient. Examples will include tablets in capsule and multiunits in capsule in which each unit contains drug dispersed within the matrix of the excipient. The drug release can be diffusion- or dissolution-controlled or both. If drug release is only diffusion-controlled, the rate of drug release is dependent on the drug diffusion and can be represented by the Higuchi equation (Equation 3.1) [98].

$$Q = \left[\frac{D\varepsilon}{T(2A - \varepsilon C_s)C_s t} \right]^{1/2} \quad \text{or} \quad Q = kt^{1/2}, \tag{3.1}$$

where Q = weight in grams of drug released per unit surface area; D = diffusion coefficient of drug in the release medium; ε = porosity of the matrix; T = tortuosity of the matrix; C_s = solubility of the drug in the medium; and A = concentration of drug in the unit (e.g., tablet).

Assumptions include sink condition, $C = 0$; diffusion coefficient remains constant; no interaction between drug and matrix; and a pseudo-steady state is maintained during drug release.

If the drug release is dissolution-controlled, the rate of drug release is controlled by the rate of flow of fluid into the matrix, which, in turn, can be determined by the nature of the excipients and wettability of the unit or tablet surface. The drug release can follow zero order or non-zero order depending on variables such as polymer type and pH-dependent or pH-independent drug release.

A matrix system was presented by two studies from two sets of authors that showed that, based on the formulation variables in the formula for verapamil, the drug release may be non-zero-order or zero-order drug release. In one study, sodium alginate that is pH-dependent was used [99]. In another study, a pH-independent polymer such as HPMC was used, as depicted in Figure 3.20a and b [100]. The release in the former study shows a non-zero order while a zero order was observed in the latter study.

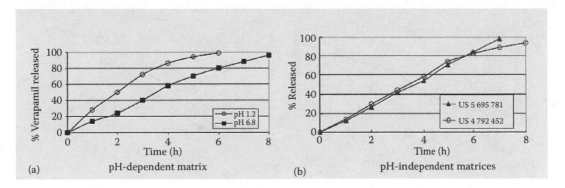

FIGURE 3.20 Drug release from different Verapamil matrix modified release. (a) Non-zero- or zero-order release; (b) zero-order release. (From Baiz E, Einig H. Alginate-based Verapamil-containing depot drug form. *US Patent 5 132 295* [1992]. United States Patent and Trademark Office (www.uspto.gov); and Howard JR, Timmins P. Controlled release formulation. *US Patent 4 792 452* [1988]. United States Patent and Trademark Office [www.uspto.gov].)

RESERVOIR CAPSULAR SYSTEMS

These are dosage forms in which a polymer encloses the drug core. An example of hard shell system is a capsule containing multiunits in which each unit contains drug that is in the core encased by polymer. In this case, the drug partitions across the membrane and is exchanged with dissolved drug through diffusion across the membrane with surrounding medium.

As shown in Fick's law (Equation 3.2), the flux of drug, J (amount/time), across the membrane along a concentration gradient is defined as

$$J = -D\,\frac{dC}{dx} \quad \text{or} \quad \frac{dM}{dt} = ADK\Delta\frac{C}{t}. \tag{3.2}$$

D = diffusion coefficient on area/time and dC/dx is the change in concentration C with distance x or dM/dt = amount of drug released; A = area; D = diffusion coefficient; K = partition coefficient of drug between the membrane and the core; l = diffusional path length (e.g., thickness of the polymer coat), and ΔC is the concentration gradient across the membrane.

If the partition coefficient is high, the drug in the core will be depleted fast and a zero-order release will be observed over a short time. However, based on variables such as polymer type in a modified-release system, a non-zero order may be observed. An extended-release verapamil hydrochloride capsule (Verelan) containing 20% of uncoated beads and 80% of the membrane-coated beads was reported by Panoz and Geoghegan [101] to exhibit release profiles that showed that the system is pH-independent (Figure 3.21a and b).

OSMOTIC SYSTEMS

Examples of capsular systems that exhibit this type of release are monolithic tablets or tablets contained in capsule, layered tablets, and multiunits in capsule. The drug release is driven by the osmotic pressure. When the system is in the dissolution medium or biological fluid, water flows into the osmotic system due to osmotic pressure difference across the membrane. The volume of water that flows into the system into the core reservoir, dV/dt, is defined and represented by Equation 3.3.

$$\frac{dV}{dt} = \left(\frac{Ak}{h}\right)(\Delta\pi - \Delta P) \tag{3.3}$$

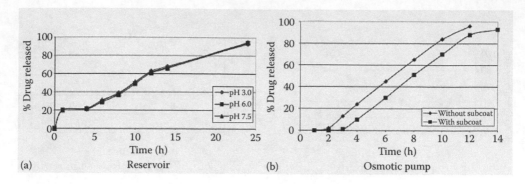

FIGURE 3.21   Drug release from different Verapamil modified release. (a) Reservoir release; (b) osmotic pump release. (From Panoz DE, Geoghegan EJ. Controlled absorption pharmaceutical composition. *US Patent 4 863 742* [1989]. United States Patent and Trademark Office [www.uspto.gov].)

A, k, and h are the area, membrane permeability, and thickness of membrane, respectively; $\Delta\pi$ is osmotic pressure difference; and ΔP is the hydrostatic pressure difference. The release is pH-independent and maintains a constant rate or zero order.

PULSATILE RELEASE SYSTEMS

Examples of this system are multiunits in capsule and coated capsules. Pulsatile delivery systems can be used for drugs such as those that develop biological tolerance; those that have extensive first-pass metabolism; those targeted to a specific site in the intestinal tract, for example, to the colon (to protect the drug from degradation); and those that need to be adapted for their circadian rhythms or for body functions or diseases [102–104].

Most pulsatile delivery dosage forms are reservoir-type devices in which the dosage form is covered with a barrier coating that can dissolve, erode, or rupture during or after a certain period, after which the drug is released rapidly from the inner reservoir core. Unlike a matrix-type device that releases the drug over time in a linear manner, drug release in a reservoir system is nonlinear. The osmotic system, intended for dosing at bedtime for releasing drugs such as verapamil to coincide with natural morning rise of blood pressure, has been documented in different reports [105,106].

Amidon and Leesman [82] observed a pulsatile drug release that follows nonlinear kinetics in the propranolol (a drug that is metabolized by first pass) bead or multiunit formulations referred to earlier. The *in vitro* pulse or release time for the drug (T_p) from the pH-dependent formulation is represented by Equation 3.4:

$$T_p = 36.9 + 0.113T + 1.27E - 0.0019\ (T*E). \tag{3.4}$$

For the osmotic system of the same drug, the T_p is represented by Equation 3.5:

$$T_p = 8.13 + 0.0645N - 0.312P + 0.0130\ (N*P). \tag{3.5}$$

N and P are the optimized concentration of the viscosity enhancer in the formulation and the plasticizer used to make the polymer coat film more compliant.

QbD APPROACH AND ENCAPSULATION FOR CLINICAL TRIALS

Overview

QbD has been defined as a science- and risk-based approach to drug product development that encompasses some set of formulation, manufacturing, and control procedures for guaranteeing a finished product that possesses a predetermined and measurable level of physical and biopharmaceutical qualities [107]. It is a holistic and proactive approach to pharmaceutical development that involves deliberate design efforts from product conception through development to commercialization. The aim is to gain a full understanding of how product attributes and processing methods affect product performance [108].

After the US FDA launched an initiative for Pharmaceutical Quality for the 21st Century in 2002, with the object of modernizing pharmaceutical manufacturing and improving product quality, QbD becomes recognized as a methodology for producing pharmaceutical ingredients and drug products that meet predetermined quality specifications. In order to design processes that are consistent with QbD principles, scientific understandings of product and processes supported with risk assessment have to be leveraged using rational experimental design [108]. Data generated through DOE will support specifications and manufacturing ranges that could enhance the implementation of post-approval changes.

According to Gassmann and von Zedtwitz, application of QbD to development process could

- Fast-track the development and introduction of new drug products to the market
- Facilitate compliance with regulatory requirements and provide supportive data to demonstrate that drug products are safe, effective, and stable
- Improve efficiency of research and development activities
- Provide regulatory relief and flexibility
- Provide important business benefits throughout the product's life cycle [109]

The US FDA initiative consists of four parts: the International Conference on Harmonization (ICH) guidance Q9, Quality Risk Management (ICH guidance Q10), Pharmaceutical Quality System (FDA Process Analytical Technology guidance), and ICH guidance Q8 (R2).

The ultimate goal of FDA and industry partnership in QbD implementation is to produce an agile, highly efficient, and flexible pharmaceutical manufacturing sector that will consistently and reliably produce high-quality drug products without extensive regulatory oversight [110]. In light of the current initiative, the FDA regulatory framework is focused on the following aspects:

- Encouraging industry early adoption of new technological advances
- Facilitating adoption of modern quality management techniques
- Encouraging implementation of risk-based approaches that focus on critical areas
- Basing regulatory review, compliance, and inspection policies on state-of-the-art pharmaceutical science
- Enhancing consistency and coordination of FDA's drug quality regulatory programs

The International Society of Pharmaceutical Engineering has undertaken an initiative known as the Product Quality Lifecycle Implementation (PQLI) to clarify the requirements for implementing QbD [109].

Elements of QbD in Development of Capsules for Clinical Trial

The ultimate aim of clinical trials is to evaluate drug product performance in humans to confirm efficacy and establish freedom from toxicity. Generally, clinical trials are conducted at four levels:

preclinical (animal) studies and Phase I to IV (human) studies. Phase I trials are targeted at healthy volunteers while Phases II through IV are run in specific disease populations as active comparator (active control) or placebo control studies. Phase I trials are closely monitored, enroll a relatively small number (20–50) of healthy subjects, and are focused on product safety. This phase may be designed as a dose-escalation study to identify appropriate therapeutic doses, usually fraction of doses that caused harm in animal studies. Phase II trials are designed to demonstrate efficacy and tolerance, and are administered on a larger number of subjects, usually 20–300 with target disease [111]. This phase should provide the first evidence that the drug is effective in patients with the specific disease and safe in patients as well as healthy subjects. Phase I and II trials are quite time-sensitive, with the object of removing less viable drug candidates from the development plan and redirecting of resources and research capacity to a higher number of and more promising molecular entities [112]. A larger number of participants from a broader demography were recruited in the Phase III trial. Depending on the disease, enrolment could range from 300 to 3000 or more. This phase confirms and consolidates product safety, dosing appropriateness, efficacy, side effects, and cost-effectiveness over a wide range of population characteristics. Marketing authorization by relevant regulatory agencies including US FDA, EMEA (Europe), and TGA (Australia) require at least two successful Phase III trials. Following marketing authorization, Phase IV trials investigate variations in specific populations of different genetic composition, overweight and underweight, children and elderly. This phase may also address long-term safety, cost-effectiveness, interactions with other drugs and diet compositions, further assessment of toxicity, and new indications for the drug product.

The number of dosage units required in Phases I through III are much fewer than the likely commercial batches at full capacity. Variations in initial number of dosage units together with the need for dose escalation studies in Phase I trials necessitate product and process flexibility and robustness that will guarantee sustainable product and process attributes across the clinical trial spectrum. The versatility of capsule and the flexibility of dose sizes that can be filled make it easier to scale up than tablets and could thus make clinical batches more representative of full-scale capacity. Capsule design should consider the available manufacturing capability that matches the clinical batch size and which could achieve robust process performance while ensuring product quality. While working with laboratory-scale batches, attention should be paid to demonstrating scalability to downstream full-scale operations. Direct filling of API into hard gelatin capsule shells (PIC) is perhaps the quickest approach for clinical batch production because it requires few or no excipients and avoids the need for preformulation compatibility and stability studies as stated in the earlier section. The Xcelodose 600S Precision Micro-Dosing System (ALMAC) has the capacity for filling powder into hard gelatin capsule shells in the size range 3 to 0 while IMA Lab 16 is capable of filling powder and formulations into hard gelatin capsule sizes 4 to 0, 0el, and 00 plus DBcaps sizes B and C. Although PIC technology could expedite Phase I clinical trials, the QbD approach that should be included beyond Phase I is excluded in the use of PIC. Although QbD need not be applied in the clinical research stages, many companies include QbD in investigational drug application submission. Therefore, despite the simplicity of PIC, risk assessment should be included.

A number of capsule micro-dosing and filling technologies have been reviewed by Edwards. Machines employing dosator technology include ModU C capsule filling and closing machine (Harro Hofliger, Germany) and the G250 Capsule filler (Mg2, Italy). These machines have capacities for filling from 10- to 500-mg dose units into sizes 5 to 0 capsule shells at the rate of 3000 to 200,000 capsules per hour. This makes the technology particularly suited to small-scale Phase I clinical studies through to full-scale manufacturing [113,114].

Drug and Excipient Characteristics

A comprehensive documentation of the functional properties of drug substance to be encapsulated and the usual excipients should be prepared. This information can be obtained from raw material manufacturers, official monographs (USP, BP, *Handbook of Pharmaceutical Excipients*, HPE, etc.) or generated in-house through preformulation studies.

Solubility and permeability are the two most important properties of drug substances. They determine, to a significant extent, drug release and bioavailability potential. Understanding drug solubility and permeability characteristics is critical to successful formulation. The BCS introduced by Amidon et al. [115] classifies drug substances into four major groups based on their solubility and permeability characteristics: Class 1: high solubility–high permeability; Class II: low solubility–low permeability; Class 3: high solubility–low permeability; and Class 4: low solubility–low permeability. Classes 2 and 4 are particularly difficult to formulate for systemic absorption. Various formulation techniques can be used to support capsule development of Classes 2 and 4 drugs for oral absorption. Other important drug substance variables include particle morphology, hydrophobicity, moisture content, particle size distribution, bulk density, cohesiveness, adhesiveness, and flow characteristics. For powder mixture, critical properties include blend uniformity, agglomeration and segregation tendencies, blend density, compressibility, and hydrophobicity imparted by formulation additives (e.g., lubricants).

Manufacturing Process and Process Control

Powder Blending

Powder mixing equipment for clinical batch manufacturing include Turbula T2F shaker blender (up to 2 L), Erweka Y Cone (2.5–5 L), Erweka Double Cone (4–8 L), Manesty Drum Blender (10 kg), Pharmatech blending system (Model 1 MB400 and 1 ATEX, capacities 15–200 L), and Pharmtech MB15 (1–5 kg). Implementation of QbD in capsule production embraces the deployment of process analytical technology (PAT). When PAT is linked with rational DOEs, it will be possible to understand the dynamic events within the process that affect product outcome, identify parameters that need more detailed studies, and provide a means of mapping the design space of the process. Hammond [116] discussed the application of PAT in mapping the design space of Dilantin capsule. Using near-infrared (NIR) spectrometric analysis, it was possible to monitor blend uniformity of phenytoin with excipients (magnesium stearate, lactose, sugar, and talc) in a 3 × 3 factorial design. Capsule dissolution was found to decrease with length of blending time, obviously as a result of the hydrophobic magnesium stearate spreading more intimately over particulate surfaces.

QbD requires a systematic, risk-based, and multivariate experimental design rather than the traditional one-factor-at-a-time approach. This is expected to provide confidence that a target capsule product of desired quality is obtained. First, critical quality attributes (CQAs) and critical process parameters (CPPs) for the desired capsule should be identified using prior knowledge (e.g., material properties, official specifications, and acceptance limits for parameters) and risk assessments (i.e., likelihood and implication of product failure). The number of variables and levels of study can be quite huge at the CQA identification stage. Lower-resolution DOE can be used to reduce the number of parameters to practical levels. Next, elements of the control strategy are identified (e.g., how to monitor, preferably, real-time changes in raw material and in-process behavior during mixing, granulation, drying, and pelletization) and control strategies are established (Figure 3.22). Multivariate experimental studies are then designed to define the manufacturing space using a more powerful and higher-resolution DOE that would produce clearer understanding of the manufacturing process and identification of parameters with the greatest effect on CQAs [ALMAC GRP]. The design should consider the available manufacturing capability that matches the clinical batch size and could achieve robust process performance while ensuring product quality.

While working with laboratory-scale batches, attention should be paid to demonstrating scalability to downstream full-scale operations. The versatility of capsule and the flexibility of dose sizes make it easier to scale up than tablets and could thus make clinical batches more representative of full-scale capacity [117].

Application of artificial intelligence (AI) for identifying and mitigating risk in a design space has been proposed by York [118]. AI is supportive of the early formulation objective of controlling

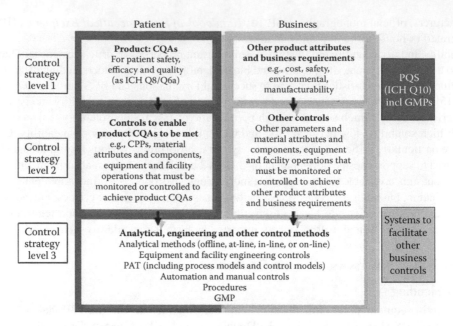

FIGURE 3.22   (See color insert.) Proposed model for control strategy. (From Garcia T, Cook G, Nosal R. PQLI key topics—Criticality, design space, and control strategy. *J Pharm Innov* 2008; 3: 60–68. With permission.)

clinical quality and minimizing toxicity and of the final product that demonstrates consistent *in vivo* performance to the specified standards. AI enables the understanding and prediction of complex relationships in processes (particularly multistage and multivariate processes) and formulations through data mining and *in silico* simulation studies. The application of molecular simulations to process technology enabled the understanding of the effect of particle size and shape on capsule filling, and the mechanisms of powder packing in mixtures and pellets filling into capsules. The knowledge gained was applied in estimating volume capacity of hard shell capsules, solving problems related to variability in filling process, establishing equipment batch capacity, determining API/excipient ratios, overcoming mixing problems, and ensuring blend homogeneity.

Capsule Filling

Although simple fill capsules are less complex than tablets, the preparation of capsules requires considerable skill [119]. Process variables can have a significant impact on the quality of the finished capsule. Mixer speed, blender fill level, powder loading mode, degree of shearing imparted by the blender parts, and RH are critical to the homogeneity, porosity, and microstructure of the mixed product. Through QbD, PAT could be used to implement feedback and feed forward adjustment mechanisms through the real-time monitoring of product and process performance. PAT was introduced by the US FDA in 2004. Its application is still limited by lack of suitable and reliable methods for determining some critical raw material attributes. To date, there are no official universally accepted criteria for defining material hydrophobicity, powder density, powder cohesion/adhesion, tensile strength, and fluidity. The empiricism of the currently available techniques implies potential for inconsistent application across the industry. Despite these limitations, critical material properties generated through preformulation studies could provide useful input to the design of clinical trial batches and serve as the input variables for a multivariate experimental design study. Invasive, nondestructive methods of powder mixture characterization are needed for measuring critical in-process product characteristics. Methods such as NIR spectrometry and scanning electron microscopy have been found suitable for monitoring in-process blend homogeneity [120]. From clinical batches through scale-up to full capacity, flexible and adjustable processes that are based on experimental and data-driven design space should be used.

Another crucial process is the filling of capsule with drug powder or formulation mixture. The design of capsule filling machine (whether tamping or dosator type) and the presence and type of device that support filling (rotary, suction or vibratory) are important components of the variable map [121]. For dosator filler, the surface texture of the dosator can affect the flow of formulation by adhesive and electrostatic forces. Hence, some dosators are coated to reduce these problems [112].

CQA AND RISK ASSESSMENT

Some of the quality attributes of hard shell capsules that are considered obligatory include uniformity of weight, content of active ingredients, disintegration time, and dissolution rate, all of which will directly affect quality of performance *in vivo*. These must fall within the normal operating ranges (Figure 3.23). Others are not so easy to identify but must not fall outside of design space. Depending on API, stability and potential for degradation during processing can constitute critical attributes. A risk assessment tool could be developed for ranking and filtering critical attributes using a scoring matrix for each variable. The criticality (risk score) is then determined by multiplying the degree or impact of an attribute on safety or efficacy by the degree of confidence that the impact is known using the following expression:

$$\text{Criticality} = \text{impact} \times \text{uncertainty} \tag{3.6}$$

The degree to which a variable is known in relation to its potential impact on process or product performance will enable its progression from knowledge space through design space to the specification (normal operating ranges) space (Figure 3.24). Ulmschneider [120] proposed a decision tree to determine degree of criticality and Zhang et al. investigated the applicability of a physiologically based absorption model to QbD in drug development [122]. An identical classical particle dissolution equation was observed for immediate-release suspensions, capsules, and tablets. However, tablets require longer transit time and the effect of food was formulation-dependent.

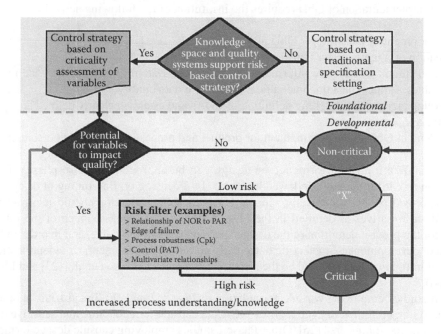

FIGURE 3.23 (See color insert.) Decision tree to define levels of criticality. (From Garcia T, Cook G, Nosal R. PQLI key topics—Criticality, design space, and control strategy. *J Pharm Innov* 2008; 3: 60–68. With permission.)

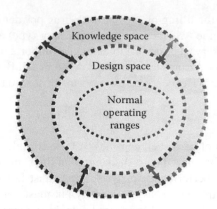

FIGURE 3.24 **(See color insert.)** Relationship between design space and normal operating ranges. (From Garcia T, Cook G, Nosal R. PQLI key topics—Criticality, design space, and control strategy. *J Pharm Innov* 2008; 3: 60–68. With permission.)

Finished Capsule Attributes

Design quality attributes of finished capsules for clinical trial include the officially recognized tests and some unofficial parameters. Capsule fill weight and weight uniformity, disintegration time, and dissolution rate are official tests with established protocols and acceptance criteria (USP 35/NF 30). Other measures of quality such as capsule microstructure, porosity, and tensile strength can provide additional variables for defining the design space and ensuring clinical batch performance on a consistent basis.

Implementation of QbD in Hard Shell Capsule Formulation for Clinical Trials

Successful implementation of QbD requires the institution of the following activities:

- Development of the strategic QbD plan
- Creation of a template for QbD implementation
- Establishment of effective information management system to capture the wide range of variables, support data documentation, and ensure data quality
- Develop an excellent working definition of CQAs and establish clearly defined acceptance criteria
- Implement QbD skills development for product and process development personnel

Operationalization of performance by design can be approached in two phases: Phase I—Focusing on risk minimization, followed by Phase II—Focusing on fine-tuning of design space in the post-approval phases. Practically, clinical batch capsule production should focus on the risk-minimization initiatives as detailed in the FDA ICHQ9. At this phase, much of the information required for the precise definition of the design space may not be available, and in order to facilitate the speed of development characteristic of the early phases of development, risk identification, evaluation, and mitigation plans should be the primary focus (see Dickinson et al. [123] and Lionberger et al. [124]).

Several studies employing capsule formulation in Phases I and II clinical trials abound in the literature. Young et al. investigated a novel 13C-Urea capsule for economic and sensitive diagnosis of *H. pylori* in six volunteers [125]. Other Phase I studies employing capsule dosage forms include a clinical trial of plant sterol esters in 16 human subjects in a double-blind, placebo-controlled sequential study over 4 weeks, with 2 weeks washout period in-between [126]; lansoprazole 30-mg delayed-release capsules (Mylan Pharm. Inc.); tofacitinib open-label, randomized, single-dose crossover bioequivalence study in fasting 50 healthy volunteers by Pfizer (2012); cefdinir 300-mg capsule trial in non-fasting 32 healthy volunteers by Tera Pharmaceuticals USA (2009); and Marinol (dronabinol) 2.5-, 5-, and 10-mg capsules for loss-of-appetite-associated weight loss in AIDS patients.

Examples of drug in capsules in Phase II trials include the Pentasa (mesalamine) capsule study in 450 patients by Shire US Mfg Inc. (PillCam Express Capsule Endoscopy Delivery System by Given Imaging Ltd), while the study on meloxicam capsules for the treatment of osteoarthritis pain in a randomized, parallel assignment, double-blind trial by Iroko Pharm. LLC illustrates the use of capsule dosage forms in a Phase III, multicenter, randomized and double-blind, double-dummy placebo-controlled study.

IN VITRO AND IN VIVO PERFORMANCE OF HARD SHELL: REGULATORY PERSPECTIVES

Different hard shells such as Coni-Snap and DBcaps for overencapsulation are often used in bio-equivalence studies or dissolution testing with the goal of obtaining a biowaiver for the product. In blinding clinical trials, the reference product could be contained in hard shell in ground form, or as single or multiple tablets, multiunits pellets, or capsules. For targeted oral delivery, hard shell capsules have been used in comparison to immediate-release products to prove that the targeted delivery has better therapeutic outcomes; that is, the drug was released at the desired site or in pulses for disease states such as ulcerative colitis and inflammatory bowel disease or for drugs with circadian rhythm.

In clinical studies involving overencapsulation of immediate-release dosage forms where blinding has to be done by placing the tablet, granules, suspension, or capsule in capsule, the questions can be asked; will the overencapsulation affect the biopharmaceutic and pharmacokinetic parameters such as dissolution, absorption, or bioavailability or will a generic hard shell capsule be bio-equivalent with an innovator tablet dosage form of the same drug [8]? Some of the questions will be addressed in "*In Vitro–In Vivo* Performance" section.

IN VITRO–IN VIVO PERFORMANCE

Capsules versus Tablets

The dissolution data of highly soluble and highly permeable, rapidly dissolving orally administered drug products (Class I drugs) can be used to demonstrate and document product quality bioavailability and bioequivalence (BA/BE) based on the BCS [127]. The BCS can be used to obtain a biowaiver and it is often exploited to the advantage of the manufacturer. Studies to measure BA and/or establish BE of a product are important elements in support of Investigational NDAs (INDs), NDAs, Abbreviated NDAs (ANDAs), and their supplements. From a reported FDA case study, a Class drug I substance was formulated as a tablet, but at the late development phase, the formulation was changed to capsule formulation [128]. The dissolution profiles of the highest strength of the tablet, the overencapsulated tablet in a hard gelatin capsule, and the new capsule formulation were not similar.

Subsequently, the similarity factor F_2 was less than 50 and the F_2 values of >50 are required for the biowaiver of *in vivo* studies if the drug release is less than 85% at 15 min at physiological pHs. Despite the lack of similarity, the sponsors were able to prove bioequivalence and apply for a biowaiver. This was based on the probe and definitive bioavailability (BA) studies conducted by the sponsors.

The probe BA/BE (which involved 18 subjects) showed bioinequivalence using the overencapsulated tablet as reference product; the geometric mean ratios at 90% confidence interval (CI) for AUC did not meet the FDA specification for the capsule formulation—0.96–1.27 versus the tablet 90% CI of 0.8–1.25 that complied with the specification. This was reported to be attributed to the higher C_{max} and shorter T_{max} for one subject. The data confirmed the fact that pharmacokinetics parameters are more sensitive to formulation changes and higher intersubject variability. The definitive BA/BE was conducted using 90 subjects in a crossover study. It was found out that the two tablet and capsule formulations are bioequivalent with 90% CI near unity despite the fact that the early T_{max} observed at the probe study was also confirmed in the definitive BE.

Dissolution could also be affected by low capsule fill weight, capsule shell [129], type of filler, and the solubility of the drug [130]. Using the right capsule size and excipients (backfill) similar to those in the tablet formulation could reduce the effect on dissolution. The solubility of the drug should be factored into the blinding trials.

In comparative pharmacokinetic trials, the encapsulation of esomeprazole multiple-unit-pellet system or 40-mg tablets using hard gelatin capsules did not influence the rate (C_{max}) and extent (AUC) of absorption in a study involving 49 volunteers [131]. Other *in vivo* studies have shown the equivalence of *in-vivo* disintegration time using gamma scintigraphy and therapeutic effect onset time between encapsulated and non-encapsulated sumatriptan tablets [132]. However, some studies have shown that although encapsulation of tablets may not affect *in vitro* dissolution studies, it could delay absorption within 0 to 2 h after dosing and *in vivo* efficacy of drugs. The importance of this is underscored for drugs that are intended for fast onset of action such as demonstrated in an open trial design with patient scoring the headache pain response to a migraine drug [133].

In a randomized two-way crossover study that compared mifepristone in capsules with tablets in nonpregnant women, the authors reported that there was no significant difference in the major pharmacokinetic parameters, and the relative bioavailability was 109.4% ± 34.8% [134]. Another group of investigators compared the pharmacokinetic properties and bioequivalence of the capsule (test) and tablet (reference) formulations of meclofenoxate hydrochloride 200 mg in healthy Chinese volunteers [135]. They reported that the 90% CIs with and without log-transformed ratios of chlorophenoxyacetic acid (the active and detectable metabolite) were between 80% and 125%, in agreement with the FDA specifications.

Capsule versus Granules

Chun et al. compared the bioavailability of lansoprazole granules administered in two types of juice and a soft food with that of the intact capsule administered with water [136]. The single-dose, randomized, open-label, four-period crossover study involved the use of healthy adult volunteers. The authors reported that the 90% CIs for all three test regimens were within the acceptable bioequivalence range of 0.80 to 1.25. The study demonstrated that for patients who may not be able to swallow, the drugs could be administered in liquids and soft foods without compromising the bioavailability.

Capsules versus Suspensions

Comparative BA/BE of ceftibuten, a new third-generation cephalosporin antibiotic given orally once daily, in capsule and suspension dosage forms, was assessed in healthy male subjects. In three separate studies, the subjects were administered either a 400-mg dose as a suspension or one laboratory-batch, 400-mg capsule; one laboratory-batch, 400-mg capsule or two laboratory-batch, 200-mg capsules; or one production-batch, 400-mg capsule or two laboratory-batch, 200-mg capsules. The randomized crossover study showed that the 90% CIs were within 80–125% of the guidelines [137]. The authors concluded bioequivalence of the suspension and capsule dosage form in each of the three studies.

REGULATORY PERSPECTIVES ON DISSOLUTION AND *IN VIVO* RELEASE FROM HARD SHELLS

The regulatory requirement for biowaivers stemmed from the BCS classification as stated earlier. Examples of useful FDA documents that can serve as a guide include Guidance for Industry:

Dissolution Testing of Immediate Release Solid Oral Dosage Forms [138] and Bioavailability and Bioequivalence Studies for Orally Administered Drug Products—General Considerations [139]. The purpose of the former guidance is to act as supplement to the SUPAC-IR guidance for industry: Immediate Release Solid Oral Dosage Forms: Scale-up and Post-Approval Changes: Chemistry, Manufacturing and Controls, *In Vitro* Dissolution Testing, and *In Vivo* Bioequivalence Documentation with specific emphasis on comparative dissolution profiles. Because of the dependence of absorption on the release of the drug substance from the drug product and the dissolution or solubilization of the drug under physiological conditions, *in vitro* dissolution becomes an essential data for assessment of lot-to-lot quality of duct immediate-release solid dosage forms such as hard shell capsules. The data would also serve in the development of new formulations. The BCS can serve, for example, in setting *in vitro* dissolution specification and predicting the likelihood of achieving *in vitro–in vivo* correlation. The dissolution testing conditions and the basis for biowaivers are contained in the reference.

The latter guidance [139] contains recommendations that the applicant will need to provide as evidence in dissolution testing that the drug is BCS Class I and dissolution is sufficient enough to be granted a waiver from conducting an *in vivo* bioequivalence study. The latter document guides the sponsor or applicant organization regarding the data that should be submitted for orally administered drug products for INDs, NDAs, or ANDAs. The BA studies focus on understanding the process by which a drug is released from the oral dosage form and moves to the site of action, estimate of fraction absorbed, and subsequent distribution and elimination. BE studies compare the systemic exposure profile of a test drug product to that of a reference or comparator drug product. It establishes that the API in the test product exhibits the same rate and extent of absorption as the comparator drug product. These considerations are very important in hard shell capsules and use in clinical trials because as highlighted in the chapter, hard shell capsules are often used in preclinical and clinical studies using miniaturization technology at the early stage to establish some or all of the considerations stated above.

CONCLUSIONS

Use of hard shells in clinical trials has been established, and more interest has been generated based on new technologies such as miniaturization and capsule engineering. This has resulted in choice from a library of different hard shells to meet a delivery goal, clinical objectives, and cultural preferences. Equipment engineering has also advanced to meet opportunities. Whether immediate-release oral drug delivery or targeted site-specific delivery, the containment of the formulation in hard shells and specialty shells and the approach to design of formulations such as QbD have been emphasized. The regulatory guidance has served to stimulate frequency of dialogues between the regulatory authorities and the pharmaceutical industry [140]. The ultimate goal is to embrace the challenge and create opportunities for scientific understanding that is needed in blinding clinical trials or bioequivalence studies involving hard shells and to ensure that a quality product that is safe and effective is developed.

REFERENCES

1. Li P, Zhao L. Developing early formulations: Practice and perspective. *Int J Pharmace* 2007; 341: 1–19.
2. Hansch C, Leo AJ. *Substituent Constants for Correlation Analysis in Chemistry and Biology.* New York: Wiley, 1979.
3. Lipinski CA, Lombardo F, Dominy BW et al. Experimental and computational approaches to estimate solubility and permeability in drug discovery and development settings. *Adv Drug Deliv Rev* 1997; 23: 3–25.
4. PCcaps™. To speed-up pre-clinical trials. *Capsugel Library*: BAS 180 E 1998.
5. Shen HR, Zhong MK. Preparation and evaluation of self-microemulsifying drug delivery systems (SMEDDS) containing atorvastatin. *J Pharm Pharmacol* 2006; 58: 1183–1191.

6. Serajuddin ATM, Sheen PC, Mufson D et al. Effect of vehicle amphiphilicity on the dissolution and bioavailability of the poorly water-soluble drug from solid dispersion. *J Pharm Sci* 1988; 414–417.
7. Sherif I, Badawy F, Ghorab MM, Adeyeye CM. Bioavailability of Danazol–hydroxypropyl-β-cyclodextrin complex by different route of administration. *Int J Pharm* 1996; 145: 137–143.
8. Esseku F, Lesher L, Bijlani V et al. The effect of overencapsulation on disintegration and dissolution. *Pharm Technol* 2010; 34: 104–111.
9. Brodniewicz T, Grynkiewicz G. Preclinical drug development. *Acta Poloniae Pharmaceutica—Drug Research* 2010; 67: 579–586.
10. Ku MS, Li W, Dulina W et al. Performance qualification of a new hypromellose capsule: Part I. Comparative evaluation of physical, mechanical and processability quality attributes of Vcaps Plus, Quali-V and gelatin capsules. *Int J Pharm* 2010; 386: 30–41.
11. Vilivalam VD, Illum L, Iqbal K. Starch capsules: An alternative system for oral drug delivery. *Pharmaceutical Science & Technology Today* 2000; 3(2): 64–69.
12. Xu C, Zhang JS, Mo Y, Tan RX. Calcium pectinate capsules for colon-specific drug delivery. *Drug Dev Ind Pharm* 2005; 31: 127–134.
13. Tozaki M, Odoriba T, Fujita T. Chitosan capsules for colon-specific drug delivery: Enhanced localization of 5-aminosalicylic acid in the large intestine accelerates healing of TNBS-induced colitis in rats. *Life Sci* 1999; 64: 1155.
14. Esseku F, Adeyeye MC. Bacteria and pH-sensitive polysaccharide-polymer films for colon targeted delivery. *Crit Rev Ther Drug Carrier Syst* 2011; 28: 395–445.
15. Dvorakova K, Rabiskova M, Gajdziok J et al. Coated capsules for drug targeting to proximal and distal part of human intestine. *Acta Poloniae Pharmaceutica—Drug Research* 2010; 67: 191–199.
16. Bain DF, Fagan PG. Miniaturisation in pharmaceutics—Addressing product development demands of the 21st century. *Business Briefing: Pharma Outsourcing* 2011; 1–4.
17. Micro-dosing equipment fills niche in R&D, clinical trial materials. *Tablets & Capsules* 2009; 22–24.
18. Kadri BV. Recent Options for Phase 1 Formulation Development and Clinical Trial Material Supply. http://www.pharmtech.com/pharmtech/Formulation+Article/Recent-Options-for-Phase-1-Formulation -Development/ArticleStandard/Article/detail/541994 02/15/2013.
19. Ruff MD. *Formulation: Rethinking Neat-API Capsule Filling for Phase I Clinical Trials*. Minnesota: CSC Publishing: Tablets and Capsules. 2011: 1–5.
20. Anon. *Health Informatics into the 21st Century*, HealthCare Reports, Reuters Business Insight, 1999: 1–4.
21. Ruff M, Xian G, Vinson R. The case against powder (active only) in capsule Phase I formulations for poorly soluble drugs: A comparison of in-vitro dissolution. *The AAPS J* 2009; abstract 3145.
22. Daviau T. API in capsule vs. the lost art of formulation development, website: 02/15/2013.
23. DBcaps® Capsules: A complete line of capsules for double-blind clinical trials. www.capsugel.com: 02/15/2013.
24. Al-Tabakha MM. HPMC capsules: Current status and future prospects. *J Pharm Pharm Sci* 2010; 13(3): 428–442.
25. Perkins AC, Wilson CG, Blackshaw PE et al. Impaired oesophageal transit of capsule versus tablet formulations in the elderly. *Gut* 1994; 35: 1363–1367.
26. Cole ET, Scott RA, Cade D et al. *In vitro* and *in vivo* pharmacoscintigraphic evaluation of ibuprofen hypromellose and gelatin capsules. *Pharm Res* 2004; 21: 793–798.
27. McCargar L, Crail D, Dansereau R et al. The *in-vitro* porcine adhesion model is not predictive of the esophageal transit of risedronate tablets in humans. *Int J Pharm* 2001; 222: 191–197.
28. Osmanoglou E, Van Der Voort IR, Fach KO et al. Oesophageal transport of solid dosage forms depends on body position, swallowing volume and pharyngeal propulsion velocity. *Neurogastroenterol Motil* 2004; 16: 547–556.
29. Honkanen O. Biopharmaceutical Evaluation of Orally and Rectally Administered Hard Hydroxypropyl Methylcellulose Capsules. Academic Dissertation, University of Helsinki, Finland, 2004.
30. Honkanen O, Seppä H, Eerikäinen S et al. Bioavailability of ibuprofen from orally and rectally administered hydroxypropyl methylcellulose capsules compared to corresponding gelatine capsules. *STP Pharma Sci* 2001; 11: 181–185.
31. Tuleu C, Khela MK, Evans DF et al. A scintigraphic investigation of the disintegration behaviour of capsules in fasting subjects: A comparison of hypromellose capsules containing carrageenan as a gelling agent and standard gelatin capsules. *Eur J Pharm Sci* 2007; 30: 251–255.
32. Cade D. Dissolution and disintegration methods for gelatin capsules, including dietary supplements. *AAPS Suppl.* October 18, 2012.

33. Plantcaps: Capsugel @ www.capsugel.com: 02/15/2013.
34. Bhat A, Chowdary KPR, Shobarani RH, Narasu L. Formulation and evaluation of chronopharmaceutical drug delivery of theophylline for nocturnal asthma. *Intl J Pharm Pharm Sci* 2011; 3: 204–208.
35. Zhang Z, Wu F, Zhang Y et al. A novel pulsed-release system based on swelling and osmotic pumping mechanism. *J Controlled Release* 2003; 89: 47–55.
36. Bikiaris D, Karavas E, Georgarakis E. Application of PVP/HPMC miscible blends with enhanced mucoadhesive properties for adjusting drug release in predictable pulsatile chronotherapeutics. *Eur J Pharm Biopharm* 2006; 64: 115–126.
37. Ali J, Qureshi J, Amir M et al. Chronomodulated Drug delivery system of salbutamol sulphate for the treatment of nocturnal asthma. *Indian J Pharm Sci* 2008; 70: 351–356.
38. Bodmeier R, Krogel I. Development of a multifunctional matrix drug delivery system surrounded by an impermeable cylinder. *J Controlled Release* 1999; 61: 43–50.
39. Samantaray DG, Rao VN, Namballa RK et al. Oral Pharmaceutica; Paricalcitol. *US Patent 2011/0033529 A1.*
40. Acid-resistant DRCaps. www.capsugel.com: 02/15/2013.
41. Romano C, Cuccihiara S, Barabino A et al. Usefulness of ω-3 fatty acid supplementation in addition to mesalazine in maintaining remission in pediatric Crohn's disease: A double-blind, randomized placebo-controlled study. *World J Gastroenterol* 2005; 11: 7118–7121.
42. Kadri BV, Greene MB. Enteric coating and stability of aqueous enteric systems on HPMC capsules. *AAPS Suppl* November, 2008.
43. Cole ET, Scott RA, Connor AL et al. Enteric coated HPMC capsules designed to achieve intestinal targeting. *Int J Pharm* 2002; 231: 83–95.
44. McConnell EL, Basit AW. Targeting the colon using COLALTM: A novel bacteria-sensitive drug delivery system. In: Rathbone MJ, Hadgraft J, Roberts MS, Lane ME, eds. (2nd ed.) *Modified-Release Drug Delivery Technology.* New York: Informa Healthcare; 2008: 343–348.
45. Study of COLAL-PRED® in the treatment of moderate acute ulcerative colitis. *ClinicalTrials.gov.* 2009.
46. McConnell EL, Liu F, Basit AW. Colonic treatments and targets: Issues and opportunities. *J Drug Target* 2009; 17: 335–363.
47. Han M, Fang QL, Zhan HW et al. *In vitro* and *in vivo* evaluation of a novel capsule for colon-specific drug delivery. *J Pharm Sci* 2009; 98: 2626–2635.
48. Vilivalam VD, Illum L, Iqbal K. Enteric coating and drug release evaluation of starch capsules in the development of colon specific drug delivery systems. *Pharm Res* 1997; 14: S-659.
49. Watts PJ, Illum L. Colonic drug delivery. *Drug Dev Ind Pharm* 1997; 23: 893–913.
50. Davis SS, Hardy JG, Newman SP et al. Gamma scintigraphy in the evaluation of pharmaceutical dosage forms. *Eur J Nucl Med* 1992; 19: 971–986.
51. Doll WJ, Sandefer EP, Page RC et al. A scintigraphic and pharmacokinetic evaluation of a novel capsule manufactured from potato starch compared with a conventional hard gelatin capsule in normal and in normal subjects administered omperazole. *Pharm Res* 1993; 10: S-213.
52. Wilding IR, Hardy JG, Sparrow RA et al. Enteric coated starch capsules: A new approach for targeted intestinal delivery. *Pharm Res* 1993; 10: S-183.
53. Kenyon CJ, Cole ET, Wilding IR. The effect of food on the in vivo behaviour of enteric coated starch capsules. *Int J Pharm* 1994; 112: 207–213.
54. Watts P, Smith A. TARGIT technology: Coated starch capsules for site-specific drug delivery into the lower gastrointestinal tract. *Expert Opin Drug Deliv* 2005; 2: 159–167.
55. Waterman KC, Goeken, GS, Konagurthu S et al. Osmotic capsules: A universal oral, controlled-release drug delivery dosage form. *J Controlled Release* 2011; 152: 264–269.
56. Crison JR, Siersma PR, Taylor MD et al. Programmable oral release technology, PORT Systems™: A novel dosage form for time and site specific oral drug delivery, *Proceed Intl Symp Control Rel Bioact Matter* 1995; 22: 278–279.
57. Lee WW, O'Mahony B, Bar-Shalom D et al. Scintigraphic characterisation of a novel injection-moulded dosage form. *Proceed Intl Symp Control Rel Bioact Matter* 2000; 27: 1288–1289.
58. Chacko A, Szaz KF, Howard J et al. Non-invasive method for delivery of tracer substances or small quantities of other materials to the colon. *Gut* 1990; 31: 106–110.
59. Capsugel Xcelodose® System Precision Powder Micro-dosing System Brochure: 2/15/2013.
60. Capsugel Xcelolab TM Powder Dispenser Brochure: http://capsugel.com/en/products-services/products/equipment/xcelodose/02/15/2013
61. Xcelodose product brochure, accessed on January 19, 2007, from http://www.capsugel.com/equipment/xcelodose_brochure.php 02/15/2013.

62. Cole E, Cadé D, Benameur H. Challenges and opportunities in the encapsulation of liquid and semi-solid formulations into capsules for oral administration *Adv Drug Del Rev* 2008; 60: 747–756.

63. Myers RG, Cratty CM. Blinding clinical supplies utilizing overencapsulation. *Pharmaceutical Engineering* 2003; Vol. 23.

64. Faust MB. Effect of variations in backfill on dissolution for an over-encapsulated comparator product. *Pharmaceutical Engineering* 1999; 19(3): 48–54.

65. Huynh-Ba K, Aubry AF. Analytical development strategies for comparator products. *American Pharmaceutical Review* 2003; 6(2): 92–97.

66. Khan MN, Suresh J, Hemant KS et al. Formulation and evaluation of antistress polyherbal capsule. *Pelagia Research Library Der Pharmacia Sinica* 2012; 3: 177–184.

67. Zick SM, Blume A, Normolle D et al. Challenges in herbal research: A randomized clinical trial to assess blinding with ginger. *Complementary Therapies in Medicine* 2005; 13: 101–106.

68. Shah J, Goyal R. Comparative clinical evaluation of herbal formulation with multivitamin formulation for learning and memory enhancement. *Asian J Pharmaceutical Clin Res* 2010; 3: 69–75.

69. Tasawar Z, Siraj Z, Ahmad N et al. The effects of *Nigella sativa* (Kalonji) on lipid profile in patients with stable coronary artery disease in Multan, Pakistan. *Pakistan J Nutr* 2011; 10: 162–167.

70. Sawicki W. Pharmacokinetics of verapamil and norverapamil from controlled release floating pellets in humans. *Eur J Pharm Biopharm* 2002; 53: 29–35.

71. Dhaliwal S, Jain S, Singh HP et al. Mucoadhesive microspheres for gastroretentive delivery of acyclovir: In vitro and in vivo evaluation. *AAPS J* 2008; 10: 322–330.

72. Sakr FM. A programmable drug delivery system for oral administration. *Int J Pharm* 1999; 184: 131–139.

73. Schellekens RCA, Stellaard F, Mitrovic D et al. Pulsatile drug delivery to ileo-colonic segments by structured incorporation of disintegrants in pH-responsive polymer coatings. *J Controlled Release* 2008; 132: 91–98.

74. Hinderling PH, Karara AH, Tao B et al. Systemic availability of the active metabolite hydroxy-fasudil after administration of fasudil to different sites of the human gastrointestinal tract. *J Clin Pharmacol* 2007; 47: 19–25.

75. Ishibashi T, Pitcairn GR, Yoshimo H et al. Scintigraphic evaluation of a new capsule-type colon specific drug delivery system in healthy volunteers. *J Pharm Sci* 1998; 87: 31–35.

76. Pinto JF. Site-specific drug delivery systems within the gastro-intestinal tract: From the mouth to the colon. *Intl J Pharmace* 2010; 395: 44–52.

77. Ishibashi T, Hatano H, Kobayashi M et al. *In vivo* drug release behavior in dogs from a new colon-targeted delivery system. *J Controlled Release* 1999; 57: 45–53.

78. Ishibashi T, Ikegami K, Kubo H et al. Evaluation of colonic absorbability of drugs in dogs using a novel colon-targeted delivery capsule (CTDC). *J Controlled Release* 1999; 59: 361–376.

79. Abdul B, Bloor J. Perspectives on Colonic Drug Delivery. Business Briefing, *Pharmatech* 2003; 185–190.

80. McConville JT, Ross AC, Florence AJ et al. Erosion characteristics of an erodible tablet incorporated in a time-delayed capsule device. *Drug Dev Ind Pharm* 2003; 31: 79–89.

81. Gong Y, Zha Q, Li L et al. Efficacy and safety of Fufangkushen colon-coated capsule in the treatment of ulcerative colitis compared with mesalazine: A double-blinded and randomized study. *J Ethnopharmacol* 2012; 141: 592–598.

82. Amidon GI, Leesman GD. Pulsatile Drug Delivery System. *US Patent 5 229 131.* July 20, 1993.

83. Saffran M, Field JB, Pena J et al. Oral insulin in diabetic dogs. *J Endocrinol* 1991; 131: 267–278.

84. Bronsted H, Kopecek J. Hydrogels for site-specific oral drug delivery: Synthesis and characterization. *Biomaterials* 1991; 12: 584–592.

85. Tozaki H, Komoike J, Tada C et al. Chitosan capsule for colon-specific drug delivery: Improvement of insulin absorption from the rat colon. *J Pharm Sci* 1997; 86: 1016–1021.

86. Yamamoto A, Tozaki H, Okada N et al. Colon-specific delivery of peptide drugs and anti-inflammatory drugs using chitosan capsules. *STP Pharma Sci* 2000; 10: 23–34.

87. Ritschel WA. Microemulsions for improved peptide absorption from the gastrointestinal tract. *Methods Find Exp Clin Pharmacol* 1991; 13: 205–220.

88. Kraeling MEK, Ritschel WA. Development of a colonic release capsule dosage form and the absorption of insulin. *Methods Find Exp Clin Pharmacol* 1992; 14: 199–209.

89. Rao S, Ritschel WA. Colonic drug delivery of small peptides. *STP Pharma Sci* 1995; 5: 19–29.

90. Youan BC. Overview of chronopharmaceutics. In: B.C. Youan, ed. *Chronopharmaceutics: Science and Technology for Biological Rhythm Guided Therapy and Prevention of Diseases*. Hoboken, NJ: John Wiley & Sons, 2009.
91. Mandal AS, Biswas N, Karim KM et al. Drug delivery system based on chronobiology—A review. *J Controlled Release* 2010; 147: 314–325.
92. Barzegar-Jalali M, Siyahi-Shadbad M. Design and evaluation of delayed release osmotic capsule of acetaminophen. *Iran J Pharma Sci Spring* 2006; 2: 65–72.
93. Cole ET. Liquid filled hard gelatin capsules. *Pharm Technol Int* Sept/Oct 1989: 1–12.
94. Cole ET. Liquid filled and sealed hard gelatin capsules. *Capsugel Library* 2000; BAS 210.
95. Seta Y, Otsuka T, Tokiwa H et al. Design of Captopril sustained-release preparation with oily semisolid matrix intended for use in human subjects. *Int J Pharm* 1988; 41: 263–269.
96. Seta Y, Higuchi F, Kawahara Y et al. Design and preparation of Captopril sustained release dosage forms and their biopharmaceutical properties. *Int J Pharm* 1988; 41: 245–254.
97. Qiu Y, Zhang G. Development of modified-release solid oral dosage forms. In: *Developing Solid Oral Dosage Forms: Pharmaceutical Theory and Practice*. Amsterdam: Elsevier, 2009; 501–515.
98. Oral Controlled Release Drug Delivery Systems. In: *Controlled Drug Delivery: Fundamentals and Applications*. JR Robinson and VHL Lee, eds. (2nd ed.). New York: Marcel Dekker, 1987.
99. Baiz E, Einig H. Alginate-based Verapamil-containing depot drug form. *US Patent 5 132 295* (1992). United States Patent and Trademark Office (www.uspto.gov).
100. Howard JR, Timmins P. Controlled release formulation. *US Patent 4 792 452* (1988). United States Patent and Trademark Office (www.uspto.gov).
101. Panoz DE, Geoghegan EJ. Controlled absorption pharmaceutical composition. *US Patent 4 863 742* (1989). United States Patent and Trademark Office (www.uspto.gov).
102. Chen X, Shou J, Yun Z et al. Calcium pectinate capsule for colon specific drug delivery. *Drug Dev Ind Pharm* 2005; 31: 127–134.
103. Chourasia MK, Jain SK. Pharmaceutical approaches to colon targeted drug delivery systems. *J Pharm Pharmaceut Sci* 2003; 6: 33–66.
104. Bussemer T, Dashevsky A, Bodmeier R. A pulsatile drug delivery system based on rupturable coated hard gelatin capsules. *J Controlled Release* 2003; 93: 331–339.
105. Jao F, Wong PS, Huynh HT et al. Verapamil therapy. *US Patent 5 190 765* (1993).
106. Jao F, Wong PS, Huynh HT et al. Verapamil therapy. *US Patent 5 252 338* (1993).
107. Somma R. Development knowledge can increase manufacturing capability and facilitate quality by design. *J Pharm Innov* 2007; 2: 87–92.
108. Martin-Moe S, Lim FJ, Wong RL et al. New roadmap for biopharmaceutical drug product development: Integrating development, validation, and quality by design. *J Pharm Sci* 100: 3031–3034.
109. Gassmann O, von Zedtwitz M. Organization of industrial R&D on a global scale. *R&D Management* 1998; 28: 147–161.
110. Woodcock J. Pharmaceutical quality in the 21st century—An integrated systems approach, *AAPS Workshop on Pharmaceutical Quality—A Science and Risk Based Approach in the 21st Century* (2005).
111. Lorimer C. Manual and Automated Filling of Powder in Capsules for Clinical Trials—*Pharmaceutical Technology* (2011) accessed at http://www.pharmtech.com/pharmtech/article/articleDetail.jsp?id=722533 (Feb. 16, 2013).
112. Edwards D. Beyond fast filling. *Therapeutic Delivery* 2010; 1: 195–201.
113. Small LE, Augsburger LL. Instrumentation of an automatic capsule-filling machine. *J Pharm Sci* 1977; 66: 504–509.
114. Cole GC, May G. The instrumentation of a Zanasi LZ/64 Capsule filling machine. *J Pharm Pharmacol* 1975; 27: 353–358.
115. Amidon GL, Lennernas H, Shah VP et al. A theoretical basis for a biopharmaceutic drug classification: The correlation of *in vitro* drug product dissolution and *in vivo* bioavailability. *Pharm Res* 1995; 12: 413–420.
116. Hammond S. PAT and the development of an advanced control system for pharmaceutical manufacturing In: *Meeting Challenges of Pharmaceutical Innovation and Quality by Design in the 21st Century: Implementation of PAT. FIP World Congress* (August 31–Sept. 4, 2008) Basel, Switzerland.
117. Garcia T, Cook G, Nosal R. PQLI key topics—Criticality, design space, and control strategy. *J Pharm Innov* 2008; 3: 60–68.

118. York P. Knowledge engineering approaches in pharmaceutical design science In: *Meeting Challenges of Pharmaceutical Innovation and Quality by Design in the 21st Century: Implementation of PAT. FIP World Congress* (August 31–Sept. 4, 2008) Basel, Switzerland.

119. Jones BE. Capsules, Hard. In: *Encyclopedia of Pharmaceutical Technology* (Swarbrick J and Boylan JC, eds.). New York: Marcel Dekker, Vol. 2. 1990.

120. Ulmschneider M. Promoting pharmaceutical excellence tools and methods for process understanding implementation of PAT. In: *Meeting Challenges of Pharmaceutical Innovation and Quality by Design in the 21st Century: Implementation of PAT. FIP World Congress* (August 31–Sept. 4, 2008) Basel, Switzerland.

121. Podczeck F, Newton JM. Filling powdered herbs into gelatin capsules. *Mfg Chem* 1999; 60: 29–31, 33.

122. Zhang X, Lionberger RA, Davit BM et al. Utility of physiologically based absorption modeling in implementing quality by design in drug development. *The AAPS J* 2011; 13: 59–71.

123. Dickinson PA, Lee WW, Stott PW et al. Clinical relevance of dissolution testing in quality by design. *The AAPS J* 2008; 10: 280–290.

124. Lionberger RA, Lee SL, Lee LL et al. Quality by design: Concepts for ANDA. *The AAPS J* 2008; 10: 268–276.

125. Young CS, Kim Y, Park SM et al. Trials of novel 13C-urea-containing capsule for more economic and sensitive diagnosis of *Helicobacter pylori* infection in human subjects. *Arch Pharm Res* 29: 879–883.

126. Acuff RV, Cai DJ, Dong Z et al. The lipid lowering effect of plant sterol ester capsules in hypercholestrolemic subjects. *Lipids in Health and Disease* 2007; 6: 11.

127. FDA guidance for industry on Waiver of *In Vivo* Bioavailability and Bioequivalence Studies for Immediate Release Solid Oral Dosage Forms Based on a Biopharmaceutics Classification System. FDA/CDER: August 2000.

128. Cook J, Addicks W, Wu YH. Application of the biopharmaceutical classification system in clinical drug development—An industrial view. *The AAPS J* 2008; 10(2).

129. Wu Y, Zhao F, Paborji M. Effect of fill weight, capsule shell, and sinker design on the dissolution behavior of capsule formulations of a weak acid drug candidate BMS-309403 *Pharmaceut Dev Tech* 2003; 8: 379–383.

130. Hogan J, Shue P, Podczeck F et al. Investigations into the relationship between drug properties, filling, and the release of drugs from hard gelatin capsules using multivariate statistical analysis. *Pharm Res* 1996; 13: 944–949.

131. Talpes S, Knoerzer D, Huber R et al. Esomeprazole MUPS 40 mg tablets and esomeprazole MUPS 40 mg tablets encapsulated in hard gelatin are bioequivalent. *Int J Clin Pharmacol Therapeut* 2005; 43: 51–56.

132. Wilding IR, Cark D, Wray H et al. *In vivo* disintegration profiles of encapsulated and nonencapsulated sumatriptan: Gamma scintigraphy in healthy volunteers. *J Clin Pharmacol* 2005; 45: 101–105.

133. Fuseau E, Petricoul O, Sabin A et al. Effect of encapsulation on absorption of sumatriptan tablets: Data from healthy volunteers and patients during a migraine. *Clin Therapeut* 2001; 23: 242–251.

134. Liao A, Pang X, Li H et al. Bioavailability of mifepristone in capsule versus tablet form in healthy non-pregnant women. *Contraception* 2008; 77: 431–434.

135. Zou J, Ji H, Wu D et al. Bioequivalence and pharmacokinetic comparison of a single 200-mg dose of meclofenoxate hydrochloride capsule and tablet formulations in healthy Chinese adult male volunteers: A randomized sequence, open-label, two-period crossover study. *Clin Therapeut* 2008; 30(9): 1651–1657.

136. Chun AHC, Erdman K, Chiu Y et al. Bioavailability of lansoprazole granules administered in juice or soft food compared with the intact capsule formulation. *Clin Therapeut* 2002; Aug:24(8): 1322–1331.

137. Lin C, Affrime M, Radwanski E et al. Comparative bioavailability of ceftibuten in capsule and suspension forms. *Clin Therapeut* 1996; 18(6): 1139–1149.

138. Guidance for the Industry: Guidance for Industry: Dissolution Testing of Immediate Release Solid Oral Dosage Forms. *FDA-CDER* (1997).

139. Guidance for the Industry: Bioavailability and Bioequivalence Studies for Orally Administered Drug Products—General Considerations. *FDA-CDER* (2003).

140. Graffner C. Regulatory aspects of drug dissolution from a European perspective. *Eur J Pharm Sci* 2006; 29: 288–293.

4 Capsule Shell Manufacture

Brian E. Jones, Fridrun Podczeck, and Paul Lukas

CONTENTS

INTRODUCTION

Both hard and soft types of capsule shells were first patented and used in France in the first half of the nineteenth century.[1] The manufacture of hard, two-piece, and soft, one-piece, capsule shells relies on the same basic phenomenon that solutions of certain polymers change their state from a liquid to a solid with a change in temperature. The polymer first used in their manufacture was gelatin, solutions of which, when their temperature drops below about 35°C, undergo a gelation process and change from a sol to a gel state, thus enabling homogeneous films to be formed rapidly on metal molds to produce hard capsules or to form sheets of material to produce soft capsules. The resulting shells are either filled with a formulated product at the point of the shell formation in the case of soft capsules or are filled in a totally separate operation in the case of hard capsules. The main formulation difference between the shells is that soft capsules contain a significant proportion of added plasticizer. This chapter describes their manufacturing processes and explains the properties of each.

HARD CAPSULES

EARLY DEVELOPMENT OF PROCESS AND MACHINES

The method of manufacture of hard two-piece capsule shells used currently is the same as that described in the patent of Lehuby granted in Paris in 1846.[1] This described the same component steps as used on modern high-speed fully automatic machines: a container with a warm solution of the shell forming polymer, into which were dipped sets of silver-plated metal molds, one for the caps and the other for the bodies mounted on wooden disks; on removal, the wet shells were trimmed to length air dried, and when ready, the shells were removed and assembled together. Each step has limitations based on mechanical issues and the physical and chemical properties of the polymer solutions being used. The challenge for chemists, engineers, and pharmacists over the years has been to increase the speed of output and to improve the dimensional and visual quality of these capsules.

The first attempts at larger-scale manufacturing were hindered by problems of fitting the two pieces together. The relationship between the cap and body mold diameters was not established until F.A. Hubel, a pharmacist in Detroit in 1874, used low-cost accurate mold pins made from standard gauged iron rod widely used in mechanical engineering.[2] Many small companies started making empty capsules. The two main players in the field were Eli Lilly & Company who started production in 1897, whose capsule division has evolved into the company Qualicaps (www.qualicaps.com), and Parke, Davis & Company who started manufacture in 1904 and evolved into Capsugel (www.cap sugel.com).[1] By the early 1900s, the process was becoming more mechanized with outputs of 8000 to 10,000 capsules per operator per day using semiautomatic machines. The first fully automatic machines were developed by the Arthur Colton Company for Eli Lilly in 1909 and 1913[3]; output per machine was 8000 capsules per hour. Capsule manufacture in the United States stopped in hot summer months because mold pins could not be kept cool enough. Eli Lilly, in 1913, was the first to install an air conditioning unit in their plant, enabling capsules to be manufactured all year round, and made the first colored capsules, a transparent pink color, which is still used in US pharmacies

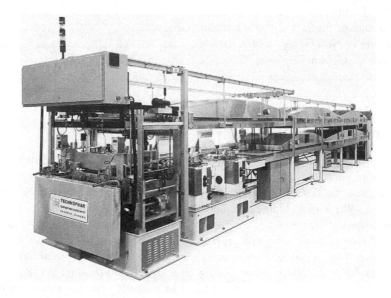

FIGURE 4.1   Photograph of the Technophar capsule manufacturing machine.

for extemporaneous dispensing of hard capsule products.[1] The next major advance was made by the Arthur Colton Company for Parke Davis in 1931.[4] They dramatically improved the rate of output by making a machine in two parts, mirror images of each other; caps were made on one side and bodies were made on the other side of the machine. Two-dipping pans enabled two-color capsules to be made for the first time. This machine design has since then been adapted as the basis for all modern machines: these machines were about 10 m long and 3 m high (see Figure 4.1).

Hard capsule shell manufacturing remained almost exclusively in the United States from the 1880s until after the Second World War. Eli Lilly Co. and Parke, Davis & Co. were leaders in this field; both opened plants in the United Kingdom in the 1950s; during the 1960s, between them, they built further plants in Europe in France, Belgium, Italy, and Spain and then in other parts of the world: Mexico, Argentina, Australia, and Japan. Since then, manufacture has become a global industry, with large companies established in India (www.acg-associatedcapsules.com), China and South Korea, and numerous smaller companies in Asia, Europe, and North and South America.

Capsule Shell Design

The standard shape for a hard gelatin capsule was established by Lehuby in his original patent. From then until the 1960s, except for a few minor exceptions, capsule design remained unaltered. This changed with the introduction of automation for filling and packaging products; handling stresses applied to filled capsules increased and they came apart shedding their contents: the need for a "self-locking" capsule to prevent reopening became a requirement. Previously, capsules were held together by powder trapped in the overlap between cap and body formed to the machine filling process. Automatic machines filled soft plugs of powder into capsules; powder was no longer present in significant amounts in this overlap. The first patent for a "self-locking" capsule in the modern era was granted to Eli Lilly & Co.[5] Their Lokcaps capsule had a circular indentation on the inside of the cap, and when the capsules were closed together after filling, this formed an interference fit with the body, increasing the force required to separate the two parts. However, capsules could not be fully closed during manufacture because the filling machines were unable to separate them. Lilly overcame this problem by adding two small rectangular indentations on the inside of the cap on opposite sides about halfway along the cylinder, called "Preloks." These held the capsule parts together, now closed to a longer length, when they were empty; avoiding separation problems during handling and transfer from manufacturer to capsule filler. Parke, Davis & Co. followed this lead later in the 1960s with the introduction of Snapfit capsules.[6] These had two oval pre-lock indentations on the cap and two circular locking features, one on each half. The body indentation was located on the outside close to its cut edge and the cap one was located on its inside surface close to the domed end, which provided a positive closure. The problem of filled capsules coming apart was increased by the speed automatic filling machines closed filled capsules; bodies entered into caps faster, resulting in more air trapped inside, increasing the internal pressure, and on storage, caps could be "blown" off their bodies. Air vents had to be included in the pin design. Eli Lilly solved the problem by introducing three lands, nonindented areas, in the circular cap groove.

Most manufactures have designed their own pins and all provide for the same set of functions. The features required are as follows: to hold empty capsules together to prevent separation on handling, to aid the entry of the body into the cap, to allow air to escape during re-closure after filling, and to hold the cap and body together after filling, (see Figure 4.2). Initially, there were two pre-lock features on capsules and it was observed that this tended to make the cap less round. Manufacturers now use multiple pre-locks, four or six, placed symmetrically round the cap, thus maintaining its circular shape. Air vents have been placed in various positions in both cap and body. Cap circular indents with unindented spaces (Eli Lilly) and on the bodies flat areas are molded on the outside surface from the cut edge crossing any circular indents (Parke Davis): both of these features provide channels for air to escape during capsule closure. The clearance between the body and the cap is very small, and rejoining the cap and body together after filling needs careful control. For good

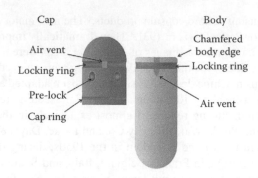

FIGURE 4.2 Drawing of a hard capsule showing the features that have been used by various manufacturers in their own preferred arrangements.

closure, the cap and the body must be in perfect alignment, and anything that prevents this must be countered. If not, the body will come into contact with the cap edge and a sliver of shell wall will be cut, which passes up the outside of the cap. This fault, in capsule makers' jargon, is called a "telescope," which is a totally wrong analogy, and would be better described as a "bad or incorrect join." It is a fault seen during capsule filling. Capsule shells have flexible walls and thus the open ends of caps and bodies can become slightly distorted, caused by poor storage or handling. The filling process also plays a part because if loose powder is present in the capsule bushings, the cap might not be seated correctly, resulting in them being tilted enough to contact the body edge. This coupled with wear of the bushings will cause this fault. Capsugel made a capsule, the Coni-Snap, which had a chamfer at the open edge of the body, reducing its effective diameter and making it easier for the body to enter the cap, thus reducing problems caused by worn bushings.[7] Elanco Qualicaps added a circular indentation close to the open end of the cap to maintain the circularity during closure.[8] The common practice for circular locking feature is to have them on both the cap and the body to provide an interference fit that increases the force to separate them to a level above those to which filled capsules are subjected to during handling.

Manufacture of Hard Gelatin Capsule Shells

This section describes the process used for gelatin. Other polymers are used and the differences in their processing behavior will be discussed in the "Gelatin Alternatives for Hard Capsule Manufacture" section.

Preparation of the Manufacturing Solutions

The first task is to make a bubble-free concentrated solution of gelatin. The simplest way to dissolve gelatin is to soak it in water at 15°C, allow it to swell and fully hydrate, and warm it to above 35°C when it will dissolve and produce a bubble-free solution. On an industrial scale, this is not a practical process because among other factors, the microbial quality of solutions could be compromised. Gelatin solutions are a good substrate for bacterial growth at ambient temperatures. In the past, preservatives such as methyl and propyl parabens and sodium metabisulfite were added into gelatin solutions to control microbial levels during production. They played no role in finished capsules because the water activity at their moisture content of 13–16% was insufficient to maintain bacterial growth.[9] Currently, preservatives are not used in gelatin capsules manufactured in Europe, and in the United States, they are only used in older products that were registered some time ago. Problems can also be avoided if the temperature of gelatin solutions is maintained at ≥45°C. The process conditions are set to maintain this temperature all through the process and equipment is designed to avoid any cooler spots. This maintains the microbial quality to the same level as the incoming gelatin.

Gelatins used are usually purchased from more than one supplier against purchasing specifications that specify in addition to standard pharmaceutical chemical and microbial purity levels two factors specific to capsule manufacture, viscosity and Bloom strength, a measure of gel rigidity.[10] Gelatins are used as single lots or blended with other lots to achieve the required quality. Solutions are prepared in large stainless steel water-jacketed pressure vessels. These are first charged with hot demineralized water at about 70°C. Gelatin is fed into the top of the tank usually by an air transport system. The concentration of gelatin is between 30% and 40% w/w. The tanks are stirred for several hours to dissolve the gelatin. When it is all dissolved, the resulting solution contains air bubbles caused either by the mixing process or by the raw material gelatin that during processing after extraction is extruded through a votator to produce small hollow tubes, which are broken up during final milling. To remove these, a vacuum suction is applied to the tank and the bubbles rise to the surface. In hot solutions, gelatin hydrolyzes with time and its Bloom strength and viscosity values fall; thus, the rate of usage on the manufacturing machines governs the lot sizes that can be manufactured.

When the solution is ready, aliquots of solutions ≥25 L are dispensed from the tank in to suitable sized containers and prepared for delivery to individual machines. First, measured quantities of dye solutions and pigment suspensions, as required to produce the correct capsule color, are added to the vessels and various process additives, such as sodium lauryl sulfate, a USP permitted wetting agent, or colloidal silicon dioxide, a substance to modify the surface structure of the film and thus reduce its frictional properties. This latter additive has been listed as a component of capsule shell formulations in products registered by the European Medicines Agency. The solution is carefully mixed with a suitable stirrer, to ensure that no air bubbles are produced. The viscosity in the individual vessels is then measured using a viscometer, usually an electromechanical one with a rotating cylinder, and the calculated amount of water is added to adjust the value to that required for the lot of capsules concerned. The target viscosity is dependent on the capsule size and whether it is for cap or body. Once the machine has been started up, subsequent deliveries to the machines have lower values than the original one made for machine setup as water is lost by evaporation during the process. Prepared solutions in their vessels are sometimes referred to as "pourings." These are delivered to the machines at regular intervals and transferred into larger water-jacketed holding vessels from which the solution is fed into the dipping container via a pipe that has a valve to regulate flow. The amount is controlled by a level sensor in the dipping container. This is a large rectangular water-jacketed vessel, inside of which is a second smaller open-top rectangular box. This is called the dip pan or dip pot. Gelatin solution is pumped up through the central box and overflows the edge, returning to the bulk of the solution below. This simple device ensures that the level of the solution in the central section is always the same during the dipping process. Baffles in the central box ensure gentle mixing of the solution as it passes through. In the outer area, at the entry end from the feeding tank, there is usually an electromechanical rotating cylinder viscometer measuring the solution viscosity. This is connected to a control system that adds hot demineralized water to keep the solution viscosity within the target limits. The viscosity of the system is always run on the slightly high side so that only water needs to be added to maintain control and not concentrated gelatin solution.

Formation of Hard Capsule Shells

The capsule manufacturing machines are housed in a carefully controlled environment: the humidity and temperature are controlled to ± 0.5% relative humidity (RH) and 0.5°C, respectively, and the air is circulated at a rate of 8 to 10 changes per hour. The process for forming hard capsules starts at the front end of the machine[11] (see Figure 4.3). Stainless steel molds, commonly known as pins, are mounted 30 in a line on metal bars. The shape of the mold pin is cylindrical with a hemispherical end; the shaft has a taper along its length toward the end of 0.1–0.3 mm cm^{-1}: this makes it easier to remove the dried films from the pins. Sets of pin bars, ≥5, are assembled in a rack above the dipping area and then are dipped into the gelatin solution. Mold pins are at about 22°C and the solution is

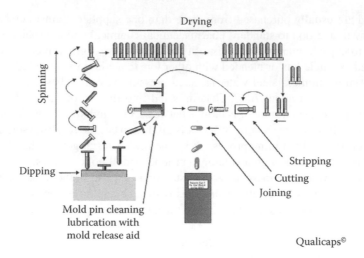

FIGURE 4.3   Outline of the hard capsule manufacturing process.

at about 45–50°C. The mold pin temperature is lower than the gelling point of the solution. When this contacts the mold pins, it changes state from a sol to a gel, forming a homogeneous film on their surface. The set of pin bars is slowly raised out of the solution and any ungelled solution drains off (see Figure 4.4). The rate of drain-off of the wet film is directly proportional to solution viscosity. The amount retained on the pin is directly related to the solution viscosity. The higher the viscosity, the greater the amount retained on the pin. This is used to control the thickness of capsule shells. When the mold pin emerges from the surface of the solution, a string-like connection forms between the pin base and the solution surface: with further movement, it gets thinner (i.e., necking), until it eventually breaks, leaving a blob of gelatin on the end of the pin. Pin bars are then rotated end over

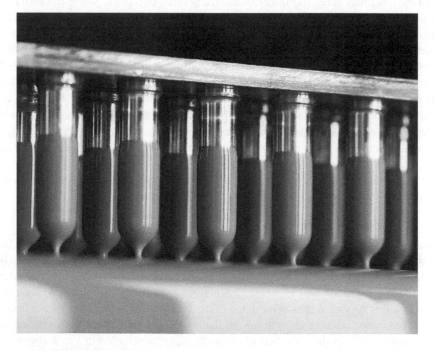

FIGURE 4.4   (See color insert.) Photograph of pins after dipping being withdrawn from the dip pan.

end as they are transferred from the dipping area to the upper deck of the machine. As this happens, the gelatin on the end of the pin flows to form a more uniform film. Cool air is blown over the pins to complete the gelling of the polymer. When the mold pins arrive on the top deck, they are now at 180° from their dipping orientation and the film is set. Pin bars are now assembled in groups, and when the table is full, this set is pushed though the drying kilns toward the rear of the machine. When sets arrive at the rear of the machine, there is a transfer elevator that lowers them down to the lower level where they are pushed forward toward the front of the machine through the remaining kilns.

The sets of pins bars as described above are passed through four or five separately controlled drying kilns in which large volumes of air at a controlled temperature and humidity and variable flow rates are directly blown over each pin. The wet films after dipping have a moisture content of about 70%, and about 80% of this needs to be removed before they emerge from the drying kilns. The air in the kilns is at different temperatures, between 0°C and 4°C above ambient conditions in the machine room. At the start of the drying process, not too much heat can be used; otherwise, the films would revert to the sol state. The temperatures later in the process are controlled so that when the mold pins exit from the kilns, they are back at 22°C, ready for the next cycle.

When the dried films emerge from the kilns, their moisture content is 15% to 18%, which is higher than the standard for empty gelatin capsules of 13.0% to 16.0% w/w. This is to enable the dried films to be easily stripped off the mold pins. There is an open area after the sets of pin bars exit the last kiln. The next part of the machine is often called the "automatic section." Before entry to this, a pair of cap and body pin bars are selected, lifted up, tipped onto their sides, and pushed into slots into the center of the automatic section. Sets of metal jaws with softer metal inserts in the open position are pushed over the mold pins. The jaws are closed and pulled backward, and in doing so, the dried films are pulled off the pins, transferring them into a matching set of four-leaf collets. The end of the film protrudes from the collet. The jaws move away and the collets are closed so that they grip the dried films. Situated above the open end of each set of collets is a knife holder with one knife for each collet. The knife bar is lowered and the collets revolve against the tip of the knife blades, cutting each capsule part to the correct length. The pieces cut off are thin and feathery and are sucked away to a collecting device. This material can be recycled.

Gelatin is a very tough material and needs a very sharp blade to cut it. These knives were originally made of steel and various grades of toughened material have been used to try and improve their performance and time between requiring sharpening. Diamond tipped blades, which cut films very well, were used at one time but proved impractical because they were very brittle and easily damaged. One of the best solutions to date has been the use of ceramic knives. These are made from the ceramic that was developed to make the heat shield tiles on US space shuttles. It is a robust material and knives made of it retain their sharpness longer than those made from other materials, giving them an increased production life.

Cut films are now pushed by rods out of the collet holders into a central joining block. The caps and bodies are joined together to form a capsule. They are closed to a specific value, the unclosed joined length, which is a position where the pre-locking features (but not the locking ones) are engaged (see the "Capsule Shell Design" section). After this, capsules are ejected from the block onto a moving conveyor belt that delivers them to a container at the machine exit.

Pin bars pass on to the next part of the machine where the mold pins are cleaned and lubricated with mold release aid. In order to be able to easily strip dried films off mold pins, it is essential to apply a release aid to their surface. The formulation for the release aid is propriety to each manufacturer and is made from food-grade materials and is listed in the manufacturer's DMFs. As the pin bars are moved to the cleaning section, a small amount of lubricant is applied to each mold pin as it passes either from a brush or from a revolving foam disc. Mold release aid is stored in a pressurized system and a pump controls the amount that is dispensed. Pins are next inserted into metal holders containing felt pads that are rotated to spread the mold release aid uniformly around them and to remove any particles on their surface. Pin bars are then assembled in groups and positioned above the dip pan for the cycle to be repeated. The cycle time is about 45 min and machines normally run 24/7.

To maintain production under control, machine operators take samples at regular intervals and check dimensions: the thickness of the shell wall near the cut open end of the capsule parts and at other places along the length of the capsule particularly at the domed end, cap and body lengths and diameters, and the unclosed joined length. Measurement gauges are now typically connected to computers, and these data are tracked and trends are displayed. These data can be used for machine validation, significantly reducing the time taken for this task.[12] This allows the machine to be controlled automatically or used by operators to make manual adjustments. Samples are also inspected for visual defects and color.

Capsule Sorting

The empty capsules go through a further series of processes in order to meet customer requirements: sorting, printing, and packaging.[11]

Capsules on leaving the machine are passed through various sorting devices in order to remove defective capsules. First, a simple mechanical device is often used, which consists of a honeycomb plate with holes the diameter of which are made so that capsules of the correct size will readily pass through and any damaged ones are retained on the plate and can be removed. Capsules with visual defects can be removed either by manual sorting on inspection belts or by the use of electronic optical devices of varying degrees of sophistication to inspect capsules individually at high speeds either by spinning them in a beam of light or by equipment with digital cameras, which use image analysis software.

Capsule Printing

In the United States and Europe, most capsules are printed by the capsule shell manufacturer with a variety of information required by their customers' pharmaceutical and nutraceutical companies, to help identify the product and other information such as the name and/or dose of API and the name of the manufacturer. Capsules are printed on machines based on the standard off-set printing process using edible inks[11] (see Figure 4.5).

The off-set printing process uses a reservoir that holds the printing ink. A cylindrical metal roto-gravure cylinder has the information to be printed (acid etched) onto its surface. This cylinder revolves in the reservoir of ink. A piece of metal with a straight edge, called a doctor blade, which is the same length as the cylinder, is in contact with it and excess ink is scrapped off. Next to the metal cylinder is a rubber off-set roller of the same dimensions and the two revolve in contact with one another. Ink in the etchings is transferred from the metal cylinder onto the rubber roller. Empty capsules held in a conveyor pass under this roller and contact it at a point where ink is transferred onto them.

Edible ink used in this process is mostly based on shellac. This is a natural polymer obtained as exudates from an insect, *Kerria lacca* (Coccideae), and is collected from trees in India and South Asia.[13] These insects live on trees and feed by sucking nourishment from them. They exude the raw shellac onto the branches where it dries; pieces are collected, liquefied by heat, and filtered to remove pieces of bark and insect parts. It is also known as "confectioner's glaze" and is widely used in the food industry. Solutions of 40% shellac in organic solvents are used as the base for ink manufacture.[11] Organic solvents are used because the ink has to dry rapidly because the time between it being applied to capsules and their exit from the machine into a container is very short. If the drying is incomplete, ink will be transferred to other capsules, making unsightly marks on their surfaces. Mixtures of solvents are used to obtain the required drying rates. The solvents used are governed by regulations that have been harmonized through the International Conference on Harmonization (ICH), which rates solvents into three toxicological classes ranging from ones to be avoided to those with low toxic potential.[14,15] Solvents in each class have been assigned a permitted daily exposure (PDE) limit. The level of residual solvents remaining in capsules is extremely low as the amount of

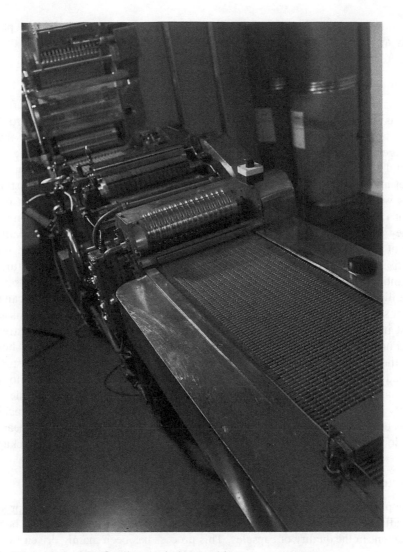

FIGURE 4.5 Photograph of the Qualicaps printing machine.

ink applied to a capsule is on the order of 1 to 3 μL and the solvents are lost as the ink dries. Inks are colored using pigments, iron oxides and titanium dioxide, and the lake form of soluble dyes. High concentrations of pigment are used in order to produce relatively stable suspensions. Other additives are used to improve the functionality of the inks such as additional suspending agents, hypromellose (required to maintain the consistency of color throughout a run), and surface active agents, such as dimethicone and lecithin, to improve the fill of the etchings and its transfer to the rubber off-set roller.

A range of ink colors is used, but the palette is much more limited than for the colors used for the hard capsule shells. The reason for this is that the print designs mostly consist of very narrow lines as large areas of ink are not good practice because chance of its transfer to other capsules increases. The human eye is less capable of distinguishing between colors of fine lines against another colored background and hence only basic colors tend to be used.

Print can be applied to the capsules in a number of ways, either axially or radially. The surface area that can be covered depends on the hardness of the rubber transfer rolls: the softer the role, the greater the potential coverage. The printing machines can rectify the capsules before printing so that specific information can be printed on caps and bodies: if not rectified, the print placement will be randomly assigned, if two designs are used. Advanced machines have systems that enable two different colors to be printed on a capsule.

Packaging and Storage

Empty hard capsules have to be packaged for shipment to customers unlike the soft capsules that rarely exist as an empty entity. Manufacturers pack their products into cardboard cuboid outer cartons with the capsules sealed inside an inner liner that is preferably heat sealed: the material of the latter ranges from polythene to aluminum foil laminates.[11] The choice is governed partly by the environmental conditions the packages are exposed to in transit from the shell manufacturer to the capsule filler and cost constraints. The packages are designed to maintain the moisture content of the capsules within their moisture content specification: for gelatin capsules, most manufacturers use a limit of 13.0% to 16.0% w/w. Empty capsules gain and lose water depending on the conditions to which they are exposed, and this causes a slight change in dimensions. For gelatin capsules, a simple rule-of-thumb calculation is that between 13% and 16% for every 1% change in moisture, there is a 0.5% change in dimensions. The packages as received from the manufacturer should not be opened until they are about to be used. This is particularly important for heat-sealed packs as resealing facilities are often not available at sampling points. Quality requirements can be met if the manufacturer sends separate sealed samples to the purchaser following supplier audits and approval.

The most important factors in storing empty capsule packages are to avoid extremes of temperature and humidity. The ideal conditions are between 15°C and 30°C, and care should be taken to maintain them at an even temperature. Temperature fluctuations will cause moisture movement inside a sealed container and, in the worst cases, could cause distortion and failure to separate on a filling machine. A potential problem often overlooked in warehouses is that capsule packages are comparatively light for their size and, as a result, are often stored at high levels on racking systems. In the rooves of warehouses, there are often space heaters or windows, which are heat sources that could cause localized heating inside a carton and moisture migration within the package.

HARD CAPSULE QUALITY

Capsules are produced on machines that operate 24/7, and like all such industrial processes, there will be a small proportion of defective capsules produced. Over the years, there has been a continuous improvement in the quality of capsules. This process has been mainly driven by the development of higher-speed capsule filling machines.[16] Up to the mid-1960s, the machines used were semiautomatic or manually operated. The operator had time in which to rectify capsule faults as the machine was running without having to stop it and filling was almost continuous. The introduction of automatic machines highlighted these capsule quality issues because they needed to be stopped to rectify blockages or other faults, and while this was being done, no capsules could be filled.

For systems that have defect levels at low levels, statistical sampling plans based on probability theory are used to reduce sample size to give an acceptable level of control. To make plans more specific, three types of capsule faults are defined: Major A, Major B, and Minor, which are sometimes named as Critical, Major, and Minor[17,18] (see Tables 4.1 through 4.3). Major A faults affect the capsule as a package for the final product or could cause a major filling problem; Major B faults cause problems on a filling machine; Minor faults are slight surface blemishes that make them visually imperfect but do not affect the performance of capsules as a package or cause filling machine problems. Each type of fault is assigned an acceptable quality level (AQL), which is defined in Military Standard MIL-STD-105E[18] as the maximum percent defective that for the purposes of sampling inspection can be considered satisfactory as a process average. A typical set of AQL values used by capsule manufacturers are Major A 0.010%, Major B 0.040%, and Minor 0.25%. In the past, a lot of time was spent in the visual inspection of capsules. However, it was realized that quality levels are not improved by this and that the way for the manufacturers to improve quality has

TABLE 4.1
Major A Faults

Cracked	Body or caps with many splits
Double cap	Capsule with additional cap covering body
Double dipping	Extra thick cap due to double dipping
Failure to separate	Cap and body may not separate properly
Hole	Irregular opening in cap or body
Joined in lock	Capsule in locked position
Long cap/body	Length cap or body 1 mm more than specification
Mashed	Mechanically damaged, squashed flat
Pinched	Cap or body damaged in collets, pinch > 3 mm
Short body	Length 0.4 mm less than specification
Short cap	Length 1 mm less than specification
Split	Split in wall starting from cap or body edge
Telescope	Closed capsule with protruding piece of cap or body
Thin spot (shoulder)	Thin area, may rupture when capsule filled
Trimming	Whole or piece of trimmed end cap or body inside capsule
Uncut cap/body	Untrimmed cap or body
Unjoined	Single cap or body

TABLE 4.2
Major B Faults

Damaged edge, large	Cap edge poorly trimmed, >1 mm into length
Dye speck	Colored spot of pigment, different from cap or body color
Grease	Visible spots of mold release aid on inside of capsule
Inverted end	Cap or body with end pushed inward
Long joined	Capsule not closed enough to engage prelock
Pinched (small)	Cap or body damaged in collets, pinch < 3 mm
Thin spot	Thin area cap or body wall may rupture when capsule filled
Turned edge	Folded over edge on body cut edge

TABLE 4.3
Minor Faults

Black speck	Noncontaminant black spot
Bubble	Air bubble in cap or body wall, with diameter > 0.4 mm
Chips, tails, string	Small fragments of shell, still attached to wall or free
Crimp	Collet damage, outside cap or body < 3 mm
Damaged edge (small)	Cap edge poorly trimmed, damage V shaped, < 1 mm into specification
Dent	Depression in end cap or body, < half diameter of part
Grease (light)	Small spots of mold release aid on inside of capsule
Scrape	Scratch mark on surface of cap or body
Starred end	Multiple small imperfections of ends of cap or body

been by concentrating on the parts of the process that produces them so that they could be eliminated by improving machine design and/or maintenance schedules.

To understand why faults are produced, it is necessary to understand how each is caused. The first part of the process is mold dipping and faults produced are as follows: Major A, thin spot; and Minor, bubble and speck. A thin spot can be attributed to either a poor distribution of the mold release aid on the pin or insufficient wetting agent being present, both resulting in an uneven coverage of the pin with a wet film of polymer. A bubble in the shell wall is attributed to one being present in the solution in the dip pan. The removal of air bubbles from this solution is a critical part of its manufacturing process, and when it is dispensed from the stock manufacturing tanks, it should be free of them. However, bubbles could be reintroduced during the addition of colorant solution or pigment suspension to this stock solution. All the mechanical operations by parts of the dip pan are designed to ensure that air entrapment is reduced to the bare minimum. A colored speck is most likely to occur as the result of small fragments of shell walls generated during the trimming process getting into the dipping area. The next part of the process is film drying and faults caused are as follows: Major A, split; and Minor, starred end. A split in a shell starts from the cut edge of the cap or body and spreads away from this point. It is caused by uneven drying or an uneven film thickness at that point. A starred end is produced when there is an excessive amount of gelled solution on the end of the pin. When the mold pins emerge from the drying kilns, they pass to the automatic section. The first operation is removal of dried films from the mold pin and faults caused are as follows: Major A, hole, caused by the stripper jaws touching the shell as it moves forward to strip it off and is attributed to mechanical problems or a poor machine setup. The second operation is the transfer of shells to the split leaf collets and faults caused are as follows: Major A, short body, large pinch > 3 mm; and Major B, minor pinch < 3 mm. A short body is caused by insufficient entry into the collet and pinches are caused by a section of the film becoming trapped in between the leaves of the collet as it is closed. This could be attributed to a drying problem, that is, a wetter area of the shell or a mechanical problem with the collet. The third operation is the cutting of the dried films to the correct length and faults caused are as follows: Major A, short body, uncut body, uncut cap; and Major B, short cap, long cap, long body, damaged edge (cap). The short cap and body are caused by insufficient penetration of the dried film into the collet for the position of the knife, the long cap and body are caused by a missing knife or a broken knife, and the damaged edge (cap) is caused by a blunt knife. The fourth operation involves joining of the two parts together and the faults caused are as follows: Major A, bad join (telescope), cracked, mashed, trimming; Major B, inverted end; and Minor, dent. The first three Major A faults are caused by mechanical problems in the joining block, the first by a misalignment of the cap and body parts and the other two by capsule parts being incorrectly transferred and the push rods distorting their shapes or breaking pieces off. The trimming inside a capsule happens if there is a problem with the extraction system to remove them or with the cutting operation and it becomes trapped in the body. Major B and Minor faults are lesser problems of the previous explanation where shells are unable to move sufficiently in the joining block and their end is dented. After being ejected from the joining block, the capsules pass along a moving belt, exit from the machine and pass through inspection systems and printing machines, and are packed for transport. During this process, faults caused are as follows: Major B, unjoined and double cap; both of these are symptoms of the same problem, with the cap separating from the body because they were joined to longer than their correct unclosed length in the joining block, and if this loose cap fits over the body of another complete capsule, a "double cap" is produced.

Modern Hard Capsule Manufacturing Machines

There are currently few specialist manufacturers who make the associated equipment used in hard capsule manufacture or supply the machinery, for example, Technophar Equipment and Services Ltd, part of the Qualicaps group (www.technophar.com), in Canada and Safrroys Machines Pvt Ltd (www.safrroys.com) in India.

The limitations to increasing the speed of output of the process are twofold. First, there are the mechanical problems of moving sets of pin bars around the machine and the precise coordination of this with the other mechanical activities such as cutting the dried films and assembling the two parts. Second, limitations are attributed to the properties of the polymers used. Drying is a significant part of the process, and typically in other fields of manufacture, to reduce drying times, higher air temperatures are used. This cannot be used in this case because at the start of the process, higher temperatures will cause the films to revert to the sol state and move out of shape and the mold pins have to be back to their dipping temperature when they have completed the cycle around the machine. There is also a limitation to the speed of drying because if it is too rapid, there will be case hardening of the surface of the films that would slow the drying process.

Mechanical problems have been overcome by changing the methods of moving bars through the drying kilns from mechanical pushers to hydraulic systems controlled by servo-motors, which can be better controlled and prevent the bars rising up over the sets in front causing a jam. As the machine speed increases, the next part of the process to cause a bottleneck is the automatic head where the shells are stripped from the mold pins and trimmed to the correct length. This has been solved by installing two automatic heads on a machine to cope with the extra throughput of pin bars.

The limitation of the maximum speed at which capsules can be dried has been solved by changing the machine design by increasing the lengths of the drying kilns and hence the overall length of the machine. This increases the passage time of the molds through the kilns, allowing the correct drying conditions to be maintained.

The original machine design of Colton relied on the use of cams to perform certain movements of the pin bars, such as during dipping or the spinning of the bars after this when they are transferred to the upper deck of the machine. Cams work well but are inflexible, because if changes are required, new cams need to be machined, which is a time-consuming process. Technophar has solved this by using servo-motors with computer control: these enable the process to be easily changed to accommodate any variations in material properties.

GELATIN ALTERNATIVES FOR HARD CAPSULE MANUFACTURE

Gelatin has been the material of choice since it was first mentioned in an addition to Lehuby's patent in 1848. However, since that time, there has been a search for an alternative material for both types of capsule, prompted first by the need to avoid existing patents, and second to find a material that had more reproducible properties than gelatin made from natural materials and more recently to improve on the pharmaceutical properties of gelatin to meet current demands. Gelatin alternatives must possess similar properties, must be widely acceptable for use in foods and medicines, must gel on a mold pin to film caused by a temperature change to enable the same manufacturing machinery to be used with minor modifications, should be stable and nonreactive, and must have similar *in vivo* release properties. A variety of substances have been used: hypromellose, methyl cellulose, and pullulan.

Cellulose compounds have been used the most and solutions of these do not gel when they are cooled. To convert them into a gelling system, two methods have been proposed, either by including network-forming additives in the polymer solution or by modifying the process to use different temperature conditions to form a film by thermal gelling of the solution.

Eli Lilly & Co. was the first large-scale manufacturer of a non-gelatin hard capsule in the early 1950s.[19] They utilized a property of cellulose solutions, the viscosity of which increases as the temperature rises (so-called thermal gelling). They reversed the conditions used for the standard process. Hot mold pins at c. 65°C were dipped into methyl cellulose (low viscosity grade) solutions at temperatures <20°C. Film formed rapidly on the pins, which were then transferred to drying kilns; in the first section, the temperature was 40°C and progressively rose to 60°C. The air was heated by infrared lamps and the transit time was about 50 min. The capsules were allowed to cool to ambient conditions before they were stripped from the pins. They were in widespread use for several years, sufficiently long enough for US Federal Specification 285A[20] to introduce a test to distinguish them from gelatin capsules: "Water resistance," in which a capsule should show no signs of disintegration when immersed in purified water at 25°C ± 1°C for 15 min. Under these conditions, only methyl cellulose capsules will dissolve, readily distinguishing them from gelatin ones. These capsules were withdrawn from use later in the 1950s after *in vivo* tests showed that capsules did not dissolve in the stomach if a patient was suffering from hypochlorhydria (lack of acid).

From the late 1980s onward, most of the work has centered on the use of hypromellose, which is widely used by the pharmaceutical industry for tablet coating and formulating tablets with prolonged-release properties. The first company to propose a successful solution was Japan Elanco (Qualicaps), which started a study in the late 1980s to try and produce hard capsules that did not have the same drawbacks as gelatin ones, namely, their high moisture content and brittleness when dried.[21] They used hypromellose and converted it into a gelling system by the addition of carrageenan, which is a network former, and potassium chloride, which is a network promoter.[22,23] The capsules were made on standard machines and were demonstrated to be less brittle than gelatin ones when stored at low humidities. The temperature of the solution at dipping was 50°C to 52°C and they commented that the speed of gelling was slower than that for gelatin. The properties of the capsules were improved by using blends of lower-viscosity hypromellose, and the disintegration time was satisfactory even in the presence of calcium ions, which form a strong network with carrageenan.[24] In a further improvement, they modified the method of dissolving hypromellose.[25] It was dispersed it in hot water at 65° to 80°C and then allowed to cool to room temperature to allow it to dissolve. The solution is then reheated to bring it to the machine dipping temperature. Solutions of carrageenan and potassium chloride were added to it either at the start of warming or when the solution has reached the correct operating temperature. This procedure improves the gelling properties of solutions, resulting in improved control of capsule formation.

Capsugel proposed an alternative gelling for hypromellose capsule production. They proposed the use of various gums as a gelling agent, gellan being the preferred one, and a sequestering agent such as ethylenediaminetetraacetic acid or citric acid and their salts as the gel promoter.[26] This solution was used in the standard hard capsule manufacturing process. In further patents, they improved the process by using a heating and cooling method for the preparation of the hypromellose solutions before dipping.[27] Hypromellose powder and solutions of the various additives were added to water at 70°C; this was stirred to mix, with the speed of the mixer reduced to allow air bubbles to be removed, and then allowed to cool to 47°C with constant mixing. This process resulted in a solution with the correct viscosity for mold pin dipping in the temperature range of 43° to 48°. If the solutions were not stirred during cooling, the solution viscosity would be too high to form capsule shells of the correct dimensions.

G.S. Technologies applied the hot mold dipping technique for the production of hypromellose capsules and were granted patents for modifications to a standard Colton-type machine.[28,29] They were able to realize the following: a method to heat pin bars to different initial temperatures to compensate for the difference in time between leaving drying kilns and entering the automatic section before dipping; a method to heat pins after dipping to aid film formation; a method to dry wet films on pins by first using humid air to slow the rate of drying and then less humid air to dry them down in closed kilns to avoid air escaping in to the machine room; a method of heating mold pins to dry films from the inside to the outside; and a modification of the machine to increase space around the dip pan to allow for a pin reheating station using isolated heating elements below the base of the pin bars. They commented in their first patent that the capsule walls were less strong than gelatin and stripping them from the mold pins was difficult. To overcome this, they increased the wall thickness of the caps and bodies to make them stronger and reduced the mold pin diameters to make shells with the same external dimensions as gelatin ones.[28] To remove the films from the mold pins, they modified the stripper mechanism to grip around the shell away from the piece to be cut off and the jaws themselves were provided with small studs to increase grip. These capsules were called Vegicaps and marketed for filling with nutraceutical products. Their literature commented that they were only suitable for running on semiautomatic machines because their dimensional control was not as good as conventional capsule shells.

Capsugel further developed the hot mold process to make pharmaceutical quality capsules, Vcaps Plus.[30] Solutions of hypromellose, USP type 2906 or 2910, were prepared by dispersing 17% to 23% w/w in water at >70°C, reducing stirrer speed to allow the removal of bubbles and then cooling it to <15°C and then stirring to dissolve. Various additives that could be added at the start or at the end of this preparation process were listed. The preferable concentrations of these were 0.01% to 3.0% w/w of a plasticizer such as glycerine or propylene glycol and 0.01% to 0.5% w/w of a preservative or flavoring agent. For use, the solution was heated to between 2°C and 6°C below its gelling temperature of approximately 34°C. The standard mold pins before dipping were heated, and their temperature was dependent on the capsule size; the smaller the size, the higher the temperature: for size 4, 80°C to 90°C, and for size 00, 70°C to 80°C. The drying process was carried out in two steps. First, the wet films were exposed to temperature between 60°C and 85°C and an RH of 20% to 60% for about 2 to 4 min and then 35°C to 55°C for 30 to 60 min. During this process, the films were dried from a moisture content of c. 80% to 7% w/w.

Pullulan is the other gelatin substitute that has been used for marketed hard capsules, originally named[31] NPcaps and afterward renamed Plantcaps by Capsugel.[32] Pullulan is made by fermentation of tapioca by the polymorphic fungus, *Aureobasidium pullulans*.[33] It has GRAS status and has been widely used in Japan since the 1980s. It has no setting properties, and to manufacture hard capsules, solutions require additives. The material recommended for use was desalted pullulan (Japanese pharmaceuticals excipient grade).[34] The preferred hydrocolloid gelling agents were kappa-carrageenan or gellan gum at a concentration of 0.03% to 1%.[35] These require the addition of a cation, and the preferred salt was potassium chloride at a concentration of 1.32%; in addition, the patent gave examples using 0.25% potassium acetate. A sequestering agent, such as ethylenediaminetetraacetic acid or citric acid and their salts, was recommended if gellan gum was used to improve the solubility of the resulting capsules. To aid the manual handling of the capsules and their performance on filling machines, a surfactant, such as sodium lauryl sulfate or sorbitan oleate, was recommended to improve their surface properties: to delay the rapid remoisturizing of the capsules when handled, which makes the capsules feel tacky, and by providing a temporary water-repellant surface to reduce the sliding friction on filling machines.[36]

Alternative Methods of Manufacture

The only manufacturing process used for hard capsules that does not rely on mold pins has been injection molding.[35,37] For this process to work, a different type of raw material had to be used because it had to have suitable thermoplastic properties. The process was developed in order to reduce the water content of the starting materials, to reduce the cost by avoiding the drying step, to avoid problems of microbial contamination, and to produce capsule with precise dimensions. Material is fed from a hopper into a tube where it is heated under pressure, gradually melting as it is transferred through the tube by a reciprocating auger, which has an increasing diameter along its length. It is then injected under high pressure, 70–200 MPa, and temperature, 120° to 180°C, into a mold, which is below the glass transition or melting temperature of the polymer. The mold is allowed to cool and the molded part is ejected. Initially, gelatin and starch were used as they have similar water absorption isotherms. To produce a capsule part with sufficient strength, the wall thickness was 0.4 mm and the resulting starch capsules, Capill, had the required pharmaceutical properties for filling, packing, and dissolution.

The other significant difference from capsules produced by dipping is that the two pieces have an entirely different shape because they cannot be joined together by fitting one inside the other. The body has a standard capsule shape. It is a cylinder with a hemispherical end that has a dimple in the bottom because of the molding process. The same diameter body is made for each capsule size and the difference between them is achieved by making them of different lengths: size 4 to size 0 varied from 6.66 mm to 17.70 mm. The cap is hemispherical in shape, with a central dimple like the body. The body and the cap have a thinner wall at the open end with an external groove on the body and an internal one on the cap. The cap acts as a lid to cover the body's open end, and after filling, they are sealed together by spraying an ethanol–water mixture on the inside rim of the cap before it is placed on the body. When dried, this forms a seal strong enough to hold the parts together.

Filling machines need to be adapted to handle these capsules because the two parts are packaged separately. Standard hard capsules are always supplied to the user pre-joined and never as separate entities. It is because when polymer capsule shells lose moisture after manufacture, there is a small change in their dimensions, and thus, when the filling machine attempts to rejoin them, there is the potential for significant problems. Their shells are flexible, and in a hopper, when in motion, there would be a tendency for halves to fit together. The injection-molded capsules are more rigid because of their thicker wall and the interlocking of parts does not occur. Bosch (Minneapolis, MN, USA) adapted a production-scale capsule filling machine, the GKF 400C, to handle these capsules. There were two separate hoppers, one for caps and one for bodies. The bodies were filled as normal into the machine bushings and passed under the filling head. The caps were rectified and guided past the sealing head where the liquid was sprayed into them immediately before it was placed on top of the filled body. This system worked well with pellets and granules but not so well with powders because if any material was present on the closure ridge of the body, then the seal was poor. Automatic capsule filling machines form soft powder plugs, at very low forces, and there will always be loose powder transferred from the dosing mechanism into the capsule.

Capsugel transferred this business to West Pharmaceutical Services in the late 1990s, which used it for preparing specialized capsule "formulations"[38]: it is no longer listed on their website. Starch capsules as described above were included in Chapter 1151 of the USP 29.[39]

SOFT CAPSULES

EARLY DEVELOPMENT OF PROCESS AND MACHINES

The first gelatin capsule described in the patent of Mothes and Dublanc in 1834 was oval in shape with a hole at one end for filling liquids, which was then sealed with a drop of gelatin solution.[1] They looked like a standard oval soft capsule, but the shells were hard and rigid like a two-piece capsule as their walls were made of gelatin, to which a variety of other materials were added such as gum, honey, and sugar. The dipping molds used were made from a variety of materials; initially, fine leather filled with mercury, but soon replaced by oval metal shapes mounted on rods. The spread in the popularity of one-piece capsules was rapid, and within a decade, they were being used in most European countries and in North America. The increased demand stimulated process improvements: the most successful was the plate and pressure method. Matching plates were made with sets of cavities in the shape of a half-capsule: thin sheets of gelatin were laid on top of the plates, which took up their form: liquids were filled into the cavities in the bottom plate, the top plate was then placed on top, and the pair passed through a press to stamp out the capsules. These capsules were very regular in shape compared to the previous manufacture and were called "perles." In 1846, Mothes and his new partner, Lamouroux, were granted a patent for a "capsulateur mecanique." This was a rotary-die device with the same format as modern soft capsule machines. Two sheets of gelatin were fed over a pair of rotating cylinders and then guided through a lower set on which the shapes of the capsules were indented. The system was not taken up, probably because the gelatin films used were not flexible when dry enough to handle. In 1850, Mothes applied for another patent using a mold-dipping process. The patent that converted these hard one-piece shells into soft gelatin capsules was granted in 1875 to M. Taetz who proposed the addition of glycerol to make "an elastic capsule … easier to swallow medicines."[1] The formulation for his shell was gelatin 1 part, glycerol 1½ parts and water 2½ parts. In the United States, in the 1890s, there was large-scale manufacture of soft capsules using the mold-dipping technique. A machine was developed that had 200 to 250 olive-shaped molds set onto metal plates.[11] The molds were dipped, moved to a cutter to remove the waste, and then transferred automatically back to the start where they were cleaned, stripped from the molds, and tipped into bins. During this process, the shells were dried. The process that brought the capsules into the modern era was the rotary-die process devised by Robert P. Scherer, a German-American, and patented in 1934[40] (see Figure 4.6). Ribbons of molten gelatin with a controlled thickness were cast onto webs and transferred to the filling head. Here, the two sheets were guided between two counter-rotating die rolls with a single line of matching half-cavities machined in their surfaces: these had outer circular flanges around the cavities to aid sealing and each had an internal element, a plug, controlled by a cam to move it to aid removal of the filled capsules. Between the die rolls was placed an injecting block that pumped the fill liquid between the sheets just before sealing, thus avoiding trapping air within the shell. When operated by a continuous three-shift system, this machine could manufacture and fill 1,250,000 capsules in 24 h.[41] Scherer obtained two further patents in the early 1940s for improvements to his machine design.[42,43] The first described improvements to a machine to prevent leakage of fill material during filling and to exclude air from entering into the capsule during sealing[42] (see Figure 4.7). Gelatin bands were formed on rotating drums and transferred to the filling head via a series of three rollers that applied oil to both of their surfaces. The bands were held firmly in place on the die rolls and kept there by the filler head, which had a mechanism to allow it to float freely to accommodate variations in gelatin band thickness and maintain contact. The filling head had arcuate faces to match the shape of the die rolls. These had plurality of cavities spaced in such a way as to minimize the area between them into which the gelatin band could sink. In each cavity, there was a plunger that was able to reciprocate up and down by gravity. The plungers were linked in groups by a rod to ensure that they all moved together to ensure cleaning of the cavity between each capsule formation. The die cavities had ledges with a flange around each one, which were wide and flat, so that when they came together, the capsules were sealed and cut from the band. The second described further developments to improve the shape, uniformity, and strength of sealed capsules, and to increase the output by producing more per unit area of gelatin ribbon[43] (see Figures 4.8 and 4.9). The cavities on the die rolls were arranged in parallel rows, each one staggered with respect to the other and with a minimal space between them: in addition, there was a small raised area between each set of cavities to further ensure minimal sagging of the gelatin band in these spaces. Each cavity had a flange around it, and these were more complex than the previous patent; each had a cutting and a pressure sealing feature. The ledges were stepped at various levels around their length. The higher face acted as a cutting edge and the lower face acted as a pressure seal without cutting the film, and their geometry varied around the cavity. The ledges were formed eccentric to the cavities; on one side, it was spaced at a maximum distance from the cavity rim, and on the other side, it was closer to the rim. These produce two different types of seal on each capsule: a leading edge and a trailing edge one. This combination ensured that the edges of gelatin bands around the cavities were securely held and the pressure for sealing was substantially higher before cutting. This ensures no loss of the fill liquid or any air entering the shell. The filling head has a feeding tube in its outlet made of a readily deformable substance with an outlet shaped as a slit. The fill liquid is injected into the heart of the capsule as it is formed. The capsule shell is closed as the cavities come into contact and liquid is being pumped in.

In 1947, Scherer's plant in Detroit was producing about 2.5 billion capsules a year.[41] This process was only suitable for the filling of liquids and was used mainly for fish oils. He maintained a monopoly on the manufacture of rotary die machines until the early 1960s when other companies started making their own machines. One of the first was P. Leiner & Sons Ltd, a gelatin company in the United Kingdom, which started manufacturing with machines of their own design.

All the soft capsules described have a visible seal around the longitudinal axis and are referred to as "seamed capsules." R.P. Scherer was the first to patent a method for making a seamless capsule with no visible seal on their surface.[44] This process involved making droplets with a core of fill material with an outer shell of gelatin and dropping them into a column of liquid while they were still plastic. The process relied on a balance between the specific gravities (Sp. Gr.) of the liquid,

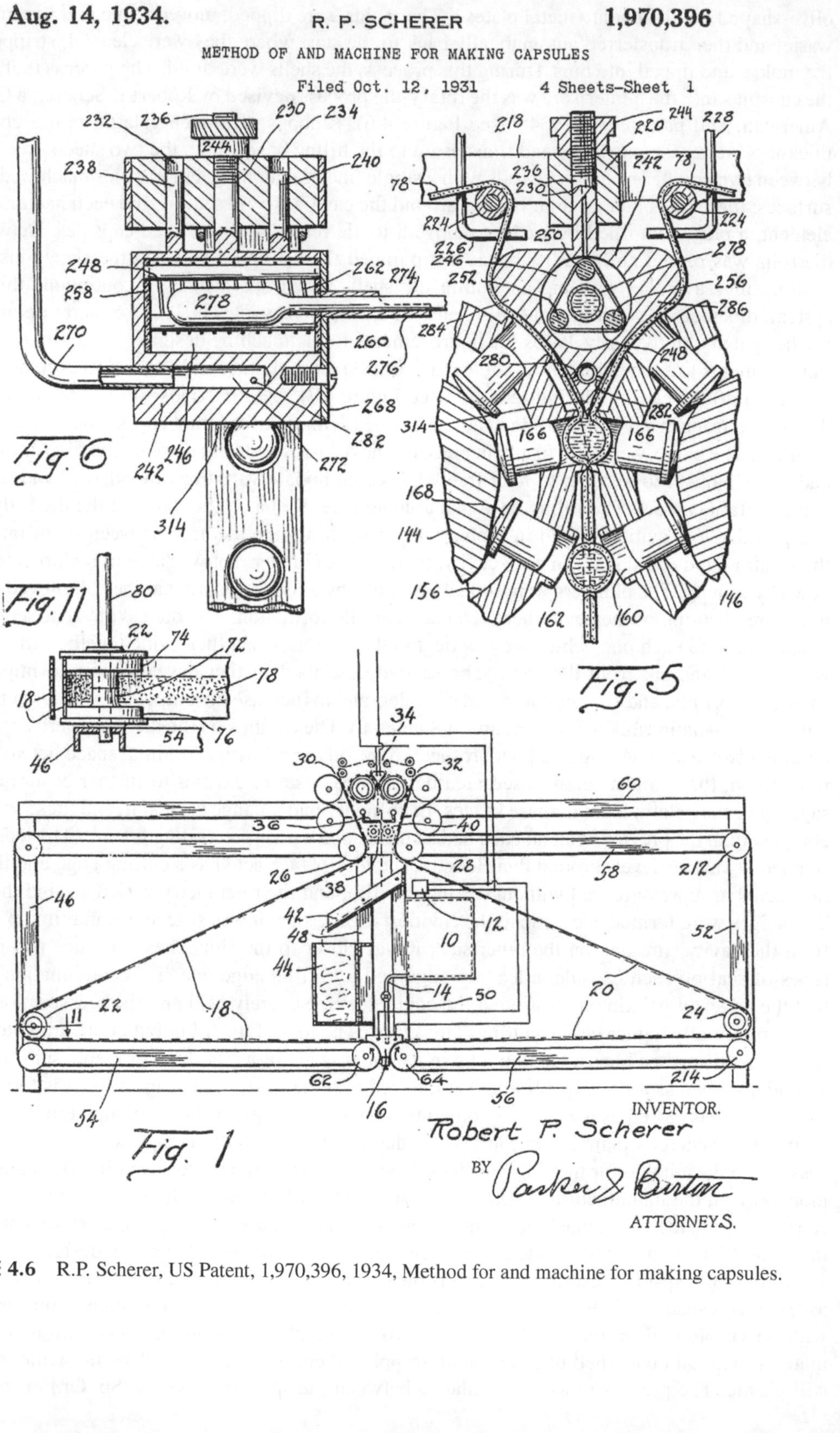

Aug. 14, 1934.   R. P. SCHERER   1,970,396

METHOD OF AND MACHINE FOR MAKING CAPSULES

Filed Oct. 12, 1931   4 Sheets—Sheet 1

FIGURE 4.6 R.P. Scherer, US Patent, 1,970,396, 1934, Method for and machine for making capsules.

June 30, 1942.   R. P. SCHERER   2,288,327
APPARATUS FOR FORMING AND FILLING CAPSULES
Original Filed Oct. 8, 1935   3 Sheets-Sheet 1

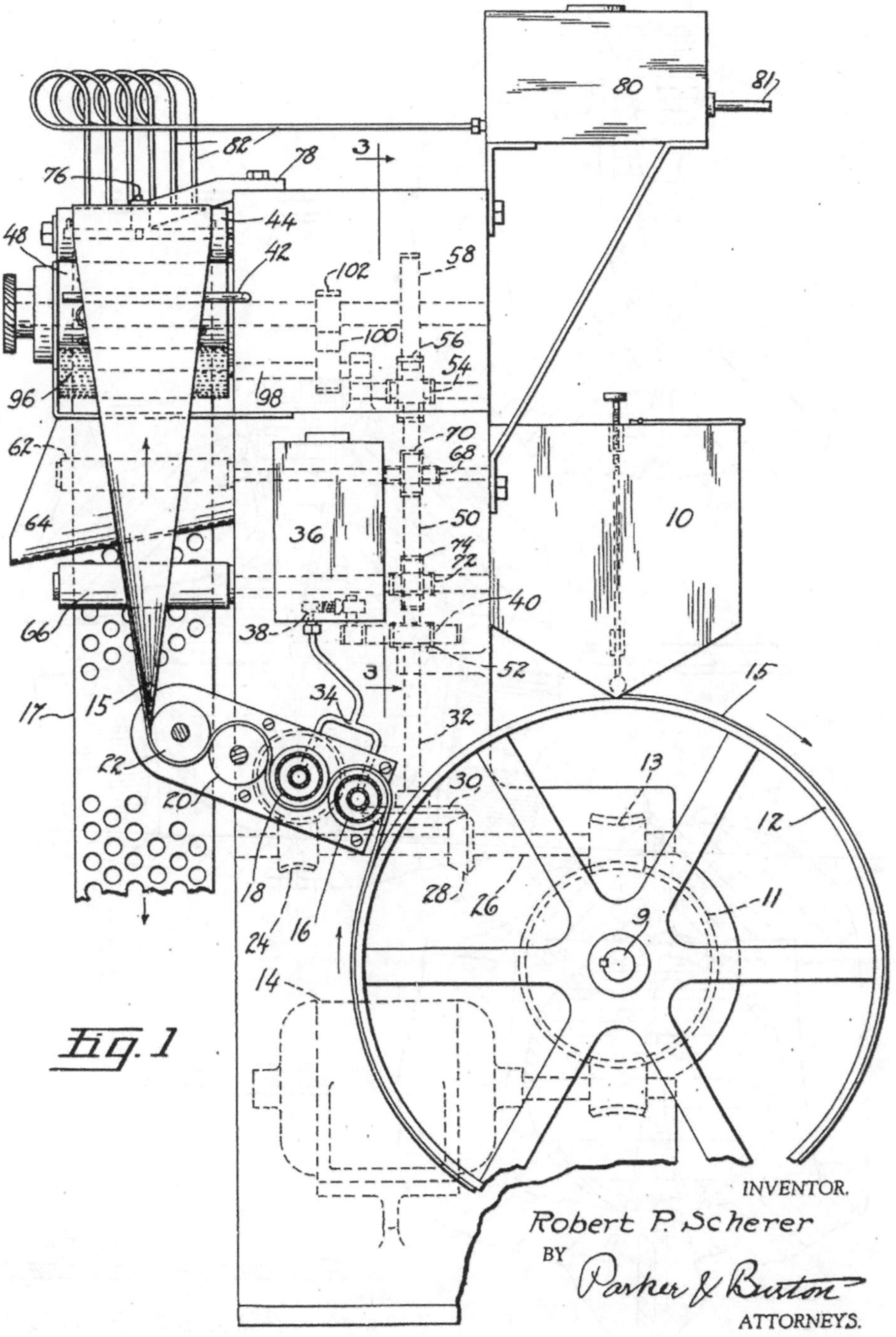

Fig. 1

INVENTOR.
Robert P. Scherer
BY
Parker & Burton
ATTORNEYS.

FIGURE 4.7   R.P. Scherer, US Patent, 2,288,327, 1942, Apparatus for forming and filling capsules.

May 11, 1943.   R. P. SCHERER   2,318,718

METHOD AND APPARATUS OF FABRICATING FILLED CAPSULES

Filed Dec. 5, 1939   4 Sheets-Sheet 3

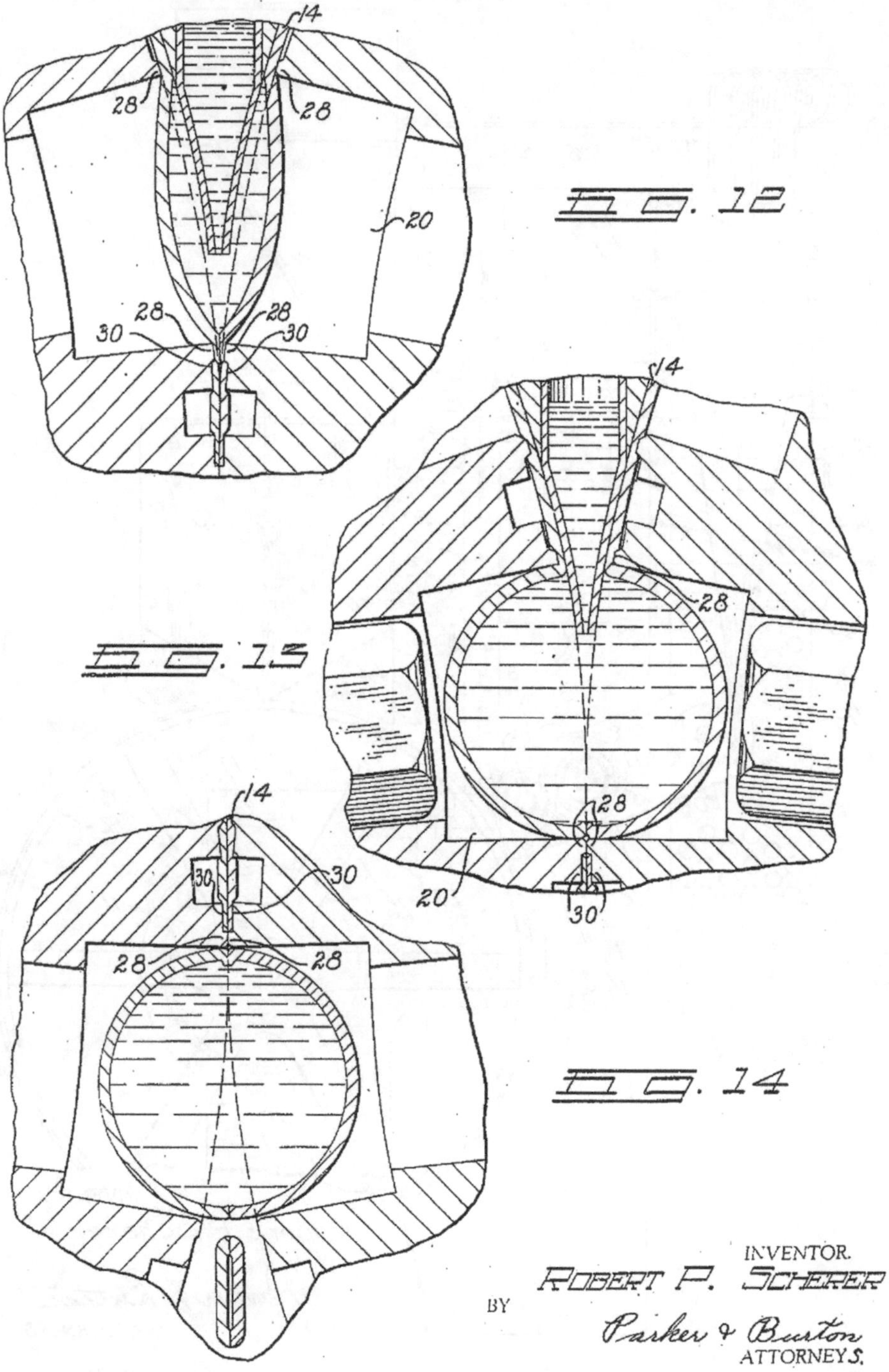

FIGURE 4.8   R.P. Scherer, US Patent 2,318,718, 1943, Method and apparatus of fabricating filled capsules.

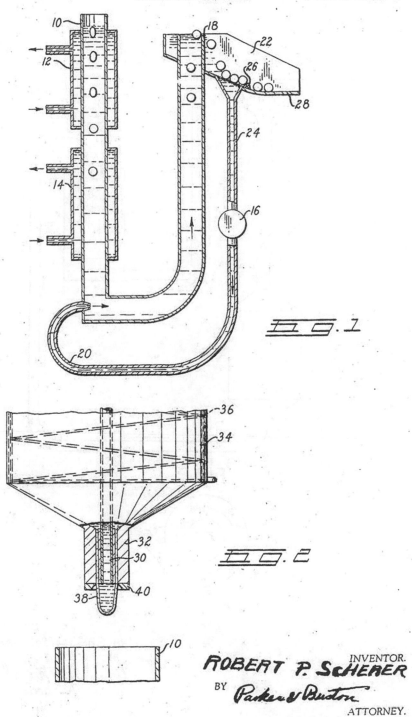

FIGURE 4.9   R.P. Scherer, US Patent 2,332,671, 1943, Fabricating of filled sealed capsules.

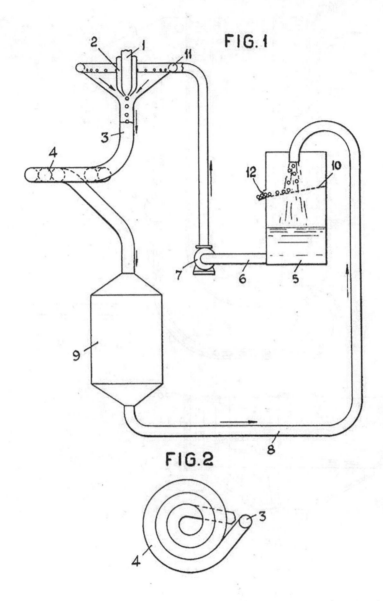

April 12, 1960   J. C. JANSEN   2,932,061

METHOD AND APPARATUS FOR PRODUCING SEAMLESS CAPSULES

Filed June 17, 1957

FIG. 1

FIG. 2

INVENTOR.

Jan Christoffel Jansen

BY

Attorneys

FIGURE 4.10   J.C. Jansen (Globex International), US Patent, 2,932,061, Method and apparatus for producing seamless capsules.

the shell wall material, and the fill and the differences in values needed to be small. Thus, in a column of liquid of a manageable height, the filled capsules would sink at a rate slow enough to allow the filled capsule by its surface tension to form a wall with a uniform thickness and a spherical shape. The difference in the Sp. Gr. between water (1.0) and gelatin (1.15) would require additions as well as the fill to satisfy this requirement. Examples were given of adding oils to gelatin to reduce its Sp. Gr. and low- and high-density powders to the fill. The patent did not disclose how the gelatin fill drops were formed. The first patent for a viable seamless capsule was awarded in 1957 to Globex International Ltd, UK[45] (see Figure 4.10). Filled capsules were formed by pumping through concentric nozzles the fill and shell wall materials into a cooling liquid in a pulsed stream in such a way that drops formed with a core of fill surrounded by an enveloping wall and the liquid temperature was low enough to produce a rapid gelling of the shell material. The Sp. Gr. of the drops is slightly higher than that of the cooling liquid such that the capsules slowly sink. For the process to work, it needs the correct interfacial tension between the cooling fluid and the wall material and the wall material and the fill. To produce capsules with the correct shape, they are guided to roll along the wall of the cooling column so that they are rotated end over end, thus producing a spherical shape. This company was selling machines based on this principle after 2000.[46] The chief application for this process has been for filling cosmetic products such as bath oils. This makes the process simpler because the oils form droplets more readily and the machines have a less complicated structure.[47]

MANUFACTURE OF SOFT GELATIN CAPSULES

Preparation of Gelatin Manufacturing Solutions and Fill Formulations

The requirement for a soft capsule is that the films produced during the process must have sufficient mechanical strength and elasticity when wet to be handled without being damaged. The gelatin blends used for this purpose have different characteristics from those used for hard capsules.[47–49] They are typically blends of high-Bloom (180–210) and low-Bloom (160–175) materials from a variety of types: limed bone, hide, acid bone, and pigskin. The use of fish gelatin has also been reported.[48,49] The high-Bloom gelatins contribute to the mechanical strength of the shell wall and the lower-Bloom ones allow for the ready melting of the films when the capsules are sealed.[47,49] For non-pharmaceutical uses, succinylated gelatins are used because they block reactions with traces of aldehydes found in natural product extracts, avoiding shell hardening, which would otherwise occur.[47] The viscosity of the gelatin solution is used to control the whole process and needs to be within specified limits: the viscosity of a 6.66% solution at 60°C should be between 2.8 and 4.5 mPa s. There is a practical limit on the particle size of the gelatin that must be small enough so that they can be dissolved readily with a limit on the amount below 500 μm. This is because the rate of addition to the reactor vessels is critical as it causes problems during processing (i.e., formation of lumps and foaming).

The process for preparing the gelatin solution and the fill formulation results in liquid masses that are bubble free.[50,51] The shell mixture is made by dissolving the gelatin in water at 80°C in a stainless steel pressure vessel with a water jacket and a built-in stirrer. When the gelatin is dissolved, the other ingredients are added. Plasticizers are chosen in relation to the properties of fill formulation (e.g., its hygroscopicity) and the required shell properties. For standard materials, glycerol is the most widely used: it is nonvolatile, has high plasticizer efficiency, and is a humectant (prevents capsules from drying out). It has a drawback as it is a good solvent for some actives. Various grades of sorbitol are used, especially those with a high content of sorbitans.[51] These hold moisture in the shell and are used with hygroscopic formulations, for example, those based on polyethylene glycol 400. Other additives (colorants, soluble dyes, pigments, flavors, and preservatives) are used. After these have been mixed, a vacuum is applied to the vessel to deaerate the solution, which is then transferred to jacketed kettles and stored for 24–28 h before transfer to the capsule manufacturing machines.

Manufacture of Seamed Soft Gelatin Capsules with Liquid Products

The modern manufacturing machines can either be fixed units requiring static fittings plumbed to exterior services or stand-alone units that can be moved easily from one position to another (see Figure 4.11). This shows two stand-alone machines: the one on the left-hand side is used to prepare the gelatin solution and the one on the right-hand is a dual-function machine producing the capsules that are transferred directly to the rotary drier at its side. The machines are controlled through an Allan Bradley Programmable Logic Controller using a touch screen to control the production and process parameters.

The first stage in the process is the formation of the gelatin ribbons.[51,52] Prepared hot gelatin solutions are stored in heated tanks kept at 58°C to 60°C. From there, they are fed via a ball valve outlet into a spreader box (see Figure 4.12). This fits over a revolving stainless steel drum. This box is held by an articulated bracket that allows it to "float" on the drums. Gelatin is fed onto the revolving casting drums where it gels to forms a ribbon (see Figure 4.13). The temperature of the drums is controlled either by circulating chilled water through them or by using an air-blower system, which uses filtered room air that is chilled using a coil system. At start-up, the casting drums are at 17°C to 22°C to ensure good ribbon formation. During the running of a lot, the temperature may be increased to improve performance. The thickness of the cast film is controlled by the position of a gate on the spreader box. The gap between it and the drum can be set to produce a ribbon thickness of between 0.63 and 1.15 mm. A sensor in the spreader box monitors the gelatin solution level and sends a signal to control the amount passing through the ball valve on the gelatin storage tank. There are two casting drums on a single rotating shaft, thus ensuring that the gelatin ribbons are formed at the same speed (see Figure 4.11).

When the drum has almost completed a full revolution, the ribbon is peeled from its surface and guided between the oil rolls onto the ribbon roller with its guiding system. The oil roll assembly consists of two units on each side of the machine. Their function is to lubricate each surface of the ribbon with a lubricating liquid, typically mineral oil: the lower one treats the surface that comes into contact with the casting drum, which forms the inner surface of the capsule, and the other lubricates the outer surface of the capsule. The ribbons are guided to the space between the die rolls and then through a divider into the mangle rolls that help to control the rate at which the ribbon

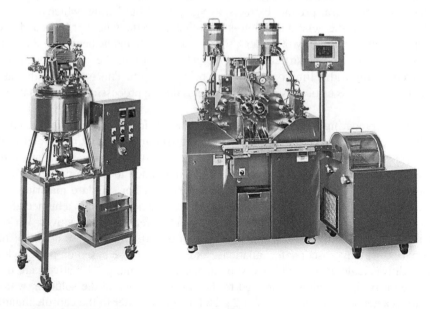

FIGURE 4.11   Technophar SGM610, stand-alone units. (Left) Gelatin solution manufacturing vessel. (Right) Capsule manufacturing machine connected to a rotary drier.

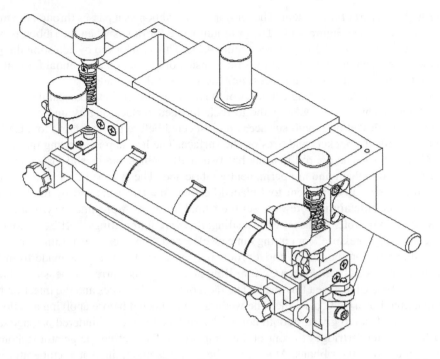

FIGURE 4.12   Technophar SGM610 machine, diagram of spreader box, which controls thickness of the gelatin ribbons.

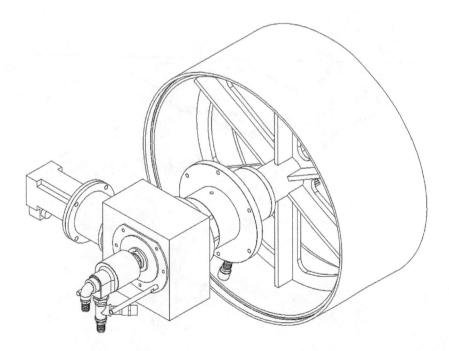

FIGURE 4.13   Technophar SGM610 machine, diagram of casting drum.

passes through this part of the system. The tension on the ribbon as it passes through the machine is a critical adjustment (see Figure 4.14). The optimum value for this is when the ribbon is peeled off the casting drum in a vertical position (see Figure 4.15). This is achieved by adjusting the gear ratio between the drums and the die rolls. The correct tension of the ribbon is essential for making good capsules as it influences the sealing process and the shape of the capsules.

The die rolls are made by cutting cylinders of the required dimension from stainless steel blanks. These are then machined on a CNC lathe to their finished surface quality and dimensions. The locating holes are drilled onto both surfaces and inspected before they progress to a CNC milling machine that forms the pockets and tires on the surface. The last step is grinding the rolls to their final outside diameter. The die roll housing has two shafts, which can be slid forward to allow the dies to be attached to them and are permanently lubricated. The attached dies are set to their correct position by using an alignment tool placed between the two rolls and by the loosening and tightening of a set of retaining screws to set their final position. A pneumatic system controls the pressure applied to the rolls to ensure good sealing: there are four settings: "off"; "inactive," that is, not connected; "high pressure" for cutting out capsules; and "low pressure" for machine setup with ribbons passing between the rolls without producing capsules. The wedge is made from brass cut from a material blank and milled on a CNC milling machine to the correct dimensions. The wedge, if required, is subjected to a heat treatment. The radii of the wedge faces and the injection holes and slots are machined on a CNC machine. The wedges are inspected before applying a Teflon coating to the required surfaces to give a smooth non-sticky surface to give unhindered passage to the ribbons and have heater cartridges to control the temperature for heating the gelatin ribbons as they come into contact with the ribbons. At start-up, the wedge is maintained at a temperature of 35°C, which is just below the liquefaction temperature of the ribbon, and this may be raised during the filling process. The lower surface of the block is radiused to match the contour of the die rolls and to take into account the thickness of the gelatin ribbon. The wedge block and die rolls need to be

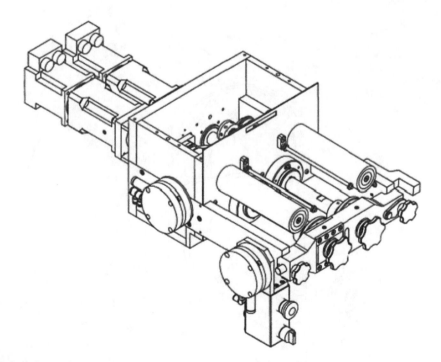

FIGURE 4.14   Technophar SGM610 machine, die roll housing and die roll pressure system.

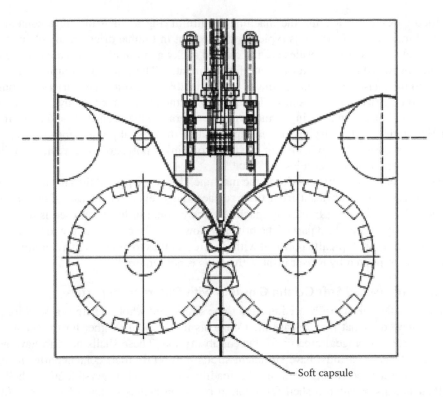

Soft capsule

FIGURE 4.15 Technophar SGM610 machine, diagram of front of machine showing how gelatin ribbon passes from the casting drum to the die.

set in a position so that the die cavities come into line at the correct moment for filling and sealing. This is achieved by lining up timing marks on the die rolls and wedge. The wedge block directs fill material though openings at its crest into the cavities formed as the ribbons are brought together by the die rolls. There are two types of injection, from the bottom or side of the wedge. The pressure from the liquid fill forces the gelatin ribbon to take up the shape of the die roll cavities.

The medicine hopper, which contains the liquid formulation to be filled, is positioned above the wedge block. At its base is a three-way valve that controls the injection process. In the operating position, the valve is open and material flows to the medicine pump via a shut-off valve into the wedge. When filling is stopped, the material passes through the three-way valve back into the hopper. The medicine pump measures the material with a positive displacement piston system and delivers it to the wedge for encapsulation. The pump is capable of delivering a wide range of fill volumes (weights) achieved by using different sizes of pistons, also known as plungers. For successful filling, the die roll speed, the piston speed, and the opening and closing of the supply valve need to be synchronized.

When the ribbon with the filled capsules comes out of the die rolls, it passes into the divider section. This removes any filled capsules still attached to the die rolls with a pair of rubber stripper brushes. Capsules still attached to the ribbon are dislodged by the stripper rollers. Filled capsules fall onto two chutes that guide them onto a conveyor belt that discharges them from the machine. The ribbon, now full of holes where the capsules were formed, is known as the "net" and passes into the mangle rolls assembly. The mangle rolls have surfaces with machined grooves that grip the net and pull it down so that it falls into a net container. The rollers apply a pressure to the net by means of spring-loading. When full, the container is removed, and the net is discarded if used with pharmaceuticals and reworked if used in the production of paint balls.

The filled capsules on leaving the machine require drying as their moisture content is about 40%.[53] The initial stage of drying is typically carried out in tumble driers, available in a range of sizes. The "wet" soft gelatin capsules are flaccid and sticky and tumble dryers are critical to maintain capsule shape and avoid the formation of agglomerates. The driers use warm air at controlled humidity, and the moisture content is reduced to 19% to 20%. The time in the driers is about 2 to 4 h and depends on the size of the capsules. The capsules are then transferred to trays, which are loaded onto gantries, and placed in a drying tunnel with a temperature between 20°C and 21°C and an RH between 19% and 20%. The drying time is dependent on the type of product formulation filled: for oils, 18–21 h; for pastes, 24–26 h; and for products containing polyethylene glycol, about 36 h. The final moisture content of the capsules is 7% to 9%.

In the past, when filled capsules exited the machine, they were passed through a washing device to remove excess ribbon lubricant from their surface. This relied on the use of organic solvents, such as methylene chloride.[54] In current machines, the amount of lubricant used is minimal; thus, this step is no longer a standard part of the process. However, if the capsules are to be printed by an off-set process, they are typically polished with lint-free clothes to remove any remaining lubricant. If the capsules are printed by a laser printer, then this is not required.

Manufacture of Seamed Soft Gelatin Capsules with Different Properties

Not all soft capsules taken orally are intended to be swallowed whole. There is a need for products that can be chewed so that they release their contents in the mouth, either for treatment of a condition in the oral–pharyngeal area or for buccal absorption. These shells need to have good oral sensory characteristics: it must have sufficient strength to retain their contents after manufacture until taken, have a good mouth feel, and be readily soluble and dispersible after shell rupture. Banner Pharmacaps patented a shell formulation based on blends of low-Bloom (80–100 g) and medium-Bloom (150–175 g) gelatins.[55] Standard plasticizers were used because they contribute to the sensation of softness and flexibility in the mouth. However, when soft capsules dry out, they tend to become leathery, and to overcome this, Banner Pharmacaps proposed the addition of moisture-retaining agents, humectants, to stabilize the shell moisture content. They recommended various celluloses and starches for this purpose and, if required, taste modifiers such as non-reducing sugars, for example, xylitol, maltitol, and Lycasin (Roquette America, Inc.).

Manufacture of Seamed Soft Gelatin Capsules with Dry Products

The filling of powders into soft capsules was made possible by the American Cyanamid Company, which adapted the rotary die principle.[56] Powders were compressed on tablet machines to form various shapes of compacts: round, oval, and elliptical long oval, which were cylindrical in shape with hemispherical ends (in current parlance, a "caplet"). The machine had a pair of rotary dies: one with a set of cavities with a shape large enough to accommodate most of the plug and the other with shallower cavities. Gelatin ribbons were fed over the two die rolls. In place of the wedge block is a device that transfers the compacts directly into the cavities on the left die roll, termed the feeding roll. The other roll is the sealing roll, and its temperature is higher than the other one to heat the gelatin ribbon to make a better seal. Suction is applied to the base of each cavity before the filling position to draw the ribbon into its shape, and this is released just before compact transfer to make sealing easier.

Since the late 1980s, after the Tylenol hard capsule tampering incident, there has been a need to produce tamper-evident dosage forms. Soft capsules have been used for this application. One example is the process patented by Banner Gelatin Products Corp.[57] Their Soflet Gelcap technology is a process for covering a tablet in an elastic gelatin film that can be either securely bonded to it or peelable in such a way as not to expose the tablet to moisture and high temperatures. The tablets, referred to as preforms or cores, can be either caplet or round concave in shape and are produced on standard tableting machines. They are typically film coated to enhance adhesion between the gelatin coat and the core surface. The rotary die machines are adapted to feed the cores into the nip position between a pair of die rolls and oriented in the correct axis for sealing. If uncoated, the cores are dedusted during their passage through the feeder. The cavities in the die rolls are differently shaped from liquid filling; their size is such that there is ample room, both in width and in length, so that the cores do not touch the sides or bottom of the recesses. Ribbons of two colors are used with a higher concentration of gelatin compared to standard soft capsules: the preferred formulation was 45% w/w gelatin, preferably 150 to 180 Bloom, with 9% w/w glycerin and water plus colorants to 100% w/w. The die rolls have extra features: each cavity has a raised rim around its circumference that comes into contact with the other die roll during its revolution and the edges of the cylinder have a series of protrusion designs to grip the gelatin ribbon to maintain the correct tension in the film. The cores are removed from the stack held in the feeder mechanism by contact with the adhesive surface of the two ribbons simultaneously as they pass the outlet. The film tension over the die recesses enables it to stretch in all directions without rupture, because of its thickness, temperature, and composition, and fully cover the cores. The film thickness is from 500 μm to 1 mm (0.02 to 0.04"), and the film temperature is between 38°C and 88°C (between 100°F and 190°F). The films are sealed around the periphery of the cores: in the case of caplets, along the mid-axis of the tablet belly band. The sealed cores either fall from the gelatin web or are forcibly extracted from it and then washed and dried. As the films dry, they become an integral part of the tablet core. One of the claims of the patent was to minimize the temperature and moisture exposure of the cores during the process unlike the hard capsule dipping process that had been used previously for Tylenol tablets, thereby not affecting the stability of the cores.

Manufacture of Seamless Soft Capsules

Several companies in the 1990s patented improvements to the production of seamless gelatin capsules. Alfatec Pharma GmbH in 1993 proposed using the standard method of producing drops with a central core of material surrounded by a gelatin mass but using a cooling bath with a very low temperature with the objective of avoiding residues of cooling oil, liquid paraffin used in cooling baths, being left on the capsules.[54] The gelatin mass and the fill material are held in separate containers and pumped through a double-tube system, either as pulses or intermittently to form a drop. The filled capsules are then fed into an insulated freezer containing liquid nitrogen at a temperature of −70° to −220°C. The temperature difference between the capsule and the liquid nitrogen causes it to evaporate and surround the gelatin-covered drops with a gas layer, which provides an even pressure on the capsules to form uniform spheres that freeze. The capsules are transported on a conveyor belt to a heating system, where they are dried. They also proposed that if the fill consisted of incompatible APIs, one could be incorporated into the gelatin film.

Seamed Modified-Gelatin Capsules

The move to replace gelatin in soft capsules started in the early 1990s and was stimulated by the need to reduce the costs by finding a cheaper alternative and to avoid the problems caused by bovine spongiform encephalopathy (BSE) and to expand the usage into other fields. Pharmacaps Inc. developed a chewable gelatin-based soft capsule by the addition of a hydrogenated starch hydrolysate.[58] This capsule was claimed to be easy to chew and dissolved quickly in the mouth without leaving a sticky residue. An example w/w formulation for the shell was gelatin 32%, glycerin 25%, hydrogenated starch hydrolysate 20%, and water 23%. R.P. Scherer Corporation in 1992 patented the use of soft capsules containing a high-amylose starch.[59] They claimed that the capsules had an improved surface finish, did not stick together, had strong seals, were resistant to shape change, and were cheaper to manufacture because of the lower raw material cost. Starches with high amylose content, preferably greater than 90%, were used to substitute up to 85% of the gelatin content. Solutions of gelatin and glycerin and suspensions of starch and glycerin were prepared, blended together, and heated. The capsules were manufactured on standard rotary die machines. The capsule surfaces had a frosted or satin finish and were rougher than gelatin ones, which was why they did not tend to stick together. A special application for gelatin/starch capsules was the subject of a further patent in 1996.[60] This was for a capsule to contain medicaments to be applied external or administered by the rectal route. A requirement for this usage is for the patients to be easily able to grip them firmly and thus the surface texture of the capsule shells needed to be modified because standard capsules have a smooth slippery surface. The shell formulations consisted of blends of gelatin types (e.g., hydrolyzed or acetylated), starch derivatives (e.g., high amylose, esterified), polysaccharide thickening agents (e.g., carrageenan gellan gum), thickening agents (e.g., chitosan derivatives, cellulose derivatives), and plasticizers (e.g., polyglycerols, maltitol). An example of a w/w formulation was acetylated gelatin 49.6%, glycerol 26.1%, hydrogenated starch 14.0%, hydrolyzed gelatin 5.5%, and high-amylose starch 4.8%. This formulation was used on a standard soft capsule machine that had die rolls with special shaped cavities: the main body being oval with a tube from one end attached to a round knob-like structure. The medicament is released by turning the "knob," which breaks off. The knurled surface of the capsules is applied to the films by means of special texturing rollers, which are applied to the outer surface of the ribbons after casting while they are still moldable and before passing between the rotary dies.[61]

Soft Capsule Quality

The physical quality attributes of filled capsules are measured, giving an indication of how they will stand up to handling on packaging equipment and the transportation to the patient. For both types of capsule, seamed and seamless, the prime concern is the potential for product leakage (leakers). For the seamed capsules, tests are carried out to determine the strength of the seal because if this is low, the potential for leaking will be high. Various instruments are available to measure how well the capsule will deform under compression and to determine the force to burst the seam.

Dr. Schleuniger Pharmatron, Inc. manufacture a soft gelatin tester model 6D (SG) (www .pharmatron.com).[62] This is based on their well-known tablet tester used to measure crushing strength. The test capsule is placed on a flat plate between two platens attached to load cells. These are driven together by a motor at a set rate and apply a force to the capsule. The force applied is displayed together with the distance between the platens. The measurements that are used are taken from the moment that the platens contact the capsule, and this point is taken as the diameter of the capsule in the uncompressed state. Various measurements can be taken: the force to compress a preselected distance and to burst the capsules and the amount of deflection for a preselected force. These values can be used to assess the integrity of the seal. Brookfield Engineering has a texture analyzer that can be used to measure similar values with a different setup (www.brookfieldengineering.com).[63]

There are many different types of visual inspection machines to control the quality of finished soft capsules. Currently, most machines are systems built around the use of high-speed cameras and imaging analyzing software. After inspection, the capsules are packaged into containers that will maintain their moisture content.

Gelatin Alternatives for Soft Capsule Manufacture

Manufacture of Non-Gelatin Soft Capsules

A gelatin-free soft capsule was first patented by Merck & Co. in 1994 to meet the need for a non-animal encapsulating polymer.[64] It was based on blends of gellan gum, κ-carrageenan and locust bean gum, and a gelling agent such as potassium citrate. The blend of polymers was chosen so that the processing temperature could be <100°C. These were mixed in cold deionized water at 20°C to 30°C; sorbitol, glycerin, and corn syrup were added; and the mixture was heated to 90°C with stirring for 10 min before it was transferred to a standard rotary die machine. Films, with a thickness of 0.76 to 1.02 mm (30 to 40 mil), were cast onto steel drums and passed through the rotary dies, where they were filled, cut, and sealed. The finished capsules were washed and dried: the final moisture content was 3% to 4%. No details of the manufacturing process were given. Banner Pharmacaps

Inc. obtained a patent for such a capsule also based on κ-carrageenan but using different additives.[65] κ-carrageenan was chosen because it produces a thermo-reversible gel and other polymers used had to have the same property: the proportion of κ-carrageenan had to be at least 50% of the total polymers. Materials such as maltodextrin increase the shell mass, and because they increase the tackiness of the wet films, they aid the capsule sealing process, and gums such as locust bean gum can be used to improve the gel strength and elasticity of the ribbons. An example of a % w/w formulation is κ-carrageenan 4%, maltitol syrup 20%, glycerin 11%, and deionized water 65%. The solution was prepared by dispersing the κ-carrageenan in the glycerin at room temperature, adding maltitol syrup and water, heating the solution, and cooling to gel. Polymer ribbons were cast in the standard fashion and fed through a pair of rotary dies to fill and form capsules.

In 2002, R.P. Scherer Technologies, Inc. proposed the use of carrageenan mixtures to produce soft capsules using a standard rotary die machine.[66] The film composition was a mixture of iota-carrageenan and a modified starch, which was required to have a hydration temperature <90°C. The mixture ratio of these two materials was critical to produce a wet film with the correct characteristics: a fusion pressure of >207 kPa at a temperature from 25°C to 80°C with a film melting temperature of preferably 4°C to 9°C above its fusion temperature, which is when the films are brought into contact will blend to form a solid structure. The preferred modified starch was a hydroxypropylated acid modified grade. The dry shell w/w composition was iota-carrageenan 12–24%, modified starch 30–60%, plasticizer (glycerin) 10–60%, and a dibasic sodium phosphate buffer 1–4%. It was noted that the sealing of these capsules occurred at a substantially lower pressure than for mammalian gelatin and that this would result in less wear and tear on the machines and in energy cost savings. The iota-carrageenan acts to make the starch film more elastic, resulting in capsules with good mechanical properties. The main difference in the machine settings between these capsules and gelatin is that their ribbon casting and the wedge sealing are carried out at higher temperatures. These capsules are sold under the trademark Vegicaps Soft by Catalent.[67] Their advantage over conventional gelatin soft capsules was that they could be filled with materials at significantly higher temperatures. This enabled excipients such as polyethylene glycol 6000, which is solid below 60°C, to be used as an excipient for liquid-filling. In a following patent, Scherer described a method of improving the process of producing films from this mass to accommodate the higher casting temperatures required for iota-carrageenan/starch films.[68] The film forming material was prepared and then was chilled and stored if it is not required immediately. When required, this material was transferred to a melt-on-demand device and heated to the correct temperature in 15 to 30 min. These film-forming materials have a high viscosity compared to gelatin, up to 20 MPa s. When ready, it is pumped under pressure into an extrusion device. This could either have the form of a "coat-hanger" die with an extrusion slot or a valved injection wedge. The extruded ribbon is applied to the casting drum at a tilt angle of c. 5°. The system was enclosed, thus reducing water loss compared to a standard spreader box, able to be operated at higher temperatures, up to 90°C, which could be easily regulated.

In soft gelatin capsules, the formulation of the shell is related to the nature of the fill materials, typically by using alternative plasticizers. The Australian affiliate of R.P. Scherer patented a method to limit fill migration into the shell.[69] They proposed that the shell and fill should be in a hydrophilic/hydrophobic balance to minimize this. They ranked suitable film-forming polymers, natural, semi-synthetic, and synthetic, into three groups: lower, mid, and higher, based on their relative water solubility. The formulations contained standard plasticizers as used in gelatin capsules. They proposed the use of mixtures with carrageenan, a relatively hydrophobic material with hydroxypropyl starch, which is hydrophilic. If the fill material was reactive, that is, contains aldehyde groups, they recommended a mixture of hydroxypropylstarch, furcelleran (12CFR172.6651), and glycerol.

The first capsule with starch as the only polymer was patented in 2004 by Swisscaps.[70] The base formulation was amorphous starch at least 45%, organic softener at least 12%, water, lubricant, or releasing aid, and a variety of normal capsule additives (e.g., colorants, preservatives, and antioxidants). An example formulation of a finished dried capsule film consisted of starch (water free) 55.15%, glycerin 38.77%, calcium carbonate 7.76%, and lecithin 1.11%. Calcium carbonate was described as a "decomposing agent" to aid capsule shell disintegration. The starch mass is produced in a double worm-type extruder that consists of 12 individual blocks. Their temperature can be individually adjusted: raised by the use of electrical heating or lowered with circulating cold water. The extruder described was 2.1 m in length. The first block is cooled with water to 20°C and has a power feeder for starch. Blocks 2 and 3 are heated to 100°C, and in between the two, there is a set of kneading discs to mix the mass. Attached to block 3 is a nozzle to pump in glycerin. Blocks 4, 5, and 6 are heated to 140°C. In block 5, there is an additional set of kneading discs to move the material backward for the screws to move it forward again to ensure mixing. Blocks 7 to 12 are maintained at 110°C. Block 7 has an outlet to which a vacuum (10 bar) is applied to remove water. Block 8 has a power feed for the addition of a powder such as calcium carbonate, and the worm has attached kneading discs for mixing in the material. Block 9 has an injection nozzle for adding more glycerin. Block 10 has several types of kneading disks similar to block 5. Block 11 has an outlet to apply a vacuum (10 bar) to remove water. In block 12, the worm has conveying kneading disks and has two possible setups. One is to extrude the mass through an end plate, which has 12×2-mm-diameter holes. This extrudate can be processed into granules and stored for future use. The other is to pump the mass through a nozzle to form a film to be transferred directly to the capsule machine. This setup shows that it is possible to make multilayer capsules because more than one film can be fed from each side of the machine and at least two of these films must have a different chemical composition. It would be possible for the inner side of the film to have an easily weldable coating and for the outer side to be the one that delayed the disintegration of the capsule. These capsules have wall thicknesses between 0.2 and 0.6 mm, and the tests reported in the patent show that they have good mechanical strengths.

The most recent patent granted for seamed non-gelatin soft capsules describes the use of starch/carrageenan mixtures. It was filed by R.P. Scherer Technologies, LLC in November 2004 and was granted on July 31, 2012.[71] The pH of liquid fills for soft gelatin capsules must be less than 7.5; otherwise, there is an interaction with the shell wall causing leakage. They had declared previously in a series of formulation patents a method of increasing the solubility of active pharmaceutical ingredients by dispersing them in polyethylene glycol solutions and titrating them with an appropriate acid or alkali to neutralize them.[72] The pH of the resulting solutions was often >7.5, and these were not suitable for gelatin capsules. Scherer found that starch/iota-carrageenan films with a composition ratio of 3:1 had a high resistance to alkali fills from pH 8.0 to 12.0: an example of a fill formulation was acetaminophen that required sodium or potassium hydroxide to neutralize the solution.[73] The film formulation contained additional components to those described in Reference 60. A proposed w/w formulation for the shell mass contained hydroxypropylated starch 23.5%, iota-carrageenan 7.5%, glycerol 12.5%, Polysorb 12.5%, disodium phosphate, and water 43.3%.

Seamless Non-Gelatin Capsules

Morishita Jintan Co., Ltd of Japan introduced a modification to the production of seamless capsules by modifying the dual-tube injection system by adding a third outer coaxial tube through which heated fluids could be pumped to prevent premature solidification of meltable solid fills.[74] In a further patent in conjunction with Fujisawa Pharmaceutical Co. Ltd., this setup was used for the production of capsules with shells made from polymers other than gelatin.[75] It was proposed for the production of capsules that had more than one API, which were not compatible, or for making combination capsules that had different release rates *in vivo*. The polymers that could be used were gelatins, alginates, pectins, and carrageenans plus water-soluble magnesium and calcium salts. The process could be used to form a filled capsule within a filled capsule. The capsules were formed by pumping with perturbations multi-jet liquid streams into a cooling liquid, such as vegetable oil, at 9°C.

Warner Lambert Co. filed four patents between 1997 and 2002 to use improvements to the drop method in the manufacture of glassy carbohydrates.[76–79] One of the objectives of the process was to avoid the use of water to save the energy costs in removing it from the capsules. The shell material was a mixture of isomalt 90% and xylitol 10%, melted together at 155°C and then stored at 148°C. The shell material had a density of 1.0 g/mL and the fill one had a density of <1.0 g/mL.[76] The coaxial jet of shell and fill material was extruded into a duct supplied with a hot liquid: the temperature of which was higher than the melting point of the shell solution. This duct was positioned inside a second duct with a cooling liquid, coconut oil at 20°C. Capsules were formed in the first one and solidified in the second one. In the next patent, one of the embodiments, the coaxial jet, extruded the shell/fill stream into a space supplied with air heated to 200°C.[77] The capsules form as they fall and drop 10 cm into a column of coconut oil cooled to 20°C. One of the problems in forming seamless capsules in moving liquid columns is that if the flow becomes turbulent, they could be damaged. However, if laminar flow systems are used, heat conduction is slow, and in the apparatus described above, when using two ducts, the second one would need to be long, >9 m. In the patent, the shell/fill material is extruded into a hot liquid and the capsules formed fall almost vertically into a duct tube, set on an incline.[78] In this duct, there are two laminar flows of liquid, one hot and one cold. The capsules as they fall pass from the hot steam to the cold stream where they solidify and do not come into contact with the duct wall and hence are not damaged. The final patent defined the optimum setting for the critical parameters: length of the second duct, angle of inclination, cooled–heated liquid flow rate, and cooled liquid temperature.[79] A shorter length, c. 500 μm to 1.0 mm, at an angle of 6° to 7° for the second duct gave more capsule exposure to the cooled liquid carrier, which must be ≤30°C for isomalt, and if the duct had a rectangular or square cross section, better results were obtained because this limits the mixing of the adjacent liquid streams. Coconut oil was given as an example of a liquid carrier: when hot, it was at 100°C, and when used cold, it was at 0°C.

ACKNOWLEDGMENT

The authors thank Dr. Al Brzeczko, V.P. Global Pharmaceutical R&D, ISP, for helpful advice with the soft capsule gelatin processes.

REFERENCES

1. Jones BE. The history of the medicinal capsule. In Podczeck F, Jones BE, eds. *Pharmaceutical Capsules*, 2nd edition. London: Pharmaceutical Press, 2004:1–22.
2. Wilkie W. The manufacture of gelatin capsules. *Bull Pharm Detroit* 1913;27:382–384.
3. Scott BW. Apparatus for forming capsules. *US Patent No.* 943,608, 1909; *US Patent No.* 1,076,459, 1913.
4. Colton A. Capsule machine. *US Patent No.* 1,787,777, 1931.
5. Eli Lilly & Co. Capsule resisting separation. *French Patent No.* 1,343,698, 1963; Separation-resistant capsule. *British Patent No.* 970,761, 1964; *US Patent No.* 3,173,840, 1965; Capsule with an integral locking band. *US Patent No.* 3,285,408, 1966.
6. Parke, Davis & Co. Hard shell capsules. *British Patent No.* 1,108,629, 1966; Self-locking medicament capsules. *US Patent No.* 3,339,803, 1968; Locking capsule. *US Patent No.* 3,508,678, 678, 1970.
7. Warner-Lambert Co. Container. *US Patent No.* 5,769,267, 1998.
8. Lilly Industries Ltd. Improvements in capsules. *European Patent Application No.* 0 246 804 A2, 1987.
9. Croda Gelatin Ltd, Equilibrium moisture content and its significance for microbiological stability. In *Gelfax, a Series of Useful Facts on All Aspects of Gelatin Stability*, No. 20, Croda Gelatin Ltd, Widnes, UK, 1980, p. 3.
10. Jones RT. Gelatin: Manufacture and physico-chemical properties. In Podczeck F, Jones BE, eds. *Pharmaceutical Capsules*, 2nd edition. London: Pharmaceutical Press, 2004:23–60.
11. Jones BE. The manufacture and properties of two-piece hard capsules. In Podczeck F, Jones BE, eds. *Pharmaceutical Capsules*, 2nd edition. London: Pharmaceutical Press, 2004:79–100.

12. Hannon JT, Markowski MJ. Using new techniques for reducing system validation time and cost. *Pharm Tech*. 1996;x:40, 42, 44, 46, 48, 50, 52, 54.
13. Jasti BR, Leopold CS, Li X et al. Shellac. In Rowe RC, Shesky PJ, Cook WG, Fenton ME, eds. *Handbook of Pharmaceutical Excipients*, 7th edition. London: Pharmaceutical Press, 2012:704–707.
14. Committee for medicinal products for human use. ICH Topic Q3C(R5) Impurities: Guideline for residual solvents step 4. *European Medicines Agency*. EMA/CHMP/82260/2006, March 2011, p. 26.
15. USDHH (US Department of Health and Human Services), Food and Drug Administration, Center for Drug Evaluation and Research (CDER), Center for Biologics Evaluation and Research (CBER). *Guidance for industry* Q3C—Tables and list, revision 2, February 2012.
16. Jones BE. Evolution of the technology for filling two-piece hard capsules with powder. *Tablets & Capsules* 2006;4:10–12, 14, 16–20.
17. Jones BE. Capsule standards. In Podczeck F, Jones BE, eds. *Pharmaceutical Capsules*, 2nd edition. London: Pharmaceutical Press, 2004:239–259.
18. Military standard MIL-STD-105E, www.archive.org/public/domain/mark/1.0/
19. Murphy, HW. Methyl cellulose capsules and process of manufacture. *US Patent No*. 2,526,693, 1950.
20. US government printing office. Water resistance. *Federal standard capsules (for medicinal purposes) 285A*, Amendment-2, July 1, 1977, p. 11.
21. Ogura T, Furuya Y, Matsuura S. HPMC capsules—An alternative to gelatin. *Pharm Tech Eur* 1998;10(11):32, 34, 36, 40, 42.
22. Japan Elanco Co., Ltd. Hard capsules for pharmaceutical drugs and a method for producing the same. *US Patent No*. 5,264,223, 1993; *US Patent No*. 5,431, 1995.
23. Japan Elanco Co. Ltd. Hard capsules. *European Patent Application* 595,130, 1993.
24. Japan Elanco Co., Ltd. Capsule shell. *US Patent No*. 5,756,123, 1998.
25. Shionogi Qualicaps Co., Ltd. Process for producing hard capsule. *US Patent No*. 6,413,463, 2002.
26. Warner Lambert Co. Polymer film compositions for capsules. *European Patent Application EP* 1,057,862, 1997; *International Publication No*. WO 98/27151, 1998; *US Patent No*. 6,517,865, 2003.
27. Pfizer Products Inc. Process for manufacturing films. *European Patent Application EP* 1,949,461, 2006; *International Publication No*. WO 2007/122465, 2007.
28. GS Technologies, Inc. Method for the manufacture of pharmaceutical cellulose capsules. *US Patent No*. 5,756,036, 1997; *US Patent No*. 5,698,155, 1998.
29. GS Technologies, Inc. Apparatus for the manufacture of pharmaceutical cellulose capsules. *US Patent No*. 5,756,036, 1998.
30. Pfizer Products Inc. Hydroxypropyl methylcellulose hard capsules and a process of manufacture. *US Patent Application Publication No*. 2010/0168410.
31. Capsugel brochure. NPcaps™ premium vegetarian capsules. Downloaded from www.capsugel.com 10.15.2008.
32. Capsugel press release. Capsugel launches Plantcaps™ capsules. A more natural alternative pullulan capsule. March 12 2012. Downloaded from www.capsugel.com 8.21.2012.
33. Rowe RC, Shesky PJ, Cook WG, Fenton ME, eds. *Handbook of Pharmaceutical Excipients*, 7th edition. London: Pharmaceutical Press, 2012:704–707.
34. Warner-Lambert Company LLC. Improved pullulan capsules. *European Patent Application EP* 1,593,376, 2004; *International Publication No*. WO 2005/105051, 2005.
35. Eith L, Stepto RFT, Tomka I et al. The injection-moulded capsules. *Drug Dev Ind Pharm* 1986;12(11–13):2113–2126 and *Mfg Chem* 1987;58(1):21, 23, 25.
36. Warner-Lambert Company LLC. Pullulan film compositions. *US Patent No*. 6,887,307, 2005; *US Patent No*. 7,267,718, 2007.
37. Warner-Lambert Co. Method for forming pharmaceutical capsules from starch compositions. *US Patent No*. 4,738,724, 1988.
38. Vilvalam D, Illum L, Iqbal K. Starch capsules: An alternative system for drug delivery. *Pharm Sci Tech Today* 2000;3(2):64–69.
39. *United States Pharmacopeia 31*. Capsules, Chapter 1151.
40. Scherer RP. Method of and machine for making capsules. *US Patent No*. 1,970,396, 1934.
41. Williams, G. He did it with capsules. *The Saturday Evening Post* 1949, The Curtis Publishing Company, p. 4.
42. Scherer RP. Apparatus for forming and filling capsules. *US Patent No*. 2,288,327, 1942.
43. Scherer RP. Method and apparatus of fabricating filled capsules. *US Patent No*. 2,318,718, 1943.
44. Scherer RP. Fabrication of filled sealed capsules. *US Patent No*. 2,332,671, 1943.

45. Globex International Ltd. Method and apparatus for producing seamless capsules. *US Patent No.* 2,932,061, 1960.
46. Podczeck FP. Technology to manufacture soft capsules. In Podczeck F, Jones BE, eds. *Pharmaceutical Capsules*, 2nd edition. London: Pharmaceutical Press, 2004:195–199.
47. Schreiber R, Gareis H. Gelatine applications, property profile for capsule gelatin. In Schreiber R, Gareis H, eds. *Gelatine Handbook*. Weinheim: Wiley-VCH, 2007:247–251.
48. Jones RT. Gelatin: Manufacture and physico-chemical properties. In Podczeck F, Jones BE, eds. *Pharmaceutical Capsules*, 2nd edition. London: Pharmaceutical Press, 2004:23–60.
49. Reich G. Formulation and physical properties of soft capsules. In Podczeck F, Jones BE, eds. *Pharmaceutical Capsules*, 2nd edition. London: Pharmaceutical Press, 2004:201–212.
50. Bauer KH. Die Herstellung von Hart- und Weichgelatinekapseln. In Fahrig W, Hofer U, eds. *Die Kapsel, Grundlagen, Technologie und Biopharmacie einer modernen Arzneiform*. Stuttgart: Wissenlichte Verlagsgesellschaft mbH, 1983:58–82.
51. Hutchinson KG, Ferdinando J. Soft gelatin capsules. In Aulton ME, and Taylor KMG, eds. *Aulton's Pharmaceutics, the Design and Manufacture of Medicines*, 4th edition. Edinburgh, UK: Churchill Livingstone Elsevier, 2013:597–610.
52. Technophar Equipment & Services Ltd. Soft gelatin encapsulation laboratory machine SGL 107, 2007, p. 57, www.technophar.com/softcapsule/softcapsulemachines
53. Fang Q, Hu Y, Yu N et al. Characterization and modeling of softgel drying process. *Tablets & Capsules* 2011;9(4):24–28, 30, 32–33.
54. Alfatec Pharma GmbH. Soft gelatin capsules. *US Patent No.* 5,254,294, 1993.
55. Banner Pharmacaps, Inc. Chewable soft capsule. *US Patent No.* 6,258,380, 2001.
56. American Cyanamid Company. Improvements relating to method of and apparatus for forming plastic film-covered pre-compacted powder-filled capsules. *British Patent No.* 755,993, 1956.
57. Banner Gelatin Products Corp. Film-enrobed unitary-core medicament and the like. *US Patent No.* 5,146,730, 1992.
58. Pharmacaps, Inc. Chewable, edible soft gelatin capsule. *US Patent No.* 4,935,243, 1990.
59. R.P. Scherer Corporation. High amylose starch substituted gelatin capsules. *International Publication No.* WO 92/09724, 1992; *US Patent No.* 5,554,385, 1996.
60. R.P. Scherer Corporation. Method and apparatus for the manufacture of textured softgels. *US Patent No.* 5,246,635, 1993.
61. R.P. Scherer Corporation. Soft gelatin medicament capsules with gripping constructions. *US Patent No.* 5,484,598, 1996.
62. Dr Schleuniger Pharmatron Inc., www.pharmatron.com
63. Brookfield Engineering Ametek, Inc., www.brookfieldengineering.com
64. Merck & Co., Inc. Composition and process for gelatin-free soft capsules. *US Patent No.* 5,342,626, 1994.
65. Banner Pharmacaps, Inc. Non-gelatin substitutes for oral-delivery capsules, their composition and process of manufacture. *U.S. Patent No.* 6,214,376, 2001.
66. R.P. Scherer Technologies, Inc. Film forming compositions comprising modified starches and iota-carrageenan and methods for manufacturing soft capsules using same. *European Patent Application EP* 1,598,062 A1, 2000; *International Publication No.* WO 01/03677, 2001; *US Patent No.* 6,340,473, 2002; *US Patent No.* 6,582,727, 2003.
67. Catalent. Vegicaps® capsules, an innovative solution for encapsulation challenges.
68. R.P. Scherer Technologies, Inc. Apparatus for manufacturing encapsulated products. *US Patent No.* 6,884,060, 2005.
69. R.P. Scherer Holdings, Pty Ltd. Non-gelatin based capsules. *International Patent No.* WO 03/009823, 2003.
70. Greither P. Method for manufacturing a shape body containing starch and a device for manufacturing a soft capsule. *US Patent No.* 6,790,495, 2004.
71. R.P. Scherer Technologies, LLC. Non-gelatin soft capsule system. *US Patent No.* 8,231,896, 2012.
72. R.P. Scherer Corporation. Solvent system enhancing the solubility of pharmaceuticals for encapsulation. *US Patent No.* 5,071,64, 1991; *US Patent No.* 5,360,615, 1994.
73. R.P. Scherer Corporation. Gelatin capsules containing a highly concentrated acetaminophen solution. *US Patent No.* 5,505,961, 1996.
74. Morishita Jintan Co., Ltd. Method and apparatus for encapsulation of a liquid or meltable solid material. *US Patent No.* 4,422,985, 1983.

75. Morishita Jintan, Co., Ltd and Fujisawa Pharmaceutical Co. Ltd, Osaka, Japan. *US Patent No.* 4,695,466, 1987.
76. Warner-Lambert Company. Seamless capsules. *US Patent No.* 5,595,757, 1997.
77. Warner-Lambert Company. Method and apparatus for making seamless capsules. *US Patent No.* 5,888,538, 1999.
78. Warner-Lambert Company. Method for making seamless capsules. *US Patent No.* 6,174,446, 2001.
79. Warner-Lambert Company. Method and apparatus for making seamless capsules. *US Patent No.* 6,361,298, 2002.

5 Non-Gelatin-Based Capsules

Sven Stegemann

CONTENTS

INTRODUCTION

Two-piece hard capsules are one of the most established dosage forms for pharmaceutical products. The concept of using hard capsules to deliver drugs was described as far back as 1846, when Jules César Lehuby was granted a patent for his "medicine coverings." The patent described the manufacturing of two-piece capsules by dipping silver-coated metal pins into a gelatin solution and then drying them (Dorvault 1923). However, it wasn't until 1931 that Arthur Colton, on behalf of Parke, Davis & Co., succeeded in designing a machine that simultaneously manufactured both halves of the gelatin capsule body and cap and fitted them together to produce a two-piece hard gelatin capsule (Colton 1931). This invention can be considered the starting point for one of the most important dosage form innovations used for pharmaceutical drug products, which is still being used to develop innovative solutions for a variety of different drug delivery systems and platforms.

Two-piece hard capsules have been traditionally made of gelatin, which exhibits unique physicochemical properties of gel and film formation within a very narrow temperature range. This feature is important for manufacturing purposes. Additionally, gelatin provides other important properties and characteristics for oral dosage forms such as fast capsule opening and dissolution *in vivo*, which are required for immediate-release dosage forms. Hard gelatin capsules are now an established pharmaceutical dosage form that are used as a delivery vehicle in 20% of all oral pharmaceutical products, several of which have been blockbuster drugs for many years. Through continuous improvements and advances in hard gelatin capsule manufacturing, these hard gelatin capsules are a state-of-the-art pharmaceutical delivery vehicle that are suited for modern Quality by Design-based pharmaceutical product development and manufacturing (Stegemann et al. 2014a).

In parallel to using gelatin for hard capsule production, scientists investigated the use of polymer-based two-piece hard capsules to broaden the applications of capsule technology for drug delivery. These resulting polymers had to display characteristics that can overcome some of the challenges associated with the delivery of specific drug molecules or that exhibit specific physicochemical characteristics. These new materials had to demonstrate utility with special drugs or delivery systems but at the same time be pharmaceutically acceptable. They also had to have manufacturing reproducibility and high capsule quality, be economically viability with respect to commercial-scale manufacturing, and be capable of being used in existing high-speed capsule filling machines. This polymer research led to the introduction of two-piece capsules made of two additional base polymers, HPMC (hypromellose, hydroxypropylmethyl-cellulose) and a polysaccharide, pullulan, which displays properties similar to those of gelatin. From these two polymers, HPMC capsules have gained regulatory approval for the formulation of orally as well as pulmonary delivered pharmaceutical products that are marketed in all major countries around the world. Furthermore, HPMC-based capsules have been developed for specific applications and with different release profiles.

TWO-PIECE HARD CAPSULES AND THEIR MANUFACTURING

Two-piece hard capsules consist of two cylindrical parts, with each half having a hemispherical closed end and an open end. The open end of the body part of the capsule is slightly smaller in diameter so that the cap part can be slipped over to close the capsule. Both parts have integrated design features that are essential for the quality performance of the capsules during transport and processing on high-speed filling machines, as well as the integrity of the filled capsule.

Manufacturing is based on the principle of dipping specifically designed metal pins into an aqueous solution of the polymer. On retraction from the solution, the pins are coated with a thin film of the polymer, which solidifies to form the body and the cap parts of the capsule in two separate sections. The "dipping process" requires the rapid and homogeneous gelation or solidification of the polymer solution on the dipping pins after they are retracted from the solution. This gelation process can be triggered either by self-gelling properties that a pure polymer displays in solution within a narrow temperature range or by the addition of additives to the polymer solution to act as a gelling system. After the polymer solution has settled as a thin film on the dipping pins, the wet films are passed through a controlled drying process to remove water until the targeted water content is achieved and the solid shells are formed. After drying, the formed shells are stripped off the pins and cut to the specific length before the cap and body part is joined to the two-piece capsule in a pre-lock position. If required, these empty capsules can be printed in a separate process before shipment.

HPMC (HYPROMELLOSE)-BASED CAPSULES

The first attempts to develop cellulose-based capsules were made by Eli Lilly in 1950 using methyl cellulose as the base polymer. However, because of the slow disintegration and dissolution of the methyl-cellulose capsules *in vivo*, the capsules were withdrawn from the market just a few years later. With the introduction of HPMC, new attempts were made to develop and manufacture cellulose-based capsules. In 1989, GS Technologies introduced the first HPMC capsules followed by additional HPMC capsules reaching the market in 1996. Today, there are a variety of different commercially available HPMC capsules, which differ from each other in respect of their performance, specific release profile, or route of administration.

HPMC CAPSULES FOR IMMEDIATE RELEASE

HPMC is a cellulose ether derived through a synthetic hydroxypropyl and methoxy substitution of pulp cellulose. A variety of different HPMC products exist that differ with regard to the degree of substitution, viscosity as a 2% solution, and grade (Li et al. 2005). The United States Pharmacopeia (USP) lists three different types of HPMC according to the different chemical substitution of the ether. These are E-types (hypromellose 2910), F-types (hypromellose 2906), and K-types (hypromellose 2208). HPMC is an excipient with a very good safety profile that is recognized by a GRAS (generally recognized as safe) status and monographs in all major Pharmacopoeias. As a result, HPMC is widely used in pharmaceutical products as a hydrophilic binder, a matrix forming agent, and coating material in tableting, and as a solubilizing agent, a crystallization inhibitor, and a viscolizing agent in liquid formulations. HPMC has been identified as a suitable polymer for the manufacture of two-piece capsules through the dipping process. It is recognized as a two-piece capsule polymer in the USP monograph on Pharmaceutical Dosage Forms, which states that "Two-piece gelatin capsules usually are formed from blends of gelatins ... or from hypromellose" (USP monograph ⟨1151⟩ Pharmaceutical Dosage Forms). Similarly but not specific for any polymer, the European Pharmacopoeia states that "capsule shells are made of gelatin or other substances" (European Pharmacopoeia 8.0 Monograph "Capsules"). The European Pharmacopoeia requires capsules to show the conformity with the specification set in "Uniformity of dose units," "Uniformity of content," "Uniformity of mass," "Dissolution," and "Disintegration."

As with the gelatin capsules, HPMC capsules are offered in different sizes with equivalent dimensional and weight specifications required to run on the existing capsule filling machines. Dependent on the processing conditions, capsules are manufactured either from a pure aqueous HPMC solution or from HPMC blend solutions containing a gelling system. Capsules that are manufactured by the different processes and made of different HPMC blend solutions show significant variation in their visual appearance and *in vitro* and *in vivo* performance. Because of these variations, different types of HPMC capsules are not interchangeable.

HPMC Capsule Manufacturing

The manufacture of two-piece capsules is based on the formation of a thin and consistent film formation on the surface of the dipping pins occurring within seconds of the pins being removed from the polymer solution. To achieve this film formation with HPMC, capsules can be manufactured by two basic principles:

- Thermo-gelation
- Gelation through gelling systems

Thermo-gelation

When compared with gelatin, which is liquid at high temperature and transforms to a gel when passed through a lower temperature (Djabourov et al. 1995), pure HPMC solutions exhibit a sol–gel transformation within a narrow temperature range at higher temperature, referred to as thermo- or thermal gelation (Sarkar 1979; Silva et al. 2008). The exact temperature range of thermo-gelation is dependent on the type of HPMC used (Haque et al. 1993), the polymer concentration, the ion content in solution, and the processing conditions (Joshi 2011; Silva et al. 2008). To achieve thermo-gelation with HPMC, the traditional capsule manufacturing process has to be reversed, and instead of dipping cold pins into a hot gelatin solution, hot pins have now to be dipped into a cold HPMC solution. Since capsule manufacturers have developed proprietary HPMC compositions along with process technology to manufacture capsules made of pure HPMC reliably on a commercial scale (Cade and He 2008), these capsules are being used widely in product development and manufacturing. HPMC capsules manufactured by thermo-gelation (e.g., Vcaps® Plus) are referred to as tg-HPMC.

Gelation through Gelling Systems

In order to use the traditional capsule manufacturing process of cold pins dipping into a hot polymer solution, gelling systems have to be added to the polymer solution. One gelling system is kappa-carrageenan; a high-molecular-weight polysaccharide made of galactose units and derived from seaweed. It is used widely in the food industry as a gelling and thickening agent. In the presence of cations and specifically potassium, kappa-carrageenan forms aggregates of carrageenan helices to form a cohesive gel network (Morris et al. 1980). Kappa-carrageenan forms strong gels in the presence of low levels of potassium chloride (0.1 M) with a thermal hysteresis between sol-to-gel and gel-to-sol transitions (Funami et al. 2007) in a suitable range for manufacturing capsules, which means that it can be used in the dipping process where cold pins dip into a hot solution of the polymer and upon retraction undergoes a sol-to-gel transformation. Gellan gum is another water-soluble polysaccharide produced by *Sphingomonas elodea* and is used for its gelling and thickening properties in the food industry as well as microbiological culturing material. Similar characteristics have been described for gellan gum as for kappa-carrageenan (Moritaka et al. 1995).

When kappa-carrageenan or gellan gum is added as a gelling agent to an HPMC solution together with ions as gelling promoters in very small concentrations, gel formation can be obtained using cold dipping pins and warm polymer solutions. HPMC capsules made using carrageenan (e.g., Quali-V®) are referred to as c-HPMC and those produced with gellan gum (e.g., Vcaps®) are known as g-HPMC.

Physicochemical Properties

HPMC is a material that is widely used in pharmaceutical product development and manufacturing. When HPMC is used as a base polymer in capsule manufacturing, the empty capsule shells effectively represent an excipient and has to fulfill the functional criteria for its use in capsule filling processes, as well as performance criteria for the specific drug and its formulation.

HPMC capsules are available in the same sizes as gelatin capsules and have the same dimensional specifications. Colorants can be added to the polymer solution to manufacture mono- and bichromatic capsules in a wide range of colors. After manufacturing of the empty capsules, they can be printed in the same way as gelatin capsules to provide product differentiation and branding. The visual appearance of the HPMC capsules depends on the shell composition and manufacturing process. Capsules manufactured by thermo-gelation have a smooth, glossy surface and the transparency of a gelatin capsule. When gelling systems are used, the shells have a rough surface that also affects the transparency of an opacifier free shell composition. The typical shell wall thickness of two-piece capsules is in the range of 100–110 µm, with HPMC capsules being toward the lower end of the range and gelatin capsules at the higher end (Ku et al. 2010).

Irrespective of the composition and manufacturing process of the HPMC capsules, HPMC polymer typically accounts for 98–100% w/w of the base polymer material in the capsules. The equilibrium water content of the capsules is therefore equivalent to the water content of HPMC (Nokhodchi et al. 1997). The absorption and desorption curves of the capsules show similar hysteresis characteristics to gelatin capsules, with a typical water content being between 3% water (at around 30% relative humidity [RH]) and 9% water (at around 65% RH). The sorption isotherm data of HPMC and gelatin capsules are shown in Figure 5.1.

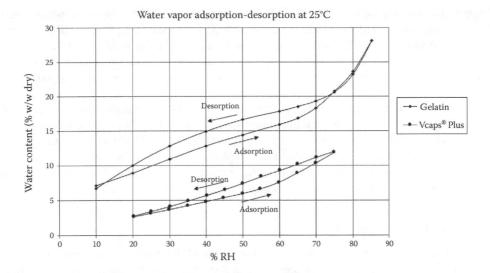

FIGURE 5.1 Sorption isotherm data (absorption and desorption) of gelatin and HPMC (Vcaps® Plus) capsules stored at different RH values. (Courtesy of Capsugel.)

The mechanical resistance and stiffness of two-piece capsules are important for its machinability and robustness in processing and handling. The mechanical resistance is dependent on the moisture content of the capsules (see Figure 5.2) and softening is observed with increasing moisture content in both types of capsules. In general, HPMC capsules tend to be less strong and more elastic compared to gelatin capsules, especially at higher moisture levels (Kuentz et al. 2006; Missaghi and Fassihi 2006). However, under dry conditions, HPMC capsules are more resistant to breakage compared to gelatin capsules and remain sufficiently flexible even at very low humidity (below 30% RH) where a gradual increase of breakage under mechanical stress conditions is observed for gelatin capsules (Ku et al. 2010). Because of this characteristic, HPMC capsules are used for products that are sensitive to moisture or which require low moisture levels during processing or storage.

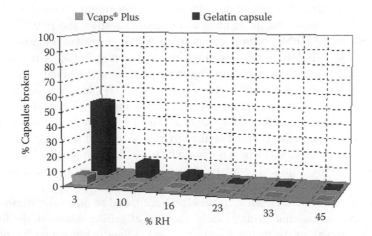

FIGURE 5.2 Mechanical properties of HPMC capsules (Vcaps® Plus) and gelatin capsules measured by the tube test method after storage at different RH values. (From Ku MS, Lu Q, Li W et al. Performance qualification of a new hypromellose capsule: Part II. Disintegration and dissolution comparison between two types of hypromellose capsules. *Int J Pharm* 2011; 416: 16–24.)

Despite the slightly higher elasticity and lower strength of HPMC capsules, when compared with gelatin capsules, HPMC capsules have a similar performance on high-speed filling machines. However, tests in which the different capsule types were run on filling machines from laboratory to commercial scale and at different machine speeds revealed that capsules manufactured by thermo-gelation have a superior performance compared to HPMC capsules containing a gelling system (Ku et al. 2010).

Accelerated stability testing has in addition shown that HPMC capsules are more inert in and resistant to residual solvents, higher temperature storage, and higher humidity conditions. In these tests, exposure of HPMC capsules to a 25-ppm (parts per million) aldehyde containing lactose blend for 1 week did not change the dissolution profile of capsules. Short-term storage at a high temperature of up to 90°C had no impact on the mechanical properties of the HPMC capsules or their disintegration and dissolution performance (Ku et al. 2010).

DISSOLUTION AND DISINTEGRATION

Capsule rupture and disintegration as well as dissolution of the empty capsule are important characteristics of the two-piece capsule dosage form as they determine the release and exposure of the drug formulation into the dissolution media. One of the basic differences between gelatin and HPMC capsules is a temperature-dependent dissolution profile of the gelatin capsule. Gelatin requires a temperature of 30°C to exhibit rapid disintegration and dissolution behavior, while HPMC dissolves independently of the temperature (Chiwele et al. 2000). By using a newly developed "dynamic open flow through test apparatus" that mimics flow rates, intragastric temperature, and gastric motility in fasted state conditions, no difference in the *in vitro* dissolution is seen between gelatin and tg-HPMC capsules when increasing the temperature slowly from 24°C to 37°C, mimicking the administration of a drug product with a glass of water. However, the application of the dynamic open flow through test apparatus also provided evidence for the importance of the intraluminal pressure caused by physiological gastric motility on capsule rupture and dissolution. Applying a short intragastric motility event after 10 min triggered product release from HPMC capsules (Garbacz et al. 2014).

The disintegration test according to the Pharmacopoeia requires the capsules to disintegrate in less than 15 min. As the disintegration test is quite unspecific, different researchers have investigated rupture time using a dissolution apparatus II with an in-line UV detector as a more precise method to determine the time point when the capsule opens and releases the content. The results from these studies confirm that gelatin capsules have a rapid rupture time of as little as 2 min in gastric or simulated intestinal media. In contrast to gelatin capsules, the HPMC capsule rupturing time is dependent on the HPMC capsule composition. HPMC capsules containing carrageenan as a gelling agent show a slightly faster rupturing time of 3–4 min in the gastric fluid compared to 6–8 min for HPMC capsules manufactured by thermo-gelation (El-Malah et al. 2007; Ku et al. 2011). However, in the study published by El-Malah et al. (2007), longer disintegration times were seen in simulated gastric fluids for the carrageenan containing HPMC capsules (6–10 min), which was not the case in the study performed by Ku et al. The longer rupturing time of HPMC capsules compared to the gelatin capsules is based on the different base polymer properties. HPMC requires more time to hydrate and dissolve, which is caused by the 3–5 min rupturing lag time. The lag time in the rupturing of HPMC capsules compared to gelatin capsules is also seen in the dissolution test (Figure 5.3).

The dissolution of different HPMC capsules has been found to differ significantly from type to type, depending on the manufacturing process, the type of gelling system in the formula, and the pH and the ionic strength of the media. Figure 5.4a shows the dissolution profile of a carrageenan gelling system containing c-HPMC capsule in different media. In a pH 6.8 USP phosphate buffer, the capsule shows a slow dissolution and simulated milk fluid, and the capsule rupture and release were delayed to about 30 min. These results are in accordance with the dissolution results of a previous study where the USP 7.2 phosphate buffer was considered as unsuitable for c-HPMC capsules

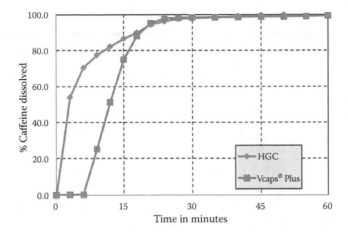

FIGURE 5.3 Dissolution profile of a fast-dissolving caffeine blend in gelatin (HGC) and HPMC (Vcaps® Plus) capsules at pH 1.2. (Courtesy of Capsugel.)

because of its slow release and was replaced by a pH 7.0 tribasic sodium phosphate buffer at 150 rpm in a USP basket dissolution test system (Honkanen et al. 2001). The delayed dissolution could also be observed in pH 1.2 media containing a high potassium concentration. The delayed dissolution profiles are believed to be caused by the interaction of the potassium cations and the carrageenan gelling polysaccharide and the pH dependence of the gel formation (Doyle et al. 2002). In Figure 5.4b, the dissolution profile of the pure HPMC capsule manufactured by thermo-gelation is shown. The rupture and dissolution time of these capsules are independent from the pH and cationic strength of the media and release occurs after 6–10 min consistently.

The dissolution profile of the c-HPMC capsules in a high-pH medium also shows a high variability between capsule types (Figure 5.5). These results are comparable to the results from the study by Ku et al. (2011) for a poorly soluble free acid compound that is ionized beyond the pKa of 4.7

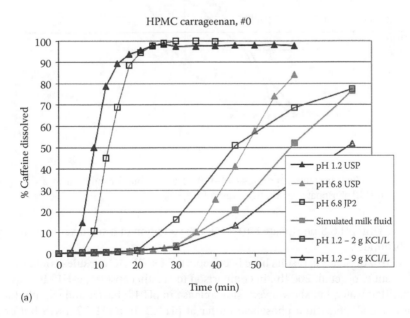

(a)

FIGURE 5.4 (See color insert.) Dissolution of a fast-dissolving caffeine formulation in different types of HPMC capsules. (a) HPMC capsule containing carrageenan as a gelling system. *(Continued)*

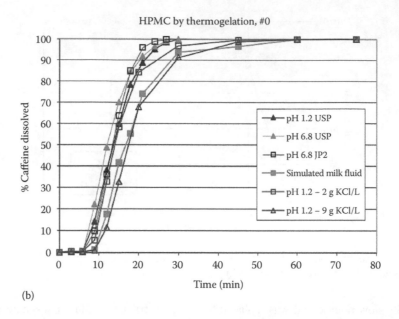

(b)

FIGURE 5.4 (CONTINUED) **(See color insert.)** Dissolution of a fast-dissolving caffeine formulation in different types of HPMC capsules. (b) HPMC capsule manufactured by thermo-gelation without any gelling system (Vcaps® Plus). (Courtesy of Capsugel.)

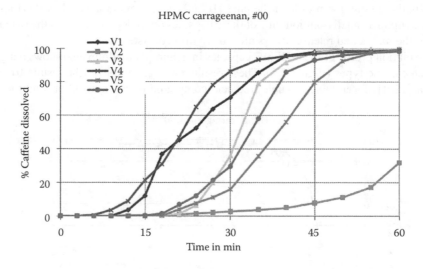

FIGURE 5.5 Individual dissolution profiles (V1–V6) of a caffeine formulation in a carrageenan HPMC capsules in pH 6.8 USP phosphate buffer. (Courtesy of Capsugel.)

when using the USP pH 6.8 phosphate buffer with the addition of a surfactant (hexadecyl trimethyl ammonium bromide).

Similar *in vitro* dissolution results have been reported for HPMC capsules containing gellan gum as a gelling agent (Cole et al. 2004b). In comparison to gelatin capsules, g-HPMC capsules dissolve rapidly in distilled water, but show a very slow release in pH 1.2 buffer and slightly longer dissolution time in the USP potassium phosphate buffer at pH 7.2. In a pH 7.2 TRIS buffer system, the g-HPMC capsules demonstrate the typical HPMC capsule lag time with a dissolution equivalent to the gelatin capsules starting somewhere in between 5 and 10 min (Cole et al. 2004b).

In Vivo Performance of HPMC Capsules

The first HPMC capsules introduced 20 years ago were manufactured by the traditional hard capsule process and contained either carrageenan (c-HPMC) or gellan gum (g-HPMC) as a gelling system. Since the introduction in 2007 of tg-HPMC capsules manufactured by thermo-gelation, the use of HPMC capsules in pharmaceutical development has gained substantial interest because of its demonstrated *in vivo* performance.

Investigations centered on the esophageal transit time of HPMC capsules have been performed with HPMC capsules containing carrageenan and gellan gum. A study by Honkanen et al. investigated the detachment forces of c-HPMC capsules and gelatin capsules *in vitro* using esophageal tissue derived from slaughterhouses (Honkanen et al. 2002). The results suggest that the detachment of gelatin capsules adhered to the isolated mucosa requires 2.5 times higher forces compared to the HPMC capsules. When the same group investigated the esophageal transit of a size 0 c-HPMC capsule in six healthy volunteers after two administrations each, the results showed that for four of the capsule administrations, there were esophageal residence times ranging from 22 to 143 min (Honkanen et al. 2004). However, these results have not been seen in other studies using gamma scintigraphy with either size 0 c-HPMC (Tuleu et al. 2007) or size 1 g-HPMC (Cole et al. 2004b). These studies found esophageal transit times for both types of HPMC capsules in the range of 10–20 s, which is also in agreement with the reported esophageal transit times of gelatin capsules. It should be noted that the esophageal transit of any solid dosage form depends on the size and shape of the dosage form, the position of the volunteer, and the amount of water provided upon administration (Stegemann et al. 2012). Honkanen suggested that the reason for the observation in their study might the incorrect water intake upon capsule administration by the four volunteers on the first day (Honkanen et al. 2004). Moreover, the protocol required capsule intake in a sitting position and then laying down in a supine position 30 s after administration, which could also have contributed to the long capsule residence times on four occasions.

The first *in vivo* studies performed with HPMC capsules were published in 2001 using c-HPMC capsules. Gelatin capsules and c-HPMC were filled with a 200-mg ibuprofen-containing lactose blend in size 0 capsules and compared in a single-dose, crossover bioequivalence test (Honkanen et al. 2001). The major pharmacokinetic parameters, AUC and C_{max}, were comparable for gelatin and c-HPMC capsules (AUC, 109 vs. 111 mg h/L; C_{max}, 39.7 vs. 38.6 mg/L) and t_{max} slightly increased from 1.19 h to 1.5 h, which is not statistically significant. Similar pharmacokinetic results have been observed for g-HPMC capsules when compared with gelatin capsules filled with 200 mg of ibuprofen formulated with a blend of microcrystalline cellulose and Mg-stearate in size 1 capsules administered in fasted and fed conditions (Cole et al. 2004b).

To understand the *in vivo* disintegration of HPMC capsules, gamma scintigraphy studies have been performed with c-HPMC and g-HPMC capsules. The initial disintegration time of c-HPMC capsules in a fasted state was investigated with powder fills of two different HPMC grades and found to be similar with 49 and 53 min (Honkanen et al. 2004). These times are longer than the times found for g-HPMC capsules with an initial disintegration time of 28 min (Cole et al. 2004b). As expected, the initial disintegration was increased in the fed state (standardized high-fat meal, 1300 kcal) for gelatin, as well as g-HPMC capsules to 23.4 min and 1, respectively. In contrast to these findings, recent studies suggest very short initial disintegration times for gelatin and c-HPMC capsules administered in fasted and fed conditions. In the fasted state, the initial disintegration time for gelatin and c-HPMC capsules was reported to be 7 min compared to 9 min in the fasted state (Tuleu et al. 2007) and 12 min compared to 16 min in the fed state. However, in these studies, the fed state was a breakfast of not more than 500 kcal and no information was provided about the time elapsed between breakfast and when the capsule was administered (Jones et al. 2012).

A comparative *in vivo* performance investigation between tg-HPMC capsules and gelatin capsules using a fast-releasing tablet (Excedrin Extra Strength caplets) with three different BDDCS class 1 drugs (acetylsalicylic acid, acetaminophen, and caffeine) as a marker has recently been reported. The study was a randomized, crossover study in 24 healthy and fasted subjects receiving either two Excedrin Extra Strength caplets overencapsulated in gelatin or tg-HPMC capsules. Despite the *in vitro* dissolution lag-time of 5–10 min between the gelatin and tg-HPMC capsules, the statistical analysis confirmed that the 90% confidence intervals for C_{max}, AUC_{0-t}, and $AUC_{0-\infty}$ are well within the range of 80–125.00% acetaminophen, aspirin (acetylsalicylic acid, total salicylates), and caffeine for comparison of the gelatin overencapsulated caplet and the HPMC capsule overencapsulated caplet (Stegemann et al. 2015).

Clinical studies have investigated tg-HPMC capsules for dabrafenib, a BCS class 2 compound and a weak base with pH-dependent dissolution characteristics, for its *in vitro* and *in vivo* performance in comparison to gelatin capsules. The *in vitro* dissolution of dabrafenib in FaSSGF at pH 1.6 measure over 24 h shows a three- to fourfold increase in the peak dissolution for the tg-HPMC capsule compared to gelatin and even though precipitation occurred after 2 to 3 h, the steady state above the drug dissolved with gelatin capsules. This higher solubility related to the precipitation inhibition effect of the tg-HPMC was reproduced *in vivo* under fasted conditions, which led to a 1.8- to 2.0-fold increase in the bioavailability of dabrafenib after a single dose in HPMC capsules compared to gelatin capsules (Ouellet et al. 2013).

A 180-subject crossover bioequivalence study carried out in 2013 compared the administration of a commercial 150-mg immediate-release formulation of dabigatran filled in either c-HPMC capsules containing a gelling system or tg-HPMC capsules manufactured by thermo-gelation (National Institutes of Health 2013). The dabigatran formulation filled in tg-HPMC capsule reached 125% of bioavailability of the c-HPMC capsules and reduced the geometric coefficient of variation from an average of 50% to 32%. As the main difference between the two HPMC capsules was the presence or absence of a gelling system (carrageenan), the results reflect the important *in vitro* findings of the pH- and ionic strength-dependent dissolution of the gelling system capsules *in vivo*.

SPECIAL APPLICATIONS OF HPMC CAPSULES

COATING OF HPMC CAPSULES

To achieve targeted intestinal drug delivery, capsule coating is being considered as a suitable option. Aqueous-based coating systems on HPMC capsules have been shown to achieve high performing functional coats because of their adhesion properties and resistance with regard to capsule softening or brittleness during processing. A recent study using scintigraphy to investigate coating performance described the coating of HPMC capsules based on two different types of coatings (Eudragit L 30 D-55 or Eudragit FS 30D at coating thicknesses of 6, 8, 10, and 12 mg/cm^2) (Cole et al. 2002).

In vitro dissolution test results confirm that the capsule coated with 6 and 8 mg/cm^2 Eudragit L 30 D-55 and 6, 8, and 10 mg/cm^2 Eudragit FS 30 D did not release the drug acetaminophen over 2 h at pH 1.2, but released rapidly at pH 6.8. The intestinal targeting of the coatings was demonstrated in a gamma-scintigraphy study in human volunteers whereby Eudragit L 30 D-55-coated capsules disintegrated completely in the small bowel and Eudragit FS 30 D-coated HPMC capsules disintegrated between the mid distal small intestine and the proximal colon while no release was seen in the stomach for either coating. This study establishes the *in vitro–in vivo* correlation and hence possibility for intestinal targeting through coated HPMC capsules (Cole et al. 2002).

HPMC CAPSULES FOR DRY POWDER INHALATION

Capsule-based dry powder inhalation (DPI) systems were introduced for the treatment of respiratory diseases approximately 45 years ago. The main elements of these drug delivery systems are the fine drug particles or drug particle–carrier interactive mixtures that are filled as a pre-metered dose into a capsule. For administration, the capsules containing the low therapeutic dose are administered directly to the respiratory system via an inhalation device. Because of the simplicity and cost-effectiveness of these platforms, capsule-based DPI systems remain the pulmonary delivery method of choice for new drugs and are gaining increasing popularity for the delivery of generic versions and new products launched in emerging markets (Stegemann et al. 2013).

In pulmonary DPI systems, the two-piece capsule plays an equally important role in product stability and performance as the drug or drug carrier interactive powder mixture and the device component. In general, the drug formulation is developed in a defined DPI device using a prequalified inhalation grade gelatin or HPMC capsule, which is then further optimized to achieve the desired fine particle drug release profile or product stability. With the introduction of HPMC capsules for DPI, several technological advantages that substantially extended the design space of capsule-based DPI systems were achieved.

Since fine drug particles of less than 5 μm size are normally very cohesive, interactive powder mixtures of the drug particles on coarse carriers of 30–100 μm size are used, whereby the fine drug particles are attached to the surface of the carrier. Upon activation, the fine drug particles have to detach from the coarse particles to be delivered to the deepest parts of the lungs. To develop capsules suitable for this application, the major quality attributes of the capsules to consider are moisture content, powder retention, and opening performance under shear force, piercing, or cutting.

The ability to adjustable moisture content of HPMC capsules at lower humidity levels, while maintaining shell flexibility upon mechanical impact, is one of the main features of HPMC capsules for DPI applications. The lower humidity levels prevent moisture affecting the formulations' stability and dispersibility over the capsule's shelf life. To minimize powder retention of the adhesive fine drug particles, the electrostatic charges can be reduced to a certain moisture level with the HPMC capsule. For each drug formulation and device combination, the optimal moisture range of the HPMC capsules can be determined and adjusted on a commercial scale. Further reduction of powder retention can be achieved by modifying manufacturing process parameters such as lubrication to achieve powder retention levels below 0.1% (Stegemann et al. 2014b).

CONCLUSION

The first HPMC capsules were introduced into the pharmaceutical market 20 years ago; since then, HPMC capsule technology has been applied to both pharmaceutical development and marketed products. The first types of HPMC capsules were manufactured using the traditional capsule manufacturing process, requiring the use of a gelling system within the HPMC shell formulation. The major limitation of gelling systems containing HPMC capsules is the capsule dissolution characteristic that is affected by pH, cations, and the ionic strength of the dissolution media and gastric and intestinal juice *in vivo*. In 2007, a new HPMC capsule that was manufactured with a modified hard capsule manufacturing technology became commercially available, which allowed the production of HPMC capsules by thermo-gelation. These HPMC capsules are manufactured from a pure aqueous HPMC solution without the addition of other components or gelling systems. HPMC capsules manufactured by thermo-gelation dissolve in all media according to the solubility characteristics of HPMC and dissolve consistently across all dissolution media. Compared to gelatin capsules, the initial rupture time of HPMC capsules has a lag time of approximately 5 min, normally releasing the content after 5–10 min, whereas release from gelatin capsules occurs after 2–3 min.

In vivo studies have confirmed rapid capsule dissolution of HPMC capsules in the gastrointestinal (GI) tract measured by gamma scintigraphy and bioavailability. There is some evidence that HPMC capsules manufactured by thermo-gelatin without the use of gelling systems can inhibit drug precipitation in the GI tract, increasing bioavailability as well as variability for certain drugs (National Institutes of Health 2013; Ouellet et al. 2013).

HPMC CAPSULES FOR DELAYED RELEASE

INTRODUCTION

Commercially available two-piece capsules have been developed for immediate-release applications as this is the requirement for most encapsulated drug products. With the increasing popularity and use of neutraceutical and dietary supplement products, there is a growing need for a delayed-release delivery in the stomach owing to the nature of these products that are either liquids such as fish oil or that cannot be processed or compressed, for example, probiotics.

IN VITRO DISSOLUTION OF DELAYED-RELEASE CAPSULES

The effect of gellan gum as a gelling system affecting the dissolution properties of an HPMC capsule has been further harnessed as a capsule that does not dissolve at a gastric pH of 1.2 over 2 h followed by a quick release in an intestinal pH of 6.8. Figure 5.6 shows the release of acetaminophen from delayed-release capsules (DRcaps™) using the dissolution test method described for extended-release dosage forms.

To demonstrate the protective effect of the delayed-release capsules on probiotic bacteria that are moisture and pH sensitive, gelatin and delayed-release HPMC capsules were filled with a strain of *Bifidobacterium longum* and investigated using the Simulator of the Human Intestinal Microbial Ecosystem (SHIME®) technology. The filled capsules were exposed to standardized simulated gastric conditions for 60 min and then gradually switched to small intestinal conditions for 3 h. The survival rate of the bacteria, determined as intact colony-forming units (CFU), revealed a fast dissolution inactivated *Bifidobacterium* under conditions found in the stomach within the first 30 min, whereas the delayed-release capsules protected the bacteria in the gastric mimic conditions and released approximately 60% active *Bifidobacterium* in conditions found in the small intestinal (Figure 5.7).

IN VIVO PERFORMANCE OF DELAYED-RELEASE CAPSULES

The *in vitro* performance of the delayed-release capsules suggests that the capsules remain sufficiently intact in the acidic environment of the stomach and dissolve only when they move to the

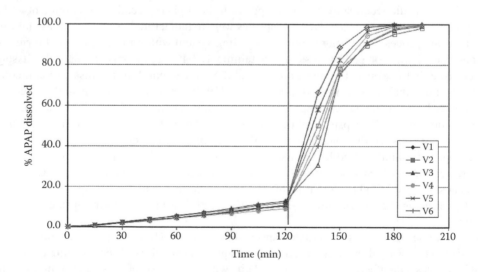

FIGURE 5.6 Individual capsule dissolution profiles (V1–V6) of acetaminophen (APAP) in DRcaps™ ($n = 6$) exposed for 2 h to pH 1.2 followed by exposure to a pH 6.8 phosphate buffer. (Courtesy of Capsugel.)

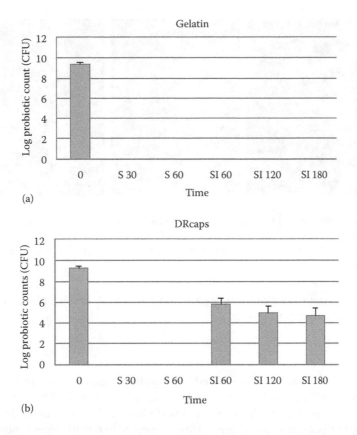

FIGURE 5.7 *Bifidobacterium longum* stability in (a) gelatin and (b) delayed-release capsules (DRcaps) incubated for 30 and 60 min in conditions found in the stomach (S) and then for 60, 120, and 180 min in conditions found in the small intestinal (SI).

intestine. To evaluate the impact of potential release through the space between cap and body under *in vivo* conditions, a preliminary gamma scintigraphy study was performed. For this study, filled delayed-release HPMC capsules [DRcaps™] were radiolabeled and either closed or closed and banded with cellulose acetate phthalate. The delayed-release capsules were administered 30 min after a light meal (~500 kcal) in a crossover design to assure sufficient residence of the capsules in the stomach, and scintigrams were taken every 5 min for up to 4 h post-dosing. The first release from the unbanded capsules was observed after 51.9 ± 16.6 min and that from the banded capsules was observed after 82.3 ± 33.2 min, suggesting that capsule banding maintains capsule integrity in the GI tract, preventing capsule caps and bodies from separating or releasing their contents through the cap and body overlap. Release from the capsules began in the stomach of five subjects in the unbanded delayed-release group. A complete release of capsule contents in the stomach was seen in only two of these subjects, and for the other six subjects, complete release of capsule contents took place in the intestine (Figure 5.8). For the banded capsules, the results showed two subjects with complete dissolution in the intestine, while one had onset of release in the stomach but complete release in the intestine and five had onset and complete release in the intestine (Hodges et al. 2014).

A 2014 study evaluated the protective effect of delayed-release HPMC capsules on fecal microflora of healthy volunteers when administered to patients with recurrent and refractory *Clostridium difficile* infection. For the fecal microbiota transplantation, the healthy fecal microflora were suspended, filled into delayed-release capsules, and frozen to –80°C. An *in vitro* evaluation confirmed that the delayed-release capsules remained intact for 115 min in up to pH 3 media. Confirmation of

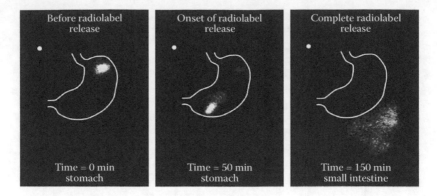

FIGURE 5.8   (See color insert.) Gammascintigraphy images of delayed-release capsules (DRcaps™, banded). (From Hodges LA, Connolly S, Cade D et al. Novel HPMC Capsules Display Acid Resistance Behaviour—A Scintigraphic Imaging Study: A Joint Presentation with Capsugel and Bio-Images. 2014. AAPS Annual Meeting, Poster W5137.)

the delivery of the intact microflora was confirmed by an overall ceasing of diarrhea in 90% of the patients (Youngster et al. 2014).

CONCLUSION

Delayed-release capsules have been developed to delay the release of the product in the GI tract. The capsules are based on the slow dissolution and release at low pH of HPMC capsules using gelling systems. *In vitro* and *in vivo* investigations into performance show that unbanded delayed-release capsules remain undissolved for more than 50 min compared to 80 min when banded. *In vitro* and *in vivo* studies confirm the protective effect of this capsule type on living organisms such as probiotics and fecal microflora. The capsules remain intact in the low pH of the stomach environment and only release their contents in the higher pH conditions of the small intestine.

PULLULAN-BASED TWO-PIECE CAPSULES

INTRODUCTION

Pullulan is polysaccharide derived by fermentation of starch. It is recognized as safe by the US Food and Drug Administration for use in food and pharmaceutical products (GRAS status). Pullulan has been identified as a suitable polymer for the commercial manufacturing of two-piece capsules using the traditional capsule manufacturing process of the addition of a gelling system.

Pullulan is a saccharide polymer that is derived from starch by a fermentation process using the fungus *Aureobasidium pullulans*. The fermentation leads to maltotriose units that are consecutively connected to each other by an α-1,6 glycosidic bond. Pullulan is widely used in the food industry and for the manufacturing of orodispersible films (e.g., Listerine film strips).

PULLULAN CAPSULE PROPERTIES

Pullulan capsules (e.g., Plantcaps®) are composed of pullulan and carrageenan as a gelling system. Pullulan capsules have a water content of approximately 2% below that of gelatin capsules and follow the same trend in the sorption isotherm (Figure 5.9).

The mechanical properties of pullulan capsules similar to those of gelatin capsules are dependent on the water content of the capsule shells. When stored at dry RH conditions (below RH 30%) over a period of many days, the capsule shows a comparable gradual increase in brittleness as gelatin capsules.

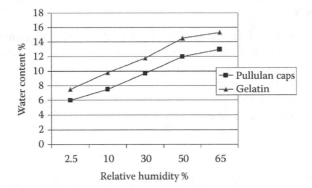

FIGURE 5.9 Sorption isotherm of gelatin and pullulan capsules (Plantcaps®) between an RH of 2.5% and 65%. (Courtesy of Capsugel.)

IN VITRO DISSOLUTION

The *in vitro* dissolution of pullulan capsules has been found to be similar to that of c-HPMC because the dissolution property is dependent on the carrageenan used as the gelling system. As can be seen in Figure 5.10, which shows dissolution times in the discriminatory buffer systems at pH 7.2, the dissolution of the pullulan capsules is mainly delayed in the potassium phosphate buffer system, which is also seen for the gelatin capsules (Figure 5.10).

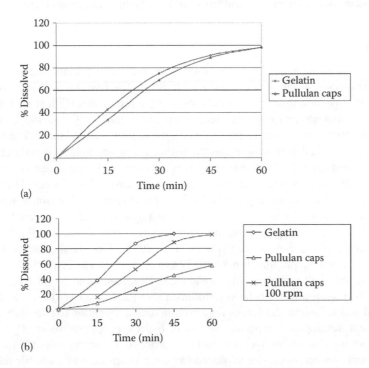

FIGURE 5.10 Dissolution profile of gelatin and pullulan capsules (Plantcaps®) in (a) sodium phosphate buffer pH 7.2 and (b) potassium phosphate buffer pH 7.2 at 50 and 100 rpm. (Courtesy of Capsugel.)

In Vivo Performance

The *in vivo* performance of pullulan capsules has been investigated with gamma scintigraphy under fasted conditions in eight healthy volunteers. The study found that the mean esophageal transit times were slightly faster for the pullulan capsules than for gelatin capsules (6.2 ± 1.4 s compared with 8.0 ± 4.6 s, respectively), while the initial disintegration time was similar between pullulan and gelatin capsules (0.15 ± 0.06 h compared with 0.13 ± 0.06 h, respectively) and occurred within 8–9 min after administration (Cole et al. 2004a).

CONCLUSION

Pullulan capsules are starch-based capsules with properties that are closely related to gelatin capsules. Pullulan capsules contain carrageenan as a gelling system, which gives the capsules a similar *in vitro* dissolution property to that of c-HPMC capsules. Initial *in vivo* studies have confirmed that pullulan capsules have a rapid esophageal transit time and *in vivo* disintegration similar to those of gelatin capsules.

INVESTIGATIONAL NON-GELATIN POLYMER CAPSULES

The traditional hard and soft capsule manufacturing was based on the unique gelling and film casting properties of gelatin that allowed hard capsule manufacturing through the traditional dip molding process as well as the soft capsule manufacturing by rotary die technology. Over the past decades, substantial research and development efforts have been invested to find alternative polymers to replace or add on the gelatin in soft or hard capsules. The major non-gelatin polymers that have been investigated for the manufacturing of hard and soft capsules are plant-derived hydrocolloids like starch, modified starch, and cellulose derivatives as well as polyvinyl alcohol, a synthetic polymer that shows relevant thermoplastic behaviors under mechanical stress under certain humidity and temperature conditions.

Hard Capsules

Injection molding is a process widely used in the manufacture of pharmaceutical components and lately in drug delivery systems as well (Zema et al. 2012). The first starch-based two-piece capsule manufacturing by injection molding was published in the mid-1980s (Eith et al. 1986, 1987). They used potato starch that was processed at a temperature between 120°C and 180°C and at a pressure between 700 and 2000 bar during the injection into the capsule-shaped mold. The molds were then cooled down and the shell forms were ejected within a few seconds (Viliviala et al. 2000). The capsules were manufactured in five different sizes, whereby only the length of the body differed from each other, allowing the use of the same cap-part dimension for all sizes. The main difference compared to the standard gelatin capsule is the different closing mechanism, whereby dip-molded gelatin capsules are closed by mechanical locking ring systems and the injected molded capsules need to be sealed by the filling machine utilizing a hydroalcoholic sealing fluid that was applied to the inner surface of the capsule cap (Burns et al. 1996). Despite the fact that these capsules were evaluated *in vitro* (Stepto and Tomka 1987) and *in vivo* (Burns et al. 1996; Doll et al. 1993), including their suitability for coating (Watts and Illum 1997) and lipid-based drug delivery systems (Burns et al. 1996), no product has been introduced into the market yet because of the remaining pharmaceutical and technical challenges for a commercial application to pharmaceutical products.

Another recent development reported the use of hydroxypropyl cellulose (HPC) for two-piece capsule manufacturing using an injection molding process. These capsules take advantage of the HPC swelling and erosion properties in order to achieve a capsule with pulsatile release characteristics. The release characteristics can be modified using different grades of HPC, and the shell wall thickness can be modified as well in a range between 300 and 900 μm. The capsules by itself, when filled with acetaminophen and sealed by application of an HPC solution on the cap and body junction, showed a thickness-dependent lag time in dissolution ranging from about 15 to 70 min for the 300- and 900-μm shell thickness, respectively (Gazzaniga et al. 2011). In a successive trial, the same group applied different levels of Eudragit L30 D 55 through spray coating to sealed and unsealed capsules, demonstrating further delay in the *in vitro* dissolution, suggesting its suitability for colonic drug delivery (Macchi et al. 2015). Further studies will be required to prove its clinical performance and technical feasibility on a commercial scale.

Soft Capsules

As for hard capsules, starch- and starch derivative–based shell compositions have been investigated for the soft capsule manufacturing using the rotary die process. This requires a polymer composition that combines film-forming properties with sealing or fusion capabilities in the rotary die process, for example, by temperature-dependent gel/sol transformation.

Potato starch has been used as the base polymer in a starch, amylopectin, and glycerol formulation by casting a nearly water-free film by a hot melt extrusion process (Menard et al. 1999). Others have suggested modified starch, primarily hydroxypropylated acid-modified corn starch formulated with iota- (Tanner et al. 2002) or iota- and kappa-carrageenan (Fonkwe et al. 2005) for the manufacturing of soft gelatin capsules in a rotary die process. However, despite the description in patents and introduction of starch capsules to the food market in 2000 by Swiss Caps as VegaGels, no further pharmaceutical or scientific data on the evaluation or performance of these capsules have been reported in the literature.

Polyvinyl alcohol (PVA) is a water-soluble, synthetic polymer with good film-forming properties (Brown 1996). To overcome the limitation of the lack of gel formation properties that are required in the conventional rotary die process, PVA has been formulated with polyols as plasticizers like glycerol or sorbitol that allow scaling of the films in a rotary die at 140–180°C (Meier 2001). A new composition of PVA soft capsules has recently been proposed for the use of hydrophilic self-microemulsifying drug delivery systems by the addition of potato starch to the PVA thermoplastic composition. At a starch, PVA, and plasticizer ratio of 40:30:30% (w/w), ribbons were extruded at 135°C and fed into the rotary die process for capsule manufacturing (Misic et al. 2012). Even though these capsules had a superior performance in terms of water migration, preventing drug crystallization, as well as good performance in other physical drug product characteristics, the capsules did not meet the expectations in the *in vitro* drug release using biorelevant media (Misic et al. 2014).

CONCLUSION

Replacing gelatin by non-gelatin polymers for hard and soft capsule manufacturing remains a major challenge for the investigational new polymers. Progress has been made in hard capsule manufacturing through the application of injection molding technology. The development of thermoplastic film compositions based on starch, modified starch, and polyvinyl alcohols advanced non-gelatin soft capsule manufacturing. The fundamentals of these developments have already been established 20–30 years ago, but they have not yet found entry into the pharmaceutical market. The major reasons are the remaining issues in up-scaling to a commercially viable process and some remaining challenges in the consistent bioperformance of the resulting capsules and capsule products as well as potential advantages compared to the existing alternative capsules and dosage forms.

APPLICATIONS OF NON-GELATIN-BASED CAPSULES

For nearly 100 years, gelatin has been the gold standard base material for the development and manufacture of two-piece hard capsules. Two-piece hard capsules have been applied to a variety of pharmaceutical products and drug delivery technologies, including immediate-release dry forms, modified-release multiparticulates, liquid and semisolid formulations, fixed dose combinations, and pulmonary drug delivery systems. To broaden the usage and application of two-piece capsules for advanced drug delivery, product development, and manufacturing, innovative technologies and materials that offer new features and technological options have been developed and brought to market.

As a result of capsule development programs, HPMC capsules were introduced and optimized to overcome the pH- and ionic strength-dependent dissolution characteristics. HPMC capsules were initially used with neutraceuticals and dietary supplement products to increase product stability and provide animal-free options for the vegetarian sector of the population or those consumers that require gelatin-free options on religious grounds. For pharmaceutical products, HPMC capsules were initially used for developing moisture-sensitive drugs or immediate-release oral drug formulations. The advantage of reducing and maintaining moisture content in HPMC capsules at low moisture levels has also been found to be beneficial for use with modified-release multiparticulate dosage forms and sophisticated drug delivery technologies. With the increasing focus on capsule-based DPI systems, HPMC capsules have gained substantial popularity as they can be customized to provide the optimal performance combination of low dose and fine particle delivery to the lungs.

Delayed-release capsules have been applied for development and manufacturing of nutraceuticals and dietary supplement products and particularly to prevent the regurgitation of products that taste or smell unpleasant, and to protect acid-sensitive products such as probiotics. For the latter, delayed-release HPMC capsules provide a dual advantage owing to the possibility of low moisture required for the stability of probiotics and acid protection after administration for the survival in the gastric environment of the stomach. Even though there is not a marketed pharmaceutical product developed in delayed-release capsules to date, the capsules have been used successfully in the early development of new products.

Pullulan capsules are the latest addition to the range of commercially available two-piece non-gelatin capsules. Currently, they are used primarily in the nutraceuticals and dietary supplement market.

ACKNOWLEDGMENT

I would like to thank Dominique Cade (Director Chemical R&D, Capsugel) and Keith Hutchison (Senior Vice President R&D, Capsugel) for their scientific support of this manuscript.

REFERENCES

Brown MD. 1996. WO 1997035537.
Burns SJ, Corness D, Hay G et al. An in vitro assessment of liquid-filled Capill potato starch capsules with biphasic release characteristics. *Int J Pharm* 1996; 134: 223–230.
Cade D, He X. 2008. Patent WO 2008/050209 A1.
Chiwele I, Jones BE, Podczeck F. The shell dissolution of various empty hard capsules. *Chem Pharm Bull* 2000; 48(7): 951–956.
Cole ET, He X, Scott RA et al. In vivo characteristics of pullulan, a new material for two-piece capsules. 2004a. AAPS poster.
Cole ET, Scott RA, Cade D et al. In vitro and in vivo pharmacoscintigraphic evaluation of ibuprofen hypromellose and gelatin capsules. *Pharm Res* 2004b; 21(5): 793–798.
Cole ET, Scott RA, Connor AL et al. Enteric coated HPMC capsules designed to achieve intestinal targeting. *Int J Pharm* 2002; 231: 83–95.
Colton A. 1931. U.S. Patent 1,787,777 and British Patent 360,427.
Djabourov M, Grillon Y, Leblond J. The sol–gel transition in gelatin viewed by diffusing colloidal probes. *Polym Gels Netw* 1995; 3: 407–428.
Doll WJ, Sandefer EP, Page RC et al. A scintigraphic and pharmacokinetic evaluation of a novel capsule manufactured from potato starch compared with a conventional hard gelatin capsule in normal and in normal subjects administered omeprazole. *Pharm Res* 1993; 10 (10 Suppl): S213.

Dorvault SLM. 1923. L'officine ou répertoire général de pharmacie pratique, Paris, Vigot Fères, 504.

Doyle J, Giannouli P, Philp K et al. 2002. Effect of K^+ and Ca^{2+} cations on gelation of k-carrageenan. In GO Phillips and PA Williams (eds.), *Gums and Stabilisers for the Food Industry 11*, Royal Society of Chemistry, Cambridge, UK, 158–164.

Eith L, Stepto RFT, Tomka I et al. The injection-moulded capsule. *Drug Dev Ind Pharm* 1986; 12: 2113–2126.

Eith L, Stepto RFT, Tomka I. Injection moulded drug-delivery systems. *Manuf Chem* 1987; 58(1): 21–25.

El-Malah Y, Nazzal S, Bottom CB. Hard gelatin and hypromellose (HPMC) capsules: Estimation of rupture time by real-time dissolution spectroscopy. *Drug Dev Ind Pharm* 2007; 33(1): 27–34.

Fonkwe LG, Archibald DA, Gennadios A. 2005. Patent US6949256.

Funami T, Hiroe M, Noda S et al. Influence of molecular structure imaged with atomic force microscopy on the rheological behavior of carrageenan aqueous systems in the presence or absence of cations. *Food Hydrocolloids* 2007; 21: 617–629.

Garbacz G, Cade D, Benameur H et al. Bio-relevant dissolution testing of hard capsules prepared from different shell materials using the dynamic open flow through test apparatus. *Eur J Pharm Sci* 2014; 57: 264–272.

Gazzaniga A, Cerea M, Cozzi A et al. A novel injection-molded capsular device for oral pulsatile delivery based on swellable/erodible polymers. *AAPS PharmSciTech* 2011; 12(1): 295–303.

Haque A, Richardson RK, Morris ER et al. Thermogelation of methylcellulose. Part II: Effect of hydroxypropyl substitution. *Carbohydr Polym* 1993; 22: 175–186.

Hodges LA, Connolly S, Cade D et al. Novel HPMC Capsules Display Acid Resistance Behaviour— A Scintigraphic Imaging Study: A Joint Presentation with Capsugel and Bio-Images. 2014. AAPS Annual Meeting, Poster W5137.

Honkanen O, Janne M, Kanerva H et al. Gamma scintigraphy evaluation of the fate of hydroxypropyl methylcellulose capsules in the human gastrointestinal tract. *Eur J Pharm Sci* 2004; 21: 671–678.

Honkanen O, Laaksonen P, Marvola J et al. Bioavailability and in vitro oesophageal sticking tendency of hydroxypropyl methylcellulose capsule formulations and corresponding gelatin capsule formulation. *Eur J Pharm Sci* 2002; 15: 479–488.

Honkanen O, Seppä H, Erikäinen S, Tuominen et al. Bioavailability of ibuprofen from orally and rectally administered hydroxypropyl methyl cellulose capsules compared to corresponding gelatine capsules. *STP Pharma Sci* 2001; 11: 181–185.

Jones BE, Basit AW, Tuleu C. The disintegration behavior of capsules in fed subjects: A comparison of hypromellose (carrageenan) capsules and standard gelatin capsules. *Int J Pharm* 2012; 424: 40–43.

Joshi SC. Sol-gel behavior of hydroxypropyl methylcellulose (HPMC) in ionic media including drug release. *Materials* 2011; 4: 1891–1905.

Ku MS, Li W, Dulin W et al. Performance qualification of a new hypromellose capsule: Part I. Comparative evaluation of physical, mechanical and processability quality attributes of Vcaps Plus, Quali-V and gelatin capsules. *Int J Pharm* 2010; 386: 30–41.

Ku MS, Lu Q, Li W et al. Performance qualification of a new hypromellose capsule: Part II. Disintegration and dissolution comparison between two types of hypromellose capsules. *Int J Pharm* 2011; 416: 16–24.

Kuentz M, Rothenhäusler B, Röthlisberger D. Time domain H NMR as a new method to monitor softening of gelatin and HPMC capsule shells. *Drug Dev Ind Pharm* 2006; 32(10): 1165–1173.

Li CL, Martini LG, Ford JL et al. The use of hypromellose in oral drug delivery. *J Pharm Pharmacol* 2005; 57: 533–546.

Macchi E, Zema L, Maroni A et al. Enteric-coating of pulsatile-release capsules prepared by injection molding. *Eur J Pharm Sci* 2015; 70: 1–11.

Meier H-J. 2001. Patent WO 2001066082.

Menard R, Tomka I, Engel WD et al. 1999. Patent WO 0 137 817.

Misic Z, Muffler K, Sydow et al. Novel starch-based PVA thermoplastic capsules for hydrophilic lipid-based formulations. *J Pharm Sci* 2012; 101(12): 4516–4528.

Misic Z, Urbani R, Pfohl T, Muffler et al. Understanding biorelevant drug release from a novel thermoplastic capsule by considering microstructural formulation changes during hydration. *Pharm Res* 2014; 31: 194–203.

Missaghi S, Fassihi R. Evaluation and comparison of physicomechanical characteristics of gelatin and hypromellose capsules. *Drug Dev Ind Pharm* 2006; 32(7): 829–838.

Moritaka H, Nishinari K, Taki M et al. Effects of pH, potassium chloride, and sodium chloride on the thermal and rheological properties of gellan gum gels. *J Agric Food Chem* 1995; 43(6): 1685–1689.

Morris ER, Rees DA, Robinson G. Cation-specific aggregation of carrageenan helices: Domain model of polymer gel structure. *J Mol Biol* 1980; 138: 349–362.

National Institutes of Health. 2013. Clinical trials NCT 01290757: Bioequivalence of two different capsule types of dabigatran. http://clinicaltrials.gov/ct2/show/NCT01290757

Nokhodchi A, Ford JL, Rubinstein MH. Studies on the interaction between water and (hydroxypropyl)methylcellulose. *J Pharm Sci* 1997; 86(5): 608–615.

Ouellet D, Grossmann KF, Limentani G et al. Effects of particle size, food, and capsule shell composition on the oral bioavailability of dabrafenib, a BRAF inhibitor, in patients with BRAF mutation-positive tumors. *J Pharm Sci* 2013; 102(9): 3100–3109.

Sarkar N. Thermal gelation properties of methyl and hydroxypropyl methylcellulose. *J Appl Polym Sci* 1979; 1073–1087.

Silva SM, Pinto FV, Antunes FE et al. Aggregation and gelation in hydroxypropylmethyl cellulose aqueous solutions. *J Colloid Interface Sci* 2008; 327(2): 333–340.

Stegemann S, Cade D, Tardy C. Improving pulmonary drug delivery in capsule inhaler systems: Optimizing capsules based on formulation–capsule-device interactions. *Respiratory Drug Delivery Asia* 2014b; 1: 25–32.

Stegemann S, Connolly P, Matthew W et al. Application of QbD principles for the evaluation of capsules in formulation development and manufacturing. *PharmSciTech* 2014a; 15(3): 542–549.

Stegemann S, Gosch M, Breitkreutz J. Swallowing dysfunction and dysphagia is an unrecognized challenge for oral drug therapy. *Int J Pharm* 2012; 430: 197–206.

Stegemann S, Kopp S, Borchard G et al. Developing and advancing dry powder inhalation towards enhanced therapeutics. *Eur J Pharm Sci* 2013; 48: 181–194.

Stegemann S, Vishwanath S, Kumar R et al. Comparative human in-vivo dissolution of an immediate release tablet over-encapsulated by gelatin and hydroxypropyl methyl cellulose capsules—Impact of dissolution rate on bioequivalence. *Am Pharm Rev* 2015; 11/12: 38–45.

Stepto RFT, Tomka I. Injection moulding of natural hydrophilic polymers in the presence of water. *Chimia* 1987; 41: 76–81.

Tanner KE, Drapper PB, Getz JJ et al. 2002. Patent US6340473.

Tuleu C, Khela MK, Evans DF, Jones BE et al. A scintigraphic investigation of the disintegration behaviour of capsules in fasting subjects: A comparison of hypromellose capsules containing carrageenan as a gelling agent and standard gelatin capsules. *Eur J Pharm Sci* 2007; 30: 251–255.

Viliviala VD, Illum L, Iqbal K. Starch capsules: An alternative system for oral drug delivery. *PSTT* 2000; 3(2): 64–69.

Watts PJ, Illum L. Colonic drug delivery. *Drug Dev Ind Pharm* 1997; 23: 893–913.

Youngster I, Russel GH, Pindar C et al. Oral, capsulized, frozen fecal microbiota transplantation for relapsing clostridium difficile infection. *JAMA* 2014; 312: 1772–1778.

Zema L, Loreti G, Melocchi A et al. Injection molding and its application to drug delivery. *J Contr Rel* 2012; 159: 324–331.

6 Hard Shell Capsule Filling Machines

Donald K. Lightfoot

CONTENTS

INTRODUCTION

The history of capsule filling started in the United States around 1900 as a result of the development of large-scale manufacture of hard gelatin capsules. Many US pharmacists began manually filling capsules using devices composed of a funnel to fill the powder into the capsule body and a spring-loaded plunger to compact the powder. Modern high-speed capsule filling machines evolved from these devices.[1]

This chapter will describe the various types of capsule filling machines, their operations, processes and capabilities, and various types of capsule filling support equipment currently in use.

OPERATIONS COMMON TO ALL CAPSULE FILLING MACHINES[2]

FEEDING AND RECTIFICATION

Capsules fall by gravity into feeding tubes or chutes (Figure 6.1). The capsules are uniformly aligned by mechanically gauging the diameter differences between the cap and the body. The rectified capsules are then fed, in proper orientation, into a two-section housing or bushing.

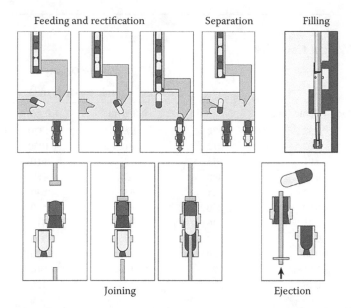

Feeding and rectification Separation Filling

Joining Ejection

FIGURE 6.1 Basic operations common to all filling machines. (Courtesy of IMA ACTIVE division, Bologna, Italy.)

Separation

The diameter of the upper bushing or housing is larger than the diameter of the capsule body bushing; therefore, the capsule cap is retained within the upper bushing while the body is pulled into the lower bushing by vacuum. Once the capsule is opened/separated, the upper and lower housing or bushing is separated to position the capsule body for filling.

Filling

The open capsule body is then dosed with the medicament. The various types of filling mechanisms are described in detail in "Capsule Filling Machine Dosing Systems" section.

Joining and Ejection

The cap and body housings or bushings are then realigned for capsule closing. An upper plate or pin will hold the cap stationary in the housing while lower closing shaft rods will push the bodies upward into the caps until the capsules are completely joined, engaging the locking mechanism of the capsule shell. The lower closing rod or shaft will ascend, ejecting the capsule from the housing or bushing into an exit chute. Compressed air nozzles are frequently used to assist the ejection of capsules from the machine, particularly with fully automatic filling machines.

CAPSULE FILLING MACHINE DOSING SYSTEMS

Capsule filling machines employ a variety of mechanisms to handle the various dosage ingredients. In every case, the dosing systems are based on volumetric fills governed by the capsule size and capacity of the capsule body. The empty capsule manufacturers provide reference tables (e.g., Table 6.1[3]) that indicate the volume capacity of their capsule body and the maximum fill weight for each capsule size based on the density of the fill material.

TABLE 6.1
Calculated Fill Weight Capacity

Capsule Size	Body Volume (mL)	Powder Density Capsule Capacity (mg)			
		0.6 g/mL	0.8 g/mL	1.0 g/mL	1.2 g/mL
000	1.37	822	1096	1370	1644
00el	1.02	612	816	1020	1224
00	0.91	546	728	910	1092
0	0.78	468	624	780	936
1el	0.54	324	432	540	648
1	0.50	300	400	500	600
2el	0.41	246	328	410	492
2	0.37	222	296	370	444
3	0.30	180	240	300	360
4	0.21	126	168	210	252
5	0.13	78	104	130	156

Source: Capsugel. Coni-Snap Hard Gelatin Capsules. 2011. Brochure: Data obtained from p. 16.

POWDERS

When calculating maximum fill weights for powder fills, the tapped density values for the specified powder should be used. The following dosing methods are employed.

Auger Fill Method

The auger fill method (Figure 6.2[4]) is employed by most of the semiautomatic capsule filling machines. A rotating auger blade at the discharge of the drug hopper forces the powder through a feed shoe into the open capsule bodies housed in a rotating ring beneath the drug hopper. The filling of the capsule is primarily volumetric.[5] The factors controlling the dosing volume are the rotation speed of the body ring, the rotation speed and design or pitch of the auger, and the level of powder within the drug hopper reservoir.

Mechanical Vibration Filling Method

The mechanical vibration method (Figure 6.3[6]) is employed specifically by Qualicaps filling machines. A level sensor located in the powder supply chute maintains a stable powder layer that fills directly into the capsule body facilitated by a vibration plate. The accuracy of the filled powder is improved by the use of an adjustable spring plunger that removes air from the powder, creating uniform density. A scraper removes any excess fill material before capsule joining.

Dosator Method

The dosator principle (Figure 6.4) is employed by numerous fully automatic capsule filling machines. The dosator consists of a hollow metal tube with a spring-loaded adjustable piston that is volumetrically adjusted to capture the powder dose. The dosator descends into a rotating dosing bowl of powder that is being maintained at a constant level. Once the dosator reaches the bottom of the powder bed, the powder dose is pre-compressed and then the piston moves downward, compressing the powder to form a plug. The dosator moves out of the powder bed and then aligns over the open capsule body. The piston descends to the bottom of the dosing tube, discharging the dosage plug into the capsule body.[7] In the case of the IMA ACTIVE dosator system, the rotary dosing bowl can be configured with a patented vacuum system for pre-compacting fine powders to create a uniform powder bed density.[8]

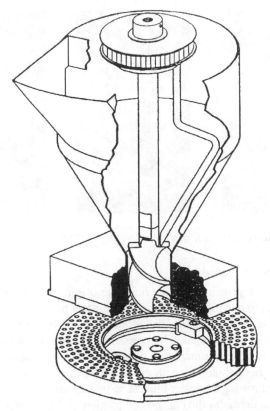

FIGURE 6.2   Auger fill method. (From Warner Lambert Co. Capsugel Division. Operation and Maintenance of the Type 8 Capsule Filling Machine. Capsugel Publication. Morris Plains, NJ; 1989.)

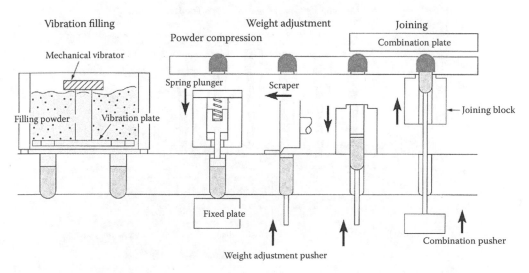

FIGURE 6.3   **(See color insert.)** Mechanical vibration filling method. (From Qualicaps. LIQFIL super 40. Brochure. Whitsett, NC; 2011.)

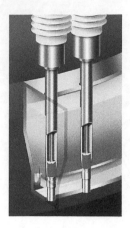
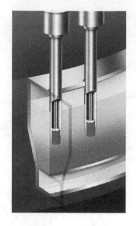
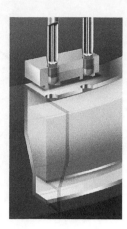

FIGURE 6.4 **(See color insert.)** Dosator method. (Courtesy of IMA ACTIVE division, Bologna, Italy.)

Tamping Pin/Dosing Disc Method

The tamping pin/dosing disc principle (Figure 6.5[9]) was originally developed by Höfliger and Karg and is now utilized on numerous fully automatic, intermittent motion capsule filling machines. The method consists of a rotating steel dosing disc mounted at the base of a dosing bowl. The dosing disc has six sets of precisely bored holes. The powder is metered into the dosing bowl via an auger from a powder supply hopper to maintain a consistent powder level above the dosing disc. As the rotating dosing disc indexes the holes beneath five sets of spring-loaded tamping pins, the powder is compressed in the bores, forming a powder plug. A stationary tamping ring seated below the dosing disc retains the powder in the holes during the compaction of the powder plug. After five tamps, a deflector isolates the powder from the disc as the holes index directly over the open capsule bodies. A set of transfer pins push the powder plug out of the holes into the capsule bodies.[10] Weight control on a tamping pin machine is controlled by three basic steps: (1) selecting the proper thickness of the dosing disc for the density and fill weight of the powder being run, (2) proper tamping penetration station settings, and (3) the height of the powder within the dosing bowl.

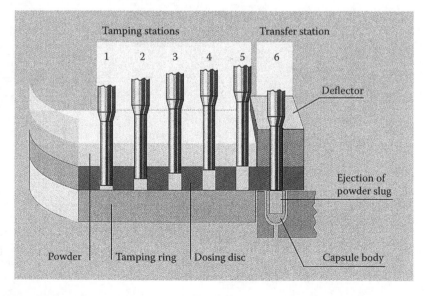

FIGURE 6.5 Tamping pin/dosing disc method. (From Harro Hofliger Packaging Systems. Modular filling and closing machine for capsules. Modu-C Mid-Speed (MS). 2010. Brochure.)

Drum Filler Method

The dose of powder is metered by dosing bores in a vacuum drum, which is rotating at the base of a powder bed (Figure 6.6[9]). A scraper blade removes any excess powder on the drum surface as it exits the powder bed. The powder dose is retained in the dosing bores by vacuum until it is discharged into the capsule body. This method is employed by the Harro Höfliger capsule filling machines for dosing powders in the micro-dose filling range with a fill amount of 1 mg and upward.

Compression Filling Method

The compression filling method (Figure 6.7[11]) is employed by certain models of Qualicaps filling machines. It is a modified version of the Tamping Pin/Dosing Disc method that employs four

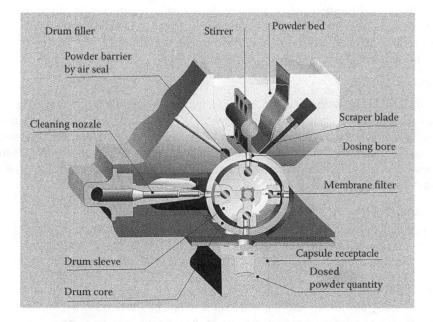

FIGURE 6.6 **(See color insert.)** Drum filler method. (From Harro Hofliger Packaging Systems. Modular filling and closing machine for capsules. Modu-C Mid-Speed (MS). 2010. Brochure.)

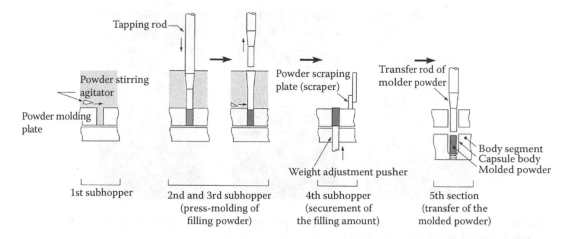

FIGURE 6.7 Compression filling method. (From Qualicaps. LIQFIL super 40. Brochure. Whitsett, NC; 2010.)

subhoppers, tapping rods, and a powder molding plate. In the first subhopper, a powder stirring agitator feeds the powder into the bores of the molding plate. In the second and third subhoppers, tapping rods compress the filling powder into the molding plate, forming a powder slug. In the fourth subhopper, a weight adjustment pusher raises the molded slug to a set height above the plate, and the excess powder is scraped away. At the fifth section, a transfer rod places the finished slug into the capsule body.[12]

Beads and Granules/Pellets

When calculating maximum fill weights for beads and granules fills, bulk density values should be used.

Direct Fill

The direct fill method is employed by most of the semiautomatic capsule filling machines. The beads/granules flow from a drug hopper (with the auger blade removed) through a feed shoe into the open capsule bodies housed in a rotating ring beneath the feed shoe. The factors controlling the dosing are the aperture of the feed shoe and the rotation speed of the body ring.

Vacuum Dosator Method

The vacuum dosator method (Figure 6.8[13]) is employed by Imatic and Zanasi capsule filling machines, which are manufactured by the IMA ACTIVE division. The dosator descends partway into the pellet layer in the dosing bowl, picking up the pellets with an aspiration vacuum. Excess pellets on the dosator tip are removed by either a brush or an air-jet. The pellet product is then dosed into the capsule body by reducing the vacuum and lowering the dosator piston.[13] This system is also used in the dosing of microtablets.

Dosing Chamber

The dosing chamber principle (Figure 6.9) is employed by numerous fully automatic capsule filling machines. It consists of various configurations of vertical or horizontal adjustable chambers that pre-measure the dose volume of beads/pellets or granules and discharge them into the capsule body.

Dosing Disc Method

Dosing pellets using the dosing disc method was developed by Bosch Packaging Technology and is similar to the powder dosing disc method, except the tamping pins are removed, and a slide gate (Figure 6.10) is installed below the dosing disc. Pellets flow into the dosing disc holes, the slide gate opens between indexes, and the pellets drop into the open capsule bodies with the assistance of the transfer pins that purge the pellets from the disc bores.[14]

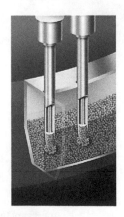 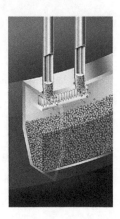 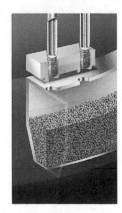

FIGURE 6.8 (See color insert.) Vacuum dosator method. (From IMA ACTIVE. IMATIC High Speed Capsule Filling Machine. 2011. Brochure.)

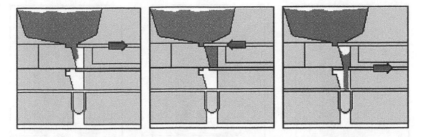

FIGURE 6.9   Dosage chamber. (Courtesy of Robert Bosch GmbH Packaging Technology, Waiblingen, Germany.)

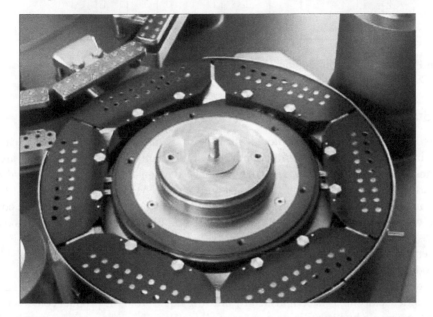

FIGURE 6.10   Slide gate. (Courtesy of Robert Bosch GmbH Packaging Technology, Waiblingen, Germany.)

TABLET AND CAPSULE OVERENCAPSULATION

Overencapsulation is the most widely used method of blinding clinical supplies, performed by placing the product or products (i.e., tablets, caplets, or capsules) into an opaque capsule. This prevents the clinical investigators and subjects from differentiating between the active, placebo, or comparator drug within double-blind studies.[15] Overencapsulation is also used in the manufacture of combination products.

Capsules

When overencapsulating a filled capsule, the receiving capsule shell should be two capsule sizes larger.

Tablets

There are different types of capsule filling machine dosing units used to handle single tablets, multiple tablets, or microtablets. The basic design of the tablet dosing units (Figure 6.11[16]) consists of a feed tube or flexible spring attached to the base of the tablet feed hopper. The tablets drop into a bushing, which transfers the tablet into the capsule body. An electromechanical device, or sensor, verifies proper dosing of the tablet within the capsule body. To assure proper handling by the dosing mechanisms, tablets should ideally be spherical or have beveled edges and coated to avoid dusting. Also, the overall tablet dimensions and hardness specifications should be kept within strict tolerances.[17]

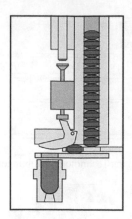
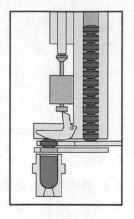
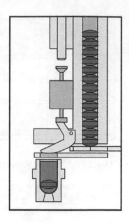

FIGURE 6.11 Tablet dosing unit. (From IMA ACTIVE division. Zanasi Low-medium speed capsule filling machines. 2011. Brochure.)

LIQUIDS/SEMISOLIDS

There has been a re-emergence of liquid-filled capsules for several reasons: They can be used for active ingredients with low melting points; they are effective for compounds that are unstable when exposed to moisture or oxygen[18]; they enhance the content uniformity of low dose drugs; they address safety concerns when handling highly potent APIs such as cytotoxins; they allow formulations with fewer excipients; they reduce manufacturing and plant infrastructure costs[19]; they overcome poor aqueous solubility; and they improve oral bioavailability.[20] To note, about 60% of compounds in development exhibit poor solubility.[21]

When calculating maximum fill volume for liquid/semisolid fills, use a target of 85–90% of the capsule body volume.

Liquid dosing systems (Figure 6.12) employ piston pumps or a series of pumping syringes. Precise volumetric dosing is accomplished by drawing liquid from the product container and pushing it into the capsule bodies utilizing a series of slide valves. Liquid containers may be fitted with a mixer and a heating and temperature control system for thixotropic or thermosetting products.[22]

MULTICOMPONENT DOSING

Many capsule filling machines can be equipped with more than one type of dosing unit to provide for filling different dosage combinations into a capsule as illustrated in Figure 6.13.[23]

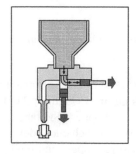
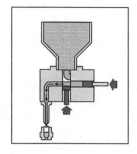
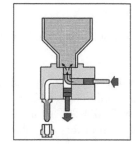

FIGURE 6.12 Liquid dosing system. (From IMA ACTIVE Division. ZANASI LAB. 2011. Brochure.)

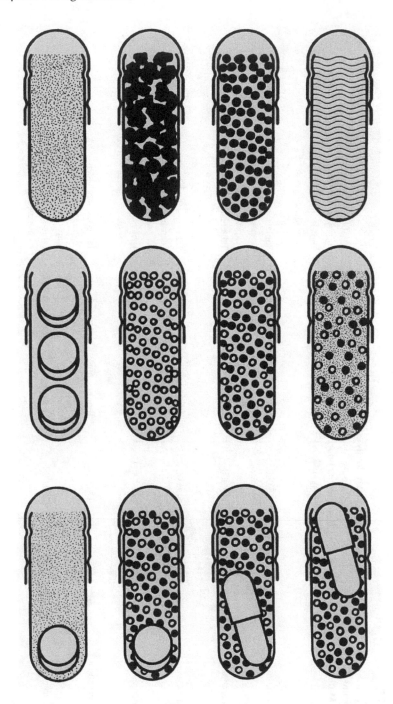

FIGURE 6.13 Multicomponent dosing. (From Warner-Lambert Company, Capsugel Division. All About the Hard Gelatin Capsule. Capsugel Publication. Morris Plains, NJ; 1991. Report No. CAP 126E.)

CAPSULE FILLING MACHINERY

The commercially available capsule filling machines are summarized in Table 6.2. Capsule filling machines can be categorized by their level of automation or their special filling capabilities described in this section.

TABLE 6.2
Capsule Filling Machinery

Manufacturer	Machine Type/ Motion	Model	Maximum Hourly Output (capsules per hour)	Method of Dosing		Other Dosing Capabilities	Other
				Powder	Granules		
ACG-pam ACG Worldwide Mumbai, India	Intermittent	AFT Lab	6,000	Tamping pin	Dosing chamber	Tablets, microtablets, capsule/softgel in capsule	
	Intermittent	AF 25T	25,000	Tamping pin	Dosing chamber	Tablets, microtablets, capsule/softgel in capsule	
	Intermittent	AF 40T	40,000	Tamping pin	Dosing chamber	Tablets, microtablets, capsule/softgel in capsule	
	Intermittent	AF 40D	40,000	Dosator	Dosing chamber	Tablets, microtablets, capsule/softgel in capsule	
	Intermittent	AF 90T	90,000	Tamping pin	Dosing chamber	Tablets, microtablets, capsule/softgel in capsule	
	Intermittent	AF 150T	150,000	Tamping pin	Dosing chamber	Tablets, microtablets, capsule/softgel in capsule	
	Intermittent	AF 200T	200,000	Tamping pin	Dosing chamber	Tablets, microtablets, capsule/softgel in capsule	ZRM technology

(Continued)

TABLE 6.2 (CONTINUED)
Capsule Filling Machinery

Manufacturer	Machine Type/Motion	Model	Maximum Hourly Output (capsules per hour)	Method of Dosing		Other Dosing Capabilities	Other
				Powder	Granules		
Bosch Packaging Technology Waiblingen, Germany	Automatic/Intermittent	GKF 700	42,000	Tamping pin	–	–	Designed for nutraceuticals
	Automatic/Intermittent	GKF 702	42,000	Tamping pin, dosator	Dosing chamber/dosing disk/dosator	R&D mini-bowl, tablets, liquids, micro-dosing, combinations	Mini-bowl, lab kit
	Automatic/Intermittent	GKF 1400	84,000 72,000—liquids	Tamping pin	Dosing chamber/dosing disk	Tablets, liquids, combinations	GKF 1400L liquid
	Automatic/Intermittent	GKF HiProTect 1700	100,000 72,000—tablets	Tamping pin	Dosing disk or dosing chamber	Tablets, liquids, combinations	Containment for processing potent substances
	Automatic/Intermittent	GKF Capsylon 705 1505 3005	42,000 92,000 175,000	Tamping pin	Dosing disk	Powder or pellets	Designed for nutraceuticals
	Automatic/Intermittent	GKF 2000	150,000	Tamping pin	Dosing chamber	Powders/pellets	
	Automatic/Intermittent	GKF 2500	150,000	Tamping pin	Dosing chamber/dosing disk	Tablets, combinations, liquids, micro-dosing	
	Automatic/Intermittent	GKF 2500ASB	150,000	Tamping pin	Dosing chamber/dosing disk	Tablets, combinations, liquids, micro-dosing	Automatic troubleshooting
	Automatic/Intermittent	GKF 2500 ABS IPK	150,000	Tamping pin	Dosing chamber/dosing disk	Tablets, combinations, liquids, micro-dosing	In-process statistical weight control
	Automatic/Intermittent	GKF 2500 ASB 100%	150,000	Tamping pin	Dosing chamber/dosing disk	Tablets, combinations, liquids, micro-dosing	Integrated checkweigher
	Automatic/Intermittent	GKF 3000	175,000	Tamping pin	Dosing disk	–	–

(Continued)

TABLE 6.2 (CONTINUED)
Capsule Filling Machinery

Manufacturer	Machine Type/Motion	Model	Maximum Hourly Output (capsules per hour)	Method of Dosing		Other Dosing Capabilities	Other
				Powder	Granules		
Capsugel Greenwood, South Carolina USA	Semiautomatic	Cap8	Up to 29,000 Dependent on capsule size	Auger	Direct fill Feed shoe	Tablets, capsules (using TFR 8)	
	Semiautomatic	Ultra 8 II	Up to 33,000 Dependent on capsule size	Auger	Direct fill Feed shoe	Tablets, capsules (using TFR 8)	
	Semiautomatic	Xcelodose 120	200	"Pepper-pot"	n/a	Other small dose containers	Precise dosing of drug substance weights from 100 µg to 100+ mg
	Automatic	Xcelodose 600	600+	"Pepper-pot"	n/a	Capsules only	Precise dosing of drug substance weights from 100 µg to 100+ mg
	Automatic	CFS1200	1,200	n/a	n/a	Liquids	Benchtop unit Filler and sealer
	Automatic	CFS 1500C	1,500	n/a	n/a	Liquids	Floor standing machine designed for containment Filler and sealer
	Manual	ProFiller 100	2,000–3,000	Manual	Manual		
	Manual	ProFill DB Overencapsulation	1,000–1,500	Manual	Manual	Overencapsulation of tablets, caplets, capsules	Designed specifically for filling DB caps capsules for double-blind studies
	Semiautomatic	Xcelolab	200	"Pepper-pot"	n/a	Small dose containers	
	Manual	ProFiller 3000	4,500–9,000	Manual	Manual		

(*Continued*)

TABLE 6.2 (CONTINUED)
Capsule Filling Machinery

Manufacturer	Machine Type/ Motion	Model	Maximum Hourly Output (capsules per hour)	Method of Dosing		Other Dosing Capabilities	Other
				Powder	Granules		
Harro Höfliger Packaging Systems Doylestown, Pennsylvania, USA	Automatic/ Intermittent	Modu-C LS (low speed)	24,000	Dosator Tamping pin Drum filler	Dosing chamber	Microtablets, tablets, capsules, liquids, combinations	Laboratory operations and production Quick-changeable (trolleys) for powder, pellets, and tablets
	Automatic/ Intermittent	Modu-C MS (mid speed)	100,000	Dosator Tamping pin Drum filler	Dosing chamber	Microtablets, tablets, capsules, liquids, combinations	Quick-changeable (trolleys) for powder, pellets and tablets Optional weight checking system for determination of the total and net weight
	Automatic Intermittent	Modu-C HS (high speed)	200,000	Dosator Tamping pin Drum filler	Dosing chamber	Microtablets, tablets, capsules, liquids, combinations	Quick-changeable (trolleys) for powder, pellets and tablets Optional weight checking system for determination of the total and net weight
	Semiautomatic Intermittent	OmniDose	100–300	Dosator Drum filler			Lab use Mounted on interchangeable trolleys *(Continued)*

TABLE 6.2 (CONTINUED)
Capsule Filling Machinery

Manufacturer	Machine Type/ Motion	Model	Maximum Hourly Output (capsules per hour)	Method of Dosing		Other Dosing Capabilities	Other
				Powder	Granules		
IMA Active Bologna, Italy	Intermittent	Zanasi Lab 8 Zanasi Lab 16	8,000 16,000	Dosators or tamping pin	Dosators (vacuum)	Liquids, microtablets, combinations	R&D production
	Intermittent	Zanasi 6 E Zanasi 12 E	6,000 12,000	Dosators	Dosators (vacuum)	Liquids, tablets, combinations	Statistic weight checking unit for production monitoring
	Intermittent	Zanasi 25E/F Zanasi 40/EF	25,000 40,000	Dosators	Dosators (vacuum)	Liquids, tablets, combinations	E-versions are equipped with a statistic weight checking unit for production monitoring
	Intermittent	Zanasi Plus 48 Zanasi Plus 70 Zanasi Plus 85	48,000 70,000 85,000	Dosators	Dosators (vacuum)	Liquids, tablets, microtablets, combinations	Statistical weight check and adjustment 100% in-line net weight control for powders (compaction force measurement)
	Intermittent	Zanasi 70C	55,000	–	–	Gelatin-coated tablet	Exclusively used for production of Press-Fit and XPress-Fit Gelcaps
	Continuous	IMATIC 100 IMATIC 150 IMATIC 200	100,000 150,000 200,000	Dosators	Dosators (vacuum)		The machine can be fitted with a wide range of devices, allowing operator unattended production
	Intermittent	ADAPTA 100 ADAPTA 200	100,000 200,000	Dosators	Dosators (vacuum)	Liquids, tablets, microtablets, capsules, combinations (up to 3–5 products)	Interchangeable dosing units make for flexible configuration Total in-process control: 100% control of gross and/or net weight

(Continued)

TABLE 6.2 (CONTINUED)
Capsule Filling Machinery

Manufacturer	Machine Type/ Motion	Model	Maximum Hourly Output (capsules per hour)	Method of Dosing			Other Dosing Capabilities	Other
				Powder	Granules			
MG2 Bologna, Italy	Continuous motion—intermittent (depending on the type of dosing unit installed)	"Labby"	3,000	Dosators (standard and low dosage) or dosing disk	Dosing chamber		Liquids, tablets, microtablets, capsules, caplets, micro-dosing	R&D capsule filler (single dosing station)
	Continuous motion—intermittent (depending on the type of dosing unit installed)	"FlexaLab"	3,000	Dosators (standard and low dosage) or dosing disk	Dosing chamber		Liquids, tablets, microtablets, capsules, caplets, micro-dosing, combinations	R&D capsule filler Up to two dosing units can be fitted on machine Potent compound Containment option
	Continuous motion	Planeta	6,000–50,000	Dosators (standard and low dosage)	Dosing chamber (up to 4 types)		Liquids, tablets, microtablets, capsules, caplets, micro-dosing, combinations	Up to two dosing units can be fitted on machine Can be fitted with "MG2 Nett Weight" control systems Lights-out version available
	Continuous motion	Planeta 100	100,000	Dosators (standard and low dosage)	Dosing chamber (up to 4 types)		Liquids, tablets, microtablets, capsules, caplets, micro-dosing, combinations	Up to two dosing units can be fitted on machine Can be fitted with "MG2 Nett Weight" control systems Lights-out version available

(Continued)

TABLE 6.2 (CONTINUED)
Capsule Filling Machinery

Manufacturer	Machine Type/ Motion	Model	Maximum Hourly Output (capsules per hour)	Method of Dosing		Other Dosing Capabilities	Other
				Powder	Granules		
MG2 Bologna, Italy	Continuous motion	Planeta 100 Pre-weight	100,000	Dosators (low dosage)	Dosing chamber (up to 4 types)	Liquids, tablets, microtablets, capsules, caplets, micro-dosing, combinations	Can be fitted with "MG2 Multi-Nett Weight" control systems
	Intermittent motion	Alterna70	70,000	Tamping pin	Dosing chamber	Tablets	Up to three dosing stations
	Intermittent motion	Alternova	105,000–180,000	Tamping pin	Dosing chamber	Tablets	Up to three dosing stations
	Continuous motion	G-70 G-140	70,000 140,000	Dosators (standard and low dosage)	Dosing chamber	Tablets, microtablets, combinations	Can be fitted with MG2 "Nett Weight" control systems Lights-out version available
	Continuous motion	G-250	200,000	Dosators (standard and low dosage)	Dosing chamber (up to 2 types)	Tablets (2 types), microtablets, combinations	Can be fitted with MG2 "Nett Weight" control systems Lights-out version available
	Continuous motion	MultiFlexa	250,000	Dosators (standard and low dosage)	Dosing chamber (up to 2 types)		Containment for processing potent substances WIP/CIP Can be fitted with MG2 "Multi-Nett Weight" control systems Lights-out version available

(Continued)

TABLE 6.2 (CONTINUED)
Capsule Filling Machinery

Manufacturer	Machine Type/Motion	Model	Maximum Hourly Output (capsules per hour)	Method of Dosing		Other Dosing Capabilities	Other
				Powder	Granules		
Qualicaps Whitsett, North Carolina, USA	Automatic/Intermittent	FS3	3,000	—	—	Liquids	Liquid filler and sealer
	Automatic/Intermittent	LIQFIL Super LABO	1,000–2,600	Dosing disk	Dosing chamber	Liquids, tablets	Lab unit for drug formulation
	Automatic/Intermittent	F-5	5,000	Compression/tamping	Dosing chamber	Liquids, tablets, microtablets, capsules, combinations	
	Automatic/Intermittent	F-40	40,000	Compression/tamping Dosing disk Vibration	Dosing chamber	Liquids, tablets, microtablets, capsules, combinations	
	Automatic/Intermittent	JCF-40	40,000	Auger	Auger	—	
	Automatic/Intermittent	F-80	80,000	Compression/tamping Dosing disk	Dosing chamber	Liquids, tablets, microtablets, capsules, combinations	
	Automatic/Intermittent	F-100	100,000	Vibration	Vibration	Liquids, tablets, microtablets, capsules, combinations	
	Automatic/Intermittent	F-120	120,000	Compression/tamping Dosing disk	Dosing chamber	Liquids, tablets, microtablets, capsules, combinations	
	Automatic/Intermittent	F-150	150,000	Compression/tamping	Dosing chamber	Liquids, tablets, microtablets, capsules, combinations	

(Continued)

TABLE 6.2 (CONTINUED)
Capsule Filling Machinery

Manufacturer	Machine Type/ Motion	Model	Maximum Hourly Output (capsules per hour)	Method of Dosing		Other Dosing Capabilities	Other
				Powder	Granules		
Romaco S.r.l. Bologna, Italy	Automatic/ Intermittent	Macofar CD25	25,000	Vacuum dosators	Dosing chamber	Tablets	Double station of capsule opening
	Automatic/ Intermittent	Macofar CD40	40,000	Vacuum dosators	Dosing chamber	Tablets	Optional statistical weight control (SWC)
	Automatic/ Intermittent	Macofar CD60	60,000	Vacuum dosators	Dosing chamber	Tablets	Double station of capsule opening Automatic adjustment of powder/pellet dosing with feedback from SWCI
Schaefer Technologies Indianapolis, Indiana, USA	Semiautomatic	Model 8 S	15,000	Auger	Direct fill Feed shoe	Tablets, capsules (using insertion ring)	
	Semiautomatic	STI Model 10	25,000	Auger	Direct fill Feed shoe	Tablets, capsules (using insertion ring)	
	Semiautomatic	STI LF10	10,000–25,000 Dependent on capsule size/ formulation	n/a	n/a	Designed for liquid filling	8 L heated hopper Will fill products with viscosities 100–1000 cps
	Automatic	Dott.Bonapace IN-CAP	3,000	Tamping pin Dosator	Dosing chamber	Tablets, liquids	
	Automatic	Dott.Bonapace IN-CAP HS	7,000	Tamping pin	Dosing chamber		

HAND-OPERATED FILLING DEVICES

These machines require an operator to manually feed, open, fill, join, and eject the capsules. The encapsulation process and machine components are as follows (see Figure 6.14a through c):

1. Empty capsules are hand fed into an orienter, which rectifies the capsules.
2. The orienter is positioned over a two-part filler plate to house the oriented cap and body. The body section has a locking mechanism to secure the capsule body while the caps are removed into the upper section cap tray. The locking mechanism is then released, allowing the bodies to drop flush into the lower filler plate.
3. A powder tray is positioned on top of the lower filler plate. Premeasured powder is poured into the powder tray and a powder spreader manually dispenses the powder into the capsule bodies.
4. A tamper plate packs the powder into the capsule bodies.
5. The cap tray is then placed over the filled capsule bodies, and the cap and body plates are manually pressed together to join and eject the capsules.
6. Some of the devices are available as benchtop fillers with a semiautomatic orienter and an optional vibrator for faster filling of powders.

The throughput of the hand filling devices depends on the number of holes in the filler plate, which can vary from 100 to 300 holes.

SEMIAUTOMATIC CAPSULE FILLING MACHINES

These machines require an operator to manually transport the capsules through the various machine operations (Figure 6.15). The machines automatically feed, rectify, and separate the capsules into a two-part plate or ring, housing the capsule cap in the upper part and the capsule body in the lower

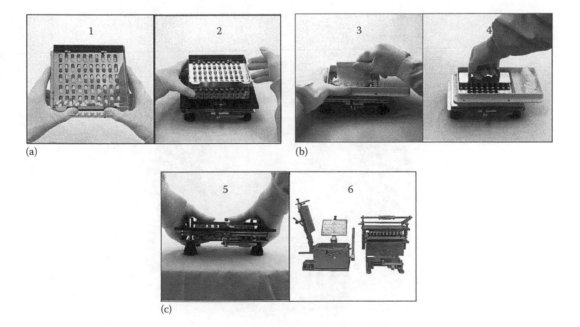

(a)

(b)

(c)

FIGURE 6.14 (a through c) Hand fillers. (Courtesy of Torpac, Fairfield, New Jersey.)

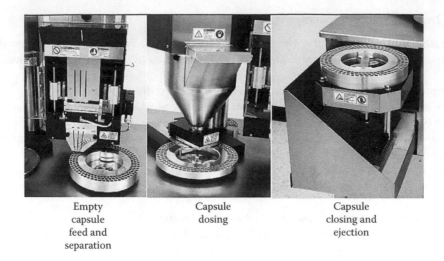

| Empty capsule feed and separation | Capsule dosing | Capsule closing and ejection |

FIGURE 6.15   Semiautomatic machine operations. (Courtesy of Schaefer Technologies Inc., Indianapolis, Indiana.)

part (Figure 6.16). The cap plate is manually removed, and the body plate is manually placed in the dosing station where the capsule bodies are automatically filled. The cap plate is then manually reassembled on the body plate and the plate is manually placed in the machine's joining station. The capsules are automatically joined and ejected from the capsule plate onto a discharge chute. Semiautomatic machines can be configured to fill powders, pellets, and liquids (Figure 6.17), and are frequently used for overencapsulation of capsules, tablets, and caplets using specially designed dispensing rings or plates.

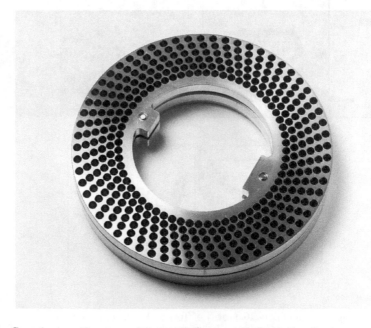

FIGURE 6.16   Capsule ring. (Courtesy of Capsugel, Greenwood, South Carolina.)

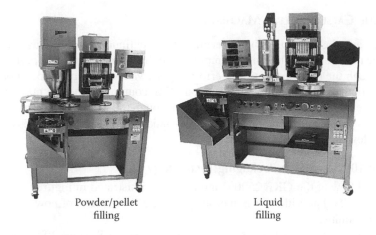

Powder/pellet
filling

Liquid
filling

FIGURE 6.17 STI Model 10. (Courtesy of Schaefer Technologies Inc., Indianapolis, Indiana.)

The output of semiautomatic machines is mainly dependent on capsule size. The larger capsule diameters will result in a reduced number of capsules per ring. Also, the operator skill level and the density and type of material being filled can affect production capacity.[24]

Models of semiautomatic capsule filling machines listed in Table 6.2 are illustrated in Figures 6.17 and 6.18.

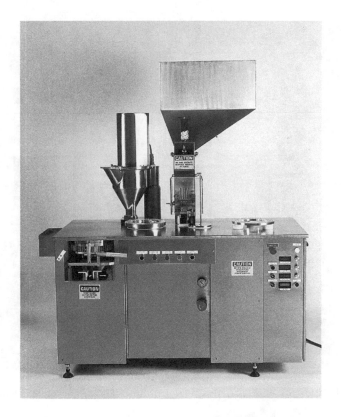

FIGURE 6.18 Ultra 8 II. (Courtesy of Capsugel, Greenwood, South Carolina.)

Fully Automatic Capsule Filling Machines

These machines are classified as either intermittent or continuous motion based on the indexing movement of the machine. The intermittent motion machine capsule transport parts rotate in a start/stop motion through the machine stations performing the various machine operations, that is, capsule feed, separation, dosing, joining, and ejection. With continuous motion machines, the capsule transport parts are constantly moving as they rotate through the machine stations.

Unique features of some of the models of fully automatic capsule filling machines listed in Table 6.2 are described below.

GKF 2500 ASB 100%—Bosch Packaging Technology

The function workflow of the GKF 2500 (Figure 6.19) is illustrated in Figure 6.20.[25] The modular design of the GKF 2500 provides for numerous product combinations of powders, pellets, tablets/microtablets, and liquids.

This machine is equipped with a KKE 2500 checkweigher at Stations 10 and 11, which weighs 100% of the filled capsules. The analysis software calculates an average fill weight from the checkweigher results and the checkweigher rejects capsules outside the tolerance range. It also controls the fill weight with a pneumatic adjustment of the tamping pin compression settings. All the weight information is stored and documented in a production report.

The ASB function is an automatic troubleshooting feature. A mechanical capsule sensor at Station 3 identifies any blockages in the empty capsule in-feed and purges the deformed capsules with a compressed air blast. A second capsule body scanner at Station 9 detects incomplete capsules and rejects the empty capsules during ejection phase at Stations 10 and 11.[25]

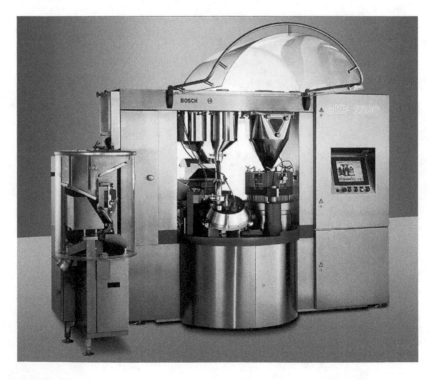

FIGURE 6.19   GKF 2500 ASB 100%. (Courtesy of Robert Bosch GmbH Packaging Technology, Waiblingen, Germany.)

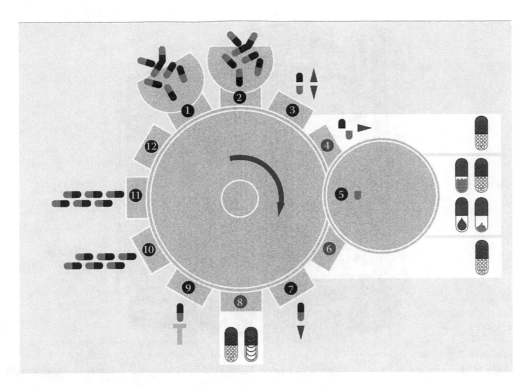

FIGURE 6.20 GKF 2500 Workflow. (1 and 2) Capsule orientation and separation; (3) capsule cap scanner; (4) open for optional pellet station; (5) dosing station for powder or pellets with dosing disk; (6) open for optional pellet station; (7) faulty capsule rejection; (8) open for optional pellet or tablet station; (9) capsule closing w/capsule body scanner; (10 and 11) capsule ejection; (12) segment cleaning. (From Robert Bosch GmbH Packaging Tecnology. GKF 2500 Capsule Filling Machine. 2012. Brochure. pp. 4–9.)

Modu-C—Harro Höfliger

The function workflow of the Modu-C (Figure 6.21) is illustrated in Figure 6.22.[26]

Modu-C provides a wide variety of product combinations for multicomponent dosing of capsules. The various dosing elements for powders/liquids or pellets/tablets are mounted on trolleys (Figure 6.23[27]). This provides a flexible exchange of dosing systems, allowing a variety of machine dosing configurations. There are three dosing systems for powders: tamping pin, dosators with compaction, and drum filler for microdosing.

The Modu-C has a size part-free tablet dosing unit that can handle a variety of tablet shapes and sizes (Figure 6.24).

The dosing systems for uniform solids (i.e., powders, pellets, capsules, or tablets) can be equipped with the Visio AMV System (Figure 6.25). This system provides for in-line mass verification, with the sensors detecting the products in flight. The system makes up to 1000 measurements per minute and can be calibrated on a mass ("weight") basis. Visio AMV can detect single doses as low as 1 mg. The system can provide in-process control up to 100,000 capsules per hour on a Modu-C machine.[28]

ADAPTA—IMA ACTIVE Solid Dose Solutions

The function workflow of the ADAPTA (Figure 6.26) is illustrated in Figure 6.27.[29]

The ADAPTA is designed to dose various combinations of up to three products in a capsule. Two of the dosing stations can be removed and interchanged, providing the possibility of a plug-and-play

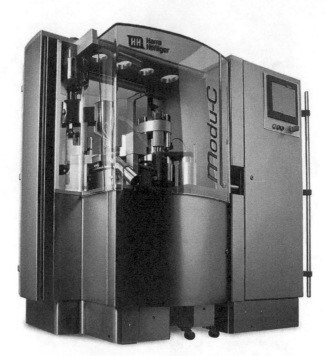

FIGURE 6.21   Modu-C—Harro Höfliger. (Courtesy of Harro Höfliger Packaging Systems, Doylestown, PA.)

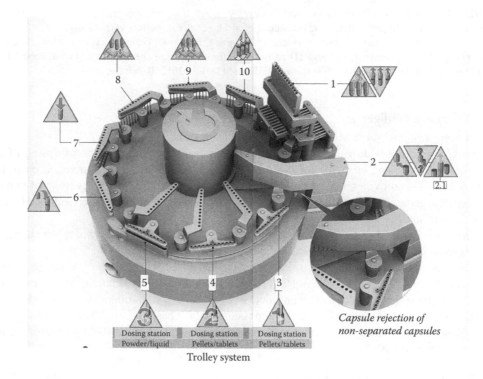

FIGURE 6.22   Modu-C Workflow. (1) Inserting and separating capsule cap and body; (2) rejection of non-separated capsules; (3) dosing station 1 [tablets, pellets, or microtablets]; (4) dosing station 2 [tablets, pellets, or microtablets]; (5) dosing station 3 [powder or liquid]; (6) empty station; (7) capsule closing station; (8) bad capsule rejection; (9) capsule discharge; (10) segment cleaning. (From Harro Höfliger Packaging Systems Inc. Modular Filling and closing machine for capsules Modu-C Mid Speed (MS). 2011. Brochure.)

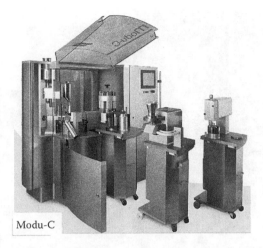

FIGURE 6.23 Modu-C dosing station trolley system. (From Harro Hifliger Packaging Systems Inc. Modular filling and closing machine for capsules Modu-C Low Speed (LS). 2011. Brochure.)

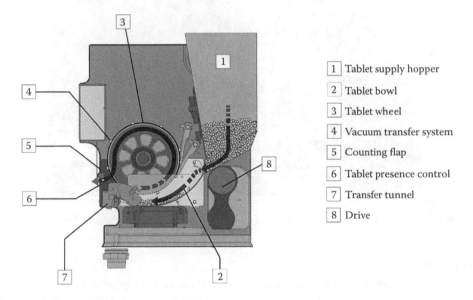

1	Tablet supply hopper
2	Tablet bowl
3	Tablet wheel
4	Vacuum transfer system
5	Counting flap
6	Tablet presence control
7	Transfer tunnel
8	Drive

FIGURE 6.24 **(See color insert.)** Modu-C size part-free tablet dosing unit. (Courtesy of Harro Höfliger Packaging Systems, Doylestown, PA.)

shift between different machine configurations. The machine has the capability to be specially designed to fill up to five products in the same capsule.

The dosage control systems at Stations 4, 6, and 8 provide the following types of 100% in-process control and rejection of "out of limit" capsules:

- Strain gauges on powder dosators measuring compaction force to determine dosing weight
- LVDT sensors mounted on pushers monitoring pellet dosage fill volume (Figure 6.28[22])
- Cameras fitted on the microtablets dosing drum to check the exact number/count of microtablets filled into each capsule[29]

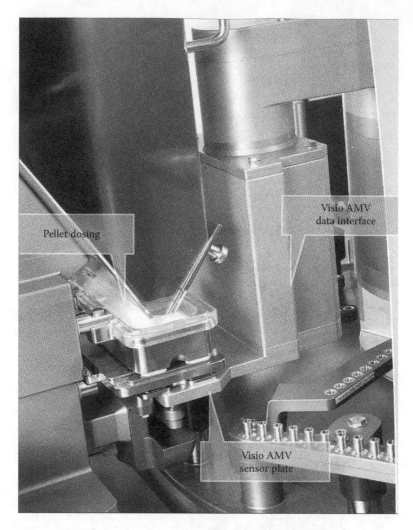

FIGURE 6.25 Visio AMV System. (Courtesy of Harro Höfliger Packaging Systems, Doylestown, PA.)

Planeta—MG2

The function workflow of the Planeta (Figure 6.29) is illustrated in Figure 6.30.

The modular design of this machine allows for different types of dosage units to be fitted at the same time at both Stations C and E. This could provide for the filling of two different types of powders, up to four different types of pellets, and various combinations of tablets, microtablets, and liquids. The machine can be fitted with a varying number of capsule transport and dosing elements, providing the flexibility to be used in R&D laboratories and scaled up to production output.[30]

The machine can be equipped with a variety of weight control systems providing capability for "lights-out operation." The MG2 NETT system (Figure 6.31) is a unique capacitive sensor system that can be built into their capsule filling machines. The NETT consists of two capacitive sensors that check the capsules before and after filling to determine net fill weight. A PC with specially designed application software monitors and stores the net weight of each capsule and rejects any capsules outside acceptable limits at the out-feed of the machine. The system corrects any variations in net weight by automatically adjusting the dosing elements to quickly bring the weight as close as possible to the required value. If the number of underdosed or overdosed capsules rejected by NETT exceeds a preset value, the machine is stopped. The system automatically calibrates the capacitive

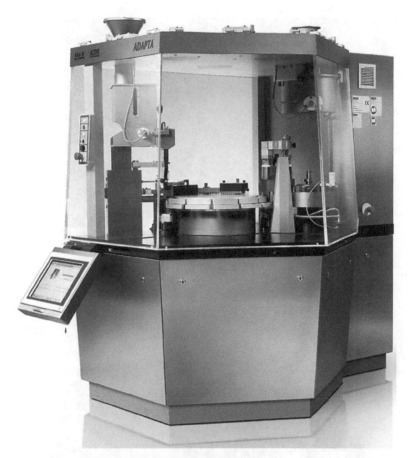

FIGURE 6.26 ADAPTA. (Courtesy of IMA Active, Bologna, Italy.)

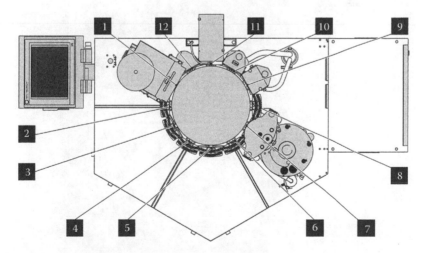

FIGURE 6.27 ADAPTA workflow. (1) Capsule in feed and opening; (2) capsule presence control–optional; (3) dosing station [powders, pellets, tablets, microtablets, or liquids]—optional; (4) dosage control system or dosing station—optional; (5) dosing station [powders, pellets, tablets, microtablets, or liquids]—optional; (6) dosage control system or dosing station—optional; (7) standard dosing station [powders, pellets, or tablets]; (8) dosage control system—optional; (9) unopened capsule selection; (10) closing; (11) capsule discharge; (12) bushing cleaning. (From IMA ACTIVE division. ADAPTA THE EVOLVING CAPSULE FILLER. 2011. Brochure.)

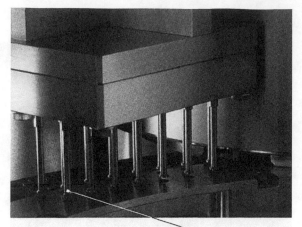

Pushers with LVDT sensors

FIGURE 6.28 Pellet control with LVDT sensors. (From IMA ACTIVE Division. ZANASI LAB. 2011. Brochure.)

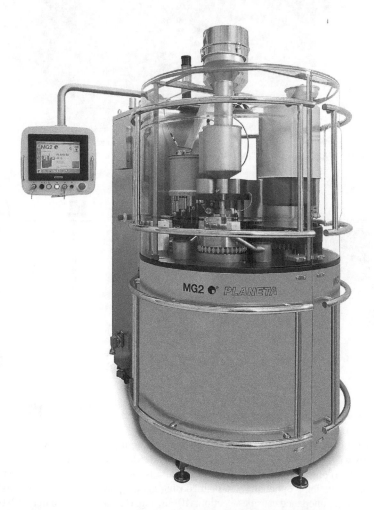

FIGURE 6.29 PLANETA. (Courtesy of MG America, Inc., Fairfield, New Jersey.)

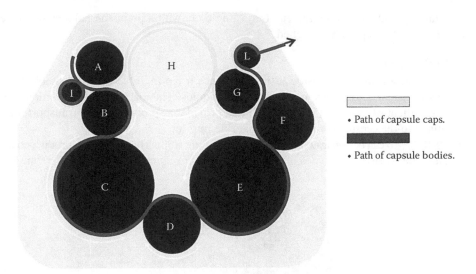

FIGURE 6.30 (See color insert.) PLANETA Workflow. (Courtesy of MG America, Inc., Fairfield, New Jersey.)

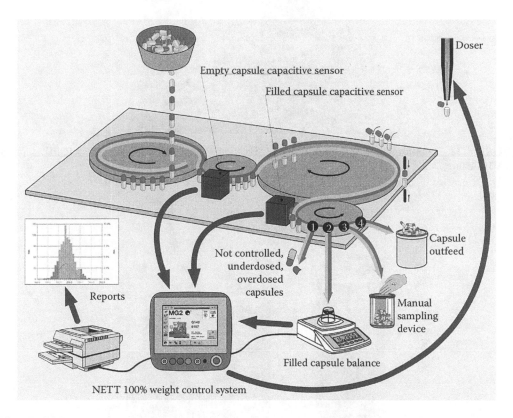

FIGURE 6.31 NETT 100% weight control system. (From MG2. NETT. 2006. Brochure.)

sensors at start-up and throughout the run by testing them with a precision balance that resets the sensors every time the capsule is weighed.[31]

LIQFILsuper80—Qualicaps

The Qualicaps fully automatic capsule filling machines listed in Table 6.2 are suitable for encapsulating powders, pellets, granules, pastes, oils, and liquids. The machines have a unique patented three-drum rectification system (Figure 6.32[12]) that provides a smooth capsule transport, minimizing any damage to the capsules or peel of the capsule imprint.

The LIQFILsuper80 can be separated into two units (Figure 6.33). This facilitates product changeover when switching between the two types of dosing units that are connected to the capsule transfer unit.[32]

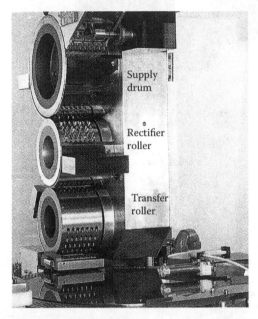

FIGURE 6.32 Qualicaps patented three-drum rectification system. (From Qualicaps. LIQFIL super 40. 2010. Brochure.)

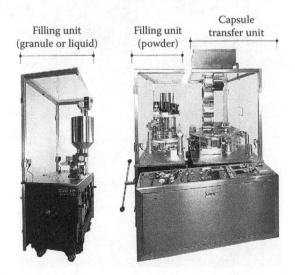

FIGURE 6.33 LIQFILsuper80. (Courtesy of Qualicaps.)

AF 200T—ACG-pam

The AF 200T (Figure 6.34) features Zero Relative Motion (ZRM) technology. This mechanism, developed and patented by ACG Worldwide, ensures that there is virtually no gap between the dosing disc and tamping ring during the tamping stroke. This eliminates the loss of powder through the gap between dosing disc and tamping ring that can occur with tamping pin machines when dosing fine powder formulations. ZRM technology improves manufacturing efficiency by minimizing powder loss and dusting during operation and is suitable for full filling operations and partial filling for quantities as low as 15 (±2) mg.[33]

SPECIALTY FILLERS

Specialty fillers are designed to dose two-piece capsules or other containers with a precise amount of drug substance or formulated material. These fillers are frequently used to create small batches for preclinical animal studies or early-phase clinical supplies. They can also be configured for various levels of containment when filling high potency materials.

Examples of specialty fillers are provided in the subsequent subsections.

Mettler Quantos QB5

The Quantos dosing system (Figure 6.35[34]) automatically fills different capsule sizes, vials, and containers up to a diameter of 28 mm. The Quantos "Connect" application software allows for a fill quantity to be determined for each capsule and checks the data records against the study protocol. The dosing head doses all free-flowing powders. Its algorithm learns the powder characteristics and registers deviations in the particle size. The system saves all substance relevant data to secure traceability. The dosing head reliably doses powder quantities of 1 mg with repeatability of 0.007 mg.[34]

Capsugel Xcelodose

The Xcelodose precision powder micro-dosing systems use the "pepper-pot" principle (Figure 6.36[35]) to dispense dose weights as low as 100 μg, and can precisely, accurately, and repeatedly fill capsules and other small dose containers without excipients or bulking agents. Most blends, or formulated

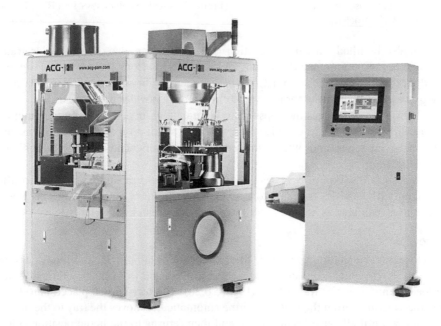

FIGURE 6.34   AF 200T. (Courtesy of ACG-pam, Mumbai.)

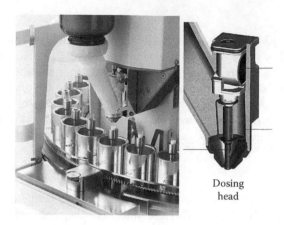

FIGURE 6.35 Mettler Quantos QB5. (From Mettler Toledo. Automatic and precise individual capsule filling. Brochure. Greifensee: Mettler Toledo AG, Laboratory & Weighing Technologies; 2011. Report No. 30008325.)

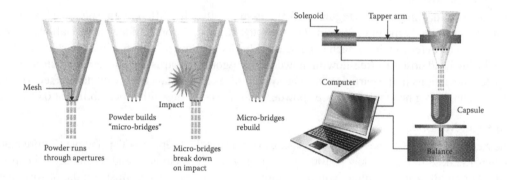

FIGURE 6.36 Xcelodose "pepper pot" principle. (From Capsugel. Xcelodose S Precision Powder Micro-dosing Systems. 2011. Brochure.)

products, can also be filled without segregation. The system can also dose beads or granules. The Xcelodose utilizes programmable dispensing of dose weights from 100 μg to 100 mg and beyond with recording to allow traceability for GMP requirements. The software automatically optimizes the filling process, compensating for any variability in drug powder properties.

The Xcelodose 120S requires the capsules to be manually loaded with semiautomatic indexing and automatic filling. This model can also fill a variety of small dose containers such as vials, tubes, blisters, cartridge cassettes, and other compact dose containers. The machine throughput is up to 200 capsules per hour.

The Xcelodose 600S (Figure 6.37) employs fully automatic capsule handling and filling. This machine can only fill capsules (sizes 00 to 4) with a throughput of 600+ capsules per hour. A high-throughput unit is available as an option for long runs and greater fill weights.[35]

OmniDose

The OmniDose is a semiautomatic capsule filler intended for lab use. It can fill powders for clinical trials in a GMP environment. It also doses powders into a variety of other containers. The capsules are hand loaded into a carrier tray offline (Figure 6.38). The tray is then placed onto the transport unit inside the machine. From there, the machine automatically moves the tray to the dosing station, indexes each row until all capsules are filled, and then returns to the home position (Figure 6.39).

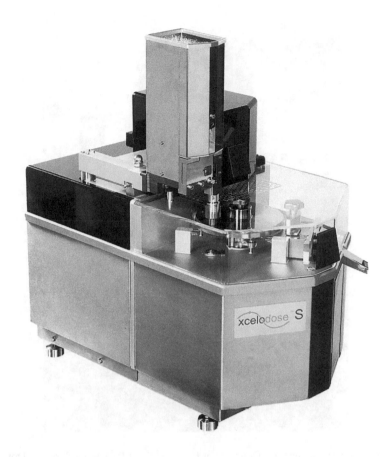

FIGURE 6.37 Xcelodose 600S. (Courtesy of Capsugel, Greenwood, South Carolina.)

For capsules, a tray would typically hold 60 capsules (10 × 6 arrays). Speeds for this system are typically 100 to 300 capsules per hour, depending on the characteristics of the powder and the number of capsules per tray. The OmniDose has interchangeable powder dosing systems, including a vacuum drum that can accurately fill within a range of 0.5–50 mg and a dosator with compaction that can accurately fill within a range of 10–600 mg. The systems are mounted on interchangeable trolleys much like the Modu-C capsule filler concept. The machine can be set up with integrated tare/gross weigh cell and can also be designed for containment when dosing high potency materials.[36]

Powdernium Powder Dispensing Workstation

Powdernium powder dispensing technology (Figure 6.40[37]) has been developed by Symyx Technologies. The system automates the weighing and dispensing of a broad range of pharmaceutical powders with various flow characteristics. The dispensing unit is coupled with a robotic system that dispenses powders into capsules that have been manually loaded into an XY table. The workstation can precisely dispense submilligram to gram quantities into capsules and up to 5 g when dispensing into other containers such as vials and bottles.[37] The Powdernium Easy-Dose software provides real-time data about the dispensing cycle and uses optimization algorithms to monitor and control any variability in the powder properties. The workstation is designed for unattended operation and can perform up to 600 different weighing operations in a single day.[38]

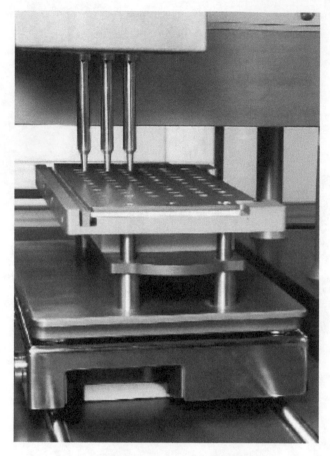

FIGURE 6.38   OmniDose carrier tray. (Courtesy of Harro Höfliger Packaging Systems, Doylestown, PA.)

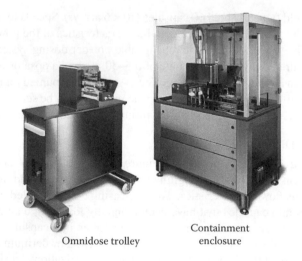

Omnidose trolley   Containment
                                    enclosure

FIGURE 6.39   OmniDose transport unit inside machine. (Courtesy of Harro Höfliger Packaging Systems, Doylestown, PA.)

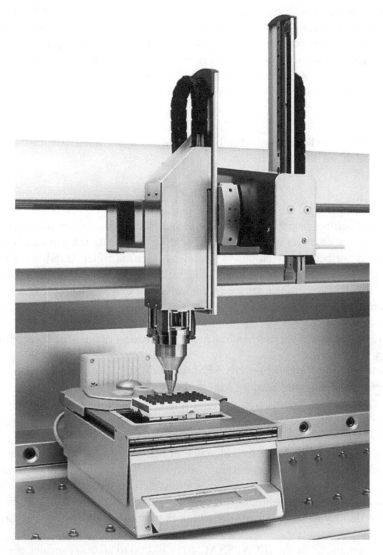

FIGURE 6.40 Powdernium powder dispensing workstation. (From Manufacturing Chemist.com. [Online]; 7-Jan 2009.)

SEALING TECHNOLOGY AND MACHINES

There are three basic purposes for the sealing of two-piece hard shell capsules:

- To create a leak-proof closure for the encapsulation of oils, pastes, and liquids.
- To create a tamper-evident dosage form that cannot be opened without visible signs of damage.[39]
- To comply with regulatory requirements for OTC capsule products for the US market as specified in FDA (US Food and Drug Administration) Compliance Policy Guide 400.500.[40] This policy states: "For two-piece, hard gelatin capsule products subject to this requirement, a minimum of two tamper-evident packaging features is required, unless the capsules are sealed by a tamper-evident technology, in which case only one tamper-evident

packaging feature is required. Technologies for sealing two-piece hard gelatin capsules are available that provide evidence if the capsules have been tampered with after filling. Such sealing technologies currently in use include sonic welding, banding, and sealing techniques employing solvents and/or low temperature heating. These examples are not intended to rule out the development and use of other capsule sealing technologies. Manufacturers may consult with FDA if they are considering alternative capsule sealing processes."

Sealing of capsules can be accomplished by banding machines, liquid sealing machines, or ultrasonic welding, which are described below.

BANDING MACHINES

Capsule banding machines orient the filled capsule and place it in a carrier slat that exposes the cap edge area. An application roller applies a film of sealing solution to the cap and body seam. Some of the machines described below employ a second application roller. Capillary action will cause some of the sealing solution to migrate into the interstitial space between the cap and body, sealing these surfaces as well. The capsules are then transferred to a carrier that moves the capsule through a drying section of the machine to set up the exposed band before the capsule is discharged into a receiving container.

Description and features of various banding machines are described in the succeeding paragraphs.

Qualicaps Band Sealing Machines—HICAPSEAL 40/100
Fully Automatic Hard Capsule Sealing Machines

Capsules pass from the hopper through the feed roller, the rectifier roller, and the transfer roller. They are fed continuously into pockets in the conveyor belt slats. The slats in the conveyor accurately position the capsules over the sealing discs (Figure 6.41). The first sealing disc applies a band of sealing solution around the circumference of the capsule cap and body seam. The second sealing disc applies a second band to ensure a good seal. The sealing solution is maintained at a constant preset temperature and is continuously circulated between the supply pans and sealing pans to maintain uniformity of conditions. Sealed capsules are transferred from the conveyor belt slat to carriers in the drying unit. The drying unit uses filtered air under room conditions to dry the capsule seals.

The production capacity of the HICAPSEAL 40 is 40,000 to 50,000 capsules per hour. The production capacity can be doubled by using the HICAPSEAL 100 drying unit (Figure 6.42[41]).

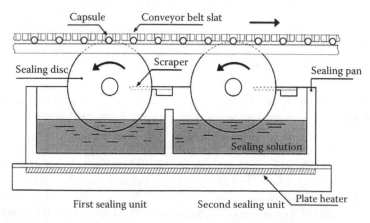

FIGURE 6.41 Band sealing diagram. (Courtesy of Qualicaps, Whitsett, NC.)

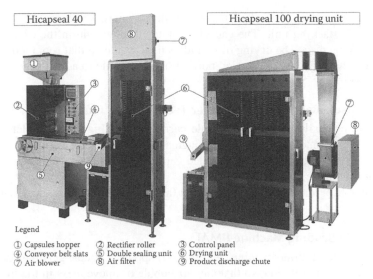

FIGURE 6.42 HICAPSEAL 40/100 Sealing Machine. (From Qualicaps. HICAPSEAL Fully Automatic Hard Capsule Sealing Machine 40/100. 2010. Brochure.)

Qualicaps Lab-Scale Filling/Sealing Machine FS3

This is a small-scale R&D integrated liquid filling and band sealing machine capable of filling and sealing 3000 capsules per hour (Figure 6.43[42]). The machine has a single cap disc and body segments capable of filling sizes 00 to 4 capsules without additional change parts. The body segments lift the capsules up into the filling nozzles to eliminate splashing of low-viscosity liquids and stringing of high-viscosity material. The sealing section uses the same technology as Qualicaps high-speed band sealing equipment. The joined filled capsules are discharged from the liquid filler and immediately

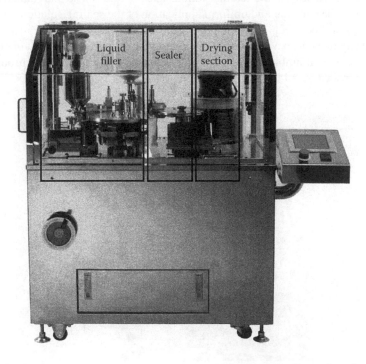

FIGURE 6.43 Qualicaps lab-scale filling/sealing machine FS3. (From Qualicaps, Inc. Qualicaps Lab-Scale Filling/Sealing Machine. Brochure.)

fed into cavities in the sealing disc, which band-seals the capsules. The capsules are then transferred into the drying disc stacking unit. The capsules rotate 10 times within the drying disc and then drop to a lower drying disc. The drying disc cradles the capsule so that room temperature filtered air from a fan unit flows around the sealed portion of the capsule to adequately dry the band seal before exiting the unit.[42]

S-1 Benchtop Capsule Band-Sealer [Schaefer Technologies, Qualicaps]

Filled capsules are manually loaded into capsule-carrying slats (Figure 6.44). Slats are then placed on feed tracks of the benchtop unit and pass through a band-sealing process identical to commercial-scale machines. Slats containing the band-sealed capsules are transferred to the drying rack. The capsules are dried at ambient conditions.[43]

The unit is capable of sealing between 100 and 1,000 capsules per hour depending on the capsule size and change parts.[44]

Hermetica Capsule Banding Machine [IMA]

The Hermetica capsule banding machine (Figure 6.45) applies a double gelatin band by two rollers with independent speed regulation, so that any air bubble or unevenness in the first band is overcome by the second application. Each roller is housed in a separate gelatin bowl with the capability to adjust gelatin temperature and viscosity independently in each bowl. A pre-drying unit (Figure 6.46) guarantees fast fixing of the gelatin band before the capsule is transferred in the drying box for final drying. A 100% checking system via a camera can be additionally fitted, to control and select each individual banded capsule.[45]

Dott.Bonapace BD-3000

The BD-3000 (Figure 6.47) is a fully automatic banding machine with an output of 3000 sealed capsules per hour. The filled capsules are rectified and positioned into the cavities of a rotating disc that transports them to cavities in the sealing station. The capsule is held and rotated three complete revolutions to assure the constant and uniform application of the sealing solution on all the circumference of the capsule body–cap junction. After sealing, the capsules are transferred in vertical position with the cap down into a second disc for drying for over 4 min. The drying is facilitated by air fans that circulate air at ambient temperature. Finally, capsules are ejected through a chute. All operations are controlled by a PLC (Programmable Logic Controller).[46]

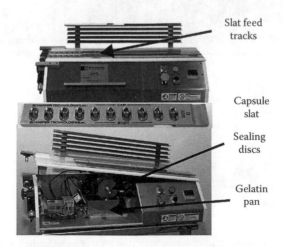

Slat feed tracks

Capsule slat

Sealing discs

Gelatin pan

FIGURE 6.44   S-1 Benchtop capsule band-sealer. (Courtesy of Schaefer Technologies Inc., Indianapolis.)

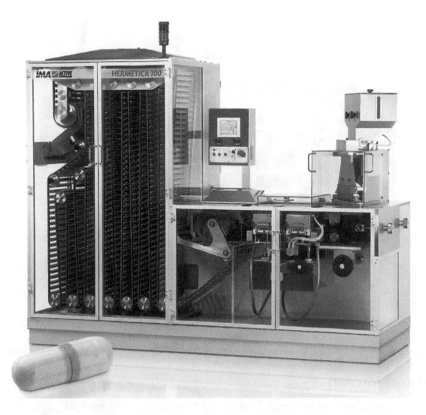

FIGURE 6.45 Hermetica capsule banding machine. (Courtesy of IMA ACTIVE division, Bologna, Italy.)

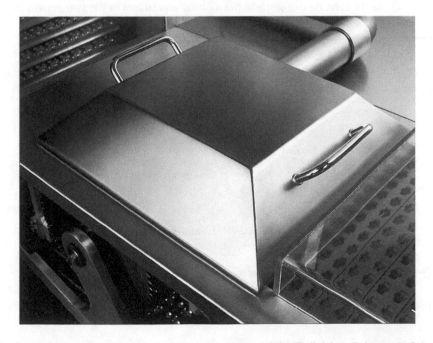

FIGURE 6.46 Hermetica pre-drying unit. (Courtesy of IMA ACTIVE division, Bologna, Italy.)

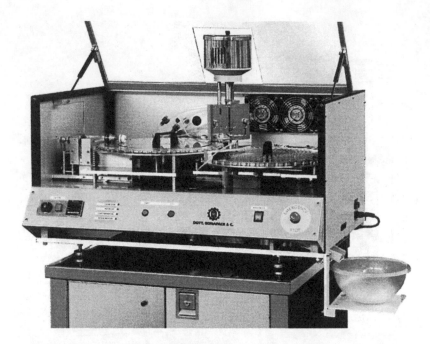

FIGURE 6.47   Dott.Bonapace BD-3000. (Courtesy of Schaefer Technologies Inc., Indianapolis, Indiana.)

LIQUID SEALING MACHINES

The Liquid Encapsulation Microspray Sealing (LEMS) system (Figure 6.48), offered by Capsugel Inc., converts two-piece capsules into one-piece fused capsules. In the first stage of this process, sealing fluid (water/alcohol solution) is micro-sprayed into the joint between the cap and the body. Capillary action draws the fluid into the interstitial space between the cap and the body. Suction removes excess solution from the capsule surface. During the second stage, air heated to 40–60°C is gently blown across the capsule to complete the melting and fusion of the two gelatin layers to form an impervious and completely fused seal. In the third and final stage, gelatin setting is complete when the product returns to room temperature.[47]

The seal integrity of the LEMS technology has been verified by X-ray tomography.[48] The LEMS sealing process achieves a tamper-evident seal. Efforts to manipulate a LEMS sealed capsule yield readily apparent evidence of tampering as well as loss of capsule integrity.

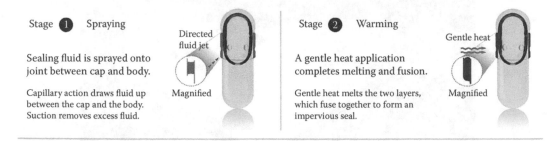

Stage ❶ Spraying

Directed fluid jet

Sealing fluid is sprayed onto joint between cap and body.

Capillary action draws fluid up between the cap and the body. Suction removes excess fluid.

Magnified

Stage ❷ Warming

Gentle heat

A gentle heat application completes melting and fusion.

Gentle heat melts the two layers, which fuse together to form an impervious seal.

Magnified

Stage ❸ Setting   Capsules equilibrate at room temperature.

FIGURE 6.48   (See color insert.) LEMS three-stage process. (Courtesy of Capsugel, Greenwood, South Carolina.)

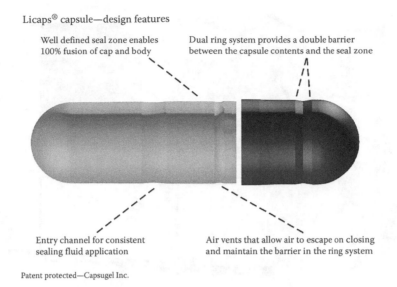

Licaps® capsule—design features

Well defined seal zone enables
100% fusion of cap and body

Dual ring system provides a double barrier
between the capsule contents and the seal zone

Entry channel for consistent
sealing fluid application

Air vents that allow air to escape on closing
and maintain the barrier in the ring system

Patent protected—Capsugel Inc.

FIGURE 6.49 Licaps capsules. (Courtesy of Capsugel, Greenwood, South Carolina.)

Capsugel also offers Licaps capsules (Figure 6.49) that are specifically designed for secure and robust containment of liquids and semisolids. Compared to standard capsules, Licaps capsules utilize a number of proprietary design features that result in a much larger contiguous seal zone. The sealing area extends along the length of the capsule above its midpoint, as compared to the narrow body/cap junction, which is the sole focus of traditional capsule banding methodologies.

Incorporated into the Licaps capsule design are full circumference rings that not only define this expanded sealing zone but also serve to isolate and contain the liquid contained in the capsule. To further enhance sealing productivity rates, the capsule design includes both a liquid entry channel that assures consistent sealing conditions and air vents that allow for rapid air escape that is critical for high-speed encapsulation.[49]

The Capsugel machines described in the subsequent paragraphs have been developed for the LEMS process.

cfs 1200

The cfs 1200 (Figure 6.50[50]) is a benchtop machine suitable for R&D labs and capable of GMP manufacturing of clinical supplies. It is a combined liquid filling and sealing machine with an output of up to 1200 capsules per hour. It can handle both liquids and semisolids using a robust temperature-controlled filling pump with a dosing accuracy of 0.1 to 1.2 mL. The CFS 1200 is scalable to commercial-scale LEMS manufacturing equipment.[51]

cfs 1500 C

The cfs 1500 C (Figure 6.51) functionality is similar to the cfs 1200; however, it is designed with containment features to provide for safe liquid filling and sealing of capsules with potent compounds used in early-phase clinical trials. The CFS 1500 C has an increased output of 1500 capsules per hour.[52] Some of the other unique features of this machine include the following: the weight of every capsule is recorded and accepted or rejected according to set weight, and an intuitive software interface saves machine settings and stores method development work for later recall. Most importantly, it is designed for ease of cleaning with easily removable parts and a verification system that prevents cleaning fluid from entering the working elements of the machine.[53]

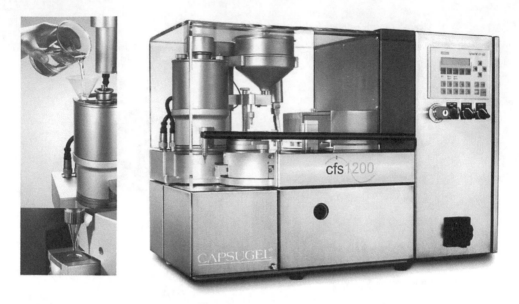

FIGURE 6.50   cfs 1200. (From Capsugel. cfs 1200 Capsule Liquid Filling and Sealing Machine. 2006. Brochure.)

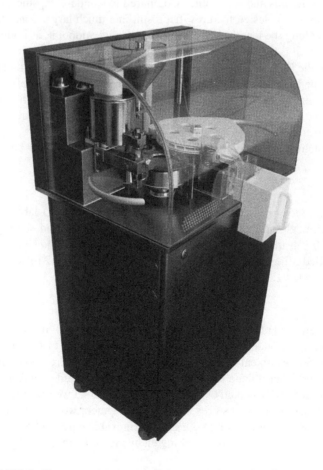

FIGURE 6.51   cfs 1500 C. (Courtesy of Capsugel, Greenwood, South Carolina.)

LEMS 70

The LEMS 70 system (Figure 6.52) is a high-speed production-scale sealing system with an output speed up to 70,000 capsules per hour. Key components include the high-capacity micro-spray bars and a contiguous tumble dryer fitted with a rotating air lock. It is constructed with FDA-approved materials and utilizes software that is compliant with 21CFR Part 11 requirements. The sealing range covers viscosity levels of 30 to 30,000 cps.

In commercial installations, the LEMS sealing machine is connected downstream from a standard capsule filling machine with a liquid filling head. Additional process equipment typically includes inspection stations.[54]

ULTRASONIC WELDING OF CAPSULE-BASED SYSTEMS

The term *ultrasonic* applies to sound waves whose frequencies are >20 kHz.

The elements of an ultrasonic welding system consist of four basic components:

- A generator or power supply that changes electrical power into electrical energy
- A transducer that converts the energy into vertical, low-amplitude mechanical motion known as vibrations
- A booster that modulates the vibrations from the transducer
- A sonotrode or horn that applies the vibrations to the material being welded

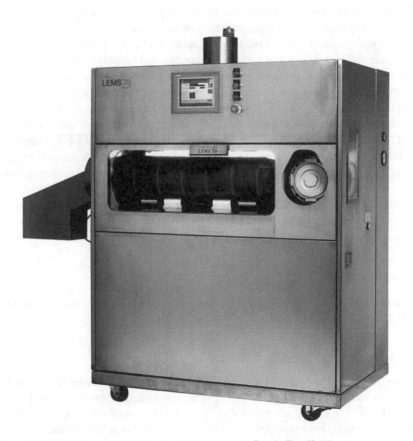

FIGURE 6.52   LEMS 70. (Courtesy of Capsugel, Greenwood, South Carolina.)

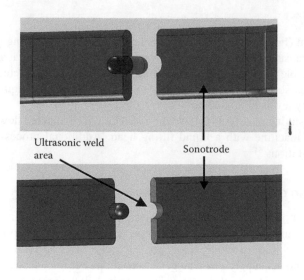

FIGURE 6.53   Ultrasonic welding diagram. (Courtesy of Rainbow Medical Engineering Ltd., Letchworth.)

Ultrasonic welding involves the application of a vibrating sonotrode to a thermoplastic/thermoplastic interface, which induces a high degree of localized frictional heat that causes the thermoplastic to melt and form a molecular bond at the interface. The key to the success of this process lies chiefly in the short welding times that are required for joining, typically 0.1–1 s.

Thermoplastic polymers have two properties that make them particularly suited to ultrasonic welding: low thermal conductivity and melting temperatures between 100°C and 200°C. Most pharmaceutical polymers, for example, the celluloses/starches and biopolymers such as gelatin, do have these thermoplastic properties. By their very nature, these polymers are often molded or extruded into capsule-shaped components for a number of drug delivery applications.

As illustrated in Figure 6.53, the capsule components are positively located within a suitable fixture that positions a sonotrode around the circumference of the cap/body interface. Upon contact and application of the ultrasound, the capsule parts will be mechanically vibrated between 20,000 and 40,000 cycles per second. The high degree of localized friction between the two capsule sections will cause molecular melting, resulting in the fusion between the capsule parts.[55]

Rainbow Medical Engineering Ltd. has devised a quick, clean method of ultrasonic sealing hard gelatin capsules that show clear evidence of tampering if the capsule body is separated from the cap, with the production of "half-moon" perforations in the capsule body.[56]

CAPSULE INSPECTION

The two basic methods of inspecting capsules for defect removal are visual inspection and vision systems. The equipment and processes are described below.

VISUAL INSPECTION

Visual inspection is facilitated through the use of capsule inspection tables (Figure 6.54). Capsules flow out of the product hopper and are conveyed to the integrated vibrator/vacuum system removing empty capsule shells. The capsules move forward on stainless steel rollers that rotate the capsules, and any defective capsules are manually removed by an inspector using the vacuum hose and pick-up wand.[57]

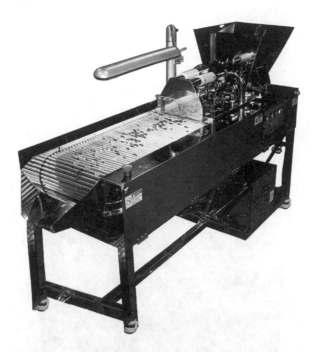

FIGURE 6.54 MCI-700 capsule inspector. (Courtesy of Mendel Company, East Hanover, NJ.)

VISION SYSTEMS

Capsule vision systems employ high-resolution cameras that pick up images of the capsule that are then compared with the corresponding image for an acceptable product, and the defective capsules are differentiated and rejected.

Viswill PAPPIS (Plug and Play Portable Inspection System)

The PAPPIS (Figure 6.55) uses four LED lighting units to illuminate the product and eight high-resolution CCD area sensor cameras for inspection (top and bottom of each row). Inspection is applied to both the top surface and the bottom surface at the same time (Figure 6.56). The system is capable of inspecting capsules, tablets, and other shapes at speeds up to 200,000 units/h (depending on product dimensions). It can detect the following product defects: dirt, foreign particles, scratches, shape, cracks, deformation, color, print blurring, or lack of printing.

CPT INSIGHT 100

The CPT Insight 100 (Figure 6.57) designed by CapPlus Technologies automatically inspects any two-piece hard shell capsule, oblong softgel, or caplet-shaped tablet. The capsule transport includes a patented drum feeder and spacing assembly. The system inspects up to 100,000 size 0 capsules per hour (28 per second) and employs a high-speed monochrome camera. An automatic speed adjustment ensures maximum production and quality control. The sensors are self-adjusting, and the system design is CFR 21 part 11 compliant.[58]

InspeCaps 150 by Proditec

The InspecCaps 150 (Figure 6.58) system performs full capsule inspection without physical rotation of the capsule. The capsules are conveyed from a centrifugal bowl onto a conveyer belt where they are held in position by vacuum as they pass through the inspection area. The inspection system employs three color cameras that create four simultaneous mirror views with overlap. The four images are merged into one flat view of the body and cap. The capsule inspection criteria include all physical

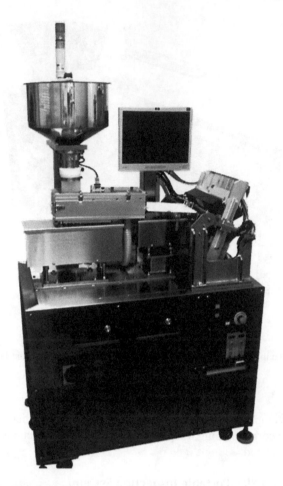

FIGURE 6.55   Viswill PAPPIS. (Courtesy of DJA-PHARMA, Wood Dale.)

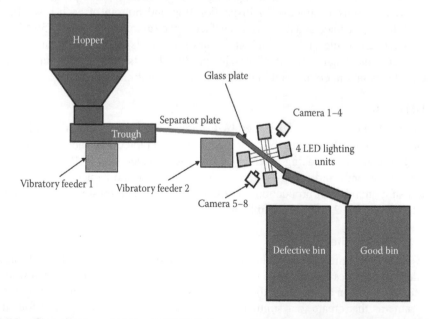

FIGURE 6.56   **(See color insert.)** Viswill PAPPIS diagram. (Courtesy of DJA-PHARMA, Wood Dale.)

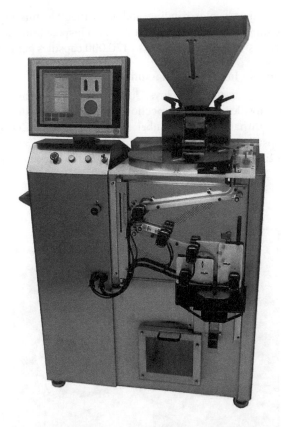

FIGURE 6.57 CPT INSIGHT 100. (Courtesy of CapPlus Technologies, Phoenix, AZ.)

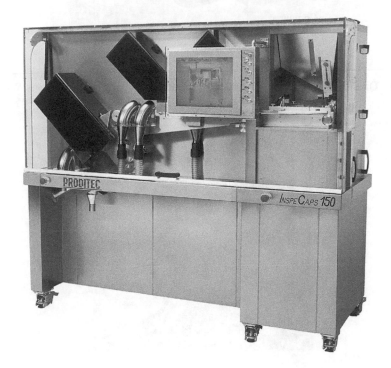

FIGURE 6.58 InspeCaps 150. (Courtesy of Proditec, Narberth, PA.)

defects, that is, appearance, shape, color, banding, and print (illegible, missing, incorrect, or smeared). In addition to inspecting standard capsule colors, it can also inspect translucent and transparent capsules, filled or empty. The inspection output is up to 120,000 capsules per hour for sizes 00 to 5.

Qualicaps CES-150 Capsule Inspection Machine

The Qualicaps CES-150 (Figure 6.59) employs Qualicaps' patented three-drum capsule transport system to feed rectified capsules into an inspection drum that turns intermittently at high speed. Using parallel lighting with halogen source fiber lights and three CCD line sensor cameras, the system inspects nine capsules in one row (Figure 6.60). During the slight stop of the inspection drum, the capsules turn 2.2 revolutions to inspect the circumference and sides without a dead angle.

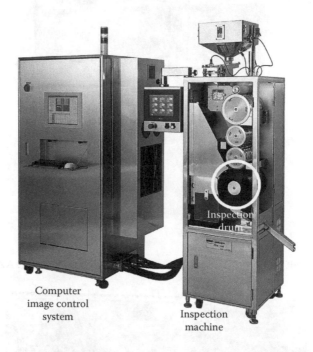

Computer
image control
system

Inspection
machine

FIGURE 6.59   Qualicaps CES-150 capsule inspection machine. (Courtesy of Qualicaps, Whitsett, NC.)

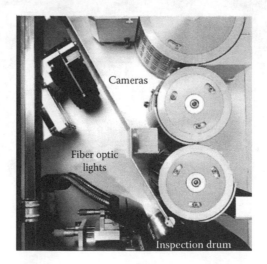

Cameras

Fiber optic
lights

Inspection drum

FIGURE 6.60   Qualicaps CES-150 inspection cameras and lighting. (Courtesy of Qualicaps, Whitsett, NC.)

The camera scans at high speed about 500 times at a fixed focal distance to input a highly accurate image of the capsule. The acceptable or reject quality is based on comparing the capsule image with a previously set up inspection threshold. The system has the capability of inspecting for the following capsule defects: foreign materials or stains greater than 100 μm, dents, splits, holes, edges, double caps, telescoped, unjoined, scrapes, short/long caps/bodies, unprinted.

The output of the CES-150 is as follows: size O capsules—103,000 capsules per hour; sizes 1 to 5—155,000 capsules per hour.[59]

OTHER CAPSULE SUPPORT EQUIPMENT

CAPSULE CHECKWEIGHERS

Unless the capsule filling machines are equipped with in-process controls to monitor the dosing of every capsule, there is always the potential for an occasional under/overfilled capsule that may not be detected by routine weight sampling of the machine output. Since many capsules are opaque, low fills would not be visually detected. Checkweighing a manufactured capsule batch is the only absolute assurance that there are no capsule out-of-weight specifications. This weight checking is critical in the manufacture of clinical supplies to assure proper dosing of all trial subjects.[60]

There are a good variety of capsule checkweighers available to suit various product/production needs that are listed in Table 6.3. Checkweighers perform gravimetric analysis using either load cells or electromagnetic force compensation balances. Unique features and illustrations of some of the checkweigher models listed in Table 6.3 are described below.

Bosch KKE 3800

The Bosch KKE 3800 (Figure 6.61) is an ultrahigh-speed checkweigher with an output up to 230,000 capsules per hour. It is ideally suited to applications with more than one capsule filling machine or for batch recovery work. The KKE 3800 and all Bosch checkweighers are equipped with Automatic Troubleshooting (ASB) function. Similar to Bosch capsule fillers, ASB automatically detects and ejects deformed capsules, eliminating unnecessary downtime.

The Bosch checkweighers have a patented "hanging weight cell" (Figure 6.62) that avoids dust or any residue buildup on the weight cell. This design also eliminates electrical interferences, that is, electrostatic fields.

Weight data from the production run are collected and evaluated by the operating system and saved on a DVD burner or can be transferred to an external system.[61]

Harro Höfliger OmniControl, Mid-Speed

This machine has a unique size part–free product in-feed (Figure 6.63[62]) that can weight sort both capsules (up to 21 mm long) and most sizes and shapes of tablets independent of geometry and dimensions. The products are picked up from the supply hopper via a vacuum wheel and are then transferred into a pocket wheel. The pocket wheel conveys the product onto the weight cell, which uses a patented rotating star concept. The star rotates to the left to divert the acceptable weights into the pass product container and rotates to the right to divert the overweight/underweight product into the bin for fail products.

MG America Anritsu KW9001AP

The Anritsu has the capability of weight sorting capsules into three separate categories: overweight, underweight, and pass at a rate of 120,000 capsules per hour (Figure 6.64[63]). It utilizes a vibration-proof weight cell and a variable cutoff digital filter to prevent floor vibrations. Monitoring systems check the rejection gate for proper operation and assure that the weight cells are in zero position.

TABLE 6.3
Capsule Checkweighers

Manufacturer	Model	Capsules per Hour (up to)	Weight Range (reproducibility)	Weighing Method[a]	Other Features
Bosch Packaging Technology Waiblingen, Germany	KKE 1,700 KKE 2,500 KKE 3,800	100,000 150,000 230,000	1–2,000 mg (±1 mg)	E	—Automatic troubleshooting mode activated when weighing cells detect a blocked capsule track —Can be coupled with GKF 1700/2500 filling machine with feedback loop for weight adjustment —Optional tablet check-weighing
Harro Höfliger Packaging Systems Doylestown, Pennsylvania, USA	Accura C (6 track) Accura C (12 track)	80,000 160,000	0–2,000 mg (±2 mg)	L	—Trend control for readjusting filling volume on Modu-C capsule filling machine —Statistical evaluation of weighing cell —Additional load cell for compensation of environmental influences such as air flow or vibration
	OmniControl (low-speed) OmniControl (mid-speed)	32,500 65,000	0–2,000 mg (±2 mg)	L	—Format free handling system that handles all capsule sizes and a wide variety of tablet shapes without changing size-parts
IMA Active Bologna, Italy	Precisa 12 Precisa 16 Precisa 18	90,000 160,000 200,000	1–5,000 mg (±1 mg)	L	—Feed channel clearance system —Possible connection to all capsule filling machines that can be stopped if produced capsules are out of limits
MG America Bologna, Italy	Anritsu KW9002AP Anritsu KW9001AP	60,000 120,000	20–1,000 mg (±2 mg)	L	—High/low/acceptable weights sorted into separate bins —Sensor on rejection gate to prevent mixing of pass and rejected product due to incorrect gate operation
MoCon Minneapolis, Minnesota, USA	AB Plus Master Module w/ 4 satellites w/ 6 satellites w/ 9 satellites	2,700 13,500 18,900 27,000	1–2,000 mg (±1 mg)	L	—Weight-sorts tablets/capsules without size parts —One computer can run master and 9 satellite units —Equipped with large capacity hopper for unattended operation
Qualicaps Whitsett, North Carolina, USA	CWI-40 CWI-90 CWI-150	40,000 90,000 150,000	20–500 mg (±2 mg) 500–1,000 mg (±3 mg)	E	—Automatic calibration —Frequent comparison check of electromagnetic force compensation balance by a built-in secondary balance —Reject confirmation device

(Continued)

TABLE 6.3 (CONTINUED)
Capsule Checkweighers

Manufacturer	Model	Capsules per Hour (up to)	Weight Range (Reproducibility)	Weighing Method[a]	Other Features
CI Precision	Sade SP-140	4,500	1–2,000 mg	L	—No change parts required
Salisbury,	Sade SP-240	9,000	(±1 mg)		—Equipped with large capacity
Wiltshire, UK	Sade SP-440	22,000			hopper designed for unattended operation
Schaefer	Dott.	3,000	1–2,000 mg	L	—Can be directly linked to the
Technologies	Bonapace		(±1 mg)		IN-CAP capsule filling machine
Indianapolis,	CW-30				
Indiana, USA					

[a] E, Electromagnetic force compensation; L, load cell.

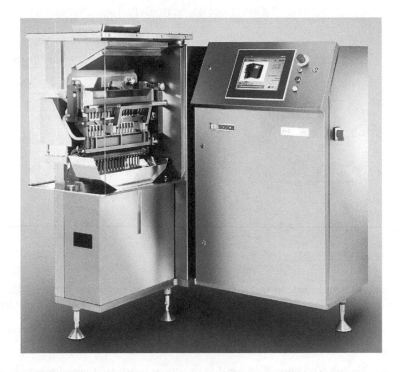

FIGURE 6.61 Bosch KKE 3800. (Courtesy of Robert Bosch Packaging Technology, Inc., Minneapolis, MN.)

CAPSULE POLISHERS

Capsule polishers are frequently used at the exit chute of the capsule filling machines to remove any excess product dust on the capsule surface and to cull out any separated capsules and loose product before the capsules are discharged into the product containers. The two types of units currently in use are brush polishers and air selection units. An older offline method of cleaning capsules is to roll the capsules in a tablet coating pan with salt.

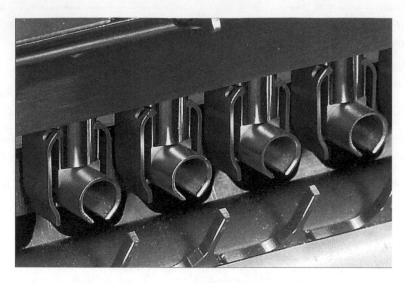

FIGURE 6.62   "Hanging weight cells." (Courtesy of Robert Bosch Packaging Technology, Inc., Minneapolis, MN.)

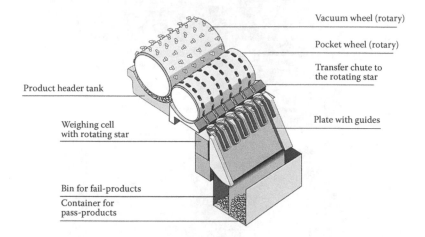

FIGURE 6.63   OmniControl Sizepart-free 100%-checking system for tablets and capsules. (From Harro Höfliger Packaging Systems, Inc. OmniControl Size part-free 100%-checking systems for tablets & capsules. 2011. Brochure.)

Brush Polishers

Brush-type units (Figure 6.65) use a motor-driven rotary brush that simultaneously conveys and dedusts the capsules.[64] A capsule separator system can be mounted to the polisher discharge chute to remove any empty, separated, or broken capsules. The units can also be fitted with a static eliminator using an ionized point conductive air probe for removal of static held dust.[65]

Air Selection Unit

The DS71 Capsule Selection Unit by IMA Active Division (Figure 6.66[66]) is designed to collect capsules from the capsule filler and separate the correctly filled capsules from the empty capsules and to remove dust or pellets from the capsule outer surface. The filled and empty capsules or capsule pieces are separated by means of a filtered air stream. The empty capsules are ejected from the cylindrical duct through an upper opening into a special container. The

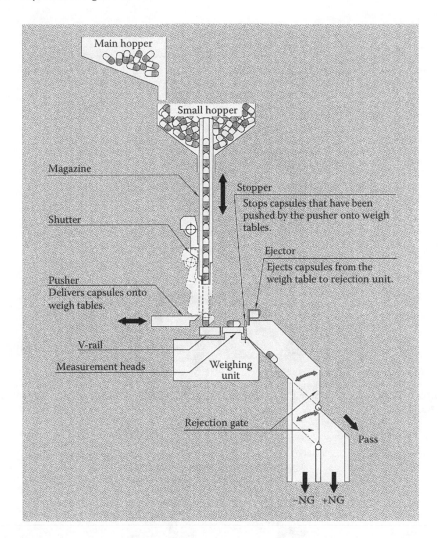

FIGURE 6.64 Process flow of Anritsu capsule checkweighers. (From Anritsu Industrial Solutions Co., LTD. KW9001AP/KW9002AP Capsule Checkweighers. Brochure provided by MG America, Fairfield, NJ; 2004–5.)

filled capsules exit through the lower opening of the cylindrical duct and are discharged from a chute into the product receiving container.

CAPSULE SEPARATORS

Capsule fill material can be automatically recovered without milling and sieving the capsules by using a capsule separator. Filled capsules are fed through a magazine of the capsule separator into holes of a raceway. As the capsules are pushed into the raceway slots, the cap and body of the capsule are pinched from both sides by the upper and lower pinching plates. The distance between the upper and lower pinching plates increases, pulling the capsule apart. Separated caps and bodies and encapsulated material are discharged through the lower chute for material recovery.

RecyCap from Harro Höfliger (Figure 6.67) is a commercially available system for recovery of product from capsules at a maximum output of 61,200 capsules per hour. The product is separated from the capsules via a screening device and discharged into separate bins for product recovery.[67]

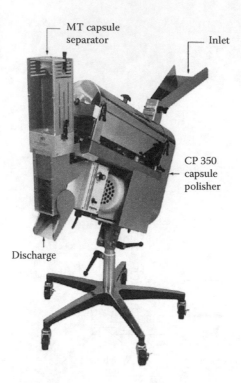

FIGURE 6.65 Turbo-Kleen Capsule Polisher Model No. CP-350-WD. (Courtesy of Key International, Inc., Cranbury, NJ.)

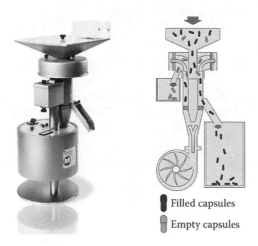

FIGURE 6.66 DS71 capsule selection unit. (From IMA Active Division. DS71 & SC System Accessories for capsule fillers. 2010. Brochure.)

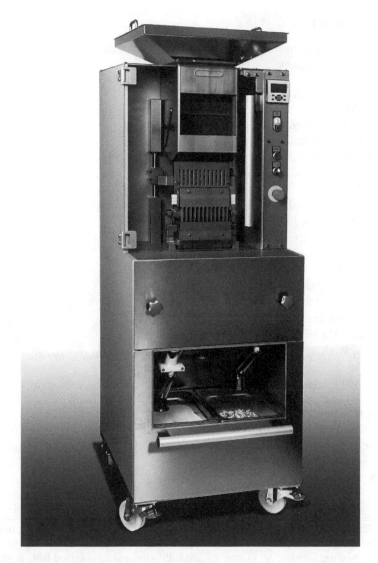

FIGURE 6.67 RecyCap. (Courtesy of Harro Höfliger Packaging Systems, Doylestown, PA.)

ACKNOWLEDGMENTS

I would like to acknowledge the following individuals for providing information on their organization's machinery and equipment:

1. Stefania Barzanti, IMA Active
2. Barry Fox, Mendel Co.
3. Ron Hayden, Key International Inc.
4. Bill Kohl, Robert Bosch Packaging Technology, Inc.
5. Frederic Le Pape, Proditec Inc.
6. Wayne Lewis, CapPlus Technologies
7. Dolphy C. Machado, ACG North America LLC
8. Glenn Martin and Claudio Radossi, MG America Inc.
9. Rusty Nelson, Daiichi Jitsugyo (America) Inc.
10. Professor Luigi G Martini, Rainbow Medical Engineering Ltd.
11. Judith Rehm, Robert Bosch GmbH
12. Paul Richer, Mettler Toledo
13. Angie Roberson, Qualicaps
14. Kevin Schaefer and Ron Silvers, Schaefer Technologies Inc.
15. Raj Tahil, Torpac Inc.
16. John Van Toll, Harro Höfliger Packaging Systems
17. Christina A. Watson, Capsugel

I would also like to acknowledge the following individuals for reviewing my manuscript:

1. Dr. David Doughty, GlaxoSmithKline
2. Matthew Knopp, *Tablets & Capsules* Magazine
3. Lewis Iler, GlaxoSmithKline

REFERENCES

1. Jones BE. Evolution of the technology for filling two-piece capsul with powderses. *Tablets & Capsules.* 2006 January.
2. Lightfoot DK. Capsule technology & encapsulation of commercial & clinical supplies. In *Bioforum Applied Knowledge Center*; 2009; Ness Ziona. pp. 57–60.
3. Capsugel. Coni-Snap Hard Gelatin Capsules. 2011. Brochure: Data obtained from p. 16.
4. Warner Lambert Co. Capsugel Division. *Operation and Maintenance of the Type 8 Capsule Filling Machine.* Capsugel Publication. Morris Plains, NJ; 1989.
5. Augsburger LL. Hard and soft shell capsules. In Banker GS, Rhodes CT, editors. *Modern Pharmaceutics, Third Edition.* New York: Marcel Dekker; 1996. p. 407.
6. Qualicaps. LIQFIL super 40. Brochure. Whitsett, NC; 2011.
7. Cole GC. History of capsule filling machinery. In Ridgway K, editor. *Hard Capsules Development & Technology.* London: The Pharmaceutical Press; 1987. pp. 95–96.
8. IMA ACTIVE division. ZANASI PLUS Medium-high speed capsule filling machines. 2011. Brochure.
9. Harro Hofliger Packaging Systems. Modular filling and closing machine for capsules. Modu-C Mid-Speed (MS). 2010. Brochure.
10. Lightfoot DK. Multiparticulate encapsulation and process. In Ghebre-Sellassie I, editor. *Multiparticulate Encapsulation and Process.* New York: Marcel Dekker; 1994. pp. 162–165.
11. Qualicaps. LIQFIL super 40. 2010. Brochure. Whitsett, NC.
12. Qualicaps. LIQFIL super 40. 2010. Brochure.
13. IMA ACTIVE. IMATIC High Speed Capsule Filling Machine. 2011. Brochure.
14. Podczeck F. Dry filling of hard capsules. In Podczeck F, Jones B, editors. *Pharmaceutical Capsules, Second Edition.* London: Pharmaceutical Press; 2004. p. 134.
15. Richardson M. Over-encapsulation: Techniques and challenges of blinding clinical supplies. *Tablets & Capsules.* 2010 March: p. 16.

16. IMA ACTIVE division. Zanasi Low-medium speed capsule filling machines. 2011. Brochure.
17. Lightfoot DK. Encapsulation equipment and process. In Ghebre-Sellassie I, editor. *Multiparticulate Oral Drug Delivery*. New York: Marcel Dekker; 1994. p. 170.
18. Smith T. The hard capsule with the soft center: The re-emergence of liquid-filled hard capsules. *Tablets & Capsules*. 2004 January: p. 15.
19. Lightfoot DK. A rising tide: Liquid filled capsules. *Tablets & Capsules*. 2008 January: Back page article.
20. Stegman MR&S. Filling two-piece hard gelatin capsules with liquids. *Tablets & Capsules*. 2007 January: p. 12.
21. Kadri BV. Delivering poorly soluble API's in liquid filled hard capsules. *Tablets & Capsules*. 2012 March: p. 16.
22. IMA ACTIVE Division. ZANASI LAB. 2011. Brochure.
23. Warner-Lambert Company, Capsugel Division. *All About the Hard Gelatin Capsule*. Capsugel Publication. Morris Plains, NJ; 1991. Report No.: CAP 126E.
24. Capsugel. Ultra 8 II Semi-Automatic Production Scale Capsule Filling Machine. 2006. Brochure.
25. Robert Bosch GmbH Packaging Tecnology. GKF 2500 Capsule Filling Machine. 2012. Brochure pp. 4–9.
26. Harro Hofliger Packaging Systems Inc. Modular Filling and closing machine for capsules Modu-C Mid Speed (MS). 2011. Brochure.
27. Harro Hifliger Packaging Systems Inc. Modular Filling and closing machine for capsules Modu-C Low Speed (LS). 2011. Brochure.
28. Harro Hofliger Packaging Systems. In-line mass verification for solids and powders VisioAMV. Brochure.
29. IMA ACTIVE division. ADAPTA THE EVOLVING CAPSULE FILLER. 2011. Brochure.
30. MG America, Inc. PLANETA/PLANETA 100. Brochure.
31. MG2. NETT. 2006. Brochure.
32. Qualicaps. Full-Automatic Capsule Filling Machine LIQFULsuper80. 2012. Brochure.
33. ACG-pam Pharma Technologies Solid Encapsulation Technologies. AF Series. Brochure.
34. Mettler Toledo. Automatic and precise Individual capsule filling. Brochure. Greifensee: Mettler Toledo AG, Laboratory & Weighing Technologies; 2011. Report No. 30008325.
35. Capsugel. Xcelodose S Precision Powder Micro-dosing Systems. 2011. Brochure.
36. Harro Hoefliger Packagong Systems. Laboratory Filler Omnidose. Brochure.
37. Manufacturing Chemist.com. [Online]; 2009.
38. Macdonald G. Pharma Technologist.com. [Online]; 2008.
39. Lightfoot D. Multiparticulate encapsulation and process. In Ghebre-Sllassie I, editor. *Multiparticulate Oral Drug Delivery*. New York: Marcel Dekker; 1994. p. 178.
40. FDA. fda.gov CPG Sec. 450.500 Tamper-Resistant Packaging Requirements for Certain Over-the-Counter Human Drug Products. [Online]. Available from: http://www.fda.gov/iceci/compliancemanuals/compliancepolicyguidancemanual/ucm074391.htm
41. Qualicaps. HICAPSEAL Fully Automatic Hard Capsule Sealing Machine 40/100. 2010. Brochure.
42. Qualicaps, Inc. Qualicaps Lab-Scale Filling/Sealing Machine. Brochure.
43. Schaefer Technologies, Inc. Laboratory Model Capsule Banding Machine. Operation and service manual, Ver. 1.00.
44. Qualicaps. Qualicaps Bench-Top Capsule Band-Sealer: The S-1. Brochure.
45. IMA ACTIVE division. Hermetica Capsule Banding Machine. 2011. Brochure.
46. DOTT.BONAPACE & C. s.r.l. BD-3000 Hard Gelatine Capsule Sealing Machine. Brochure.
47. Capsugel. Liquid filling and sealing of hard capsules cfs 1500C. 2010. Brochure.
48. S. Robin HBSVDC. X-ray Tomography to Determine Seal Integrity of Filled Capsules Sealed on Capsugel LEMS 70 and CFS 1200 Equipment. Capsugel Report. Report No. BAS 409.
49. Capsugel. Licaps. Greenwood, SC.
50. Capsugel. cfs 1200 Capsule Liquid Filling and Sealing Machine. 2006. Brochure.
51. Capsugel. Pharmaceutical Online.com CFS 1200 Liquid Capsule Filling & Sealing Machine. [Online]. [cited 2012 August 4]. Available from: http://www.pharmaceuticalonline.com/doc.mvc/CFS-1200-Liquid-Capsule-Filling-and-Sealing-M-0002
52. Capsugel. Pharmaceutical Online.com New CFS 1500 C Capsule filling and Sealing System. [Online]; 2010 [cited 2012 August 4]. Available from: http://www.pharmaceuticalonline.com/doc.mvc/New-CFS-1500-C-Capsule-Filing-And-Sealing-0001
53. Capsugel. cfs 1500 C Containment. 2010. Brochure.
54. Capsugel. LEMS 70 Production of liquid filled hard Capsules. 2008. Brochure.

55. Martini PLG,ALP. Ultrasonic welding of solid oral dosage forms: capsule based systems. 2012. Report to Donald Lightfoot.
56. Rainbow-medical. [Online]; 2006 [cited 2012 August 20]. Available from: http://www.rainbow-medical .eu/pharmaceutical.html
57. Mendel Company. MCI-700 Capsule Inspector. Brochure.
58. CapPlus Technologies. CPT Insight 100 Inspection System. Brochure.
59. Qualicaps. Qualicaps Inspection Machine CES-150. Brochure.
60. Lightfoot DK. An overview of capsule checkweighers. *Tablets & Capsules*. 2011 January.
61. Robert Bosch GmbH Packaging Technology Division. KKE 1700/KKE 2500/KKE 3800 Bosch Weighing Technology. 2011. Brochure.
62. Harro Hofliger Packaging Systems, Inc. OmniControl Sizepart-free 100%-checking systems for tablets & capsules. 2011. Brochure.
63. Anritsu Industrial Solutions Co., LTD. KW9001AP/KW9002AP Capsule Checkweighers. Brochure provided by MG America, Fairfield, NJ; 2004–5.
64. Smith TLaB. What to consider when selecting a tablet/capsule deduster. *Tablets & Capsules*. 2006 July: p. 48.
65. Key International, Inc. Turbo-Kleen Tablet Deduster/Capsule Polisher. Bulletin No. CP-350-WD.
66. IMA Active Division. DS71 & SC System Accessories for capsule fillers. 2010. Brochure.
67. Harro Hofliger. RecyCap—A system for recovery of product from capsules. Brochure.

7 Instrumented Automatic Capsule Filling Machines and Filling Machine Simulation

Larry L. Augsburger and Vikas Moolchandani

CONTENTS

The advent of research instrumented automatic capsule filling machines and filling machine simulators has ushered in a new era in formulation research for this dosage form. The ability to measure the forces involved in plug formation and ejection on actual machines or in simulators under controlled laboratory conditions has provided new insights into the interplay of formulation and machine operating variables and its effect on both the filling of capsules and the performance of encapsulated dosage forms as drug delivery systems. This information thus reduces formulators' reliance on empiricism in formulation design and supports Quality by Design (QbD).

INSTRUMENTED CAPSULE FILLING MACHINES

Today, industrially filled hard gelatin capsules are most often filled using automatic filling machines that form powder plugs by compression and eject them into the empty capsule bodies. Given the similarity of plug compression and ejection to tableting and the utility of instrumented tablet presses in the production environment and in research, it is not at all surprising that the techniques that had proved successful in the instrumentation of tablet presses have been applied to such capsule filling machines.[1,2] Table 7.1 provides a chronology of the research instrumentation of automatic capsule filling machines.

Generally, two types of plug forming machines may be distinguished. These may be described as "dosing disc machines" and "dosator machines." Zanasi, MG-2, and Macofar machines, for example, utilize a dosator that consists of a cylindrical dosing tube fitted with a moveable piston to form and eject plugs. With the piston set to a particular height in the dosing tube, the dosator assembly

TABLE 7.1

Instrumented Automatic Capsule Filling Machines

Date	Investigators	Machine	Methodology
1972, 1975	Cole and May[3,4]	Zanasi LZ-64	Strain gauged piston; planetary gear system to modify dosator motion
1975, 1977	Small and Augsburger[5,6]	Zanasi LZ-64	Strain gauged piston; mercury pool swivel
1977	Mony, Sambeat, and Cousin[7]	Zanasi RV-59	Piezoelectric load washer mounted on piston end
1980	Greenberg[8]	Zanasi AZ-60	Strain gauged piston; slip ring
1980	Mehta and Augsburger[9]	Zanasi LZ-64	Displacement transducer (LVDT) added
1983	Rowley, Hendry, Ward, and Timmins[10]	Zanasi LZ-64	Piezoelectric load washer installed on ejection knob
1983	Shah, Augsburger, Small, and Polli[11]	Hofliger & Karg GKF 330	Strain gauged pistons (two tamping stations)
1986	Shah, Augsburger, and Marshall[12]	Hofliger & Karg GKF 330	Strain gauged pistons (all tamping stations)
1986	Maury, Heraud, Etienne, Aumonier, and Casahoursat[13]	Zanasi LZ-64	Piezoelectric load cells installed in the overload mechanism and on ejection knob
1988	Cropp, Augsburger, and Marshall[14]	Hofliger & Karg GKF 330	Displacement transducers (LVDT) added to previously instrumented machine
1993	Hauer, Remmele, and Sucker[15]	Zanasi LZ-64	Strain gauged piston; differential condenser
2000	Podczek[16,17]	Bosch GKF 400S	Prototype pneumatic tamping head fitted with a piezoelectric force transducer
2010	Moolchandani[18–20]	Harro Hofliger KFM/3 dosing disc machine	Strain gauged pistons (all middle tamping stations) with SCXI chassis and Labview data acquisition software

is plunged downward into a powder bed set at a particular height. The plug initially forms through the passage of the dosator through the powder bed. As the plug forms in the open end of the dosing tube, a degree of compression against the piston develops (sometimes called "precompression"). While the dosator is in the full down position, the plug contained within may be further compressed by causing the piston itself to execute a downward displacement through contact with a downward-moving compression knob (e.g., Zanasi) or via a cam track (e.g., MG2). The dosator bearing the plug is lifted from the bed and the same piston will later eject the plug into a capsule shell similarly via a descending ejection knob or cam track movement. After each ejection (and piston compression), a piston return spring housed within the dosator returns the piston to its original position. Like dosator machines, Bosch GKF (formerly Hofliger & Karg) and Harro Höfliger machines, for example, also operate on a piston-tamp filling principle. However, unlike their dosator counterparts, these machines utilize a dosing disc and a multiple-tamp process to fill powders. The dosing disc forms the base of a dosing chamber. It has a number of holes bored through it. A solid brass "stop" plate slides along the bottom of the dosing disc to close off these holes, thus forming openings analogous to the die cavities of a tablet press. The powder or granular formulation is filled to a particular height over the dosing disc. The formulation flows into the cavities. Tamping pins (sometimes referred to as "tamping fingers") compress the formulation into the cavities. As they do so, some additional formulation from above the dosing disc is pushed into the dosing disc cavities. Plugs are built up in stages. The dosing disc rotates under several sets of tamping pins such that the plugs are built up gradually through as many as five (depending on the machine) separate compression (i.e., tamping) events. The tamping pins are spring loaded to prevent overstressing the system. Ultimately, the disc will rotate to position completed plugs under a different set of similar pins that eject the plugs from the dosing disc into capsule shells. It is not surprising that most investigators have chosen to instrument dosator and dosing disc machines by bonding strain gauges directly to the dosator pistons or the tamping and ejecting pins of dosing disc machines since they are central to the plug formation and ejection processes. A more detailed discussion of the design and operating principles of these machines may be found elsewhere in this book.

The parameters to measure which are of greatest interest are the compression forces involved in plug formation, plug ejection, and the tamping pin or piston displacement. Plug compression force can affect drug dissolution,[21–23] as well as plug formation, fill weight and weight variation.[12,24] Plug ejection force measurements allow objective decisions to be made on the type and level of lubricant to include in formulations.[25] The monitoring of piston displacement provides the information needed to program laboratory machines designed to simulate actual capsule filling machines.[9,14] Simultaneous measurement of both tamping pin force and displacement makes basic research on the plug compaction mechanism possible. Many of these points will be discussed later in this chapter.

TRANSDUCERS

Two types of force sensing devices are commonly employed in capsule filling machine instrumentation: resistive strain gauges and piezoelectric load cells. Strain gauges can be bonded directly to load-bearing components to form a force sensing transducer in situ. In other instances, strain gauge-based load cells or piezoelectric load cells can be installed in strategic locations to sense forces. The LVDT (Linear Variable Differential Transformer) displacement transducer has been installed on both dosator and dosing disc machines. Details of the characteristics and use of these transducers may be found in standard references such as Daly and Riley[26] and Ridgway Watt.[27] Because of the extensive use of resistance strain gauges in research instrumented capsule filling machines, additional information on strain gauges has been given in the example followed below.

LOCATION OF TRANSDUCERS AND SITE MODIFICATION

There are practical considerations to selecting the site of transducers. For instance, instrumentation systems for dosator machines that mount transducers on the compression knob (as opposed to the piston itself) or on the distal end of the dosator piston are incapable of registering the precompression force experienced when the dosators plunge downward into the powder bed. In these cases, a force can only be registered when the upper end of the piston comes in contact with the compression knob or ejection knob. Moreover, that limitation prevents the measurement of piston retraction or drag forces (described later) that sometimes are observed when running dosator machines. The first example of this approach was reported by Mony et al.[7] who instrumented a Zanasi RV/59 by mounting a piezoelectric load cell to the upper end of a piston. A further complication of this approach is that the force measured by this instrumentation must necessarily include the force required to compress the piston retraction spring. No attempt to correct their data for this variable was reported. Rowley et al.[10] reported the mounting of a small piezoelectric load cell to the ejection knob of a Zanasi LZ-64 machine to monitor ejection force. This approach also suffers from the disadvantage that the force measured includes the force required to compress the piston return spring. However, in this case, the authors made a "blank" run with an empty dosator and subtracted the force required to compress the dosator spring from their measurements. The method of Maury et al.[13] in which piezoelectric load cells are installed in the overload mechanism and on the ejection knob of a dosator machine is similarly disadvantaged.

The application of strain gauges may involve a modification of the piston or tamping pin at the site to which they are bonded. Depending on the situation, this modification may be undertaken to provide a convenient bonding surface and increase sensitivity by removing some of the steel and/

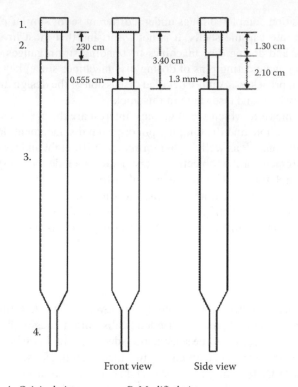

Front view   Side view

A. Original piston   B. Modified piston

1. Head; 2. Neck; 3. Upper shank; 4. Lower shank

FIGURE 7.1 A comparison of the original and modified pins of a Harro Hofliger KFM/3 capsule filling machine. (From Moolchandani V. *Functionality and Performance of Different Lactose Grades in Capsule Filling: Characterization and Evaluation of Formulation and Operating Variables on Dosing Disc Machines,* PhD Thesis, University of Maryland at Baltimore, 2010.)

or simply to provide sufficient clearance to avoid damage to the gauge and wiring during machine operation. As an example, consider the modification of the tamping pin made for the instrumentation of a Harro Hofliger KFM/3 dosing disc filling machine illustrated in Figure 7.1.[18–20] As can be seen, the size 1 tamping pin can be divided into four main regions: (1) the head, which is held in the pin holder; (2) the neck; (3) the upper shank; and (4) the lower shank, the tip of which compresses the powder. The neck and a small part of the adjoining upper shank are the only portions not occluded during the upward and downward movement of the tamping pin and plug compression. Therefore, this part of the tamping pin was chosen as the location for strain gauges. A portion of the elongated cylindrical neck was altered in each case to provide a flat rectangular section, 0.555 cm wide and 2.10 cm long, to provide a convenient site for bonding strain gauges. The thickness of this section was reduced to about 1.3 mm to enhance the sensitivity of the instrumentation. An instrumented Harro Hofliger KFM/3 tamping pin mounted in a tamping pin block is shown in Figure 7.2.

WHEATSTONE BRIDGE

Transducers are devices that convert some physical quantity (such as force) into a more conveniently measured property (such as voltage). Electrical resistance strain gages measure strain in an object based on the change in electrical resistance of an electrical conductor as a function of the strain. Strain gauges are often connected in a Wheatstone bridge circuit, often consisting of a combination

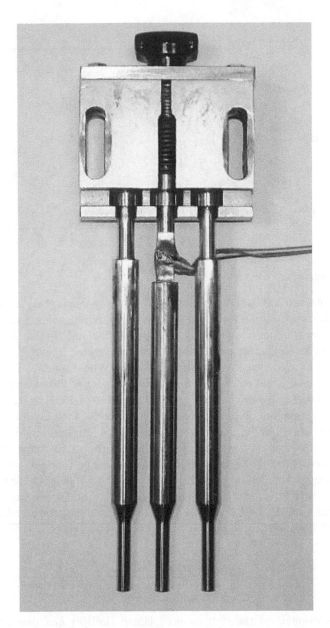

FIGURE 7.2 Image of one modified-instrumented and two original tamping pins mounted in a tamping pin block. (From Moolchandani V. *Functionality and Performance of Different Lactose Grades in Capsule Filling: Characterization and Evaluation of Formulation and Operating Variables on Dosing Disc Machines*, PhD Thesis, University of Maryland at Baltimore, 2010.)

of four active gauges (full bridge), as discussed here. As stress or load is applied, resistive changes to the bonded strain gauges take place, which unbalances the Wheatstone bridge. The result is a signal output related to the stress value. As the signal value is small (typically a few millivolts), the signal conditioning electronics provides amplification to increase the signal level to 5 to 10 V, a suitable level for external data collection systems.

It is good practice to select strain gauges with a thermal expansion coefficient that matches that of the surface to which they are applied, in this case the stainless steel of the piston or tamping pins, to compensate for possible temperature changes during operation. However, a Wheatstone bridge

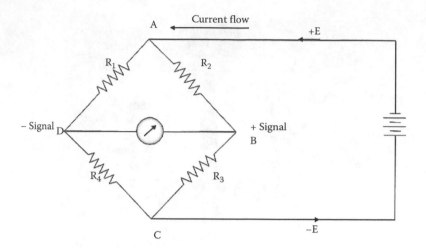

FIGURE 7.3   Wheatstone bridge.

provides an additional method to achieve temperature compensation. This technique is commonly referred to as circuit compensation with push (compression)–pull (tension) gauges. In the push–pull method, a C (compression) and T (tension) gauge are bonded side by side on the test piece (e.g., tamping pin) and wired as adjacent arms in the Wheatstone bridge (Figure 7.3).

The active gauges are connected in opposite arms of the Wheatstone bridge so that the contribution of each to the output could be expressed as a sum. A wire or foil element in the gauge under a positive strain (tension) will increase in length and decrease in diameter, resulting in increase in resistance. A compressive force will decrease the wire length, increase the diameter, and lower the resistance. Therefore, if strain gauge (R1) in arm 1 goes into tension, resulting in an increase in resistance, less current would flow through it. Whereas the strain gauge (R2) in arm 2 would undergo compression and the current in the circuit will take the path of least resistance, that is, more current will flow through arm 2 as compared to arm 1, causing a higher voltage potential at the junction between arms 2 and 3 than at the junction between arms 1 and 4. For that reason, the junction between arms 2 and 3 is called the positive signal. The change in voltage under compression load can be expressed by Equation 7.1:[26]

$$\frac{\Delta V}{V} = \text{Const.}\left(\frac{\Delta R_1}{R_1} - \frac{\Delta R_2}{R_2} + \frac{\Delta R_3}{R_3} - \frac{\Delta R_4}{R_4} \right) \tag{7.1}$$

In the previous example of the instrumented Harro Hofliger machine, one gauge pair was bonded on each side of the thinned neck portion of the modified piston. One gauge in each pair was aligned parallel to the major strain axis to form the primary active arms of a full Wheatstone bridge circuit. This resulted in the orientation of the other two gauges perpendicular to the major strain axis, which provided not only temperature compensation but also a small but significant contribution to the bridge-unbalance voltage through the Poisson effect. The circuit diagram appears in Figure 7.4.

Installation of Gauges

A great deal of care must be exercised in the proper installation of strain gauges. There are many considerations, such as cleaning, degreasing, and abrading the surface to which the gauge will be bonded, choice of adhesive, and curing. A specific procedure and technique needs to be learned and rigorously followed to assure a successful installation that exhibits reliable performance.

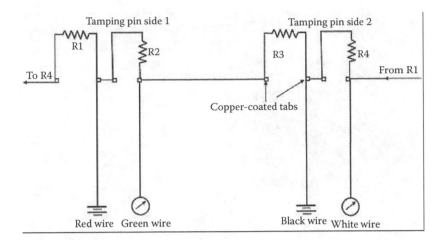

FIGURE 7.4   Circuitry diagram of Wheatstone bridge on a Harro Hofliger tamping pin. (From Moolchandani V. *Functionality and Performance of Different Lactose Grades in Capsule Filling: Characterization and Evaluation of Formulation and Operating Variables on Dosing Disc Machines*, PhD Thesis, University of Maryland at Baltimore, 2010.)

A discussion of these details is beyond the scope of this chapter, and the interested reader is referred to major strain gauge suppliers who often provide detailed guidance on strain gauge installation.

SIGNAL RETRIEVAL FROM ROTATING COMPONENTS

If pistons or other transducer sites are stationary or move only in one plane, sensing devices may be mounted directly onto them and signal retrieval is straightforward. However, when the instrumented site is rotating, there is the added complication of twisting or winding up of the connecting cables. This problem is commonly encountered with rotary tablet presses where the usual method of resolving the problem is to not instrument the actual punches, but to mount the transducer on a stationary, remote site, such as the tie rod between compression rollers, the eyebolt connecting the lower compression roller with the overload mechanism, or the compression roll pins. In such cases, the farther away the transducer is from the compaction event, the smaller the proportion of the actual punch force actually recorded.

The earliest reports (Table 7.1) of the instrumentation of automatic capsule filling machines have involved intermittent motion dosator machines in which the dosators rotate through 180° from the plug formation to the plug ejection stations and then back again (e.g., Zanasi LZ-64). Cole and May[3,4] reported on the modification of a Zanasi LZ-64 machine by the addition of a planetary gear system to prevent damage to the lead wires from an instrumented piston during such rotation. The planetary gear system keeps the same face of the instrumented dosator forward at all times by causing the dosator to rotate one full turn in the opposite direction for each rotation of the dosator assembly.

Small and Augsburger[5,6] used a mercury pool swivel to circumvent the problem of dosator rotation on an intermittent motion Zanasi machine. The mercury pool swivel is a form of slip ring. The swivel consists of a stationary plate, which is connected to the monitoring equipment, and a rotating wheel, which is connected to the rotating piston assembly. The complete bridge is assembled on the rotating component. Electrical conductivity through the swivel is by means of platinum-tipped electrodes that dip down from the stationary plate to individual mercury-filled canals in the rotating wheel. In instrumenting a Zanasi LZ-60 machine, Greenberg[8] used a traditional (non-mercury) slip ring assembly to connect the bridge to the power supply and recording instrument. The rings are mounted on a shaft attached to the rotating component such that the axis of the shaft coincides

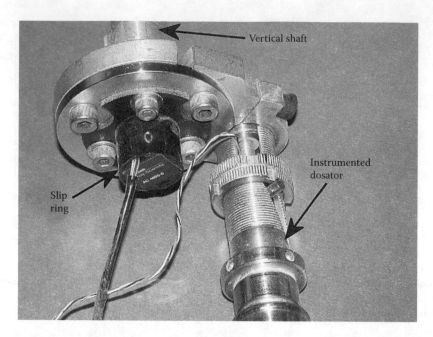

FIGURE 7.5 Zanasi dosator mounted to a slip ring assembly. During capsule filling, the vertical shaft keeps the slip ring in position while the dosator rotates.

with the axis of rotation of the rotating component. The shell of the assembly usually carries several brushes or sliding contacts for each ring. Lead wires from the bridge rotate with the specimen and are connected to the rings. Lead wires from the power supply and recording equipment are connected to the brushes. Later, the potentially hazardous mercury swivel of the earlier instrumented Zanasi LZ-64 was replaced with a similar instrument quality slip ring assembly (Figure 7.5).[22]

Hauer et al.[15] also bonded strain gauges to the piston of a Zanasi LZ-64 filling machine. They resolved the problem of dosator rotation by mounting a differential condenser in the shaft about which the dosators rotate that links the signal from the bridge with the cables to the recording system. Dosing disc machines (e.g., Hofliger-Karg and Harro Hofliger) do not require such considerations since the tamping pin assemblies move up and down in a vertical plane and do not rotate.

CALIBRATION

In all cases, calibration is essential to establish the relationship between the actual force or displacement being monitored and the output signal. The overall quality of the instrumentation depends on the accuracy and precision of the calibration and the institution of a periodic recalibration checking program. Instrumented pistons may be removed and installed in-line with a load cell of known output between the platens of a physical testing machine (e.g., Instron). The load cell thus functions as a primary standard. The outputs from the load cell and the instrumented piston or punch are monitored simultaneously during loading and unloading, preferably using a microprocessor-based digital data acquisition system (DAQ). Displacement transducers may be calibrated by direct comparison of the output against actual displacement measurements.

Following the previous example, Figure 7.6 illustrates the assembly used to calibrate instrumented tamping pins for the Harro Hofliger (H&H) filling machine using an Instron physical testing machine.[18] The test was performed in blocks. In the first block, the instrument was run in "position control" wherein the position of the hydraulic actuator was lowered at a rate of 60 mm/min until the specified load (end point) is reached. Once the specified load (e.g., 50 N) on the tamping pin was attained, the instrument would switch to the second block. In the second block, the instrument was

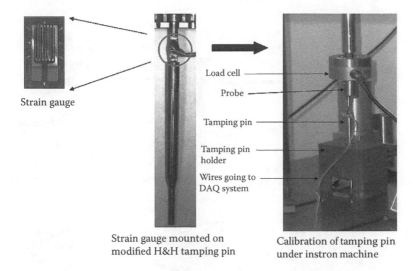

Strain gauge

Load cell

Probe

Tamping pin

Tamping pin holder

Wires going to DAQ system

Strain gauge mounted on modified H&H tamping pin

Calibration of tamping pin under instron machine

FIGURE 7.6 Calibration of instrumented tamping pins for the Harro Hofliger (H&H) filling machine using an Instron physical testing machine. (From Moolchandani V. *Functionality and Performance of Different Lactose Grades in Capsule Filling: Characterization and Evaluation of Formulation and Operating Variables on Dosing Disc Machines*, PhD Thesis, University of Maryland at Baltimore, 2010.)

run in load control, where the specified load would be maintained for 30 s (end point for the second block). After 30 s, the instrument would switch to the third block. In the third block, the instrument was run in position control, where the hydraulic actuator retracts back to about 15 mm above the tamping pin. The force was increased up to 300 N with the increment of 50 N per stage. Later, calibration force was reduced in a similar manner in order to check whether there is any hysteresis. During calibration, each tamping pin was checked for torsion loss by rotating the centering position of the pin.

MONITORING/DATA HANDLING

The output of these types of transducers is generally a DC voltage proportional to the magnitude of the property measured (force or distance). In selecting the voltage measuring and display instrument, the first criterion to be met is the frequency response. If the signal is static, the time available for recording is relatively long, and simple direct reading indicators or strip-chart recorders can be used. With dynamic signals, the time available to measure the output voltage may be very short, thus making recording more difficult.

Reading a meter or a line on a chart paper introduces a source of error and also demands a large amount of operator time and skill in transcribing the analog readout to digital numbers. Inexpensive, powerful digital microprocessors now available make unnecessary such laborious data handling and enhance the quality and quantity of the data produced. The analog signals are often multiplexed to an electronic analog-to-digital converter. The digital data may then be stored in a temporary "buffer" memory or permanently recorded on hard drive or disc. The data may be recalled for manipulation or display in either graphical or tabular form on a video monitor and/or hardcopy printer or plotter.

The mechanism that allows the interaction, via the computer, between the strain gauges and the operator is commonly referred to as a data acquisition system (DAQ). The DAQ collects and translates the signals from the different transducers mounted on a capsule filling machine, bringing these signals to a computer ready for processing, examination, storage, and other data processing. In the previous example of the instrumented Harro Hofliger machine,[18] the compression and ejection events detected by the instrumented tamping pins were monitored by measuring the bridge

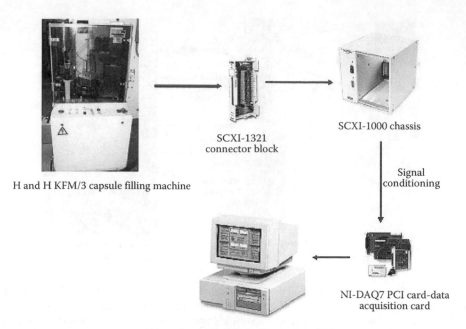

SCXI-1321
connector block

SCXI-1000 chassis

Signal
conditioning

H and H KFM/3 capsule filling machine

NI-DAQ7 PCI card-data
acquisition card

Data collected by Labview 7 on control PC

FIGURE 7.7   Signal conditioning and data acquisition schematic for the instrumented Harro Hofliger KFM/3 capsule filling machine. (From Moolchandani V. *Functionality and Performance of Different Lactose Grades in Capsule Filling: Characterization and Evaluation of Formulation and Operating Variables on Dosing Disc Machines*, PhD Thesis, University of Maryland at Baltimore, 2010.)

unbalance voltage using a carrier preamplifier SCXI 1000 chassis block and SCXI-1321 module (National Instruments, Austin, Texas), which also serves to activate the bridge. A NI-DAQ 7 PCI card (National Instruments) was the data acquisition device. The compression and ejection events were recorded continuously by means of Labview 7 software (National Instruments). A schematic of the DAQ system operation is shown in Figure 7.7.

Signal conditioning involves primarily an amplifier that provides the excitation voltage, as well as gain (a factor used in converting millivolt output of the strain gauge bridge to the volt-based range of the input of the data acquisition device). For example, the output of the Wheatstone bridge is normally expressed in millivolts per volt of excitation per unit of applied force. The sensitivity of 0.2 mV/V/kN means that, on application, a 10-kN force and a 10-V excitation will produce a 20-mV output. To utilize such output, it usually needs to be amplified several hundred times to reach units of volts. In the present example,[18] the SCXI 1000 chassis with NI SCXI-1321 module was used as a signal conditioning device.

Labview software controls the measurement system, telling the DAQ when and from which physical channels to acquire or generate data. This SCXI-1321 module supports the monitoring of four signals from the instrumentation at any one time.

APPLICATION OF INSTRUMENTED AUTOMATIC CAPSULE FILLING MACHINES IN RESEARCH AND DEVELOPMENT

Dosator Machines

Plug Compression and Ejection

The instrumentation of an automatic capsule filling machine was first reported by Cole and May[3,4] who bonded strain gauges directly to the piston of a Zanasi LZ-64 dosator machine; however, they

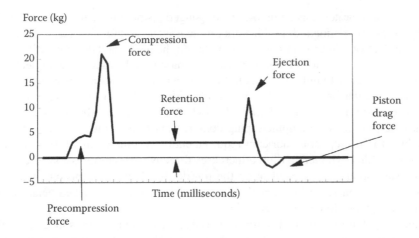

FIGURE 7.8   Representation of various features that may be found in dosator force–time traces.

did not make use of the piston compression feature of this machine. Small and Augsburger[5,6] also instrumented the piston of a Zanasi LZ-64, but their use of the compression mechanism provided a more complete evaluation of the role of the dosator in plug formation. The diagrammatic representation of the force–time traces shown in Figure 7.8 show the generation of a precompression force that typically occurs when the dosator plunges downward into the powder bed to capture a plug of powder. When the piston compression feature of the machine is utilized to apply more force to the plug, this precompression force is immediately followed by a spike, which results from the active compression of this plug by the piston when the dosing tube is at its lowest point of travel. Plug formation is then followed by a sharp spike, indicating the ejection force required to initiate the movement of the plug as it is pushed by the piston into the receiving capsule. Although plug compression forces (typically not greater than 200 N) are far lower than normally achieved in tableting, sufficient force may be developed to increase the density of the powders above their maximum tapped bulk density.

For a given formulation, the development of a precompression force depends on the piston height and the powder bed height.[28,29] For a given powder bed height, precompression force increases with decreases in the piston height. This apparently is the result of forcing smaller and smaller volumes through the same powder depth. Similarly, for a given piston height setting, the deeper the powder bed is, the greater the precompression force. Interestingly, increasing the magnesium stearate added to pregelatinized starch from 0.005% to 0.02% increases the precompression force, all other things being equal.[28,29] Two factors may contribute to this latter finding. First, an increase in the lubricant level may increase the packing density of the powder bed through the glidant effect of the lubricant. Second, the greater precompression force may in part also be attributable to reduced friction at the dosing tube wall, thereby causing less force to be lost in overcoming friction at the dosing tube wall, and more force to be transmitted to the piston during precompression.

Lubrication Requirements

A great deal of information about the state of lubrication can be learned by studying the traces produced using instrumented pistons. For example, a compression force–time trace that does not recover fully to the baseline before ejection (illustrated in Figure 7.8) may be seen with some formulations. This retention force is apparently attributed to expansion of the plug back against the end of the piston, and is mostly likely to be observed under conditions of marginal lubrication, particularly with materials that have substantial potential for elastic recovery.[4,6] With adequate lubrication, retention forces are negligible or do not appear, probably because the lubricant allows the plug to slip to relieve the residual pressure. Occasionally, a "negative trace" occurs after ejection and as the piston spring recovers to retract the piston to its initial position, as illustrated in Figure 7.8.[4,6]

This negative trace indicates tension on the strain-gauged piston during its retraction and can only be caused by excessive frictional drag. This drag force is attributed to inadequate lubrication and/or excessive accumulation/adhesion of powder particles on the piston and dosator wall.

Small and Augsburger demonstrated that instrumentation can be used to help select the type and level of lubricants.[25] They found lubricants to be effective, sometimes at unusually low concentrations: minimum ejection forces were observed at 1% with anhydrous lactose, 0.5% with microcrystalline cellulose, and 0.1% with pregelatinized starch. Moreover, they showed that, within certain limits, it may be possible to manipulate plug compression force, powder bed height, and piston height to reduce the hydrophobic lubricant requirement of a formulation while still achieving the target fill weight. Although ejection force increases directly with compression force as expected, this increase was found to be dependent on the powder bed height and piston height. At a given compression force, an increase in either the piston height or the powder bed height increases the magnitude of the ejection force, and vice versa.

Mehta and Augsburger mounted a linear variable displacement transducer (LVDT) on the Zanasi LZ-64 previously instrumented by Small and Augsburger.[9] This modification permitted the simultaneous measurement of both force and piston displacement. As expected, no displacement of the piston was observed at precompression. During piston compression, actual displacement was less than that set by adjustment of the compression knob owing to the deformation of the overload relief spring mounted in the compression knob holder. Generally, ejection force was found to rise to a maximum at the onset of the ejection displacement, indicating that sufficient force must be developed before the piston can displace the plug. In certain cases, a slight further compaction of the plug can be observed to occur during the development of the peak ejection force. Mehta used this instrumentation to estimate the work of plug ejection from the area under ejection force–piston displacement profiles.[30] Five formulations consisting of common fillers (anhydrous lactose, dicalcium phosphate, and microcrystalline cellulose) lubricated with either stearic acid or magnesium stearate were studied. Compression force and lubricant level were varied to yield similar peak ejection forces ($P = 0.05$). Yet, in most cases significant differences in the work of ejection were observed, suggesting that work measurements may be more informative than peak ejection force measurements.

It is well known that lubricants such as magnesium stearate can interfere with bonding and soften compressed tablets. Similarly, capsule plugs can also be softened, and this could adversely affect weight variation if it leads to powder loss during plug transfer. Powder could be lost from the end of the dosing tube during rotation to the ejection position or could result from plug collapse and breakup during ejection. It is interesting, however, that at certain limits, drug dissolution may be enhanced in certain formulations, presumably by a reduction in plug cohesion, as a result of increasing the magnesium stearate level[21,31] or by extending the mixing time of a given concentration magnesium stearate.[32] In one example, Mehta and Augsburger found that as the concentration of magnesium stearate increased from 0.05% to 0.75%, the time required for 60% dissolution of hydrochlorothiazide ($T_{60\%}$) decreased from 55 to 12 min and the breaking strength of these microcrystalline cellulose-based plugs measured using a three-point bending test was markedly reduced, from 85 to about 2 g.[21] The capsules were produced on an instrumented Zanasi LZ-64 machine with a standardized compression force. Interestingly, in a parallel study with the same range of magnesium stearate concentrations in a lactose-based formulation, hydrochlorothiazide $T_{60\%}$ increased slightly with the lubricant level (from 12 to 18 min) while the plug breaking force decreased slightly, although not significantly ($P = 0.05$), from 18 to 13 g.[21] In the case of microcrystalline cellulose, the initial increase in hydrophobicity with increase in magnesium stearate level may be more than offset by reduced plug cohesiveness in the concentration range studied, which probably improves moisture penetration and plug disintegration. Since dissolution markedly slowed when the magnesium stearate concentration was further increased to 2%, the hydrophobic effect of the lubricant apparently becomes overwhelming at higher levels.

Dosing Disc Machines

Plug Compression and Ejection

From the preceding discussion, it is evident that the tamping pins or the tamping assembly provides a logical location for transducers in dosing disc machines. Shah et al.[11,33] were the first investigators to report the instrumentation of the tamping pins of a dosing disc machine, a Hofliger & Karg model GKF 330 machine. Later, Cropp et al.[14] added two LVDTs to that same machine. One LVDT was connected to the ring on which the piston assemblies are mounted. Since the up and down movement of this ring provides the piston movements, this LVDT monitored the travel of the piston assemblies during the compression and decompression strokes. The distance traveled represents the actual displacement of the ejection pins, but not necessarily that of the tamping pins. Normally, a portion of the tamping piston displacement will be taken up by the compression of the overload relief springs mounted over the end of each pin. The second LVDT was thus installed to provide a measure of the movement of the overload spring. This LVDT was mounted to one pin block assembly directly above the center tamping pin, which was instrumented with strain gauges. Together, these two LVDTs made measurement of the actual penetration of the tamping pin into the dosing disc possible.

Force–time traces for plug compression events have been studied and correlated with the mechanical operation of the Hofliger & Karg GKF-type capsule filling machine.[11,12,14] Figure 7.9 shows a typical compression force–time trace for a single tamping event. It is interesting to note that this force–time trace is quite different from that reported for a Zanasi dosator capsule filler in that a decompression plateau follows the peak of compression. The decompression plateau appears only if the compression force exceeds a minimum (~50 N), and always persists for the same duration, regardless of the extent of compression.[11,33] At each tamping station except for station #1, the height of the decompression plateau was found to increase linearly with the peak compression force.[33]

An examination of machine operation at a slow speed revealed that the sustaining of the decompression plateau over a constant period resulted from a temporary halt in the upward movement of the tamping piston during the time of the decompression.[11,33] In effect, there is a halt in movement of the entire dosing unit during this time. Synchronous with this halt, the turret that houses the cap and the body bushings starts its own half of the intermittent clockwise rotation, and the halt is sustained until a set of body bushings are positioned directly under the ejection station. Compression during this halt is sustained by the partially relaxed overload spring that maintains contact of the tamping piston with the plug. Since the overload spring has to be partially compressed to maintain plug contact during the halt, the decompression plateau appears only if peak compression is great enough to activate the overload spring. The presence of a decompression plateau has an additional

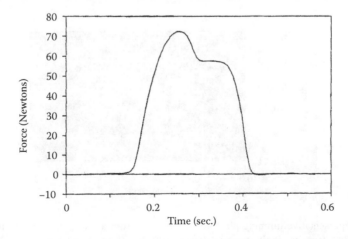

FIGURE 7.9 Representative force–time trace for a single tamping event on an H&K GKF machine.

implication in that it increases the total time under compression significantly. With an Hofliger & Karg GKF 330 running at 100 strokes per minute, the time under compression is still comparable to that obtained with a Zanasi model LZ-64 running at its typical speed of 33 revolutions per minute.

Cropp et al.[14] were able to generate tamping force–displacement profiles that provide further clarification of the GKF dosing disc filling principle. A force is detected by the piston before any powder displacement is detected owing to resistance developing against the piston as it moves through the powder bed toward the dosing disc. After the peak force is reached, powder displacement decreases slightly until the plateau is reached. Here, additional powder displacement can be seen to occur as a nearly constant force is maintained on the plug owing to the overload spring tension. From the area under the curve of a force–displacement profile for single tamps, the work of compaction was calculated for microcrystalline cellulose (0.1% magnesium stearate) and anhydrous lactose (0.5% magnesium stearate). The work of elastic recovery, as estimated by monitoring the displacement of the piston in decompression, was subtracted from the overall work. The maximum reported values were 0.40 NM for microcrystalline cellulose (peak tamp force of ~80 N) and 0.24 NM for the anhydrous lactose (peak tamp force ~150 N). Although direct comparisons are difficult, these values are about 20-fold less than values typically quoted for the tableting of various materials.

The force–time profile of the GKF-type dosing disc machine contrasts markedly with that of the Harro Hofliger KFM/3 dosing disc machine of the previous example in that there is no halt or plateau in decompression. A typical trace of tamping pin compression force during a complete compaction event under 100 N is displayed in Figure 7.10.

Generally, plug ejection occurs very rapidly in dosing disc machines. With a GKF 330 machine, the entire ejection event lasts only about 40–50 ms, with the peak ejection force developing within about 5 ms.[14] The ejection pistons are preset in a fixed but lower position than that of the tamping pistons at other stations. This is because an ejection piston must travel the entire length of the disc cavity to eject the plug completely out of the dosing disc. The peak ejection force develops before peak compression occurs at any tamping station because of the lower initial position and because ejection pistons come in contact with the fully formed plugs. This results in a time lag between the ejection and compression events, with ejection preceding. In fact, by the time the compression force peaks, which relates to completion of the downstroke, the ejection event is long completed.

A different approach to instrumenting a dosing disc machine was taken by Podczeck.[16] The goal was to develop a method that is potentially capable of providing feedback control of capsule fill weight in manufacturing similar to that which is commonly used in tablet production. To that end, Podczeck modified one of the tamping blocks of a Bosch GKF 400S machine. Like the

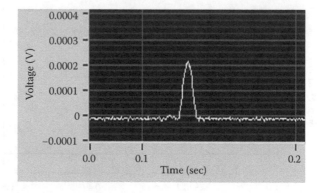

FIGURE 7.10 Representative tamping pin force–time trace from an instrumented Harro Hofliger KFM/3 dosing disc machine from a single compression at 100 N. (From Moolchandani V. *Functionality and Performance of Different Lactose Grades in Capsule Filling: Characterization and Evaluation of Formulation and Operating Variables on Dosing Disc Machines*, PhD Thesis, University of Maryland at Baltimore, 2010.)

Harro Hofliger KFM/3 tamping block shown in Figure 7.2, each GKF 400S tamping block also holds three tamping pins, each fitted with an overload spring. Podczeck replaced the springs with dashpots and a compressed air chamber that combines all three tamping pin inserts. A piezoelectric force transducer is connected at the upper part of the air chamber. The instrumentation simulates the conventional tamping process. Capsule fill weight and penetration depth of the pins and/or powder bed height are adjusted manually, as normally done, but the overload spring deflection point is simulated and can be raised or lowered continuously. For example, an increase in chamber pressure (simulating an increase in spring stiffness) leads to increased powder plug consolidation pressure. Thus, more room becomes available for powder in the dosing disc cavities at the next tamping station and fill weight increases. The spring deflection point can be manipulated during running by means of a feedback pressure valve. In practice, this system is capable only of small adjustments of up to about ±5 mg, which would provide for a coefficient of variation of about 1% for a 500-mg fill weight. In evaluating this system, Podczeck examined tamping force as a function of capsule fill weight and the cumulative tamping distance (CTD). CTD is determined from the pin penetration depth settings at each tamping station. Podczeck concluded from this analysis that tamping pins do not push all the powder situated above the dosing disc inside the dosing disc cavities; rather, the data suggest that most of the powder enters by flow during rotation of the dosing disc.

In a further study, Podczeck[17] observed that the tamping station used to measure the tamping force and that used to regulate of the pressure of the pneumatic chamber of the tamping head preferably should not be the same. Podczeck proposed the installation of the instrumented pneumatic tamping head on tamping station 4, where plugs were found to have achieved maximum length and density, and the installation of a second, non-instrumented pneumatic tamping head at station 3. The unit at station 3 would adjust fill weight according to signals from the instrumentation at station 4.

Podczeck's finding that most, but not all, powder enters the dosing disc cavities by flow during disc rotation supports the earlier conclusions of Shah et al.[12] Working with an instrumented Hofliger & Karg GKF 330 machine, Shah et al.[12] found that the time between the peak ejection force and the start of plug compression decreases with increases in tamping force. Since the ejection piston is always preset to the lowermost position, peak ejection force should always precede the start of compression. Their observation could only occur if compression started before the entry of the piston into the disc cavity. Additional powder is apparently being pushed into the dosing disc by the descending piston. It was observed that lactose fill weight increased from 279 mg, when no pin compression was applied, to 362 mg when a compression force of 240 N was applied at a single tamping station. Moreover, when a modified scrape-off bar was used to eliminate the powder bed over the disc at station 5, fill weight attributed to tamping solely at station 5 was constant, regardless of the tamping force (i.e., piston penetration setting) at that station. Force–displacement profiles later generated by Cropp et al.[14] clearly demonstrated that effective compression begins before the tamping piston enters the dosing disc. Taken together, these data suggest that powder above the dosing disc "builds up" in front of the downward plunging piston and is at least partially pushed into the dosing disc cavity.

Interrelationship of Tamping Force and Number of Tamps on Fill Weight

In a study using an instrumented Hofliger & Karg GKF 330 machine, two instrumented pistons were installed, permitting the monitoring of either two compression stations or one compression station and the ejection station.[11] By moving the instrumented piston from one station to another, the researchers looked at the effect of piston penetration setting on compression force and fill weight. At each station, the theoretical penetration of the instrumented piston was varied from 0 to 14 mm while keeping all other stations at 0 mm. The term *theoretical* is used here because a portion of the adjusted piston displacement will be taken up by the compression of the overload relief springs mounted over the end of each piston. Increases in the theoretical penetration setting resulted in greater compression force and greater final fill weight at each station. In general, the volume in a disc cavity available for filling depends on how much compression occurs at the preceding station. How much powder gets filled into that volume depends on the ability of the powder to flow into the cavity during rotation to the next station and on how much is pushed in by the piston during its downward stroke at that station. It was also found that the powder bed height over station 1 tended to be variable. The proximity of station 1 to the ejection station scrape-off bar, together with the clockwise motion of the powder container, caused the powder blend to shift away from station 1 and toward station 5 during running.

In a follow-up study, in which an instrumented piston was inserted at each tamping station of that same machine, Shah et al.[12] further examined the progressive plug formation process. On the basis of an examination of several compaction parameters measured at individual tamping stations, they concluded that all tamping stations, and all piston positions within a station, with the exception of station 1, contributed equally to plug formation.

Assuming each individual tamping station contributes equally to the plug forming process, Shah et al.[12] determined the number of tamps required to attain the target weight for a given compressive force using only the initial bulk density of the powder formulation, the disc cavity volume, and the target density (target weight/disc-cavity volume) and making several simplifying assumptions. For several lubricated fillers, the prediction based on this calculation that as few as three tamps would be sufficient to achieve the desired target fill weight was confirmed by actual filling operations. This prediction may not apply well to formulations that have flowability or densification problems. An extension of this calculation has been used to determine the appropriate dosing disc thickness required for a given target fill weight.[34]

AUTOMATIC FILLING MACHINE SIMULATION

In recent years, unique tablet compaction simulators have been designed, which at least have the capacity to mimic the action of a high-speed rotary tablet press at its operating speed under controlled laboratory conditions. Simulators consisting of tooling mounted to the cross heads of specially designed hydraulic mechanical testing machines can provide either single-ended or double-ended compression with independent control over the load, position, and velocity. The first of these was reported by Hunter et al.[35] These computer-controlled hydraulic presses are capable of compressing materials according to programmable displacement–time profiles at rates up to 3000 mm/s and loads of up to 50 kN.[36] Because they require only small samples of test materials, can mimic the punch force–displacement profiles of various machines, and provide independent control over load, position, and velocity, these machines provide a substantial advantage over instrumented tablet presses in research and development.[37] Although a suitably designed capsule filling machine simulator would be similarly advantageous over instrumented filling machines, to date, the logical extension of this concept to automatic capsule filling machines has not been fully realized. Table 7.2 summarizes the key developments in capsule machine simulation. Most of these reports describe the use of a dosator mechanism removed from an actual machine and mounted in some type of compression device. Most reported simulators are not programmable in the same sense as a tablet compaction simulator and do not allow independent control over moving elements such as pistons and dosators.

Jolliffe et al.[38] described the development of a simulator consisting of the turret of an MG2 model G-36 so modified that only the central shaft and top of the turret rotated. In effect, the dosators do not rotate, but execute their up and down movements while the cams rotate. This approach greatly simplified instrumentation since rotation was avoided and all movement of the dosators was limited to the vertical plane. Semiconductor strain gauges were bonded to a necked-down section of a piston, and two displacement transducers were mounted to record piston movement relative to the dosator and dosator movement relative to the turret itself. Only a single instrumented dosator assembly was used.

TABLE 7.2

Examples of Filling Machine Simulation

Date	Investigators	Simulation Equipment or Study
1979	Stewart, Grant, and Newton[31]	Fitted a Zanasi dosator to a moveable cross head
1982	Jolliffe, Newton, and Cooper[38]	Simulated MG-2 operation using a modified turret from a G-36 production machine
1991	Veski and Marvola[39]	Mounted an MG-2 dosing tube a on a digital balance with piston fitted to a manually operated lever system
1991, 1995	Britten and Barnett[40]; Britten, Barnett, and Armstrong[41]	Simulated a Macofar MT 13-2 machine using pneumatic pistons to operate an actual dosator mechanism in a laboratory setup
1998	Heda, Muller, and Augsburger[42]	Modified Mand tablet compaction simulator to study plug formation

Jollife and Newton used this setup to study the relationship between particle size and compression[43] and the role of dosator nozzle inner wall texture on plug retention.[44,45] Later, Tan and Newton used this system to study the relationship between flow parameters and fill weight and weight variation,[46] to further explore the relationship between dosator inner wall texture and powder retention,[47–49] and to examine the influence of compression setting on the observed plug density.[50]

Only the simulators described by Britten, Barnett, and Armstrong[40,41] and Heda et al.[42] come closest to meeting the objectives noted above for simulation. Britten, Barnett, and Armstrong's simulator employs the dosator mechanism from a Macofar MT13-2 capsule filling machine and is pneumatically operated. To simplify the assembly, rather than have the dosator plunge into a powder bed for precompression, a pneumatic cylinder brings a bowl bearing the powder bed to the dosator. Thus, "dosator speed" is in fact the rate at which the powder bowl moves toward the dosator. With the powder bowl raised, a separate pneumatic cylinder can provide active piston compression. After plug formation, the powder bowl is retracted and a third pneumatic cylinder is used to eject the plug. The speeds of these three cylinders are independently adjustable through flow control valves. LVDTs monitor the independent movement of the bowl and piston. Semiconductor strain gauges mounted on the piston and on the outer surface of the dosator tube measure both the tamping pressure and the radial pressure on the plug. The analog signals from the four transducers are digitized and the digital data are stored by a microprocessor-controlled data acquisition system. The data are downloaded to a PC for further manipulation. The system is capable of maximum dosator and pistons speeds of 500 and 600 cm/s, respectively. As such, this system was only able to attain about 75% of the full range of speeds attainable with the Macofar MT13-2, although its range nearly covered the full range of speeds of the Zanasi AZ-20, which also has a dosator mechanism. The machine can be operated in either a constant pressure mode (i.e., set to develop a preset compression pressure regardless of the piston travel) or a constant displacement mode (i.e., preset to achieve a fixed piston displacement regardless of the pressure that is generated).

Using their simulator, Britten, Barnett, and Armstrong[51] made a number of observations that often confirmed data reported by others using instrumented filling machines. But because their simulator allowed independent control over piston and dosator movement, many of their observations could not have been made with instrumented filling machines. One such finding was that the rate of plug ejection did not significantly affect average plug weight, plug density, or plug weight variation. Higher precompression speed resulted in decreased weights and plug densities when the simulator was in precompression and constant displacement modes. Two possible explanations were thought most likely: (1) at higher speeds, powder may be pushed ahead of the dosator instead of entering it, and (2) less consolidation may occur at higher velocities. The effect of speed vanished when the simulator was run in constant pressure mode, and the authors suggested that higher tamp pressures should be used to assure that uniform and predictable plug weights are achieved, provided that drug dissolution was not adversely affected by the greater compaction of the plug. Their simulator also enabled the first reported direct measurement of residual radial plug pressures.

Using this simulator, Tattawasart and Armstrong[52] later carried out a comprehensive study of the plug forming properties of lactose using a Box-Behnken experimental design. Among other conclusions from that study was the finding that magnesium stearate concentration had no significant effect on plug properties and that the lowest concentration studied (0.5%) was more than adequate for lactose under the conditions studied.

Heda et al.[42] reported the simulation of plug formation using a programmable Mand tablet compaction simulator. The simulator was fitted with tooling machined to match a No. 1 tamping pin, a special deep die to accommodate different capsule plug lengths, and load cells suitable for measuring the low forces involved in plug formation. Different constant punch speeds of 1, 10, and 100 mm/s were studied. The speed of 100 mm/s slightly exceeds the reported tamping pin movement of a GKF 330 dosing disc machine.

Their study revealed that the following compression models could be applied in the low-pressure region encountered in plug formation, if properly interpreted: (1) the exponential decay of applied force through the length of the plug could be modeled by the Shaxby–Evans relationship; (2) the Kawakita pressure–volume relationship was a very good fit for this low-pressure compression; and (3) Heckel analysis revealed apparent yield pressures (AYP) of 25–70 MPa, which were dependent on the material type, machine speed, and plug height. Given the low compression stresses involved in plug formation, Heda et al. noted that these AYP values are best interpreted as measures of resistance to compression, which is probably predominantly particle arrangement and packing, and not material deformation. The simulator of Heda et al. has been used to study the physical properties of commercial *Hypericum perforatum* extracts[53] and the plug forming properties of silicified microcrystalline cellulose.[54]

The instrumentation of capsule filling machines brought about a new era of capsule formulation and process research. The advent of capsule filling machine simulators offers a still greater opportunity to examine the plug formation and ejection under dynamic conditions comparable to production conditions using small samples and under controlled laboratory conditions. Independent control of piston and dosator speeds makes studies of compaction dynamics that cannot be studied in actual machines possible. The further development of these devices to permit programmable simulation of various machines will make it possible for one to have a much better understanding of how formulations should be developed for specific machines, to facilitate product scale-up, to help design formulations that are machine independent, and to support FDA's QbD initiative.

REFERENCES

1. Augsburger LL. Instrumented capsule-filling machines: Development and application. *Pharm Tech* 1982; 6(9): 111–119.
2. Augsburger LL. Instrumented capsule-filling machines: Development and application. Update '87. *Pharm Tech* 1987; 11(6): 156.
3. Cole GC, May G. Instrumentation of a hard shell encapsulation machine. *J Pharm Pharmacol* 1972; 24 (Suppl): 122P.
4. Cole GC, May G. The instrumentation of a zanasi LZ/64 capsule filling machine. *J Pharm Pharmacol* 1975; 27: 353–358.
5. Small LE, Augsburger LL. Instrumentation of an automatic capsule filling machine. *Abst Acad Pharm Sci* 1975; 5(2): No. 3.
6. Small LE, Augsburger LL. Instrumentation of an automatic capsule filling machine. *J Pharm Sci* 1977; 66: 504–509.
7. Mony C, Sambeat C, Cousin G. Application of the measure of force on the formation and filling of hard gelatin capsules. In *Proceedings of the 1st International Conference on Pharmaceutical Technology*. APGI, Paris, 1977; II: 98–108.
8. Greenberg R. Effects of AZ60 filling machine dosator settings upon slug hardness and dissolution of capsules. In *Proceedings of the 88th National Meeting of the American Institute of Chemical Engineers*. Session 11, Philadelphia, PA, 1980; Fiche 29.

9. Mehta AM, Augsburger LL. Simultaneous measurement of force and displacement in an automatic capsule-filling machine. *Int J Pharm* 1980; 4: 347–351.
10. Rowley DJ, Hendry R, Ward MD et al. The Instrumentation of an automatic capsule filling machine for formulation design studies. In *Proceedings of the 3rd International Conference on Pharmaceutical Technology.* APGI, Paris, 1983; V: 287–291.
11. Shah KB, Augsburger LL, Small LE, Polli GP. Instrumentation of a dosing-disc automatic capsule filling machine. *Pharm Tech* (1983); 7(4): 42–54.
12. Shah KB, Augsburger LL, Marshall K. An investigation of factors affecting plug formation and fill weight in a dosing disk-type automatic capsule filling machine. *J Pharm Sci* 1986; 75: 291–296.
13. Maury M, Heraud P, Etienne A et al. Mesures de pressions pendant le remplissage de gelules. In *Proceedings of the 4th International Conference on Pharmaceutical Technology.* APGI, Paris, 1977; 1: 384–389.
14. Cropp JW, Augsburger LL, Marshall K. Simultaneous monitoring of tamping force and piston displacement (F-D) on an Hofliger–Karg capsule filling machine. *Int J Pharm* 1991; 71: 127–136.
15. Hauer VB, Remmele T, Zuger O, Sucker, H. Rational development and optimization of capsule formulations with an instrumented dosator capsule filling machine. I: Instrumentation and influence of the filling material and the machine parameters. *Pharm Ind* 1993; 55: 509–515.
16. Podczeck F. The development of an instrumented tamp-filling capsule machine: I. Instrumentation of a Bosch GKF 400S machine. *Euro J Pharm Sci* 2000; 10: 267–274.
17. Podczeck F. The development of an instrumented tamp-filling capsule machine II. Investigations of plug development and tamping pressure at different filling stations. *Euro J Pharm Sci* 2001; 12: 515–521.
18. Moolchandani V. *Functionality and Performance of Different Lactose Grades in Capsule Filling: Characterization and Evaluation of Formulation and Operating Variables on Dosing Disc Machines*, PhD Thesis, University of Maryland at Baltimore, 2010.
19. Moolchandani V, Augsburger LL, Gupta A, Khan M, Langridge J, Hoag SW. Characterization and selection of suitable grades of lactose as functional fillers for capsule filling: Part 1. *Drug Dev Ind Pharm* 2014; 41: 1452–1463.
20. Moolchandani V, Augsburger LL, Gupta A, Khan M, Langridge J, Hoag SW. To investigate the influence of machine operating variables on formulations derived from lactose types in capsule filling: Part 2. *Drug Dev Ind Pharm* 2015; 42: 624–635.
21. Mehta AM, Augsburger LL. A preliminary study of the effect of slug hardness on drug dissolution from hard gelatin capsules filled on an automatic capsule filling machine. *Int J Pharm* 1981; 7: 327–334.
22. Botzolakis JE, Augsburger LL. The effect of disintegrants on drug dissolution from capsules filled on a dosator-type automatic filling machine. *Int J Pharm Pharm* 1982; 12: 341–349.
23. Shah KB, Augsburger LL, Marshall K. Multiple tamping effects on drug dissolution from capsules filled on a dosing-disk type automatic capsule filling machine. *J Pharm Sci* 1987; 76: 639–645.
24. Jollife IG, Newton JM. Capsule filling studies using an MG2 production machine. *J Pharm Pharmacol* 1983; 35: 74–78.
25. Small LE, Augsburger LL. Aspects of the lubrication requirements for an automatic capsule-filling machine. *Drug Devel Ind Pharm* 1978; 4: 345–372.
26. Daly JW, Riley WF. *Experimental Stress Analysis*, New York: McGraw-Hill, 1978: 153–332.
27. Ridgway Watt P. *Tablet Machine Instrumentation in Pharmaceutics*, New York: Halsted Press div. John Wiley & Sons, 1988: 27–170.
28. Small, LE. *Important Formulation Requirements for an Automatic Capsule Filling Machine and a Preliminary Study of Their Influence on In Vitro Drug Availability.* PhD Thesis, University of Maryland at Baltimore, 1980.
29. Augsburger LL. Instrumented capsule filling machines: Methodology and application to product development. *STP Pharma* 1988; 4(2): 116–122.
30. Mehta AM. *Effect of Selected Formulation and Process Variables on Slug Hardness, Drug Dissolution, and Work of Slug Ejection for a Dosator-Type Automatic Filling Machine.* PhD Thesis, University of Maryland at Baltimore, 1981.
31. Stewart AG, Grant DJW, Newton JM. The release of a model low-dose drug (riboflavin) from hard gelatin capsule formulation. *J Pharm Pharmacol* 1979; 31: 1–6.
32. Nakagwu H. Effects of particle size of rifampicin and addition of magnesium stearate in release of rifampicin from hard gelatin capsules. *Yakugaku Zasshi* 1981; 100: 1111–1117.
33. Shah KB. *The Influence of Important Machine Operating variables on Plug Formation, Fill Weight and Drug Release for a Dosing-Disk Type Automatic Capsule Filling Machine.* PhD Thesis, University of Maryland at Baltimore, 1986.

34. Davar N, Shah R, Pope DG, Augsburger LL. Rational approach to the selection of a dosing disk on a Hofliger Karg capsule filling machine. *Pharm Tech* 1997; 21: 32–48.
35. Hunter BM, Fisher DG, Prate RM, Rowe RC. A high speed compression simulator. *J Pharm Pharmacol* 1976; 28: 65P.
36. Bateman SD, Rubinstein MH, Rowe RC et al. A comparative investigation of compression simulators. *Int J Pharm* 1989; 49: 209–212.
37. Celik M, Marshall K. Use of a compaction simulator system in tabletting research, I. Introduction to and initial experiments with the system. *Drug Devel Ind Pharm* 1989; 15(5): 759–800.
38. Jolliffe IG, Newton JM, Cooper D. The design and use of an instrumented mG2 capsule filling machine simulator. *J Pharm Pharmacol* 1982; 34: 230–235.
39. Veski P, Marvola M. Design and use of equipment for simulating plug formation in hard gelatin capsule filling machines. *Acta Pharm Fennica* 1991; 100: 19–25.
40. Britten JR, Barnett MI. Development and validation of a capsule filling machine simulator. *Int J Pharm* 1991; 71: R5–R8.
41. Britten JR, Barnett MI, Armstrong NA. Construction of an intermittant-motion capsule filling machine simulator. *Pharm Res* 1995; 12: 196–200.
42. Heda PK, Muller FX, Augsburger LL. Capsule filling machine simulation. I. Low-force powder compression physics relevant to plug formation. *Pharm Dev Tech* 1998; 4(2): 209–219.
43. Jollife IG, Newton JM. Practical implications of theoretical considerations of capsule filling by the dosator nozzle system. *J Pharm Pharmacol* 1982; 34: 293–298.
44. Jollife IG, Newton JM. An investigation of the relationship between particle size and compression during capsule filling with an instrumented mG2 simulator. *J Pharm Pharmacol* 1982; 34: 415–419.
45. Jollife IG, Newton JM. The effect of dosator nozzle wall texture on capsule filling with the mG2 Simulator. *J Pharm Pharmacol* 1983; 35: 7–11.
46. Tan SB, Newton JM. Powder flowability as an indication of capsule filling performance. *Int J Pharm* 1990; 61: 145–155.
47. Tan SB, Newton JM. Influence of capsule dosator wall texture and powder properties on the angle of wall friction and powder-wall adhesion. *Int J Pharm* 1990; 64: 227–234.
48. Tan SB, Newton JM. Capsule filling performance of powders with dosator nozzles of different wall texture. *Int J Pharm* 1990; 66: 207–211.
49. Tan SB, Newton JM. Minimum compression stress requirements for arching and powder retention within a dosator nozzle during capsule filling. *Int J Pharm* 1990; 63: 275–280.
50. Tan SB, Newton JM. Observed and expected powder plug densities obtained by a capsule dosator nozzle system. *Int J Pharm* 1990; 66: 283–288.
51. Britten JR, Barnett MI, Armstrong NA. Studies on powder plug formation using a simulated capsule filling machine. *J Pharm Pharmacol* 1996; 48: 249–254.
52. Tattawasart A, Armstrong NA. The formation of lactose plugs for hard shell capsule fills. *Pharm Dev Tech* 1997; 2: 335–343.
53. Kopelman S, NguyenPho A, Zito SW, Augsburger LL. Selected physical and chemical properties of commercial *Hypericum perforatum* extracts relevant for formulated product quality and performance. *AAPS J* 2001; 3(4): 1–18.
54. Guo M, Muller FX, Augsburger LL. Evaluation of the plug formation process of silicified microcrystalline cellulose. *Int J Pharm* 2001; 233: 99–109.

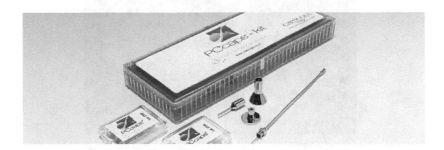

FIGURE 3.3 PCcaps for a preclinical trial study. (Courtesy of Capsugel.)

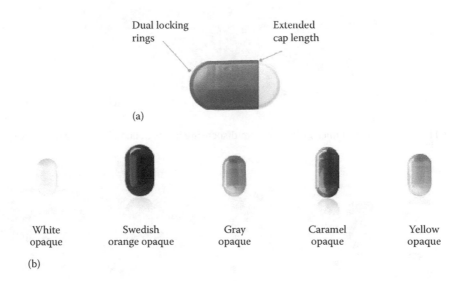

FIGURE 3.4 DBcaps showing dual locking rings and extended cap length. (a) Extended cap length of DBcaps capsules that completely covers the sidewall of the capsule body. This makes it virtually impossible to open the capsule without causing visible damage. A dual locking ring design provides a full-circumference, leak-free closure. (b) DBcaps capsules formulated in a wide array of colors. The five standard color formulations were developed based on globally accepted colorants and on sufficient opacity to ensure blinding. (Courtesy of Capsugel.)

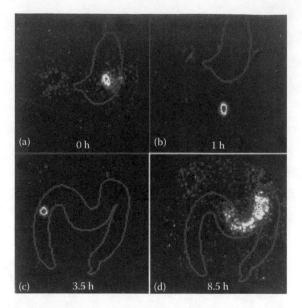

FIGURE 3.7 Scintigraphic images of a radiolabeled TARGIT capsule in a human after oral administration. At 0 h, the capsule is in the stomach (a); 1 h, small intestine (b); 3.5 h, ascending colon (c); and 8.5 h, dispersed in transverse and descending colon (d). (Courtesy of Taylor & Francis.)

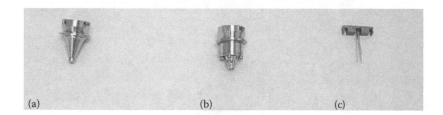

FIGURE 3.11 Xcelodose 600 micro filling system dispensing heads (a and b) and fingers (c). (Courtesy of Capsugel.)

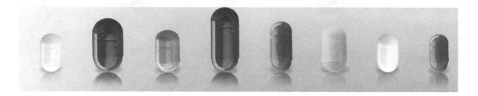

FIGURE 3.13 Different DBcaps sizes. (Courtesy of Capsugel.)

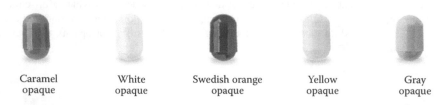

Caramel opaque   White opaque   Swedish orange opaque   Yellow opaque   Gray opaque

FIGURE 3.17 DBcaps in different colors. (Courtesy of Capsugel.)

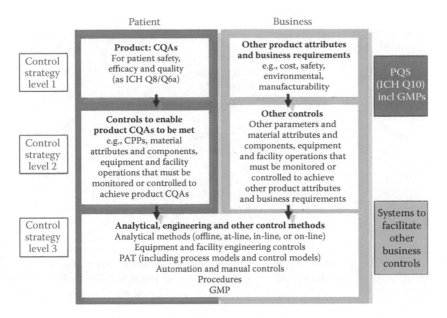

FIGURE 3.22 Proposed model for control strategy. (From Garcia T, Cook G, Nosal R. PQLI key topics—Criticality, design space, and control strategy. *J Pharm Innov* 2008; 3: 60–68. With permission.)

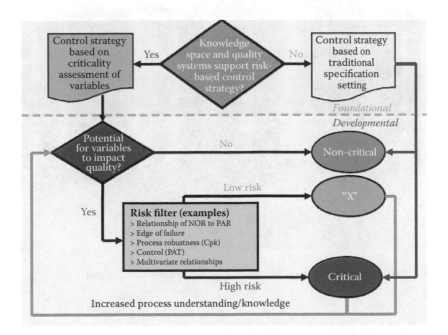

FIGURE 3.23 Decision tree to define levels of criticality. (From Garcia T, Cook G, Nosal R. PQLI key topics—Criticality, design space, and control strategy. *J Pharm Innov* 2008; 3: 60–68. With permission.)

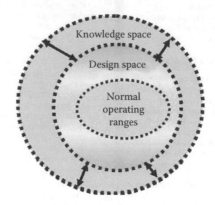

FIGURE 3.24 Relationship between design space and normal operating ranges. (From Garcia T, Cook G, Nosal R. PQLI key topics—Criticality, design space, and control strategy. *J Pharm Innov* 2008; 3: 60–68. With permission.)

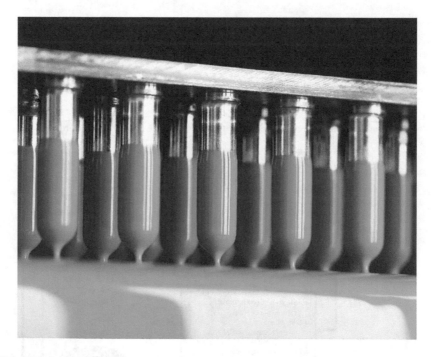

FIGURE 4.4 Photograph of pins after dipping being withdrawn from the dip pan.

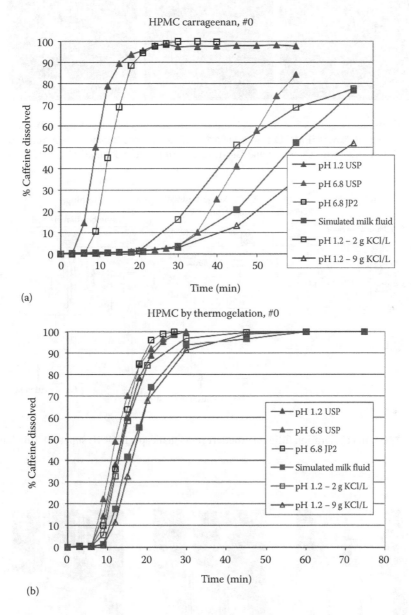

FIGURE 5.4 Dissolution of a fast-dissolving caffeine formulation in different types of HPMC capsules. (a) HPMC capsule containing carrageenan as a gelling system. (b) HPMC capsule manufactured by thermogelation without any gelling system (Vcaps® Plus). (Courtesy of Capsugel.)

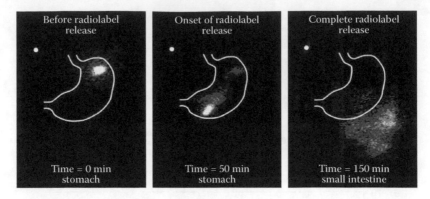

FIGURE 5.8 Gammascintigraphy images of delayed-release capsules (DRcaps™, banded). (From Hodges LA, Connolly S, Cade D et al. Novel HPMC Capsules Display Acid Resistance Behaviour—A Scintigraphic Imaging Study: A Joint Presentation with Capsugel and Bio-Images. 2014. AAPS Annual Meeting, Poster W5137.)

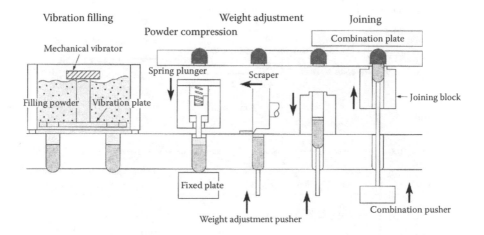

FIGURE 6.3 Mechanical vibration filling method. (From Qualicaps. LIQFIL super 40. Brochure. Whitsett, NC; 2011.)

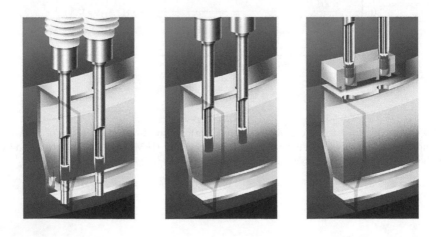

FIGURE 6.4 Dosator method. (Courtesy of IMA ACTIVE division, Bologna, Italy.)

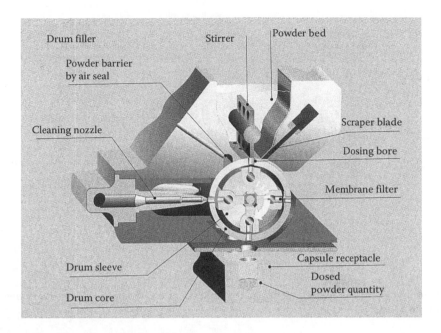

FIGURE 6.6 Drum filler method. (From Harro Hofliger Packaging Systems. Modular filling and closing machine for capsules. Modu-C Mid-Speed (MS). 2010. Brochure.)

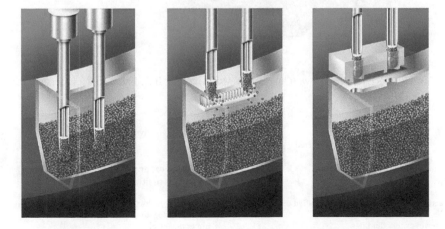

FIGURE 6.8 Vacuum dosator method. (From IMA ACTIVE. IMATIC High Speed Capsule Filling Machine. 2011. Brochure.)

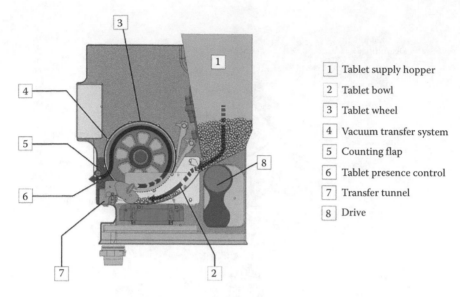

FIGURE 6.24 Modu-C size part-free tablet dosing unit. (Courtesy of Harro Höfliger Packaging Systems, Doylestown, PA.)

1	Tablet supply hopper
2	Tablet bowl
3	Tablet wheel
4	Vacuum transfer system
5	Counting flap
6	Tablet presence control
7	Transfer tunnel
8	Drive

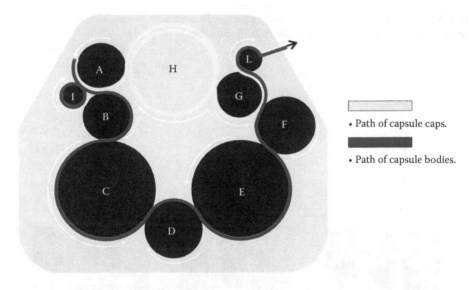

FIGURE 6.30 PLANETA Workflow. (Courtesy of MG America, Inc., Fairfield, New Jersey.)

• Path of capsule caps.

• Path of capsule bodies.

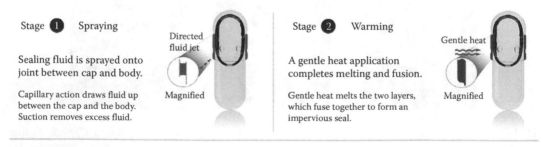

Stage ❶ Spraying

Sealing fluid is sprayed onto joint between cap and body.

Capillary action draws fluid up between the cap and the body. Suction removes excess fluid.

Directed fluid jet

Magnified

Stage ❷ Warming

A gentle heat application completes melting and fusion.

Gentle heat melts the two layers, which fuse together to form an impervious seal.

Gentle heat

Magnified

Stage ❸ Setting   Capsules equilibrate at room temperature.

FIGURE 6.48 LEMS three-stage process. (Courtesy of Capsugel, Greenwood, South Carolina.)

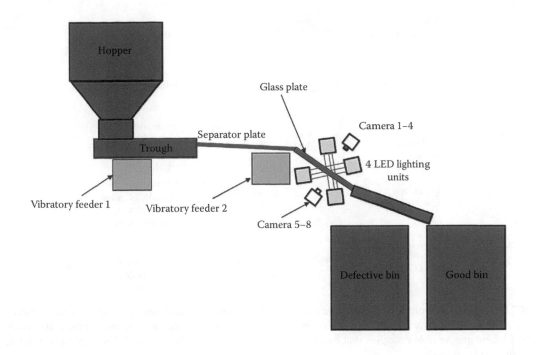

FIGURE 6.56 Viswill PAPPIS diagram. (Courtesy of DJA-PHARMA, Wood Dale.)

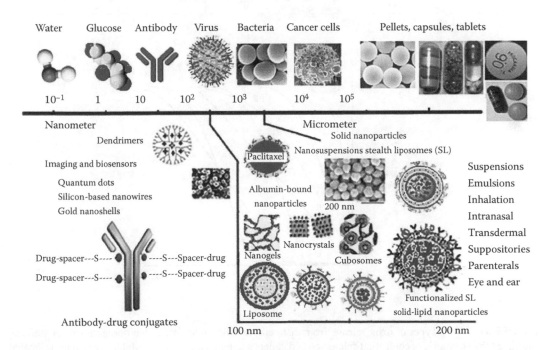

FIGURE 12.1 Approximate size spectrum showing dimensions of typical molecules, carrier types, and drug delivery systems based on the published literature and some of the commercialized nanotechnology products, conventional dosage forms, modified-release technologies, and their combinations.

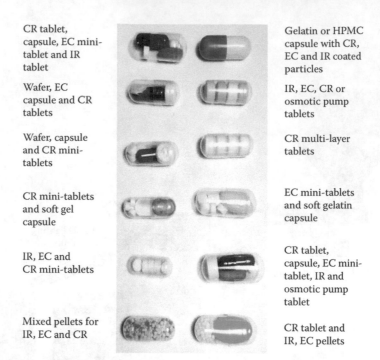

CR tablet, capsule, EC mini-tablet and IR tablet

Gelatin or HPMC capsule with CR, EC and IR coated particles

Wafer, EC capsule and CR tablets

IR, EC, CR or osmotic pump tablets

Wafer, capsule and CR mini-tablets

CR multi-layer tablets

CR mini-tablets and soft gel capsule

EC mini-tablets and soft gelatin capsule

IR, EC and CR mini-tablets

CR tablet, capsule, EC mini-tablet, IR and osmotic pump tablet

Mixed pellets for IR, EC and CR

CR tablet and IR, EC pellets

FIGURE 12.6 Controlled-release capsule drug delivery systems with different types of dosages or encapsulated formulations (transparent shell is chosen to show the content). Some of these are commercially available; others are possible examples that can be for investigation. EC, enteric coated; CR, controlled release; IR, immediate release.

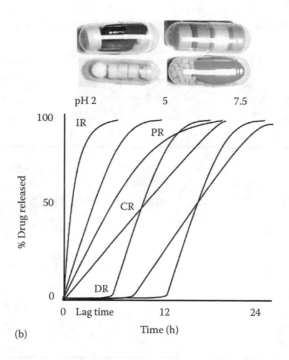

(b)

FIGURE 12.7 (b) Types of drug release from different modified-release capsule dosage forms containing multiple tablets, enteric or controlled-release coated pellets and tablets, coated mini-tablets, and enteric-coated small capsule placed in a larger capsule with different tablet combinations. Various release profiles from different combinations are possible for different time periods (i.e., 1- to 24-h duration). Systems may allow for either one drug or drug combinations. Type of release: immediate release (IR); prolonged release (PR, with or without a bolus dose); delayed release (DR): release after lapse of certain time in a desired pH environment; controlled release (CR) with zero-order kinetics.

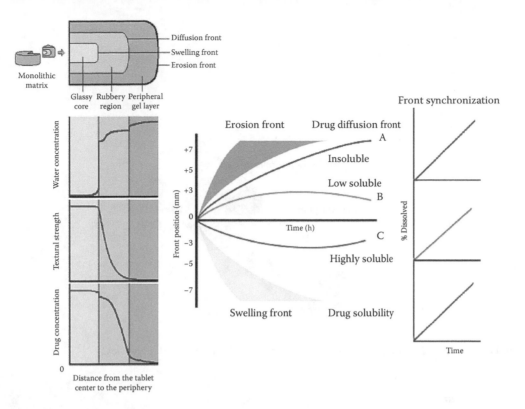

FIGURE 12.15 Graphic representation of a matrix undergoing hydration and swelling. Depending on the properties of polymer(s), drug, and excipients. Exact release is influenced by synchronization of various fronts as shown. Left panel illustrates hydration of matrix from periphery to the center of the matrix showing different fronts and dynamics of changes in matrix from tablet center to the erosion front. Middle panel shows synchronization of drug diffusion front within a hydrating matrix dominated by either swelling aspect or erosion aspect contingent upon drug solubility. The right panel shows achievement of zero-order drug release owing to front synchronization.[25,26]

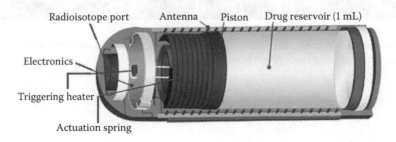

FIGURE 12.24 The Enterion capsule can be used to assess absorption of drug from modified-release formulation during product development in different clinical phases. (Courtesy of Quotient Clinical, UK.)

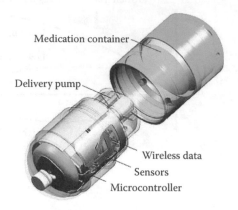

Medication container

Delivery pump

Wireless data

Sensors

Microcontroller

FIGURE 12.25 "IntelliCap" system and its components. (Courtesy of Medimetrics.)

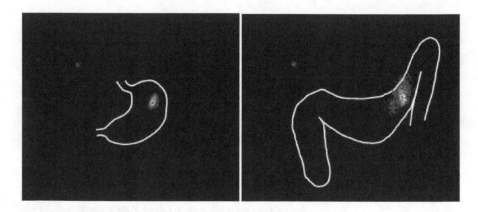

FIGURE 12.26 A scintigraphic study showing the location of IntelliCap device after oral administration. (Courtesy of Medimetrics and Bio-Images Research partnership.)

8 Dry-Fill Formulation and Filling Technology

Pavan Heda, Vikas Agarwal, and Shailesh K. Singh

CONTENTS

INTRODUCTION

Hard and soft gelatin capsules were patented more than a century ago. They are classified as either "hard" or "soft" depending on the nature of the shell. Soft gelatin capsules (sometimes referred to as "softgels") are made from a more flexible, plasticized gelatin film than hard gelatin capsules.

Their success as dosage forms can largely be attributed to the fact that they are a "container" drug delivery system. That is, the medication is packaged in gelatin shells that typically provide a tasteless/odorless dosage form without need for a secondary coating step, as may be required for tablets. Swallowing is also easy for most patients, since the shell is smooth and readily hydrates in the mouth, and the capsule often floats upon swallowing in the liquid taken with it. The availability of capsules in a wide variety of colors also makes them aesthetically pleasing and is a good way for product identification and differentiation.

There are many advantages for choosing to develop and scale up a capsule formulation over a tablet. The versatility of hard gelatin capsules means that they can be used at every step in the development cycle dependent on dose and obviates the need to switch to other dosage forms after initial studies, for example, tablets, which increases the amount of effort required for testing and validation. The use of hard gelatin capsules would appear to be a simple way to reduce the workload during development and hence speed up the scale-up process. As the development costs for new medicines continue to rise, it has become imperative to obtain international registration for these formulations. Most companies aim to achieve reproducible consistency of product quality that is acceptable worldwide. The simplicity of hard gelatin capsule formulation and manufacturing as well as the versatility of this dosage form substantially support these requirements.

When it comes to a decision at the end of phase II, which dosage form will be developed as the "to be marketed" formulation, high production costs of hard gelatin capsule products are generally assumed. This assumption is valid if the production costs are limited to the comparison of the excipient (including capsule shell) only. External perceptions of cost suggest that when taking into account total manufacturing (which includes the hidden costs coming from process equipment; GMP [Good Manufacturing Practice] space required; total production time; in-process controls; and analytical, cleaning, and validation work), the comparison easily turns out in favor of capsule formulation. Other factors such as the number of processing steps in the manufacturing train and the use of a number of excipients, as well as with respect to running compatibility tests, can also contribute to the cost. Considering these factors, the comparison of cost may show no significant differences between a tablet and a capsule. Table 8.1 shows a comparison of tablets and capsules as delivery systems.

During the formulation development stage, some have adopted what is called as "capsule-to-tablet" formulation concept. Ideally, the same formulation would be used in capsules for early clinical phases and, subsequently, in tablets for commercialization. As the excipients used are identical, the stability of the clinical capsule formula and the commercial tablets should be similar.[1]

TABLE 8.1
Comparison of Tablets and Capsule as Delivery Systems

Tablet	Capsule
Common excipients—although should not assume that a formulation will be suitable for both tablet and capsule	
More excipients in formulation	Fewer excipients
Additional processing steps for manufacture	Fewer processing steps—simplified process
High compression forces	Low forces
Mechanical viscoelastic properties of paramount importance	Low-pressure densification and packing behavior more important
Potential for higher drug loading/dose	Dose restrictions <600 mg
Higher manufacturing output (high-speed machines capable of 300,000 tablets/hour (product dependent)	Lower machine output (high-speed machines capable of 200,000 capsules/hour (product dependent)
Can be difficult to formulate	Generally, easier to formulate
Requirement for larger quantities of API for formulation	Usually requires less active to formulate
Limited potential for fill with beads	Flexibility of fill materials: beads, granules, tablets, powders, semisolids, nonaqueous liquids and suspensions; blinding
Depending on the size and surface, sometimes not easy to swallow compared to a capsule?	Perceived as easier to swallow than tablet
Product identification for patient compliance/branding	
Additional excipients/coatings required for taste masking	Easy taste/odor masking
More difficult to blind	Preferential for blinding
Tooling definition (shape, size considerations) additional cost/increase in development time/cost implication for packaging (tooling)	Capsules predefined form, shape for ease of packaging tooling selection
Perceived as less bioavailable compared to capsules	Perceived bioavailability advantage over tablets

From a technical perspective, formulation of a rapid-release hard gelatin capsule/tablet can be guided based on the physicochemical properties of the drug active; for example, a low melting point active with poor mechanical properties may impair the option for tableting. With a tablet, it is necessary to produce a compact capable of withstanding the rigors of downstream processing. For capsules, it is often necessary to form a plug for ejection into a capsule body, but it is not necessary for the plug to retain its integrity beyond the filling stage. Tablet processes operate at high compression forces (10–15 kN), and the compaction event occurs over a short time (milliseconds); therefore, the viscoelastic properties of the formulation are of paramount importance. In contrast, tamp processes operate at relatively low forces (50–150 N)—in this case, the low pressure densification and packing behavior of the material is more important. In addition, the plug is formed by a single or series of tamps and consequently over an extended period of time; hence, the time-dependent viscoelastic deformation of the material is less important. While good flow is necessary for successful manufacturing of both tablets and capsules, the filling mechanisms on production capsule machines tend to be more forgiving than those on tablet machines. These reduced demands on compressibility and flow increase the option for powder mixes, making capsules a potential dosage form for active substances that do not possess compaction properties required for direct compression tablets and are not amenable to granulation.

Capsules, as a delivery system, offer the formulator increased versatility compared to tablets. Various materials can be filled into hard gelatin capsules and tablets (e.g., dry solids: powders, pellets, granules, and tablets). In addition, capsules can also be filled with semisolids: nonaqueous liquids and suspensions. From a pharmaceutical point of view, there are several advantages in formulating liquid and semisolid fillings as hard gelatin capsules. Drug actives with certain characteristics (e.g., low melting point, low dose, critical stability, and poor bioavailability) present problems that make development in solid oral dosage form difficult, but which can be circumvented by formulation as liquid or semisolid fillings in hard gelatin capsules. Soft shell capsule technology also evolved to include enrobed granules/beads (Diamox Sequels) that were filled by the Accogel process. In addition, the enrobing process has been extended to tablets (e.g., Geltabs). However, this chapter will primarily focus on hard shell capsule formulation involving powders, granules, pellets, and mini-tabs and their combinations. Before getting into the fill formulation, it is important to understand the biopharmaceutical aspects for capsules.

BIOPHARMACEUTICAL ASPECTS FOR CAPSULES

Generally, the bioavailability of a drug from a well-formulated hard gelatin capsule dosage form will be better than or at least equal to the bioavailability of the same drug from a compressed tablet. The small particles of a drug in a capsule are not subjected to the same degree of compression and possible fusion that can reduce the effective surface area of the drug. Provided that the hard gelatin shell dissolves rapidly in the gastrointestinal (GI) fluids and the encapsulated mass disperses rapidly and efficiently, a relatively large effective surface area of drug will be exposed to the GI fluids, thereby facilitating drug dissolution. However, it is incorrect to assume that because a drug formulated as a hard gelatin capsule is in a finely divided form surrounded by a water-soluble shell, no bioavailability problems can occur. Sometimes, there are practical limitations to this approach. Micronized particles with high surface/mass ratio tend to aggregate, owing to surface cohesion, thereby reducing the overall surface area available for dissolution.

The overall rate of dissolution of drugs from capsules appears to be a complex function of the rates of different processes such as the following:

1. Dissolution rate of the gelatin shell
2. Rate of penetration of the GI fluids into the encapsulated mass
3. Rate at which the mass de-aggregates (i.e., disperses) in the GI fluids
4. Rate of dissolution of the dispersed drug particles

The inclusion of excipients (e.g., diluents, disintegrants, lubricants, and surfactants) in a capsule formulation can have a significant effect on the rate of dissolution of drugs, particularly those that are poorly soluble and hydrophobic. A hydrophilic diluent often serves to increase the rate of penetration of the aqueous GI fluids into the contents of the capsule and to aid dispersion and subsequent dissolution of the drug in these fluids. However, the diluent should exhibit no tendency to absorb or complex with the drug since either can impair absorption from the GI tract.

Magnesium stearate is commonly included as a lubricant for the capsule-filling operation. Its hydrophobic nature often retards liquid penetration so that a capsule-shaped plug often remains after the shell has dissolved in the GI fluids, especially when the contents have been machine filled as a consolidated plug. However, this effect can usually be overcome by the simultaneous addition of a wetting agent and a hydrophilic diluent to the contents.

Both the formulation and the type and conditions of the capsule-filling process can affect the packing density and liquid permeability of the capsule contents. In general, an increase in packing density (i.e., a decrease in porosity) of the encapsulated mass will probably result in a decrease in liquid permeability and dissolution rate, particularly if the drug is hydrophobic or if a hydrophilic drug is mixed with a hydrophobic lubricant such as magnesium stearate. If the encapsulated mass is tightly packed (high packing density) for a hydrophobic drug, then even with a reduction in particle size, the dissolution rate decreases, unless a surfactant is included to facilitate liquid penetration. Alternatively, wettability of poorly soluble drugs can be improved by adding a solution of a hydrophilic polymer. In this process called hydrophilization, a solution of hydrophilic polymer is spread evenly onto the drug in a high-shear mixer and the resultant granules are dried and screened before filling into capsules. Such granulations can increase the dissolution rate of a micronized hydrophobic drug by increasing the liquid permeability of the encapsulated mass.

In summary, formulation factors that can influence the bioavailability of drugs from hard gelatin capsules include the following:

- Surface area and particle size of the drug (particularly the effective surface area exhibited by the drug in the GI fluids) (A reduction in particle size is not a solution for all problems because agglomeration effects may prevail.)
- Use of the salt form of a drug in preference to the parent weak acid or base
- Crystal form of the drug
- Chemical stability of the drug (in the dosage form and GI fluids)
- Nature and quantities of the diluent, lubricant, and wetting agent
- Drug–excipient interactions (e.g., adsorption, complexation)
- Type and conditions of the filling process
- Packing density of the capsule contents
- Composition and properties of the capsule shell
- Interactions between the capsule shell and contents

The formulation of a poorly soluble, low-dose drug in a gelatin capsule presents several problems. Because of the dose of the medicament, it is necessary to add diluents in order to get the bulk required to fill the capsule. A disadvantage of this is that many diluents interfere with the release of the medicament.

A further disadvantage in the release of a poorly soluble medicament from gelatin capsules is that during the hydration, the gelatin forms a viscous barrier. This results in the formation of a plug or coagulation of the capsule ingredients, which in turn results in poor dispersion and dissolution of the active ingredient. Instead of obtaining a maximum surface area for the drug, which is one of the prerequisites for increased solubility, a minimum surface area is obtained. A very erratic dissolution rate may result.

Powder processing may induce changes in *in vitro* dissolution results. Several of these process-related factors could affect dissolution, for example, overlubrication during blending or capsule filling, changes in the filling mechanism, changes in plug strength, or changes in active pharmaceutical ingredient (API) particle size.

Dissolution issues may occur with time as a result of the cross-linking of gelatin in the shell. Cross-linking is facilitated and/or accelerated when the formulation in the capsule contains a carbonyl compound or derivatives such as aldehydes, especially formaldehydes. With the passage of time and/or under the accelerated conditions, aldehydes react with the amino acid groups within the gelatin shell to generate a cross-linked structure. This is described as a very thin, tough, and water-insoluble film observed around the capsule contents during dissolution testing in USP dissolution media without enzyme. This film does not disrupt easily by gentle agitation and is usually referred to as a pellicle. As a result, an insoluble cross-linked gel forms (pellicle formation) that water cannot easily pass through and does not rupture to release the contents. The disruption of this film seems to be the dissolution rate-limiting factor for the drug product.

It is likely that cross-linking has a much greater impact on the results of *in vitro* dissolution testing than on the *in vivo* bioavailability of drugs formulated in gelatin capsules. However, since *in vitro* dissolution testing is commonly employed as a method of measuring the stability of drug products, it is important to utilize a capsule fill that minimizes cross-linking in the capsule shell and thus minimizes the impact of time and/or stress conditions on the dissolution profile of the filled gelatin capsule, especially during accelerated stability studies wherein the capsules are subjected to high temperature and relative humidity.

It is sometimes possible to reverse the type of chemical reaction by adding compounds that are carbonyl scavengers such as lysine, phenylamine, glycine, and so on that prevent the interaction of aldehydes with gelatin and thereby inhibit the cross-linking. In other approaches, the degradation of capsule is controlled by manipulation of the pH. Carboxylic acids such as benzoic acid, fumaric acid, and citric acid have been found to be effective. Also, trials have shown that using a combination of an amino acid and a buffer can significantly prevent pellicle formation.

It has been shown, for example, that reducing the release rate *in vitro* in dissolution tests bears no relationship to the *in vivo* dissolution rate and the consequent bioavailability.[2] However, adding enzymes pepsin and pancreatin to the dissolution medium prevents the inhibitory factors from taking effect. This result has led to the assumption that inhibited dissolution is attributed to the test conditions.

The USP 24 proposes therefore that pepsin (for acid media) and pancreatin (for alkaline media) can be added to the dissolution tests aimed at establishing the likely *in vivo* dissolution properties (two-tier dissolution test). Only in cases where the enzymes have been added and the test still shows poor dissolution should a negative effect attributed to cross-linking be assumed.

Issues of cross-linking can be avoided by using hypromellose (HPMC) instead of gelatin capsules. Use of HPMC capsules may also be advantageous from a bovine spongiform encephalopathy/transmissible spongiform encephalopathy (BSE/TSE) perspective, being of vegetable origin. HPMC capsules contain less water compared to gelatin and are also more suitable for hygroscopic drugs.

FORMULATION PRINCIPLES FOR DRY-FILL (POWDER) FORMULATION

Similar formulation and processing considerations are prevalent for tablets and capsule, for example, API solubility, morphology, particle size, excipient compatibility, as are requirements for content uniformity and *in vitro*/*in vivo* bioavailability. The decision to formulate a capsule should be based on an understanding of the physicochemical properties of the API, filling machine, and capsule size to be used.

A capsule formulation may not be considered suitable for drugs that are very soluble such as salts (potassium chloride, potassium bromide, and ammonium chloride), for efflorescent or deliquescent materials, materials that react with gelatin and materials that contain a high level of free moisture. Also, formulations that exceed the volume size of a selected capsule shell should not be filled into hard gelatin capsules.

Care should be taken deriving a method for determining capsule/excipient compatibility. In the case of powder formulations, the mass inside a capsule shell is relatively porous in the order of 40–70% compared to a tablet (8–12%). For stability, it may be considered more appropriate to prepare mixtures for testing that have similar porosities because the closer they are in contact with each other, the greater the interaction between the active and excipients. Formation of compacts may be considered a worst-case scenario for stability but realistically is not representative of drug–excipient interaction within a capsule. A modified Accelerated Stability Program regime below the glass transition temperature of gelatin may be required to prevent high temperature/humidity degradation of capsule shell.

Knowledge of API moisture sensitivity should be used as a predictor for suitability for capsule development. Hygroscopic compounds can have a negative influence on the formulation of hard

TABLE 8.2
Typical Formulation Composition for Powder in Hard Gelatin Capsule

Class	Function	Examples	Comments
Diluent/filler	Increases bulk and aids plug formation	Mannitol, lactose(monohydrate and anhydrous), microcrystalline cellulose, corn starch, pre-gelatinized starch (e.g., Starch 1500), dibasic calcium phosphate	Section of diluent/filler related to solubility of active ingredient to aid and not interfere with dissolution. That is, for poorly soluble active, select a soluble excipient (e.g., lactose); for soluble active, select an insoluble excipient (e.g., starch). Choice of diluent/filler dictates plug-forming capability at low compression forces (10 to 100 N). Such fillers modified for direct compression tableting have enhanced flowability and compactibility and may be of special advantage in automatic filling machine that form plugs by tamping or compression.
Lubricant	Reduces powder-to-metal adhesion; improves flow properties	Magnesium stearate, glyceryl monostearate, stearic acid	Most frequently used lubricant in capsule formulations is magnesium stearate. It has a plate-like structure that adheres well to metal surfaces. Laminar lubricants like magnesium stearate should not be over-blended since particles delaminate under the shearing of blending to produce more hydrophobic particles in the blend.
Glidant	Improves flow properties	Colloidal silica (e.g., Aerosil, Cab-O-Sil), talc	Reduce interparticulate friction. They coat the surface of powder particles and reduce contact between them. If too much is used, they can act as an anti-glidant.
Wetting agent	Improves wetting–water penetration into powder mixture	Sodium lauryl sulfate, Tween 80	Used to assist wetting of hydrophobic surfaces and aid the penetration of the dissolution solvent into the powder mass. By far, the most commonly used wetting agent is sodium lauryl sulfate.
Disintegrant	Disrupts powder mass	Croscarmellose, crospovidone, sodium starch glycolate, Starch 1500	Disintegrants aid the breakup of the powder mass inside the capsule. Traditional disintegrants (e.g., starch) are not added to capsule formulations because of the high porosity of fill. Starch is not a very effective disintegrant in a capsule because the grains do not swell sufficiently to break up the plug. Today, such super-disintegrants as sodium starch glycolate and croscarmellose are preferred over starch to ensure that the powder mass inside the capsule is dispersed into the dissolution medium when the capsule disintegrates.
Stabilizer	Aids stability of active	Antioxidants or moisture scavengers	Depending on the stability of the active in the formulation.

gelatin capsules in a number of ways. Hygroscopic compounds can absorb water out of the shell, which normally has a water content of 13–16%. This can subsequently lead to brittleness and drying out of the shell. The rate and extent of physical shell/fill interactions depend strongly on the qualitative and quantitative composition of both the shell and the fill. As a general rule, the water content of the fill should not exceed a critical value of about 5%.

The absorption of moisture during production can lead to the buildup of a sorption film that affects the fluidity of the powder mix filling. Ideally, hygroscopic compounds should be combined with the diluent mannitol, as mannitol is relatively inert where water absorption is a concern. Also, dicalcium phosphate is very dense and may be less suitable as a capsule filler.

A suitable capsule formulation composition may include a diluent, a glidant, a lubricant, a surfactant, and a disintegrant.[3,4] Examples are presented in Table 8.2.

Dose range may limit formulation as a capsule. Doses > 600 mg in powder form are virtually impossible to fill into capsules of acceptable size. It may be possible to produce such doses in hard gelatin capsule form by increasing the density of the formulation, for instance, by granulation.

High concentrations of active usually lead to difficulties in the filling process, proportional to the concentration of the active in the formulation. Problems at this stage can be prevented by diluent selection and lubricant concentration.

The capacity of the capsule is dependent on the density and powder characteristics. Table 8.3 shows examples of typical hard gelatin capsule dimensions and their filling capacities.

The capsule size selected should be slightly larger than that needed to hold the powder to provide a full capsule (optimum fill level, 90%). Generally, smaller capsules are preferred for their perceived ease of swallowing. Typically size # 2 or less is preferred, but larger sizes may be necessary in some applications. Size # 0 capsules are often considered the largest size acceptable to patients, although these are not acceptable in some countries (e.g., Japan).

The filling mechanism will depend on the excipient choice and properties of the blend. Some of the important capsule blend properties are as follows:

1. Density: This affects fill weight and size of capsule.
2. Flow: This affects bed recovery and segregation.
3. Adhesion: This affects the fill weight uniformity, potency drop, segregation, and electrostatic interactions.
4. Water content: This can affect wettability, dissolution, and shell and content stability.

TABLE 8.3
Hard Gelatin Capsule Dimensions and Filling Capacities

Capsule Size	Capsule Volume (mL)	Capacity in mg Powder Density (mL)			
		0.6	0.8	1.0	1.2
000	1.37	822	1096	1370	1644
00 el	1.02	612	816	1020	1224
00	0.91	546	728	910	1092
0 el	0.78	468	624	780	936
0	0.68	408	544	680	816
1	0.50	300	400	500	600
2	0.37	222	296	370	444
3	0.30	180	240	300	360
4	0.21	126	168	210	252
5	0.10	78	104	130	156

5. Compactibility: This can affect fill weight uniformity, plug formation, tamp/compression pressure, plug retention in dosing tubes and dosing discs, and dissolution.
6. Compressibility: This affects fill weight, tamp/compression pressure, and capsule size selection.

While poor flow gives an angled or uneven bed in the hopper—"bed recovery," very good flow may lead to "flooding" or "splashing" with tamping machines. Similarly, high cohesivity should mean good plug formation, while low cohesivity (or good flow) would result in poor plug formation with dosator machines. Hence, for a capsule blend, both flow and cohesivity are desirable. Typically, for flow using a ring shear cell, a flow-function coefficient (ffc) range from 4 to 10 appears to be most suitable.[5–7] Suitable angles of repose for flow ranges from 25° to 30°. Similarly, certain ranges for the compressibility index (CI) have been preferred for tamping machines and dosators.[8]

High compressibility or compatibility is not crucial. It may have an impact on dissolution. Optimum densification to approximately close to the tapped density usually is sufficient to ensure good dissolution. To gauge this, CI is a good measurement. Also, Texture Analyzer can be used to determine plug height versus compression stress. The plug solid fraction might be useful for dissolution optimization.

Thus, although a high compactibility characteristic is not a requirement for a capsule formulation to form a hard compact, the selection of excipients in the formula remains critical to ensure good flow properties and content uniformity for filling on automated encapsulation equipment. A formulation should be designed based on an understanding of filling machine requirements. The two most common types of automated capsule-filling machines are the dosator type and the dosing disk machines. If the formula is to be encapsulated on a dosator-type machine, then the blend should also have sufficient binding properties to facilitate plug formation for transfer to a capsule shell. A somewhat lesser degree of cohesiveness also appears to be important when running formulations on a dosing disc machine as this is thought to promote clean, efficient transfer at ejection. A capsule formulation should have satisfactory powder fluidity, lubrication, and compactibility for a successful manufacturing operation.

Particle size of the drug substance and excipients is important to the homogeneity and fluidity of a powder blend. This is because the powder bed from which the dose of mix is measured needs to be homogeneous, packed reproducibly, in order to give uniform fill weights. Good packing is assisted by good powder flow, and this is aided by mechanical devices on the filling machine. Low-dose drugs can be made to flow well by mixing with free-flowing diluents (e.g., maize starch). For higher-dose drugs, the space available within the capsule shell for formulation aids is minimal. Small quantities (up to 5% w/w) of highly active materials are used: glidants, which improve flow by reducing interparticulate friction (e.g., fumed silicon dioxide), and lubricants, which reduce powder to metal adhesion (e.g., magnesium stearate), thus enabling the dosing devices to function properly.

For the filling of hard gelatin capsules, literature suggests a minimum particle size of 10 µm. If the particle size is more than 60 µm, the fluidity of the powder starts to deteriorate, which leads to unwanted deviations of the filling weights.[9] The size of particles should ideally measure between 10 and 150 µm. Excipients should be chosen in relation to the particle size of the drug active. Table 8.4 shows the relative impact of mean particle size on capsule filling.

A formulation strategy may be to optimize small-scale formulations using Carr's Index as a predictor for acceptability at scale. Literature suggests use of Carr's Index as a suitable guide for flow performance on tamp and dosator machines. Table 8.5 shows the relation between CI and the outcome of the automatic tamp filling outcome at scale.

API morphology should also be taken into consideration. Product flow is mainly defined by the shape of the particles as well as by interparticulate cohesion and surface films (sorption water). The fluidity of anisometric particles such as needle-shaped, plate-shaped, or prismatic particles is peculiar in so far as it follows not only the primary direction but also a secondary direction according to the orientation of the particles. This is the reason why anisometric particles result in significant differences in bulk and tap density. The mechanical vibration is strong enough to allow the particles to gain a higher grade of order.

TABLE 8.4

Effect of Mean Particle Size on Capsule Filling

Mean Particle Size	General Properties	Effect on Filling (dosator and tamp)
>150 µm	Excellent flow	No plug formation—dosator not recommended High fill weight variations No overfilling possible
100–150 µm	Plug strength is variable Add 10–20% MCC	Plug formation physically unstable
50–100 µm	Ideal for plugs Flow may need improvement	Plug form can be varied and controlled by tamping pressure Flowing properties might be improved by addition of glidant
20–50 µm	Sticking and poor flow	Increased adhesion of powder on dosing tools Poor flowing properties Flowing properties might be improved by addition of glidant and lubricant and use of low tamp force
<20 µm	Excessive adhesion and very poor flow	No filling/high adhesion Need to granulate

TABLE 8.5

Relation between Carr's Index and Filling Performance on Automatic Capsule-Filling Machines

Carr's Index (%)	Result
<15	• Best flowing properties • Water effect • High fill weight variations • Increase powder bed height
15–25	• Acceptable flowing properties • Best filling results • Powder bed angled but flat
25–35	• Bad flowing properties • Powder bed strongly angled • Additions of glidants/lubricants may be required
>35	• Worst flowing properties • Powder bed strongly angled and inhomogeneous • High fill weight variations • Granulation may be required

Isometric (e.g., round) particles are already in highly compact order, forming the densest shape. For hard gelatin capsules, the drug and excipients should preferably be isometric shapes. In the case of anisometric particles, grinding or granulation should be considered.

The tendency toward adhesion of many drug actives or excipients might lead to difficulties during capsule filling, as particles stick to the surfaces of the filling machine. The consequence of this sticking can result in breakup of the plugs, which leads to unacceptable fill weight variations. If the actives or excipients have a tendency to adhere, it is advisable to add a glidant or a combination of a glidant and lubricant such as Aerosil/magnesium stearate or talc/stearic acid. However, appropriate amounts need to be optimized based on the other physicochemical properties of the active and the excipients in relation to the primary function of the dosage form.

Diluents should be chosen based on the solubility of the API to aid release. Solubility of the active and the excipients is the major contributory factor in disintegration and dissolution. The more water soluble the formulation, the quicker it disintegrates and releases the drug substance. In the case of substances that are poorly soluble in water, the disintegration and release depend heavily on disintegrants and diluents. Insoluble drugs should ideally be mixed with soluble diluents (e.g., lactose) in order to make the mixture more hydrophilic. Soluble drugs can be mixed with insoluble diluents (e.g., starch) in order to avoid competition for solution. Primary factors influencing drug release rate from a capsule are particle size and aqueous solubility of the drug. Interactions between various components within a formulation can either accelerate or inhibit the release of drug from the capsule, for example, competition for available water between a highly soluble drug and a disintegrant with a high swelling capacity may exist, which can result in retarded dissolution.

A formulation should be designed for both machinability (machine performance) and good release properties. Some of the materials used to improve the filling performance (e.g., lubricants like magnesium stearate) are hydrophobic in nature, thus tending to slow down release. This effect can be minimized by formulation optimization or by inclusion of a wetting agent (e.g., sodium lauryl sulfate [SLS]) into the mix. In some cases, it is better to wet-granulate with a soluble binder than include SLS in the formulation.

Disintegrants (e.g., sodium glycolate, starch, or corn starch) or super-disintegrants (e.g., sodium croscarmellose and crospovidone) may often be suitable to promote API release in capsule formulation.[3,10,11] The requirement for a disintegrant should be accessed on a case-by-case basis. It also depends on the mechanism of the disintegrant. Powder plug porosity is high (50–70%) compared to tablets (10–15%); therefore, depending on the mechanism, higher concentrations may be needed. It is believed that for swelling to be effective in generating a disintegration action in the more porous capsule plugs, more disintegrant is needed. Botzolakis et al.[10] reported that as much as 4–8% concentrations were needed. In some capsule formulations, it is known to require even higher amounts. In general, addition of a disintegrant may be prevalent for high-dose, hydrophobic API formulations.

Addition of a lubricant may be required to prevent the powder adhering to the metal surfaces of an encapsulation machine as well as to optimize the powder flow and compressibility characteristics. Beside the lubricating effect, the commonly used lubricants have hydrophobic properties that reduce the dissolution significantly when used in excess. Overlubrication can result in a decreased dissolution but may also negatively impact the content uniformity, powder density, and plug formation.

The addition of lubricants should therefore be restricted to the minimum. Some diluents like Starch 1500, which are often referred to as "self-lubricating" because of their minimal lubrication requirements, do not necessarily need additional lubrication when used at high concentration. Research has shown that Starch 1500 plugs (and tablets) exhibit substantial post-compression axial relaxation, which tends to reduce contact with the confining side walls and reduce residual radial pressure.[12] Star cap is a co-processed mix of maize starch and pre-gelatinized starch designed typically for capsule filling. It has fewer fines than Starch 1500. Magnesium stearate, which is used in 80% of capsule formulations[13] as a lubricant, provides sufficient lubrication at a concentration 0.5–1% when filled on a dosator type of filling machine and even half of this concentration when filled on a dosing disk-type filling machine.[14]

The dosage form design criteria often require competitive requirements. In such cases, the formulation and process variables need to be optimized to meet all the design criteria. In this regard, instrumentation of capsule-filling machines has made it possible to measure forces involved in plug formation and ejection.[15] Also, capsule-filling machine simulators are available. Several studies utilizing statistical analysis and neural networks and expert systems have been performed.[16,17]

The role of excipients and formulation strategy in dealing with a BCS Class II drug was clearly demonstrated in a case study of piroxicam capsules from UMAB-FDA's collaborative research.[18]

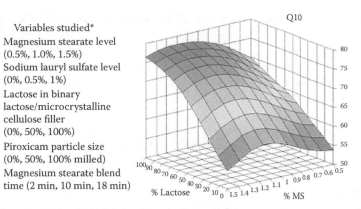

Variables studied*

- Magnesium stearate level (0.5%, 1.0%, 1.5%)
- Sodium lauryl sulfate level (0%, 0.5%, 1%)
- Lactose in binary lactose/microcrystalline cellulose filler (0%, 50%, 100%)
- Piroxicam particle size (0%, 50%, 100% milled)
- Magnesium stearate blend time (2 min, 10 min, 18 min)

*Central composite design comprising 32 batches of capsules.
Plug compression force, sodium starch glycolate and colloidal silica levels fixed.

FIGURE 8.1 The parameters studied for optimization of the formulation and process variables (18) and a representative response surface* (Q10 = percent dissolved in 10 min). (Courtesy of L. Augsburger.) *Response surface plotted from data generated under University of Maryland–Food and Drug Administration collaborative agreement No. 223-91-3401.

The purpose of this study was to determine the effect of major compositional changes on the bioavailability of piroxicam from IR formulation filled in hard gelatin capsule. The capsules were manufactured using a resolution V experimental design to study the effect of SLS level, magnesium stearate level, lactose/microcrystalline cellulose ratio, piroxicam particle size, and lubricant blend time (Figure 8.1). The SLS level and piroxicam particle size were the most important main effects affecting dissolution. The other factors were least important. Three of these formulations exhibiting slow, medium, and fast dissolution were compared to a single lot of the innovator product in a small bioavailability study. The slow formulation did not meet the USP dissolution specification for piroxicam capsules. Compositionally, these experimental formulations represented major changes to the levels. However, the results from the bioavailability study showed that the three formulations were bioequivalent to the commercial formulations and to each other. Thus, the dissolution profiles that discriminated between the formulations *in vitro* did not accurately represent the *in vivo* bioavailability results. These results were part of the research database that supports SUPAC-IR guidance that provided relaxed testing and filing requirements for scale-up and post-approval changes to IR oral solid dosage forms.

FILLING TECHNOLOGY

AUTOMATIC CAPSULE-FILLING MACHINES

The various types of filling machines available to the pharmaceutical industry may be conveniently categorized according to the manner in which the dose of the formulation is measured into the capsule body. The methods of dosing for dry powders can be divided into direct and indirect types.[19,20] In the direct type, the capsule body is used as the volumetric chamber in which the dose of the formulation is measured. In the indirect type, the quantity to be filled is measured in a chamber completely independent of the capsule body. There is a great variety of capsule-filling equipment available, which ranges in output from 1000 to more than 200,000 capsules per hour. The machines can also be grouped into two distinct types based on their motion, those that operate in an intermittent fashion (*Hofliger-Karg, Harro-Hofliger [H&H], Zanasi A Z-2 0, AZ-40, Macolar,* and *Dott.Bonapace RC-530*) and those that have a continuous motion (*MG2, Zonasi Z5000, Farmatic,*

Osaka). However, despite these differences, all machines have the following operational steps in common:

- Orientation and separation of the shell into its components—body and cap
- Dosing the material into body
- Rejoining the cap and body

Capsule-filling equipment has been previously discussed in detail by Lightfoot in Chapter 6. Three main dosing methods may be identified, and these are briefly reviewed in the subsequent paragraphs to support a discussion of their formulation requirements.

Auger Fill Principle

At one time, nearly all capsules were filled by means of semiautomatic equipment, wherein the powder is driven into the capsule bodies by means of a rotating auger. This type of filling machine is exemplified by the *Capsugel/Type 8* machine. The empty capsule bodies are held in a filling ring that rotates on a turntable under the powder hopper. The fill of the capsules is primarily volumetric. Because the auger mounted in the hopper rotates at a constant rate, the delivery of powder to the capsules tends to be at a constant rate. Consequently, the major control over fill weight is the rate of rotation of the filling ring under the hopper. A faster rate produces lighter fill weight because bodies have a shorter dwell time under the hopper.

Vibratory Fill Principle

The *Osaka* machines employ a vibratory feed mechanism. In this machine, the capsule body passes under a feed frame that holds the powder in the filling section. In the powder, a perforated resin plate is positioned that is connected to a vibrator. The powder bed tends to be fluidized by the vibration of the plate, and this assists the powder to flow into the bodies through holes in the resin plate. The fill weight is controlled by the vibrators and by setting the position of the body under the feed frame. The process affords only slight compression of the powder against the resin plates.

Piston-Tamp Principle

Today, most capsules are filled on what may be described as piston-tamp machines. These are fully automatic encapsulators in which pistons or tamping pins are employed to lightly compress the individual doses of powders into plugs (sometimes referred to as "slugs") that often resemble soft tablets in consistency and eject them into empty capsule bodies. There are two types of piston-tamp encapsulators: (1) the dosing disc type and (2) the dosator type.

Dosing Disc Machines

This type of machine is exemplified by the Bosch (formerly *Hofliger Karg*) *GKF* models and the H&H, KFM models. The dosing disc, which forms the base of the dosing or filling chamber, has a number of holes bored through it. A solid brass "stop" plate slides along the bottom of the dosing disc to close off these holes, thereby forming openings similar to the die cavities of a tablet press. The powder is maintained at a relatively constant height over the dosing disc, though the powder bed is not actually leveled. Five sets of tamping pins (in GKF machines) compress the powder into the cavities to form plugs. The dose is controlled by the thickness of the dosing disc (e.g., cavity depth), the powder depth, and the tamping pressure. These machines generally require that formulations be adequately lubricated for efficient plug ejection to prevent filming on tamping pins and to reduce friction between any sliding components that may come into contact with powder. A degree of compactibility is important, as coherent plugs appear to be desirable for clean, efficient transfer at ejection. However, there may be less dependence on formulation cohesiveness than exists for dosator machines. The H&H machine is similar to GKF machines, except that it employs only three tamping stations. However, at each station, the powder in the dosing cavities is tamped twice before rotating a quarter turn to the next station. One other difference between them is that the powder in the filling chamber of H&H machines is constantly agitated to help in the maintenance of a uniform powder bed depth.

Dosator Machines

The dosator machines are exemplified by the *Zanasi*, *MG2*, *Dott.Bonapace*, and *Macolar* machines. The dosator consists of a cylindrical dosing tube fitted with a movable piston. The end of the tube is open, and the position of the piston is preset to a particular height to define a volume that would contain the desired dose of powder. In operation, the dosator is plunged down into a powder bed maintained level at a constant preset height by agitators and scrapers. The powder bed height is generally greater that the piston height. Powder enters the open end and is slightly compressed against the piston (sometimes termed "pre-compression").[21] The dosator, bearing the plug, is withdrawn from the powder hopper and is moved over to the empty capsule body where the piston is pushed downward to eject the plug. The primary control over fill weight (for a given set of tooling) is the initial piston height in the dosing tube. A secondary control of weight is the height of the powder bed into which the dosator dips.

FORMULATION REQUIREMENTS FOR PLUG-FORMING AUTOMATIC CAPSULE-FILLING MACHINES

Usually, automatic capsule filling is carried out on either the dosator or the dosing disc types of machines. The basic requirements of a powder formulation for clean and efficient filling on these machines are as follows:

- Good fluidity
- Ability to form a cohesive plug
- Sufficient lubricity
- A reasonable bulk density

The basic requirements for a dosator type and dosing disk machine are summarized in Table 8.6.
Good flow is necessary to produce a working powder bed that can reform adequately after doses have been removed. A degree of compactibility or cohesiveness under pressure is important to prevent loss of material from the end of the plug during transport to the capsule shell. Sufficient

TABLE 8.6
Summary of Basic Requirements for a Dosator and Dosing Disk Machine

Requirements	Dosing Disk	Dosator
Lubricity	Adequate lubrication is required for efficient plug ejection, to prevent filming and reduce friction of sliding components	To ensure clean ejection
Compactibility	Coherent plugs are desirable for clean plug ejection	Necessary to ensure that the plug does not break up when the dosator is withdrawn from powder bed Since lubricants are generally hydrophobic, a poorly wettable plug may result if too much compression force is used The plug should not protrude above the capsule Overfilling of capsule
Flowability	Auger feed in hopper aids filling of formulations with poor flow	To ensure weight uniformity

lubricity in a formulation is needed to permit easy and efficient ejection of the plug and prevent or minimize adhesion to the tooling and other surfaces in contact with the formulation. The necessity for a reasonable bulk density becomes important when dealing with active ingredients that are administered in large doses, since the formulation is limited by the available or preferred capsule sizes.

The instrumentation of capsule-filling machines, which is discussed in detail in Chapter 7, has provided new insights into the interplay of formulation and machine operating variables that can affect both the manufacturability of capsules and their performance as drug delivery systems. The basic formulation requirements of the automatic capsule-filling machines operating on the piston-tamp principle as reported in the literature to date are reviewed in this section.

FLOWABILITY

Repeated extraction of powder from a previous dosing site is a common problem on automatic capsule-filling machines because of inadequate replenishment or remixing of the powder bed. This could be overcome by either mechanical or formulation means. In most machines, the powder bed is reformed by mechanical devices such as static agitators and active-stirring devices or by the application of suction to the base of the powder to densify it at the dosing point. An alternative method that is used on continuous motion dosator machines is the rotation of the dosator assembly and the powder hopper being maintained at different speeds and out of synchronization so that the dosator enters the bed in the same position only after a few rotations.

Simple powder flow measurements such as angle of repose, Hausner's ratio, flow rate, and minimum orifice diameter, although limited to the study of free-flowing powders, have been used successfully to predict the capsule-filling performance for powders. Schatz[22] characterized powders by measurements of angle of repose and changes in bulk density using a jolting volumeter. These properties were used to compare their filling performance on a dosator machine, Zanasi RV-59, and a dosing disc machine, Hofliger-Karg (H&K) GKF 70. Various blends of lactose, talc, and magnesium stearate were tested. The blends with poorest flow properties gave the worst filling performance and the more free-flowing ones gave the best fill weight uniformity. An angle of repose of less than $42°$ was proposed as the value to be used for achieving satisfactory filling. However, free-flowing powders required a higher degree of compaction to achieve satisfactory filling on the dosator machine. According to this study, the inclusion of starch in the mixture overcame this aforementioned problem because it allowed reasonable compression to be employed successfully.

Kurihara and Ichikawa,[23] working on an H&K machine, reported that variation in fill weight was closely related to the angle of repose of the formulation; however, a minimum point appeared in the plots of the angle of repose versus coefficient of variation of fill weight. Apparently, the powders with higher angles of repose did not have sufficient mobility to distribute well under the acceleration of the intermittent-indexing motion. At lower angles of repose, the powder was apparently too fluid to maintain a uniform bed. However, the investigators did not appear to make use of powder compression by tamping, and this complicates the interpretation of their findings.

Some researchers have examined the relation between formulation flow properties and weight variation on Zanasi machines. Irwin et al.[24] compared the weight variation of capsules filled on a Zanasi LZ-64 machine from formulations composed of different diluents and lubricants. The formulations had different flow properties, as judged in a recording flow meter. He showed that greater uniformity of fill weight could be achieved with powders that were more free flowing or having better flow rate. This was explained by the superior replenishment and mixing of the powder extraction sites in the powder bed. Chowhan and Chow[25] compared powder consolidation ratio with the coefficient of variation of capsule weight and found a linear relationship for a test formulation containing 5% or 15% drug, 10% starch, and 0.5% magnesium stearate, and lactose q.s. The capsules were filled on a Zanasi machine.

The bulk density (loose and tapped) of the powder has been linked to flowability, as measured by the "angle of internal flow"[26] and Carr's CI.[27] The latter parameters have significant advantage over other methods of measuring flow, such as angle of repose, and so on, because they are not limited to free-flowing powders. Carr's CI is defined as follows:

$$CI = \frac{(TBD - LBD)}{TBD} \times 100, \tag{8.1}$$

where TBD = tapped bulk density and LBD = loose bulk density.

Powders with values less than 15% are considered to have excellent flow and those with CI values greater than 40% have very bad flow.[27] The angle of internal flow is also calculated from the bulk density data. Verthalis and Pilpel[26] described a method of obtaining a straight line from the graph of bulk density as a function of the number of taps. By plotting the expression $K = E^2 \, n/(1 - E)$, where E is the porosity versus the number of taps n. If K_o is the y-intercept of this plot, a straight line passing through the origin can be obtained by plotting $K - K_o$ as a function of n. The slope of the line passing through the origin is termed as the angle of internal flow, $<p$. This angle effectively reflects the rate of change of bulk density with the number of taps.

Tan and Newton[28] using the instrumented MG2 capsule-filling machine simulator developed by Jolliffe et al.[29] studied the capsule-filling performance of five pharmaceutical excipients, Starch 1500, Avicel PH 101, calcium carbonate, maize starch, and Lactose B 170. They found a significant correlation between the coefficient of variation of the fill weights and a number of flow parameters such as Carr's CI, Hausner's ratio, angle of repose, Kawakita's constant a, and Jenike's flow factor.

The flow properties of a formulation can be improved by the addition of a glidant. Glidants are fine particles that appear to coat the particles of the bulk powder and enhance fluidity by one or more of several mechanisms:[30,31]

- Reducing roughness by filling surface irregularities
- Reducing attractive forces by physically separating the host particles
- Modifying electrostatic charges
- Acting as moisture scavengers
- Serving as ball bearings between host particles

Glidants include the colloidal silicas, cornstarch, talc, and magnesium stearate. Usually, there is an optimum concentration for flow, generally less than 1% and typically 0.1–0.5% when colloidal silicas are used. The optimum concentration may be related to the concentration sufficient to coat host particles.[32] Exceeding this concentration will usually result in no further improvement in flow and may even cause worsening of flow.

Hogan et al.[9] investigated the relationship between drug properties, filling parameters, and release of drugs from hard gelatin capsules using multivariate statistical analysis. They concluded that the optimum concentration for Aerosil (colloidal silica) appears to be 1%, with respect to both coefficient of fill weight variation and flowability, as measured by Carr's CI.

Nair et al.[33] investigated the comparison between the Carr index, Johanson flow rate, and critical orifice diameter of lubricated excipients and drug blends. The Johanson flow rate appeared to be a more discriminating method among the tests used to compare.[34,35]

More recently, Nalluri et al.[36] investigated the co-relation between powder avalanching and shear cell parameters of drug–excipient ratios to design minimal weight variation into the capsules. They concluded by running a series of binary blends of paracetamol and microcrystalline cellulose that the flow property increased until it reached a percolation threshold when abrupt changes in flow behavior were observed. This correlated well with the capsule weight variability and the angle of internal friction. On the basis of the results, they proposed a strategy to design minimal weight variability into powder-filled capsules by using the powder avalanching as a control strategy.

Osorio and Muzzio[37] investigated a wide array of powder flow measurement techniques using the more recent Freeman Technology Rheometer V.4 (FT4). Their methods have used flow parameters such as gravitational displacement rheometer, flow index, powder rheometer compressibility, basic flow energy, cohesion, and ffc measurements in a shear cell on the FT4. Their results show good co-relation between the measured parameters and weight and weight variability in the filled capsules.

Faulhammer et al.[38] recently used a predictive statistical model for filling of low–fill weight inhalation products using dosator nozzles. Using the Quality by Design Paradigm, they were able to determine the effect on the critical quality attribute (CQA), fill weight, and weight variability. They identified critical material attributes (CMAs) and critical process parameters (CPPs) that affected the CQA. The model developed was able to predict the fill weight and weight variability for the inhalation product. They validated the model and established a design space for the performance of different types of inhalation grade lactose on filling based on the CMAs and CPPs.

Lubricity

Fully automatic capsule-filling machines apply a significant amount of compression (though well below that applied in tableting), usually up to 100 N, but values as high as 300 N have also been reported. The powder is compressed into a coherent or apparently (partially) coherent plug. Apart from increasing the density of the powders above their maximum tapped bulk density, this compression may necessitate the addition of anti-adherents to the formulation to prevent the powder adhering to the metal surfaces of the tooling (dosators and pistons) used in dosing. The powder plug must also be removed cleanly from the dose-measuring device, which necessitates the inclusion of a "true lubricant" in the formulation.

Plug ejection force measurements make possible objective decisions on type and level of lubricant to be included in formulations. The earliest reported work on an instrumented capsule-filling machine by Cole and May[39] included an examination of the effect of a lubricant, magnesium stearate, on the compression and ejection forces on a dosator machine, Zanasi LZ-64. They demonstrated a considerable reduction in the forces when 0.5% magnesium stearate was added to a lactose mixture. Small and Augsburger[40] later reported a detailed study of the lubrication requirements of the Zanasi-LZ 64. Three fillers were studied (microcrystalline cellulose, pre-gelatinized starch, and anhydrous lactose). Powder bed height, piston height, compression force, and lubricant type and concentration were studied to determine their effects on ejection force. In general, anhydrous lactose exhibited higher lubrication requirements than either pre-gelatinized starch or microcrystalline cellulose. Comparing several concentrations of magnesium stearate, minimum ejection forces were recorded at 1% with anhydrous lactose, at 0.5% with microcrystalline cellulose, and at 0.1% with pre-gelatinized starch. Magnesium lauryl sulfate compared favorably with magnesium stearate for pre-gelatinized starch but was not as efficient as magnesium stearate for the other two fillers. Also, the magnitude of the ejection force was affected by machine-operating variables. Ejection force increased with the compression force. However, at a given compression force, ejection force also increased with an increase in either the piston height or the powder bed height. These results suggest the possibility of manipulating machine-operating variables to reduce the lubricant requirements in a formulation.

The lubricants may not always be beneficial to filling performance. Takagaki et al.[41] found in a study using a dosator machine that fill weight uniformity decreased at higher lubricant levels. This was explained by the loss in cohesiveness of the plug by the addition of lubricant.

Mehta and Augsburger[42] reported the effect of magnesium stearate on plug hardness and the dissolution of hydrochlorothiazide from capsules filled on a Zanasi LZ-64. The fillers were microcrystalline cellulose and anhydrous lactose. They concluded that it might be advisable to sometimes exceed the minimum lubricant concentration requirement of a capsule-filling machine with fillers such as microcrystalline cellulose. The mechanical strengths of the plugs produced in a dosator may be reduced by the amount of lubricant used, and this could have a beneficial effect on drug dissolution. Small[43] showed similar results with pre-gelatinized starch, using acetaminophen as a model drug. A similar finding was also reported by Stewart et al.[44] for the dissolution of riboflavin from microcrystalline cellulose plugs. Interestingly, hand-filled rifampicin capsules also exhibited a similar phenomenon. Nakagawa et al.[45] found that up to a limit, increasing the blending time of magnesium stearate (tantamount to increasing the concentration) improved the dissolution rate of rifampicin. The effect was most marked at the lowest lubricant levels studied.

The minimum lubricant concentration requirement of one type of filling machine might be too much for another type and could affect the final product specification (dissolution requirement). Ullah et al.[46] encountered an *in vitro* dissolution problem during scale-up of cefadroxil monohydrate, a water-soluble drug product. Initial formulation development had been carried out on a Zanasi LZ-64 with a blend containing 1% magnesium stearate as lubricant. Scale-up on a Hofliger-Karg GKF 1500 (H&K) showed a significantly slower dissolution rate for the drug when compared to the capsules produced on a Zanasi LZ-64. Analysis of the problem indicated that powder was being sheared during encapsulation on the H&K filling machine, leading to overcoating of the drug particles by magnesium stearate and a slower dissolution rate. Shear simulation studies were conducted to select the level of magnesium stearate appropriate for encapsulation on the H&K that would maintain a satisfactory *in vitro* capsule dissolution rate. A 0.3% w/w level of magnesium stearate was selected on the basis of the simulation studies. At this lubricant level, capsules were routinely produced on the H&K machine with satisfactory dissolution and encapsulation characteristics.

Tattawasart and Armstrong,[47] using the simulator developed earlier by Britten and Barnett, studied the effect of lubricant concentration on plug formation. They found that 0.5% level of magnesium stearate provides adequate lubrication for lactose plugs. The simulator was designed to simulate the operating principle of the dosator machines. Shah et al.,[48] working on an H&K GKF 330, found that the optimum level of the lubricant, magnesium stearate, was 0.1%, resulting in maximum plug strengths and fill weights, regardless of the number and intensity of the tamps used.

COMPRESSIBILITY, COMPACTIBILITY, AND COHESIVENESS

Conflicting powder properties are required for processing on automatic capsule-filling machines. A free-flowing powder is needed for a homogeneous powder bed but a cohesive powder is preferable for powder retention during transfer of the powder to the capsule shell.

Compression is applied during the capsule-filling process to consolidate the powder for a couple of reasons: (i) to increase powder density and hence maximize the amount filled into a desired capsule size, and (ii) to aid powder retention as the plug is transferred from the dosing cavities to the capsule body. The latter could be more important on dosator machines and to a somewhat lesser extent on the dosing disc machines because the plug is supported underneath until the moment of transfer on the latter.

Jolliffe et al.[49] have studied the aforementioned problem on dosator machines theoretically by the application of hopper design theory. The retention of powder during transfer requires the formation of a stable powder arch at the dosator outlet, and this depends on the angle of wall friction. Generally, theory predicts that cohesive materials will be retained with minimal compressive stress on rough dosator walls and that smoother walls provide the best conditions for retaining more freely flowing powders. On the basis of this theory, Jolliffe and Newton[50] later demonstrated that for free-flowing particles to be retained, more compressive force is needed than for cohesive particles, which sometimes could be retained with no compression.

Jolliffe and Newton,[51] using the MG2 simulator developed earlier,[29] showed that capsule fill weights obtained using fine, cohesive powders are relatively insensitive to the compression applied by the piston and are able to give uniform fill weights over a wide range of compression settings.

TABLE 8.7

Quantitative Comparison of the Fluidity, Lubricity, and Compactibility Requirements of a Dosator and Dosing Disk Encapsulation Machine

Formulation Characteristic	Dosator Type	Dosing Disc Type
Fluidity	The optimum values if Carr's Index (CI) lies between 25 and 35 for best % CV of fill weights.	The optimum range of CI for efficient encapsulation is $18 < CI < 30$.
Lubricity	The amount of lubricant necessary for clean encapsulation may be around 0.5–1% depending on the formation.	The amount of lubricant required for successful encapsulation could be as low as 50% of the level used on a dosator machine.
Compactibility/ compressibility	Higher CIs produced stronger plugs and better % CV of fill weights. In a formulation with lower CIs (<20), higher compression forces about 150–200 N could pride better retention ability of the powder in the dosator tube.	Formulations with higher CIs tend to flood near the ejection station. Although this damming of powder may not affect the overall % CV, the process is certainly not very clean. Even though strong cohesion in a formulation is not required for successful transfer of the plug from the dosing disc to the capsule body, for certain very free-flowing formulations (granulations), moderately higher compression forces around 150 N would be beneficial.

Coarse, free-flowing powders require a minimum compression to be uniformly filled and fill uniformity will only occur for small increases in compression above this. For both types of powders, compression above an optimum limit, that is, beyond its ability to pack more tightly by rearrangement, resulted in poor fill uniformity. This occurs at lower compression forces for coarse, free-flowing powders because of their lower compressibility. They validated their results obtained with the simulator using a production-scale MG2 machine. Shah et al.,[48] working on a Hofliger-Karg GKF 300 filling machine, evaluated several compression parameters and concluded that, aside from station # 1, all tamping stations and all piston positions within a station contribute equally to plug formation. The nearness of station # 1 to the scrape-off bar results in nonuniform powder bed height and a high degree of compression force variability. They also showed that increases in tamping force resulted in harder plugs, as measured with a plug mechanical strength tester. However, plug strengths did not increase in mechanical strength when additional segments were compressed over them using the same force. The authors also found that target fill weights could be achieved using as few as three tamps.

Shah et al.,[52] in a related study, observed the effects of number of tamps and tamping force on drug dissolution on the same machine, using hydrochlorothiazide as a model low-dose, poorly soluble drug. With increasing number of tamps, the dissolution rate was slower, the effect being most marked with dicalcium phosphate dihydrate as the filler. Inclusion of a disintegrant, 4% croscarmellose sodium, tended to nullify the effects of number of tamps or tamping force regardless of the filler used. Table 8.7 shows the quantitative comparison of the fluidity, lubricity, and compactibility requirements of a dosator and dosing disk encapsulation machine.

ROLE OF DENSITY IN PREDICTING CAPSULE FILL WEIGHT

The density of a powder influences its flowability and compressibility and hence it is an important parameter to consider in capsule filling. Stoyle[53] in one of the earliest reports evaluating the Zanasi machine suggested that formulations should possess a moderate bulk density. Low bulk density materials or those that contain entrapped air will not consolidate well, and capping similar to what occurs in tableting may result.

Small and Augsburger[40] studied various grades of microcrystalline cellulose and suggested a general correlation of capsule-filling performance with the tapped bulk density. As the tapped bulk density increases, capsule fill weight increases, generated compression force increases, weight variation decreases, and the overall filling performance of the material improves.

From measurements of the properties of individual components, Newton and Bader[54] were able to predict the maximum tapped bulk density of two component mixtures of a range of particle size fractions of aspirin and lactose in varying proportions. They extended their treatment to the prediction of the bulk density of such mixtures when filled into hard gelatin capsules assuming that the powders are filled at the maximum tapped bulk density. This relationship worked better for the uncompressed powders than the compressed ones since compression can cause densities greater than the maximum tapped density.

Shah et al.[48] have utilized bulk density changes to predict the filling behavior of powders on a dosing disc machine, Hofliger-Karg GKF 330. The maximum densification possible at each compression stage was calculated from the bulk density data. This enabled them to predict not only the maximum fill weights that can be accommodated for a particular dosing disc height but also the number of tamps required for achieving a target fill weight.

Davar et al.[55] developed a systematic approach to estimate the dosing disc height for achieving a target fill weight from the bulk density data of the formulation. Dosing discs representing the calculated height were then used on a capsule-filling machine (Hofliger-Karg GKF 330) to achieve the target fill weight. The target fill weight was successfully achieved using the dosing discs selected by this method with reasonable fill weight variation.

Usually, plug weight does not follow the tapped density of formulations because of the greater densification being achieved on tamping and other processing factors involved on automatic capsule-filling machines, but it is a good starting point in predicting the capsule size required for encapsulating the desired dose of a formulation.

FILLING OF GRANULATIONS INTO HARD SHELL CAPSULE

In a survey of industry practices, Heda[8] found that as a matter of policy, 46% of the firms sampled favor direct filling of powders as a first choice over granulation before filling in capsules. Thirty-six percent of firms allow formulators to make that decision at their own discretion, whereas 18% of the firms favor granulation of all formulations before encapsulation. Yet, for half of the firms responding, only 0–10% of their hard shell capsule products are direct-fill powder formulations, and only 27% of firms reported that more than 50% of their capsules were developed as direct-fill formulations. Although some of these non-direct-fill formulations may be controlled-release formulations (e.g., coated bead products), difficult direct-fill formulation problems may at least in part account for this observations.

For granulation, the standard wet and dry methods used to granulate powders before tableting are typically used. Among the firms sampled by Heda, 64% favored wet granulation for capsule formulations, 18% favored dry granulation, and the remainder had "no policy" as such.

Granulation of powder is typically done to increase density. This helps enormously as the weight of bulk that can be filled on a given size of capsule can be increased, or a smaller capsule size can be selected based on the reduced volume. However, granulations can also enhance some other processing characteristics and attributes as desired for the finished dosage form. Flow and compression properties of formulations can be improved. Dustiness and particle adhesion onto metal surfaces can be reduced. Granulation also increases the robustness by reducing the variability in the physical properties of raw materials. Wet granulation may improve wettability and drug dissolution through hydrophilization.[56] Common binders used in wet granulation such as pre-gelatinized starch and polyvinyl pyrrolidone are hydrophilic and can be expected to deposit on particle surfaces where they may enhance wettability. Granulation can improve content uniformity by holding the active particles in granules so that the formulation can be handled without loss of blend quality. Moreover, the binder liquid in wet granulation provides a convenient vehicle to introduce and uniformly disperse a very low dose drug throughout the granulated mass.

In general, the same principles applied in filling powders should be applied in filling granules, with some qualifications. For example, Podczeck et al. found that an acceptable filling performance was always achieved when different granule size fractions of sorbitol instant were filled on both a dosing disk (Bosch GKF 400) machine and a dosator (Zanasi AZ5) machine. However, the dosing disk machine, which depends less on forming firm plugs, seemed slightly better suited to the coarser granule size fractions than the dosator machine. On the other hand, the dosator machine invariably produced plugs that were denser than the formulation maximum bulk density, suggesting that this dosing principle might be more useful to form granulations where the dose is large or where smaller capsule size is desired.

CONSIDERATIONS IN SCALING-UP OF POWDER-FILLED HARD SHELL CAPSULE FORMULATION

For regulatory purposes, equipment for each unit operation is classified by class (operating principle) and subclass (design characteristics). The division of material into a hard gelatin capsule by encapsulation is an operating principle. The various methods by which machines fill the formulation into capsules represent different design characteristics and are considered subclasses. Therefore, equipment within the same class and subclass are considered to have the same design and operating principle under SUPAC. However, a change from a dosator machine to a dosing disc machine would constitute a change in subclass, but no change in the operating principle (i.e., encapsulation). According to the FDA's scale-up and post-approval changes guidance for immediate-release formulations (SUPAC-IR),[57] scale-up to and including a factor of 10 times the size of the pilot/bio-batch is considered a level 1 change if the equipment used to produce the test batch(es) is of the same design and operating principle and follows the principles of CGMP. Level 1 changes are likely to cause any detectable impact on the formulation quality or performance and need only be reported in the Annual Report. In the same situation, if the scale-up is beyond 10 times the pilot/bio-batch, that is considered a level 2 change. Level 2 changes are changes that could significantly affect formulation quality and performance and require the filing of "changes being effected supplement." However, the most significant outcome is that in neither case are *in vivo* bioequivalence data required to support the change in scale.

There are various factors that need to be considered with such scale-up situations as scaling up within the same class of machine or within the same subclass and transfer across different machine types. The reader is referred to Chapter 11 for a complete discussion of these and other considerations in scaling up powder formulations.

DIRECT FILL OF API (OR WHAT IS REFERRED TO AS "POWDER-IN-CAPSULE") WITHOUT EXCIPIENTS

Exploratory formulation approaches favor the use of the simplest formulations such as "powder-in-capsule" (PIC). In its simplest form, this would be API-in-capsule. Use of API-in-capsule has seen a large growth in popularity during the last decade or so, not the least because of arrival of systems that enable automated and accurate filling of large quantities of API-in-capsules, such as the Xcelodose (Capsugel, Cambridge, UK), Powdernium (Symyx Autodose Technologies, Sunnyvale, California), or the Quantos (Mettler Toledo, Columbus, Ohio). Direct filling of API in capsule is possibly the fastest way of entering clinical trials as this method is material sparing (use of little or no excipients), which could result in big savings on resources (time, money, and additional stability testing of samples). Also, it is not uncommon in early development to encounter differences in particle size distribution, hygroscopicity, polymorph content, or crystallinity of the API. Such changes during chemical development can have an impact on the formulation and process approach for development. This may be time consuming. Such changes can easily be accommodated by an API-in-capsule formulation.

Several approaches to delivering formulations for first-time-in-human dosing have been discussed.[58] There are also examples of the capsule-to-tablet concept where a common formulation approach could take the same formulation from a clinical capsule formulation to a commercial film-coated tablet.[1] However, there is no one-size-fits-all. PIC has been successfully been used for some time now. The Xcelodose 600 from Capsugel is a good example. This is a system for small-scale capsule filling. It is automated and programmable and provides precision metering of powdered drug in capsules. This is based on the "pepper pot" principle where the dispensing of powder simulates the action of a pepper shaker.[59] It works with capsules ranging from size 00 to 4. It can accurately weigh doses as low as 100 µg[60] and greater than 100 mg with an RSD of 1–2% weight precision. Typically ~5 g of API is required to develop Xcelodose filling parameters, such as tap frequency, pulse width, amount of slow tapping, and high-throughput unit settings. It can fill up to 600 capsules per hour, which is 10 times faster than a manual operation.

The suitability of API-in-capsule is based on assessment of some of the physicochemical properties of the API. If the API has poor physicochemical properties (e.g., poor aqueous solubility with BCS II and IV compounds), then they may not be suitable without the use of functional excipients and appropriate formulation strategy to enhance solubility. This may be required to improve bioavailability. Also, for potent low-dose API, it may be difficult to achieve the appropriate potency and uniformity without additional formulation strategy, although recent attempts have been made to show that, for low-dose potent drugs (between 5 µg and 5 mg), formulated blends of these API have been successfully filled with adequate CU using the Xcelodose.[61]

Another property to consider is the bulk density of the API, as most API-in-capsule machines do not have a "tamping" feature. Consequently, the bulk density and the packing of particle have a direct effect on the amount of API that can fit into a capsule. Dose in this case is limited by the size of the capsule. Thus, the Xcelodose may not be suitable for high-dose/low–bulk density drugs without additional formulation strategy. In these situations, the use of In-cap (Dott.Bonapace & C, Milan, Italy) as an automated tamping type of capsule filler with low output has been reportedly used.[33]

PRACTICAL CONSIDERATIONS IN FILLING OF PELLETS INTO HARD SHELL CAPSULE

Multiunit dosage forms and powders and their combinations may be poured directly into a capsule body by gravity-feed devices via delivery tubes that rely on the free-flowing nature of such materials. A good example is the Qualifill pellet filler (Schaefer Technologies Inc.). Using this approach, capsules are filled to their volumetric capacity, but partial fills for multiple dosing are not possible.

Indirect filling methods can circumvent these issues by using some of the current automatic filling machines where the required quantity of multiple-unit dosage forms are first fed into a separate volumetric metering (dosing) chamber and then the measured volume of material is transferred into the capsule body. The schematics illustrating the operational principles of these machines appear in Chapter 6. The metering chamber could be filled by gravity (e.g., Hofliger-Karg). In certain machines (e.g., Zanasi), the chamber is a modified dosator that draws and holds the pellets or beads into the open end by means of vacuum. In this technique, the dosing tube typically enters the pellet bed and, with the help of vacuum, the pellets are sucked into the dosing tube. The excess pellets are scraped off from the end of the dosing tube. The dosing tube is then lowered and the pellets are released into the capsule body. Other indirect machines have special chambers with sliding plates to give a variable volume in which to measure the material (e.g., Bosch GKF). In this process, the pellets flow from the pellet machine into the dosing chamber when the dosing plate slides open. The dosing slide is closed to separate the dosing chamber and the pellet magazine. Next, the outlet slides open to release the pellets into the capsule body. Also, Bosch has developed a variable thickness dosing disc that uses a slide underneath to hold the material before transfer. The dosing volume can be adjusted to the desired amount. Transfer of pellets or beads and/or granules to the capsule body can be done either by gravity or by assisted air pressure (e.g., the IMA and MG 2).

In general, the dose is determined by the size of the metering chamber. Products that are blends of different beads or pellets raise the issue of content uniformity especially when blend includes high- and low-dose pellet groups. These pellets should be such that they flow and pack well in the capsule body. The size of pellets is important as void space increases for larger pellets in a smaller-diameter tube. Their size should be related to the size of the capsule. In general, smaller-size pellets should be used for smaller sizes of capsules; otherwise, lower fill weights than expected will occur because of "wall effects" of particle packing.

Particle size, shape, and density of pellets and also their tendency toward electrostatic attraction can lead to segregation during the feeding or encapsulation process. Flow properties of the blend may lead to segregation of blends. This may be attributed to poor hopper design resulting in segregation. In such situations, it may be worth dosing pellet groups separately using a filling machine with multiple feeding stations (e.g., MG 2 Futura or Planeta 600). The modular design of these machines allows for flexibility and ease of use, which allows several of these combinations to be filled accurately with automatic dosing chamber adjustments and precision weight controls.

Electrostatic charges may retard the transfer of pellets from the dosing chamber to the capsule body. Film coating of pellets can typically result in pronounced electrostatic charge and thus in agglomeration, bridge formation, and blockage during the filling process. Surface roughness of pellets also hinders in the filling process. Large surface roughness can result in tribo-electrification. Friction by sliders or dosator nozzles can happen. Chopra et al. have shown that an addition of ~1% talc can help reduce this electrostatic effect.[62]

In several cases, the pellets have a functional coating that controls the release. In such cases, it is important to verify that the dosing system and the material handling systems are not abrading the coating, which could affect the product release. For typical size distribution of coated pellets, the pellets need not be perfectly spherical to be filled reproducibly into hard shell capsules. It has been demonstrated experimentally that an aspect ratio (AR) = (ratio of length to breadth) of 1.2 is the threshold value below which variations in AR have no impact on the fill weight or weight variation of the capsules.[62] This was further verified by computer simulation process on the filling accuracy for different capsule sizes.[63]

Recently, the FDA has suggested a new guidance in 2012 for certain drug products that contain beads within a capsule, in which, as indicated in the label, the capsule can be broken and the internal beads can be sprinkled on soft foods (e.g., apple sauce) and swallowed without chewing as an alternative administration technique. The agency reviewed human mastication studies that demonstrated that food is chewed to a median particle size range from 0.82 to 3.04 mm before swallowing.[64] Also, they reviewed all currently approved products labeled for sprinkle that contain beads up to 2.4 mm and found no associated safety risks or loss of efficacy associated with the bead size. On the basis of the above, the agency recommended a target bead size up to 2.5 mm with no more than 10% variation over this size, to a maximum size of 2.8 mm. The recommended bead size allowances consider the variability and differing manufacturing processes of beads. Any proposed bead sizes above this would require the applicant to justify with appropriate studies.[65]

PRACTICAL CONSIDERATIONS IN FILLING OF TABLETS INTO HARD SHELL CAPSULE

Similar to pellets, tablets can be filled into capsules with systems that can handle single and multiple additions. Typically, tablets are fed through tubes that have sensing devices, either electrical or mechanical, to check that the correct number of tablets has been dosed. A schematic of the tablet-filling process may be found in Chapter 6. The single dosing process involves the following:

Typically, a dosing slide that can accommodate exactly one tablet moves underneath the tablet feeder. The slider moves over the capsule body where the tablet simply drops into it. If properly filled, the pin dropped into the capsule body will have limited movement; the horizontal bar connected to the pin touches the sensor. If the tablet is not properly filled, then the horizontal bar will switch the sensor, indicating incorrect filling. Empty capsules can be detected and eliminated from the product.

The physical properties of these types of tablets are similar to pellets or mini-tablets. Tablets are preferably nonfriable and usually film-coated. Generally, they are convex in shape, are stackable, and have diameters that enable them to be introduced with sufficient clearance so that they do not tip on their side.

PRACTICAL CONSIDERATIONS IN FILLING OF GRANULES, PELLETS, TABLETS, AND/OR COMBINATIONS INTO HARD SHELL CAPSULE

Filling of combination of powders, pellets, and tablets in hard shells is also becoming very common. This may be attributed to several reasons. Primarily, there may be interactions between the active and the excipient components such that when given as a segregated unit, as in multiunits, the stability of the product is guaranteed. Also, the nature of the disease condition has given rise to development of multiple therapies in one dosage forms (e.g., "poly pill"). The use of several fixed-dose combinations is also very popular. Several innovative drug delivery capsule platform technologies have been developed (e.g., port capsule, pulsincap, l-oros, etc.). Also, in terms of a specific release profile like pulsed release (e.g., Elan's Codas-Prodas technology, Pulsys technology, Orbexa technology, Eurand's Minitab technology), the combination of one or more of these dosage forms is possible to create a distinct release profile and a therapeutic response. Several different automatic filling machines are currently available that have the capability to deliver one or more of these multiple units and their combinations. For example, the MG2 Planeta is a versatile machine that can do multiple combinations of four to five of such dosage forms (including liquids) using modular filling stations. It also has weight controls for all dosed capsules, integrated in the capsule filler, with automatic dosing chamber adjustment and automatic ejection of capsules outside the weight limits.

In addition to filling of pellets and tablets into hard shell capsules, alternative processes also exist, although rarely for enrobing pellets and tablets into soft shell capsules. In 1949, a rotary-die process of incorporating powder into soft gelatin capsules was made possible by Lederle Laboratories. The process commonly known as the "Accogel process" involves a measuring roll that holds the fill formulation in its cavities under vacuum and rotates directly over the elasticized sheet of gelatin ribbon. The ribbon was drawn into the capsule cavities of the capsule die roll by vacuum. The measuring rolls empty the fill material into the capsule-shaped gelatin cavities on the die roll. The die roll then converges over the rotating sealing roll covered with another sheet of elasticized gelatin. The convergence of the two rotary rolls creates pressure to seal and cut the formed capsules. A good example of use of this process was for the development of Diamox sequels at Lederle Laboratories.

Similarly, enrobed Geltabs can also be manufactured. Capsugel's Press Fit gelcaps are a unique dosage form consisting of a high-gloss gelatin coating that encases a caplet core. They use a patented cold-shrink process on a special filling and coating machine. The X-Press-Fit gelcaps are similar to the Press-Fit gelcaps but have an exposed center portion for rapid release. Soflet gelcaps (Banner Pharmacaps) are caplets filled in soft gelatin capsules. One key advantage of these dosage forms is ease of swallowing. Also, it eliminates any tablet friability and dusting issues and protects patients from exposure to potent compounds. In addition, it provides unique product identification by choosing from a range of colors. Gelatin film maintains product integrity and hermetically seals the tablet from exposure and thereby provides increased stability.

REFERENCES

1. Do N, Hansell J, Farrell TP. Narrowing the gap between clinical capsule formulations and commercial film-coated tablets. *Pharm. Tech. Europe* May 2009; 21(5): 18–23.
2. Singh S, Ramarao KV, Venugopal K et al. Alteration in dissolution characteristics of gelatin-containing formulations. *Pharm. Tech.* April 2002; 36–58.
3. Jones BE. New thoughts on capsule filling. *S.T.P. Pharma Sciences* 1988; 8: 277–283.
4. Shangraw RF, Demarest DA. A survey of current industrial practices in the formulation and manufacture of tablets and capsules. *Pharm. Tech.* 1993; 17(1): 33–44.
5. Jager PD, Bramante T, Luner PE. Assessment of pharmaceutical powder flowability using shear cell-based methods and application of Jenike's methodology. *J. Pharm. Sci.* 2015; 104: 3804–3813.
6. Jenike AW. Storage and flow of solids, Bull No. 123, *Eng. Exp. Station*, Univ. of Utah, Salt Lake City, 1964. Vol. 53, No. 26.
7. Schulze, D. Flow properties of powders and bulk solids. In Schulze, D. editor. *Powders and Bulk Solids: Behavior, Characterization, Storage and Flow*. New York: Springer-Verlag, 2008: 1–21.
8. Heda PK. A comparative study of the formulation requirements of dosator and dosing disc encapsulators. Simulation of plug formation, and creation of rules for an expert system for formulation design. PhD Dissertation, University of Maryland, Baltimore, MD, 1998.
9. Hogan J, Shue PI, Podczeck F, Newton JM. Investigations into the relationship between drug properties, filling, and release of drug from hard gelatin capsules using multivariate statistical analysis. *Pharm. Res.* 1996; 13: 944–949.
10. Botzolakis JE, Small LE, Augsburger LL. Effect of disintegration on dissolution from capsules filled on a dosator type automatic capsule filling machine. *Int. J. Pharm.* 1982; 12: 341–349.
11. Botzolakis JE, Augsburger LL. The role of disintegrants in hard-gelatin capsules. *J. Pharm. Pharmacol.* 1984; 36: 77–84.
12. Britten JR, Barnett MI, Armstrong NA. Studies on powder plug formation using a simulated capsule filling machine. *J. Pharm. Pharmacol.* 1996; 48: 249–254.
13. Jones BE. Two-piece gelatin capsules: Excipients for powder products, European practice. *Pharm. Tech. Eur.* 1995; 11: 25–34.
14. Heda PK, Muteba K, Augsburger LL. Comparison of the formulation requirements of dosator and dosing disc automatic capsule filling machines. *AAPS Pharm. Sci.* 2002; 4(3): 1–15.
15. Armstrong NA. Instrumentation of capsule filling machinery. 2004: 207–220. Available at http://www.pharmpress.com/files/docs/tablet_and_capsule_sample(1).pdf.
16. Wilson WI, Peng Y, Augsburger L. Comparison of statistical analysis and Bayesian networks in the evaluation of dissolution performance of BCS Class II model Drugs. *J. Pharm. Sci.* 2005; 94(12): 2764–2776.
17. Guo M, Kalra G, Wilson WI et al. A prototype intelligent hybrid system for hard gelatin capsule development. *Pharm. Tech.* September 2002; 44–60.
18. Piscitelli DA, Bigora S, Propst C et al. The impact of formulation and process changes on the in-vitro dissolution and bioequivalence of piroxicam capsules. *Pharm. Dev. Technol.* 1998; 3(4): 443–452.
19. Jones BE. *Encyclopedia of Pharmaceutical Technology*. New York: Marcel Dekker, 1990; 251–268.
20. Jones BE. *The Gelatin Capsule: Hard & Soft: Manufacture, Properties and Formulation*. Center for Professional Advancement, Amsterdam, June 1995.
21. Small LE, Augsburger LL. Instrumentation of automatic filling machine. *J. Pharm. Sci.* 1977; 66: 504–509.
22. Schatz B. Lilly Elanco; European Capsule Technology Symposium, Constance, Germany, Oct. 1978.
23. Kurihara K, Ichikawa I. Effect of powder flowability on capsule fill weight variation. *Chem. Pharm. Bull.* 1978; 26: 1250–1256.
24. Irwin GM, Dodson GJ, Ravin LJ. Encapsulation of clormacran phosphate I: Effect of flowability of powder blends, lot-to-lot variability and concentration of active ingredients on weight variation of capsules filled on an automatic capsule filling machine. *J. Pharm. Sci.* 1970; 59(4): 547–550.
25. Chowhan ZT, Chow YP. Powder flow studies I: Powder consolidation ratio and its relationship to capsule-filling weight variation. *Int. J. Pharm.* 1980; 4: 317–326.
26. Verthalis S, Pilpel N. Anomalies in some properties of powders. *J. Pharm. Sci.* 1976; 28: 415–419.
27. Carr RL. Evaluating flow properties of solids. *Chem. Engg.* 1965; 72: 163–168.
28. Tan SB, Newton JM. Powder flowability as an indication of capsule filling performance. *Int. J. Pharm.* 1990; 61: 145–155.

29. Jolliffe IG, Newton JM, Cooper D. The design and use of an instrumented MG2 capsule filling machine simulator. *J. Pharm. Pharmacol.* 1982; 34: 230–235.
30. Augsburger LL, Shang Raw RF. Effect of glidants on tableting. *J. Pharm. Sci.* 1966; 55: 418–423.
31. York P. Application of powder failure testing equipment in assessing effect of glidants on flowability of cohesive pharmaceutical powders. *J. Pharm. Sci.* 1975; 64: 1216–1221.
32. Sadek HM, Olsen JL, Smith HL et al. A systemic approach to glidant selection. *Pharm. Tech.* 1982; 6(2): 43–62.
33. Nair R, Vemuri M, Agrawala P et al. Investigation of various factors affecting encapsulation of the In-Cap automatic capsule-filling machine. *AAPS Pharm. Sci. Tech.* October 2004; 5(4): 1–8.
34. Johanson JR. Applying flow principles to liquids/solids processing. *Chem. Proc.* September 1986.
35. Johanson JR. Modeling flow of bulk solids. *Powder Technol.* 1972; 5(2): 93–99.
36. Nalluri V, Puchkov M, Kuentz M et al. Toward better understanding of powder avalanching and shear cell parameters of drug–excipient blends to design minimal weight variability into pharmaceutical capsules. *Int. J. Pharm.* 2013; 442: 49–56.
37. Osorio JG, Muzzio FJ. Effects of powder flow properties on capsule filling weight uniformity. *Drug Dev. Ind. Pharm.* 2013; 39: 1464–1475.
38. Faulhammer E, Llusa M, Wahl PR et al. Development of a design space and predictive statistical model for capsule filling of low-fill-weight inhalation products. *Drug Dev. Ind. Pharm.* 2015; 42(2): 221–230
39. Cole GC, May G. The instrumentation of a Zanasi LZ-64 capsule filling machine. *J. Pharm. Pharmacol.* 1975; 27: 353–358.
40. Small LE, Augsburger LL. Aspects of the lubrication requirements for an automatic capsule filling machine. *Drug Dev Ind. Pharm.* 1978; 4: 345–372.
41. Takagaki K, Sugihara M, Kimura S. Studies on filling properties in automatic filling machine. *Yakuzaigaku* 1969; 29: 245–249.
42. Mehta AM, Augsburger LL. A preliminary study of the effect of slug hardness on drug dissolution from hard gelatin capsules filled on an automatic capsule filling machine. *Int. J. Pharm.* 1981; 7: 327–334.
43. Small LE. Important formulation requirement for an automatic capsule filling machine and a preliminary study on their influence on in-vitro drug availability. PhD Dissertation, University of Maryland, Baltimore, MD, 1980.
44. Stewart AJ, Grant DWJ, Newton JM. The release of a model low-dose drug (riboflavin) from hard gelatin capsule formulations. *J. Pharm. Pharmacol.* 1979; 31: 1–6.
45. Nakagwa H, Mohri K, Nakashima K, Sugimito I. Effects of particle size of rifampicin and addition of magnesium stearate in release of rifampicin from hard gelatin capsules. *Yakugaku Zasshi* 1980; 100: 1111–1117.
46. Ullah I, Wiley GJ, Agarkar SN. Analysis and simulation of capsule dissolution problem encountered during product scale-up. *Drug Dev. Ind. Pharm.* 1992; 18(8): 895–910.
47. Tattawasart A, Armstrong NA. The formation of lactose plugs for hard shell capsule fills. *Pharm. Dev. Tech.* 1997; 2(4): 335–343.
48. Shah KB, Augsburger LL, Marshall K. An investigation of some factors influencing plug formation and fill weight in a dosing disc type automatic capsule filling machine. *J. Pharm. Sci.* 1986; 75(3): 291–296.
49. Jolliffe IG, Newton JM, Walters JK. Theoretical considerations of the filling of pharmaceutical hard gelatin capsules. *Powder Technol.* 1980; 27: 189–195.
50. Jolliffe IG, Newton JM. An investigation of the relationship between particle size and compression during filling with an instrumented MG2 simulator. *J. Pharm. Pharmacol.* 1982; 34: 415–419.
51. Jolliffe IG, Newton JM. Capsule filling studies using an MG2 production machine. *J. Pharm. Pharmacol.* 1983; 35: 74–78.
52. Shah KB, Augsburger LL, Marshall K. Multiple tamping effects on drug dissolution from capsules filled on a dosing disc type automatic capsule filling machine. *J. Pharm. Sci.* 1987; 76(8): 639–645.
53. Stoyle LE. *Evaluation of the Zanasi Automatic Capsule Machine.* American Pharmacists Association. April 1966, Dallas, TX.
54. Newton JM, Bader F. The prediction of bulk densities of powder mixtures, and its relationship to the filling of hard gelatin capsules. *J. Pharm. Pharmacol.* 1981; 33: 621–626.
55. Davar N, Shah R, Pope DG et al. Rational approach to the selection of a dosing disc on a Hofliger Karg capsule filling machine. *Pharm. Tech.* 1997; 21(2): 32–48.
56. Lerk CF, Lagas M, Fell JT et al. Effect of hydrophilization of hydrophobic drugs on the release rate from capsules. *J. Pharm. Sci.* 1978; 67: 935–939.

57. Guidance for Industry, SUPAC-IR: Immediate release oral solid dosage forms: Scale-up and post approval changes: Manufacturing and controls, in-vitro dissolution testing and in-vivo bioequivalence documentation, FDA, CDER, FDA-November 1995.
58. Hariharan M, Ganorkar LD, Amidon GL et al. Reducing the time to develop and manufacture formulations for first oral dose in humans. *Pharm. Tech.* 2003; October: 68–84.
59. Summary from Edwards D. Micro-dosing equipment fills niche in R&D, clinical trial materials. *Tablets & Capsules* 2009; March: 1–3.
60. Beale D, Woods P, Edwards D. Can automated API dose dispensing be accurate at 10 µg? An analysis of limiting factors. AAPS (poster) Nov. 8–12, 2009.
61. Bi M, Sun CC, Alvarez F et al. The manufacture of low-dose oral solid dosage form to support early clinical studies using an automated micro-filing system. *AAPS Pharm. Sci. Tech.* 2011; 12(1): 88–95.
62. Chopra R, Podczeck F, Newton JM et al. The influence of pellet shape and film coating on the filling of pellets into hard shell capsules. *Eur. J. Pharm. Biopharm.* 2002; 53: 327–333.
63. Rowe RC, York P, Colbourn EA et al. The influence of pellet shape, size and distribution on capsule filling—A preliminary evaluation of three-dimensional computer simulation using a Monte-Carlo technique. *Int. J. Pharm.* 2005; 300: 32–37.
64. Malbous-Jalabert ML, Mishellany-Dutour A, Woda A et al. Particle-size distribution in the food bolus after mastication of natural foods. *Food Quality Preference* 2007; 18: 803–812.
65. Guidance for Industry. Size of beads in drug products labelled for sprinkle, May 2012, US FDA.

9 Plug Formation

Fridrun Podczeck

CONTENTS

INTRODUCTION

The formulation and filling of powders into hard capsules requires knowledge about powder and machine properties and their interrelationships. This chapter focuses on the physics of plug formation under low-compression conditions including mathematical modeling, measurement and testing, as well as practical aspects of plug formation during automated capsule filling.

Despite numerous monographs addressing the differences between tablet and capsule formulations,[1–4] these differences are still not well understood. A powder or granule formulation to be filled into hard capsules is different from that of a tablet, and as a consequence, capsule formulations do not readily make tablets and vice versa, yet all too often pharmaceutical companies attempt to make a tablet formulation, fill it initially into hard capsules to ease the efforts needed for provision in clinical trials, yet the envisaged end product is a tablet. As a result, drug release from capsules is often not ideal, delayed, or even nonlinear owing to excessive amounts of unnecessary excipients; chosen capsule sizes are unjustifiably large; and there is the potential for the drug to fail in clinical trials because of its incorrect formulation. A successful powder formulation for filling into hard capsules has a minimum number and concentration of excipients, and if these are chosen correctly, it will be possible to provide different dose levels with one and the same formulation by choosing matching capsule sizes. In contrast to tabletting that requires the powder/granule formulation to form compacts of sufficient mechanical strength to withstand downstream processing and handling, capsule formulations only require some degree of compressibility (i.e., appropriate volume reduction). Depending on the type of filling machine, the requirements for mechanical strength of the plugs formed are limited or even negligible. As a result, a large proportion of capsule formulations on the market have no diluent at all,[5] and if a diluent is present, then it typically has no binder properties.[6] Due to the filling mechanism involved, powder/granule formulations require slightly higher amounts of lubricant,[5,7] and the type and amount of disintegrants incorporated is also different.[8–10] As will be discussed in more detail below, the porosity of the plugs formed is three to four times that of tablets. The different types and amounts of excipients used in powder formulations for hard capsules make these formulations less suitable for tabletting, but result in optimum and rapid drug release and improved bioavailability,[11] providing an advantage over tablets.

PLUGS VERSUS TABLETS

Geometry

Historically, the invention of the powder-compacted tablet and that of the hard two-piece capsule are only 3 years apart; in 1843, English entrepreneur William Brockedon[12] was granted a patent on the manufacturing of "pills" and "medicinal lozenges" from materials that he described as "in a state of granulation, dust or powder," by forming and solidifying them with pressure in dies, whereas in 1846, the Parisian pharmacist J.C. Lehuby[13] was granted a patent for the development of "medicinal covering," which was cylindrical in shape and composed of two compartments, which when fitted one inside the other formed a little box, into which the medicine was measured. The basic geometry of tablets and two-piece hard capsules has been defined in these patents, and while tablets have evolved in many ways and no longer simply resemble flat disk-shaped entities, the two-piece hard capsule still resembles the original shape and structure, but the manufacture of the shells and the filling machinery have changed dramatically over time.

In order to compare powder plugs that are filled into two-piece hard capsules with tablets, the simplest form of a tablet (i.e., a flat disk-shaped compact) has to be considered. Both the powder plugs and these compacts are cylindrical in shape, and hence their basic dimensions are that of the so-called "right circular cylinder":[14] a circular base of radius r and the cylinder height h. From these two key dimensions, the volume ($V = \pi r^2 h$), the lateral surface ($A_L = 2\pi r h$), and the total surface area ($A_O = 2\pi r(r + h)$) can be determined. The center of gravity is positioned on the axis of symmetry at a distance $x = h/2$ from the base, and the diameter of the base $D = 2r$.

In tablets, the height of the cylinder is usually considerably smaller than the diameter (i.e., $h \ll D$), except for "mini-tablets" (tablets of less than 5 mm in diameter), where $h \approx D$, and OROS Multilayer Osmotic Pump Systems, where the cylinder height of the multilayer tablet can exceed the base diameter considerably ($h > D$; e.g., Concerta XL). The powder plug contained in two-piece hard capsules, however, is always a long cylinder (i.e., $h \gg D$).

There are two main types of capsule-filling machines. Dependent-type machines, such as Auger filling,[15] filling wheel,[16] vibrating metering system,[17] and hand-filling equipment, where the powder is directly filled into the capsule body, typically do not involve the formation of a firm plug. On the other hand, independent-type machines such as dosator-nozzle[18] and tamp-filling machines[19] form a plug from powder/granules first and transfer the plug into the capsule body afterward. Vibration-assisted filling combines the filling of the powder formulation directly into the capsule body with some low-force powder compression of the filling *in situ*, thereby avoiding plug transfer from the forming tools into the capsule body.[20] The development of the independent machines resulted from the industrial demands for increased production of capsules, as new drugs were developed in the 1950s and 1960s. For example, in the 23rd Edition of Martindale's *Extra Pharmacopoeia*,[21] capsules listed in the index were predominantly soft gelatin capsules containing oil-soluble vitamin preparations with only one hard capsule product. By the 26th Edition,[22] the index listed more than 120 hard capsule preparations, several of which were major products. In the 1960s, the output rate from semiautomatic, dependent machines, the most popular of which was the Colton 8, was rated at up to 13,000 h^{-1};[19] automatic H&K Auger filling machines were capable of up to 12,000 h^{-1}.[19] These rates were notably increased by the introduction of the independent filling machines; by 1970, tamp-filling machines and dosator-nozzle machines were capable of capsule-filling production rates of up to 34,000 h^{-1} and 30,000 h^{-1}, respectively.[19] Even these, however, could not compete with rates of maximum tablet production of up to 600,000 h^{-1}.[23] However, the choice of machinery depends not only on the required output but also on the properties of the powders or granules to be filled.[24] In this chapter, only capsule filling with machinery that forms the plugs first and then transfers them is considered.

The cylinder height of the powder plugs is mainly governed by the dimensions of the empty capsule shells that are manufactured to agreed standards, and when using tamp-filling machines, also by the availability of dosing discs of defined height. On an Auger filling machine, uniformity of capsule weight can only be achieved by filling two-piece hard capsules as full as possible.[25] Newton et al.[26] suggested that this should also apply to filling principles where the plug is formed first and then transferred into the capsule body, and they suggested a minimum fill volume of 90% of the capsule body. Filling capsules as full as possible appears more economical as well. Therefore, the plug length (i.e., height of the powder cylinder) is directly related to the capsule size. Assuming a firm, nondeforming powder plug, the maximum plug length can be calculated from the dimensions of the empty capsule shells, considering the final plug length to be the sum of a cylinder fitted into cap and body each and the cylinders having each one hemispherical end. The maximum plug length ranges from 13.2 mm for capsule size 4 to 19.7 mm for capsule size 0 and 21.9 mm for capsule size 0E.[6] The corresponding plug diameters are 4.3 and 6.3 mm for capsule size 4 and 0 as well as 0E, respectively, whereby the plug diameter is less than the inner diameter of the capsule body[2] to permit frictionless transfer from the dosing mechanism into the capsule shell. For standard capsules of sizes 4 to 0, the ratio of cylinder height h ("plug length") to cylinder base diameter D ("plug diameter") hence remains fairly constant ($h/D \approx 3.1$), but for size 0E, it is increased to 3.5.

DENSITY AND POROSITY

Powders and granules for the manufacture of tablets are typically compacted to a degree, requiring extensive deformation beyond the yield strength of the powder, resulting in compact porosities typically less than 20%, and values between 2% and 10% are common.[27] The porosity of powder-filled two-piece hard capsules is at least 30%, and more typically between 40% and 60%.[28] The large porosity of the powder plugs has implications for the formulation of powder/granule-filled capsules, especially in terms of type and amount of disintegrants added. In 1975, Newton and Rowley[29] showed that the use of sodium carboxymethyl starch at concentrations of 10% and above was able to increase drug release of a range of high-dose drugs filled into capsules without addition of filler. In terms of plug disintegration, however, tablet disintegrants acting by exertion of a pressure owing to a rapid increase in volume by swelling, such as sodium carboxymethyl cellulose, sodium carboxymethyl starch, sodium starch glycolate, and cross-linked polyvinyl pyrrolidone, were found to be less effective in capsules because of lack of structure to swell against,[9] and compared to tablets, larger amounts of disintegrants were required.[10] For a rapid disintegration of the powder plug and fast drug dissolution, a higher degree of swelling of the powder plug at reduced plug porosity was required.[8] As larger proportions of the swollen disintegrants can be accommodated in the large pore space of the capsule plugs, it is also possible for the disintegrants to delay drug release because of gel formation, depending on the type of filler. This phenomenon would especially be expected to occur if the filler was a cellulose or starch type. There is also a considerable difference in capsule fill porosity when comparing dependent-type and independent-type machines.[6]

Tablets are formed by use of eccentric, rotary, or centrifugal die filling machines, and this affects the resulting density of the tablets, particularly their density distributions. On an eccentric tablet press, the tabletting force is exerted from the top punch with the bottom punch remaining stationary, whereas in the two other machine types, both top and bottom punch take part in the compression act. As a result, the density of tablets produced on rotary machines is comparatively similar at both tablet faces,[30] and this presumably also applies to tablets manufactured on centrifugal die filling machines. Tablets made on an eccentric tablet press show a density gradient decreasing from the upper face toward the lower tablet face.[31-34] In addition, there is a radial density distribution, with tablets being denser close to the corners and along the circumference owing to increased amounts of powder–metal friction.[31,33]

The formation of plugs is fundamentally different in dosator-nozzle compared to tamp-filling machines.

On a dosator machine, the plug is formed in a single step. Initially, the nozzle dips into the powder bowl. A pre-compression step occurs if the height of the piston in the nozzle is less than the depth of the powder bed,[35] whereas powder compression is achieved by an active downward movement of the piston while the nozzle is in the powder bed.[18] Adjusting the height of the powder bed to be equal to the position of the piston inside the dosing tube, to prevent any pre-compression, enables a compression ratio to be defined as $C(\%) = (h_0 - h)/h_0 \times 100$, with h_0 being the original height of the powder bed and h being the height of the powder bed after compression.[18] Compression can be applied alone or in addition to pre-compression.[36] The pre-compression rate was found to affect the plug density significantly with plug density and pre-compression rate being inversely related.[37]

In industrial-scale tamp-filling machines, the powder plug is formed as a result of several tamping steps (two to five), the most common being five. During indexing of the dosing disc, the dosing bores are filled with powder from the powder bed, which covers it. The powder is then compressed by the tamping pins to form a plug segment. With each successive indexing step, more powder enters the dosing bores. This cycle is repeated up to five times. Additionally, powder might also be pushed into the dosing bores by the tamping fingers, but it has been shown that the majority of powder forming the plug enters the dosing bores during the indexing step.[38] The plug segments formed during each tamping event do not have the same height; that is, the final plug is not equally divided into several segments of similar height and density. On the contrary, the lowest segment, which is formed first, is usually the longest segment, and each further segment is reduced in height. To this end, Davar et al.[39] developed a spreadsheet to calculate the amount of powder entering the disc cavity at each indexing step. The authors used such calculations to predict the required dosing disc height for a given target plug weight and overall plug density using five tamping steps. Their results showed that approximately 95% of the total plug weight had already been achieved within three tamps, and the fifth tamping event added less than 1% to the final plug weight. This was also observed experimentally.[40] Pore size distribution data obtained on plugs made from a mixture of hydrochlorothiazide, anhydrous lactose, and magnesium stearate indicated that, in some cases, the maximum plug density was already achieved after two tamps.[41] The successive building of the plug in five steps was found to result in lower fill weight variability because of reduced sensitivity to powder flow problems, when compared to dosator-nozzle filling.[42] The amount of tamping applied can be quantified by the cumulative tamping distance, that is, the sum of the penetration distances of the pins into the dosing disk bores (in millimeters) achieved over five tamping events.[38] Typically, at station 1, the pins penetrate the dosing disk bores to a maximum degree, and at each further station, the penetration is reduced; pins at tamping station 5 do not normally penetrate the dosing bores but are set flush with the upper surface of the dosing disk when at their lowest position. It was found that for cumulative tamping distances between zero and approximately 18 mm, the plug density achieved increased steadily with increase in cumulative tamping distance. Cumulative tamping distances above 18 mm did not result in further densification.[43] The In-Cap benchtop capsule-filling machine, which uses only four tamping stations, required a very different pin setting from that employed in industrial-scale machines using five tamping stations when filling size 0 and 00 capsules, in order to produce sufficient plug weights and densities and low variability in fill weight.[44] This might be the result of the construction of the dosing mechanism, which restricts the depth of insertion of the pins when using larger capsule sizes.

The low-compression force exerted on a powder bed in capsule filling, when using independent machines, always comes from above, similar to an eccentric tablet press, and should hence result in a similar vertical density distribution throughout the powder plug. The theoretical radial density distribution of powder plugs has been studied in more depth on small packed powder columns employing a gamma-ray attenuation technique,[45] which is able to detect small local variations in packing porosity at an accuracy of ±0.5%. The velocity and intensity of deposition were found to be the most important factors affecting the overall porosity of the powder plugs. The authors also observed that plugs typically were least porous in the center, and the porosity increased radially toward the outer diameter. This was confirmed by Wang et al.[46] and contributed to wall effects such as particle–wall friction.[47] When the powder plugs were formed in a layer-by-layer fashion, the highest degree of uniformity was found; that is, the difference between local minimum and maximum porosity was only between 3% and 5%, whereas for continuous plug formation, this difference was at least 5% and could reach up to 13%.[48] This implies that powder plugs produced in five indexing steps on tamp-filling machines are more homogeneous in terms of plug porosity than plugs formed on dosator-nozzle machines. Vibratory consolidation of powder beds, which could occur owing to machine vibrations during capsule filling, has been studied and was found to be affected by particle size and shape. Vertical vibration was more effective in packing powder beds quickly to minimum uniform porosity than horizontal vibration,[49] and the most effective vibration conditions were characterized by amplitudes similar to the modal size of the particles in the powder bed.[50] Tamp-filling machines have vertical vibrations because of the up-and-down movement of the tamping rig holding the tamping pins, and dosator-nozzle machines are more prone to horizontal vibrations because of the movement of the turret holding the nozzles. The filling of powder formulations might hence be affected by the machine vibrations during production, with tamp-filling machines reaching a constant low-porosity powder bed more quickly. Using a fine fraction of lactose monohydrate with a particle size between 18 and 27 μm and an angle of repose of 51.6°, Woodhead[51] prepared powder beds by densifying them by vertical vibration to maximum bulk density before capsule filling with a dosator-nozzle simulator. For a sample size of 50 capsules, the coefficient of fill weight variation was significantly smaller (3.62%) compared with that achieved using a poured powder bed (7.26%). Llusa et al.[52] studied the vibrations of a dosator-nozzle filling machine using laser Doppler vibrometry. They found that at very high filling speeds, when filling various grades of microcrystalline cellulose, vibrations of the powder bowl resulted in an increase in the powder bed density and a statistically significantly higher capsule fill weight. The only exception was Avicel 301, which was the grade with the smallest particle size and consequently poor flow properties. This indicates that the effect of vibrations of the powder bowl on powder bed densification and capsule fill weight depends on the flow properties of the powders. Particle size-related effects were also observed on a vibratory sieve-chute system developed for micro-dosing of powders into two-piece hard capsules.[53] Finer powders required higher amplitudes and frequencies for powder flow and correct dosing to take place. Using a combination of Discrete Element Method (DEM) and computational fluid dynamics, Guo et al.[54] demonstrated that filling of small dies from moving powder hoppers can result in particle segregation and hence in inhomogeneous powder plugs, especially if the particles of the mixture had different material densities or were different in size and/or shape. Lighter particles were found to deposit at the leading side of the dies and to migrate to the top of the die. This will result in horizontal and vertical inhomogeneities in density of powder plugs. In capsule-filling machines, the powder hopper is usually stationary, but it is conceivable that during indexing of the dosing disk in a tamp-filling machine, similar segregation could occur.

When different size fractions of granules, ranging from 150–300 to 710–1400 µm, were filled on a dosator-nozzle machine, it was found that the plugs formed were always denser than the maximum bulk ("tapped") density of the granules. However, when the same granule formulations were filled on a tamp-filling machine, for the smallest size fraction (150–300 µm), a plug density as large as the maximum bulk density could not be achieved with the settings employed.[55] The authors concluded that in situations where a low plug density was a prerequisite for drug dissolution and bioavailability, the use of a tamp-filling machine appeared more suitable, but in cases were a greater extent of compression was necessary, for example, to fill large-dose drugs or to be able to use a smaller capsule size, a dosator-nozzle filling machine would be the better option.

Using a benchtop powder plug tester, Jones[6] demonstrated that the plug density increased with an increase in mixing time, when 1% magnesium stearate had been added to either microcrystalline cellulose or pregelatinized starch. This has practical significance; in tamp-filling machines, the dosing disc determines the length of the powder plugs formed, and in dosator-nozzle machines, the plug length is controlled by the piston setting and the bed height in the powder hopper. During the capsule-filling process, the powder in the hopper is subjected to constant movement and hence further mixing occurs, which could result in an increased density of the plugs formed and consequently in an increase in capsule fill weight with time.

A two-phase relationship between a powder densification ratio obtained through pre-compression, ρ_r (defined as ratio between powder material density and density of the powder plug), and a pre-compression ratio P_r ($P_r = (H - L)/L$, where H is the height of the powder bed and L is the length of the dosing tube from its opening to the piston) was reported when filling excipients such as microcrystalline cellulose, lactose monohydrate, and corn starch on a dosator-nozzle machine.[56] When plotting ρ_r as a function of $\log_{10}P_r$, it was observed that, initially, an increase in the degree of pre-compression resulted in a rapid increase in plug density, but at a powder densification ratio close to the maximum bulk ("tapped") density, a sharp kink in this relationship was seen and pre-compression settings aiming for plug densities above the maximum bulk density resulted in a significantly reduced rate of increase in plug density. The minimum coefficient of variation in capsule fill weight was observed for $P_r = 1$, which refers to the length of a formed plug that is 50% shorter than the height of the powder bed, whereby the plug density achieved was 20–30% above the maximum bulk density. It is not clear from the paper whether the capsule-filling experiments had been undertaken using only pre-compression, or whether an additional compression force had been applied; Figure 9.1 would suggest the use of an additional compression force, but no values have been stated in the text.

For capsules that are to be filled at a plug density matching the maximum bulk ("tapped") density of the powder, it is possible to predict the maximum bulk density and hence also the capsule fill weight for mainly binary powder mixtures from the volume fractions and maximum bulk densities of the individual powders.[57] When filling mixtures of granulated powdered cellulose and magnesium stearate on a tamp-filling machine at a cumulative tamping distance of zero, that is, all pins were set to be flush with the upper surface of the dosing disc when at their lowest position during tamping, it was possible to predict the plug density and fill weight of the capsules from Carr's compressibility index[58] and the maximum bulk density of the mixtures.[59] The decrease in one and the simultaneous increase in the other bulk property with increasing magnesium stearate concentration resulted in the plug density to go through a local minimum at 0.4% magnesium stearate. Podczeck and Newton[60] reported that the maximum plug density that can be achieved on a tamp-filling machine is inversely related to the angle of internal flow,[61] indicating that during the downward movement of the tamping pins inside the dosing disk bores, particle slippage and particle rearrangement are hindered by interparticulate friction.

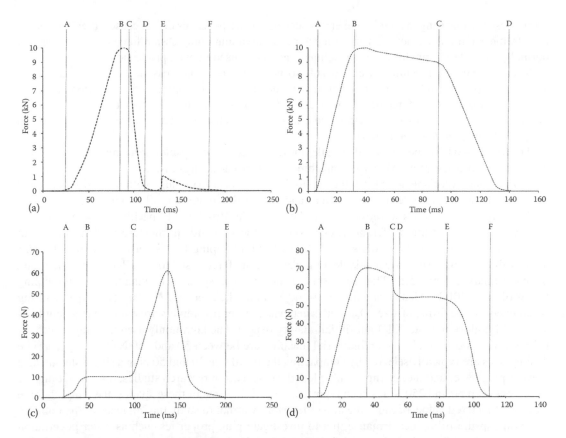

FIGURE 9.1 (a) Schematic drawing of a force–time profile that would be obtained on an eccentric tablet press, based on time calculations for a running speed of 43.6 rpm[66] and general force profiles as described by Jones.[113] (b) Schematic drawing of a force–time profile that would be obtained on the upper punch of a Fette P2 rotary tablet machine, based on measurements on pregelatinized starch.[117] (c) Schematic drawing of the force–time profile that would be obtained on a dosator nozzle capsule-filling machine, based on traces obtained for lubricated microcrystalline cellulose.[35,83] (d) Schematic drawing of the force–time profile that would be obtained on a tamp-filling machine,[68] based on traces obtained using a pneumatic tamping head, installed at tamping station 3, for pregelatinized starch.[38]

Compression Pressure Used in Development and Manufacture

As mentioned above, during tabletting, the degree of densification of the powders is much more extensive than that achieved in capsule filling. The forces that can be applied to powders using, for example, a rotary tablet machine, are only restricted by the capacity of the load frame. For example, the Fette P2 rotary tabletting machine was able to withstand compression forces up to 35 kN,[62] which translates into a theoretically possible maximum tabletting pressure of 1.2 GPa for a 6-mm punch (i.e., the plug diameter of a size 2 capsule). More recent rotary machines are able to withstand 60–80 kN of force. The reason that tabletting machines are built to withstand these high maximum compression forces is that tablet dimensions are normally larger than the diameter of a capsule plug; typical tablet dimensions are, for example, a diameter of 10 or 12 mm for round circular tablets, or 15 mm × 5 mm for capsule-shaped tablets. This is equivalent theoretically to maximum tabletting pressures of 880, 620, and 400 MPa, respectively, assuming a maximum compression force of 70 kN. The maximum compression forces and related tabletting pressures used in the mass production of tablets are, however, lower (10–15 kN;[63] 100–250 MPa[64]), depending on size and shape of the tablets, in order to produce tablets with adequate mechanical strength and disintegration as well as drug dissolution properties, and ensuring that tabletting errors such as double-pressings do not cause a breakage of the load frame.[65] On an eccentric tabletting machine, a maximum compression force of 15 kN was not normally exceeded,[66] but this type of machine is no longer used in mass production.

Rotary tabletting machines are also able to provide a pre-compression step, for example, to allow entrapped air to be vented and hence to reduce the risk of capping and lamination. The pre-compression pressure is typically set between 10% and 20% of the final tabletting pressure. The pre-compression step will also lengthen the time over which the compression pressure is exerted on the powder or granule formulation.[67]

The force used to fill powders and granules into two-piece hard capsules on a tamp-filling machine has changed over the years. Very early machines used strong springs inside the tamping heads, and these machines were able to exert forces up to 500 N to form firm plugs with defined mechanical strengths. However, in order to reduce wear and tear of the motor and all moving machine parts, in the early 90s, machines were redesigned. For example, Bosch GKF machines now provide the user with a choice of four different types of springs; the standard spring starts to deflect at about 55 N and allows filling of capsule sizes 2, 1, and 0 with tamping forces between 90 and 100 N.[38] Two further sets of springs are available for lower tamping forces used for smaller capsule sizes and filling of inhalation powders. The fourth set is a "heavy duty" spring achieving theoretical tamping forces of up to 200 N,[68] but in practice, 150–160 N cannot be exceeded.[38,43,68,69] This type of spring is intended for the filling of size 00 capsules and when larger fill weights are required (e.g., antibiotics and high-dose non-steroidal anti-inflammatory drugs). The commonly used tamping forces for filling powders or granules on an industrial machine are between 50 and 150 N.[63] The appropriate dosing discs are typically selected by compacting the powder at 20 and 50 N in a single step using a powder plug tester and measuring the plug length achieved.[6] In research studies, the use of tamping forces between 50 and 250 N has been reported.[38–41,70–76] In some of these studies, the tamping force was kept to a fixed value, because the aim of the work was not to study the influence of the tamping force on capsule-filling performance, but to investigate plug properties such as water penetration rates into hydrophilic polymer matrix plugs and drug release (200 N),[70] or to study drug dissolution under defined conditions.[75] Other studies aimed to investigate tamping forces per se; for example, Shah et al.,[40] reporting on anhydrous lactose lubricated with 0.5% magnesium stearate, found that tamping forces were low at tamping station 1, at their maximum at station 2, and were similar at tamping stations 3 and 4, but slightly reduced and were lowest at station 5. Podczeck[74] found that the tamping force recorded depended on the cumulative tamping distance and was material dependent. For pregelatinized starch, the highest tamping force was recorded at station 3, and at this station, a change in cumulative tamping distance also resulted in a maximum change in tamping force. For microcrystalline cellulose, however, the maximum force and the steepest slope of the force as a function of cumulative tamping distance were observed at station 4.

In dosator-nozzle machines, the force achieved depends on a number of factors such as type of powder or granules, powder bed height and density, pre-compression and compression settings, and strength of the overload spring. In intermittent dosator-nozzle machines, the linear up and down movement of the nozzles makes the process of force application similar to that achieved on an eccentric tabletting machine. In rotary-type dosator-nozzle machines, the movement of the turret and hence the compaction cycle appears to be more similar to a rotary tabletting machine, yet the force exerted on the powder bed is only from above, as in eccentric tabletting machines. Extensive research on plug formation using dosator-nozzles has been undertaken using instrumented production machines as well as machine simulators; instrumentations and simulators used have been reviewed by Armstrong.[77] Britten et al.[37] studied pregelatinized starch and lactose monohydrate using precompression pressures between 3 and 4.4 MPa alone or in combination with an additional compression pressure to reach either a constant plug length (displacement mode) or the maximum possible compression pressure (compression pressure mode). In displacement mode, the pressures applied were between 4.6 and 6 MPa, whereas in compression mode, the maximum pressures achieved were between 8.7 and 8.8 MPa. The findings of their research will be further discussed in the "Rates of

Compression and Ejection" section. The diameter of the dosator tube used was 6 mm.[78] Compression pressures as high as 50 MPa were reported by Tan and Newton[79] using an unlubricated size 1 nozzle in a rotary nozzle filling-simulator. Values between 5 and 8 MPa were observed by Jolliffe and Newton[80] with the same simulator using a size 3 nozzle and various size fractions of unlubricated lactose monohydrate. The surface finish and cleanliness of the nozzles have an important influence on the compression pressures[79,80] because of the interaction between powder and metal surfaces. Pre-compression forces between 40 and 140 N were observed by Hauer et al.[81] using lactose monohydrate of two different size fractions and their mixtures, and four different powder bed heights between 30 and 50 mm and a dosing tube length between 10 and 16 mm. They found that the pre-compression forces increased with an increase in the powder bed height, but decreased with an increase in the dosing tube length. When the powder bed height remains constant and the volume in the dosing tube increases with a change in piston setting, the powder is compressed less and the pre-compression force will drop. These authors also found that for all machine settings the use of microcrystalline cellulose always resulted in the lowest pre-compression force and hence microcrystalline cellulose was classed as "easily compressible."[81] In other reports, overall achieved compression forces of, for example, 5–350 N,[82] 126–159 N,[35] 35–213 N,[7] 137 N,[83] 213 N,[84] 222 N,[10] and 50–100 N[85] are quoted, often presented as kg-force values, which, for ease of comparison, have been converted into N by multiplying them by the gravitational constant (9.81 m s^{-2}). Similar to reports on tamp-filling machines, some workers have made use of the ability to control the compression forces applied by the piston in order to study problems such as the mechanical strength of plugs[84,85] or drug dissolution.[8–10] Small and Augsburger[35] compared the traces obtained when filling lubricated microcrystalline cellulose, lactose monohydrate, pregelatinized starch, and dibasic calcium phosphate dihydrate. They could clearly distinguish between the forces achieved by pre-compression and compression. Differences in the forces between materials were attributed to differences in the initial powder packing density and also to differences in the ability of the materials to reduce their volume under load. When filling unlubricated pregelatinized starch at various compression settings and unlubricated microcrystalline cellulose and lactose monohydrate at the lowest compression setting, a residual force attributed to elastic rebound against the piston was detected.

It can be concluded that the maximum achieved total force, that is, the resistance of the powder against pre-compression and compression, is fairly similar in dosator-nozzle and tamp-filling machines. This force is approximately 1–2% of the compaction force used in tabletting machines, and the comparative compression pressures range between 5% and 10% of those used in tabletting. As a result, the powder plugs are soft and of substantially higher porosity, as discussed above.

AXIAL FORCE TRANSMISSION RATIO

In tabletting, especially when using eccentric machines or compaction simulators, the stress transmission from the upper punch to the lower punch is used to assess the state of lubrication and influence of powder–die wall friction on the densification of powders. To this end, Nelson et al.[86] defined the axial force transmission ratio R as the ratio of maximum force at the lower punch (F_L) to the maximum upper punch force (F_U); ($R = F_L/F_U$). (This equation can be rewritten using the pressure equivalents P_L and P_U.) Under conditions of uniaxial compression, perfect lubrication would result in total axial force transmission, that is, $R = 1$, and R values vary with the type of lubricant and its concentration within the compact. The nature of the powder formulation, the tablet weight (effectively the dimensions for conditions of uniform material density and packing), and the type of die used all affect the value of R according to Sheinhartz et al.[87] Toor and Eagleton[88] and Hölzer and Sjögren[89] found the value of R to vary with the applied compaction force, while Lewis and Shotton,[90] using a variety of materials, noted both increased and decreased R values upon raising the "mean" compaction pressure P_M, whereby P_M had been defined as $P_M = 0.5(P_U + P_L)$.

Hölzer and Sjögren[91] demonstrated that effective use of R values to study friction and lubrication requires both constant tablet dimensions and a constant maximum compaction force, because the value of R is pressure dependent even for a constant tablet height. Increased axial pressure transmission usually results from an increase in the applied pressure or a decrease of the compaction height-to-diameter ratio.[89]

Strickland et al.[92] constructed R values versus admixed lubricant concentration curves and suggested a functional relationship of "Langmuir type" at low lubricant concentrations by assuming that the reduction in frictional force corresponds to the degree of lubricant cover of the die wall. Little increase in the values of R was obtained beyond a 1% lubricant level. After sectioning and staining compacts, the authors concluded that lubricants such as magnesium stearate and graphite coat the base material granules (starch paste granules of sulfathiazole, sodium bicarbonate, or acetyl salicylic acid) without penetrating their interior. Wolff et al.[93] reported entrapment of lubricant particles within the surface features of granules, suggesting different types of behavior for different lubricants.

Strickland et al.[94] divided lubricants into two groups, that is, boundary lubricants and hydrodynamic lubricants, and determined their R values for two granule formulations (i.e., starch paste granules of sulfathiazole and sodium bicarbonate). More than 70 different lubricants were tested. They concluded that the general theories of solid–solid lubrication[95] are applicable to the tabletting process. Excellent lubricity was defined as having an R value above 0.9 (the unlubricated controls had R values of 0.67). Lewis and Shotton[96] found that with some tabletting formulations, the axial force transmission ratio was insufficiently sensitive to distinguish between similar lubricants and that the best lubricants were those with the lowest melting point.

In capsule filling, R values cannot be obtained directly, because there is no "lower" punch or support that can be instrumented. However, R values have been obtained under low-force compression conditions similar to the capsule-filling process using compaction simulators. Heda et al.[97] used an Abacus compaction simulator, fitted with a specially designed longer die and 5.71 mm tooling equivalent to a size 1 capsule. The force was applied as single-ended saw-tooth waveform at constant speeds of 1, 10, and 100 mm s^{-1}. The speed of 100 mm s^{-1} exceeds the speed of a tamping pin in a GKF 330 tamp-filling machine slightly[68] and is three times the piston velocity measured on a Zanasi LZ-64 intermittent dosator-nozzle filling machine.[83] Heda et al.[97] produced plugs of different lengths (4, 8, and 12 mm) from a coarse-grade microcrystalline cellulose, anhydrous lactose, and pregelatinized starch and determined the axial force transmission ratio R. As expected, the values for R increased with a decrease in plug length, but compared to tablet formation, the values did not reach "acceptable" magnitudes, with $R = 0.77$ being the highest value found (microcrystalline cellulose at 4 mm plug length). For the ductile powders, microcrystalline cellulose, and pregelatinized starch, the R values decreased in general when the compression speed is increased from 1 to 10 mm s^{-1}. For microcrystalline cellulose, the R value remained constant when changing from 10 to 100 mm s^{-1}, except for the smallest plug length, where the R value increased significantly. For pregelatinized starch, the change from 10 to 100 mm s^{-1} resulted in an increase in R value at 12 and 8 mm plug length. For anhydrous lactose, no influence of compression speed was detected, and the authors attributed this to the ability of the powder to attain a relatively higher packing density upon die filling owing to better flow properties. Guo et al.[71] used a similar methodology to compare different types of microcrystalline and silicified microcrystalline cellulose, anhydrous lactose, and pregelatinized starch. The plug lengths were set to 6, 8, and 12 mm, and only two compression speeds were used (1 and 50 mm s^{-1}). In general, the R values decreased with an increase in plug length, and as before, the R values did not reach levels seen in tabletting (0.43–0.78). At plug lengths of 8 and 12 mm, most R values were found to decrease with an increase in compression speed, but for the 6-mm plugs, the dependence on compression speed was more varied. The authors[71] stated that they would have expected the R values to increase with compression speed, because the dynamic coefficient of friction between two bodies in motion relative to each other should decrease with an increase in sliding velocity. They attributed the deviations found to differences in time needed for particle packing and rearrangement, particle size distribution, particle shape and surface roughness, and particle deformation properties, which were different for the various materials studied.

When studying the low-compression properties of commercially available *Hypericum perforatum* extracts, Kopleman et al.[73] found that the axial force transmission ratio R decreased significantly when increasing the plug lengths at both 50 and 150 N maximum compression force as a result of loss of force attributed to plug-die wall friction. They found that overall the punch speed did not affect the R values. As the R values were again comparatively low (0.2–0.7), they suggested that addition of a die wall lubricant such as magnesium stearate would be beneficial.

Shaxby and Evans[98] reported that when applying a downward force to the top of a column of sand confined into a tube, it was not fully transmitted to the bottom if the height of the column exceeded its diameter. The force decay was described as approximately exponential:

$$R = \frac{F_L}{F_U} = e^{-\frac{4hK_m}{d}},$$ (9.1)

where F_L and F_U are as defined earlier, h and d are the final powder column height (i.e., plug length) and diameter, respectively, and K_m is a material constant related to the coefficient of friction between the wall of the tube and the powder. In developing this equation, Shaxby and Evans[98] made the assumption that the vertical (axial) pressure applied is uniform across the diameter of the powder column at any point along its length and that the frictional force per unit area at the outer vertical surface of the column at a given depth is given by the product of the coefficient of friction and the horizontal (radial) pressure acting on the tube wall at that position. They also pointed out that the force transmitted is a function not only of the length of the powder column but also of the initial packing of the powder bed and one should not expect that variations in the packing state will be reflected in a measurable change in powder density, because powders behave in line with continuum theory, that is, are highly incompressible.

A number of equations have been developed from that of Shaxby and Evans,[98] notably those by Spencer et al.[99] and by Toor and Eagleton.[88] Spencer et al.[99] studied powders confined into a tube and compressed by a piston. Under the assumption that the powder bed remained static and interparticulate friction was absent, they considered force transmission through the compact to be essentially hydrostatic, with a constant density of particle point contacts. The authors related the die wall friction coefficient, μ_d, to the initial powder column height h_0, the column diameter d, and the axial force transmission ratio R:

$$R = \frac{F_L}{F_U} = e^{-\frac{4\mu_d h_0}{d}}.$$ (9.2)

Toor and Eagleton[88] found deviations from this equation owing to the dependence of R on the axial pressure applied and the influence of particle size on the relationship. They introduced a correction factor α to take account of the structural rigidity of the particle bed. The value of α was defined as the ratio of radial to axial force on any particle situated at the interface to the tube wall. Assuming α to be constant, their equation took the form of

$$R = \frac{F_L}{F_U} = e^{-\frac{4\mu_d \alpha h_0}{d}}.$$ (9.3)

The values of μ_d were influenced by the amount of lubricant used and the previous history of the die in terms of duration of use and cleaning. Small amounts of lubricant (0.01–0.2%) were found to reduce the value of R, but a further increase in lubrication increased the axial force transmission ratio. Similarly, the value of μ_d increased initially and then decreased with increased amount of lubrication. Maximum R and minimum μ_d values were obtained after 8–10 successive compactions of polystyrene particles lubricated with zinc stearate powder without cleaning of the tooling. It was suggested that a gradual coating of the die wall with lubricant had occurred, reducing die wall friction.[88]

Heda et al.[97] fitted their compression data to Equation 9.1 and found that their data could be fitted fully. The proposed exponential reduction in force along the length of the powder plug was found for all three powders studied (coarse-grade microcrystalline cellulose, anhydrous lactose, and pregelatinized starch). The slopes for pregelatinized starch and anhydrous lactose were almost identical, whereas that for microcrystalline cellulose was less steep. This could be the result of a different particle size of microcrystalline cellulose, but the actual values were not reported and the authors did not discuss the outcome of their model fitting procedure further. Kopleman et al.[73] also reported excellent fit of their data, obtained with herbal extracts, to Equation 9.1. Guo et al.[71] also used Equation 9.1, but their data from microcrystalline and silicified microcrystalline cellulose, anhydrous lactose, and pregelatinized starch did not fit the model as well as described by Heda et al.,[97] and they concluded that the less favorable outcome was the result of differences in the maximum compression force used (250 N instead of 500 N), the use of a lower axial force, and their data maybe being more sensitive to small variations in the initial bulk density of the powders when filled into the die, which agrees with the remarks on the limitations of Equation 9.1 made by Shaxby and Evans.[98]

EJECTION FORCES

In the development of tablet formulations, the recording of ejection forces is very important, as it permits optimization of lubricant concentrations in the formulation. Compaction simulators are preferred for this work because of the more accurate instrumentation, but the use of piezo-electric load washers mounted directly on the lower punch of a rotary machine was reported to produce equally high-resolution force measurements with the advantage of having the data recorded on a production machine.[100] This is important because ejection forces can increase with running time of the machine owing to buildup of materials around the punch tip and at the die walls.[101] The maximum ejection force F_e and the pressure equivalent P_e will hence be modified by frictional conditions at the die wall and by the magnitude of the residual radial pressure across the compact-die interface. A linear relationship between the ejection force F_e and the ratio between loss of axial force to the die wall during the final stage of the tablet formation F_d ($F_d = F_U - F_L$) and the force recorded at the lower punch F_L was reported by Nelson et al.,[86] who also found a linear dependency of F_e on the apparent area of compact-die contact A_a, estimated from the tablet thickness. Train[102] related the maximum ejection force to the maximum compaction pressure exerted from the upper punch (P_U) via a power law equation ($F_e = c(P_U A_a)^n$). The constant c is related to the surface condition of the die wall and the power law constant n is related to the physical character of the compacted material. Lewis and Shotton[90] confirmed that this relationship was obeyed by crystalline materials. They also found that some materials exhibited an increase in value of F_e with a decrease in particle size and that this effect was eliminated by lubrication. They concluded that the effect of a lubricant on die wall friction depends on the deformation properties of the crystalline powders to be compacted.

A reduction in the value of F_e can be interpreted as an indication of lubricant efficiency, and lubricants have been assessed in this way.[94,96,103] The effectiveness of metallic stearates as boundary lubricants was shown to vary with the stearic acid content using this type of data.[104] Juslin and Krogerus[105,106] compared a range of admixed lubricants by measuring the value of F_e on an eccentric tablet press. In one experiment, the punches and die were cleaned between successive compactions, and in a second experiment, the compaction tooling was left unclean after the initial preparation. A significant difference between the two protocols was observed, with the average maximum upper punch force and ejection force values increasing when repetitive cleaning was omitted. Successive compactions exhibited decreasing values of F_e, which the authors interpreted as evidence for an accumulation of lubricant at the die wall, increasing the ratio of lubricated to unlubricated die wall contact. The ejection force was found to be dependent on the melting points of the organic lubricants, and this physical parameter was taken to represent indirectly the ability to form and retain a coherent film of lubricant at the die wall.

For capsule filling, to date, instrumentations to determine an ejection force have mainly been reported for dosator-nozzle machines, for example, by Cole and May,[107] Small and Augsburger,[35] Mehta and Augsburger,[83] Botzolakis et al.,[10] Jolliffe et al.,[36] and Hauer et al.,[81] typically with strain gauges mounted on opposing sides of the dosator piston shank and using intermittent motion machines to enable wiring of the instrumentation. Shah et al.[108] described the instrumentation of a tamp-filling machine with two tamping pins equipped with strain gauges, one kept at the ejection station to monitor plug ejection forces.

The ejection force of unlubricated microcrystalline cellulose was found to be approximately half of that of unlubricated pregelatinized starch.[35] For unlubricated pregelatinized starch, Small and Augsburger[7] reported that the ejection force slightly decreased when the filling setting was changed from using pre-compression force alone to using an additional small amount of compression force. A further increase in the compression force resulted in an increase in ejection force. The ejection force was also related to the length of the plugs produced, increasing with an increase in plug length, similar to the observations made by Nelson et al.[86] with respect to tablet thickness. When adding 0.005% magnesium stearate, the ejection force was greatly reduced. At lower compression forces, the effect of plug length on the ejection force was less pronounced, but at higher compression forces, the effect was again distinct, similar to that seen using unlubricated powder. The ejection forces were significantly higher for a powder bed height of 50 mm compared to that of 30 mm, and the authors stated that the influence of the powder bed height on ejection forces was greater than the influence of the plug length. Similar findings were made for microcrystalline cellulose and anhydrous lactose lubricated with 0.2% magnesium stearate, but the effect of plug length at the 50-mm powder bed setting was less pronounced with microcrystalline cellulose. They concluded that if uniform fill weights can be achieved at lower powder bed heights and the required compensatory increase in piston height does not negate this effect, the decrease in powder bed height might provide a means of reducing the plug ejection forces without the need for an increase in lubricant concentration. For pregelatinized starch, it was also observed that a magnesium stearate level of 0.1% resulted in the lowest ejection forces, and a similar reduction was observed for microcrystalline cellulose lubricated with 0.5% magnesium stearate. A minimum amount of 1% of magnesium stearate was required to lower the ejection forces for anhydrous lactose. The alternative lubricants magnesium dodecyl sulfate and stearic acid required comparative lubricant levels of 3% and 1%, respectively, to reduce the ejection force of anhydrous lactose to values achieved with the optimum magnesium stearate concentration. When using 0.1% of stearic acid with microcrystalline cellulose and 0.1% of stearic acid or magnesium dodecyl sulfate with pregelatinized starch, the ejection forces were only marginally larger than those obtained with magnesium stearate, but when using 0.1% of magnesium dodecyl sulfate with microcrystalline cellulose, adequate reduction of the ejection forces was not achieved, presumably because of the higher specific surface area of this powder.

For various size fractions of unlubricated lactose monohydrate filled with an instrumented mG2 simulator and size 1 nozzle, Jolliffe and Newton[80] reported ejection stresses between 0.4 and 4 MPa. The ejection stresses increased with an increase in particle size and doubled (larger size fractions) or trebled (smaller size fractions) when an initially clean nozzle received a powder coating during filling. For pregelatinized starch filled with the same simulator but a size 3 nozzle, Tan and Newton[79] found that ejection stresses dropped from 5 MPa to just above 1 MPa above a threshold particle size of 23 µm, whereas for microcrystalline cellulose, the ejection stresses decrease from 3 to 0.5 MPa with an increase in particle size from 11 to 23 µm.

Hauer et al.[81] also reported that with anhydrous lactose, the ejection force increased with an increase in powder bed height and an increase in the length of the dosing tube owing to higher piston position, and that in general, because of the stickiness of this powder, ejection forces were rather large. With microcrystalline cellulose, they observed for a powder bed height between 40 and 50 mm and a piston height of 14 and 16 mm that the ejection force increased steeply. Hauer et al.[109] also found that for anhydrous lactose and lactose monohydrate, stickiness and ejection forces could be significantly reduced with the addition of 0.5% magnesium stearate, and its addition reduced the effect of the piston height on the ejection force. A further increase in the magnesium stearate concentration did not further reduce the ejection forces but resulted in insufficient powder arching and loss of powder from the dosator-nozzle during plug transfer. These authors also investigated the addition of Precirol (a mixture of mono-, di-, and triglycerides of palmitic and stearic acid), stearic acid, and talcum powder on the ejection force of lactose monohydrate plugs. Only Precirol at concentrations between 1% and 2% was deemed a useful alternative to magnesium stearate, especially as this lubricant did not affect the dissolution properties of a model drug (anhydrous caffeine).

Guo and Augsburger[85] likewise pointed out that a reduction in the ejection force is not only a sign for reduced powder plug-wall friction but could also be due to insufficient plug formation. When filling different types of microcrystalline and silicified microcrystalline cellulose on an instrumented intermittent dosator-nozzle machine in comparison to anhydrous lactose and pregelatinized starch, they confirmed that ejection forces generally increase with an increase in compression force. They also found that anhydrous lactose required substantially more magnesium stearate to lower the ejection forces than the other powders tested, but that the ejection resistance decreased more rapidly once a threshold concentration of lubricant had been reached. More lubricant was also required for powders with smaller median particle size because of the larger surface area to be covered. When hydrophilic sodium stearyl fumarate was used as lubricant, for pregelatinized starch and an experimental grade of silicified microcrystalline cellulose, the ejection force was reduced more than when using the same concentration of magnesium stearate. For these two powders, sodium stearyl fumarate was deemed to be more effective in reducing the ejection force than magnesium stearate, but for the majority of powders at equal concentrations, the former was less effective than the latter.

Heda et al.[72] observed that ejection forces were higher for smaller particle sizes because of their greater specific surface area and more particle-dosator-nozzle wall contact points. When filling binary powder mixtures of anhydrous lactose, coarse-grade microcrystalline cellulose, pregelatinized starch, and ascorbic acid on both an instrumented dosator-nozzle and an instrumented tamp-filling machine, Heda et al.[72] were able to compare directly the ejection forces on both types of filling mechanism. In general, the ejection forces increased with an increase in the applied compression force. When using an intermittent dosator-nozzle machine, the ejection forces decreased with increasing concentrations of magnesium stearate of 0.25%, 0.5%, and 1%. However, when filling the same formulations on the tamp-filling machine, the ejection force remained constant. Based on findings reported by Ullah et al.[110] and Desai et al.,[111] Heda et al.[72] concluded that this was attributed to the presence of an Auger screw-feeder, which supposedly led to increased mixing of the lubricant and hydrophobic film formation, which, in turn, masked the influence of increasing concentrations of magnesium stearate on ejection forces. The absolute values of the ejection forces for unlubricated single powders as well as lubricated binary powder mixtures were always higher on the dosator-nozzle machine. This was attributed to differences in the elastic recovery of the plugs before ejection. As discussed by Britten et al.,[37] a larger amount of elastic recovery in axial direction is thought to lower the residual radial forces acting on the walls of a confined space such as a dosator-nozzle or dosing-disk bore, thereby reducing the ejection force, and the findings by Heda et al.[72] therefore imply that elastic recovery of plugs in axial direction is larger in tamp-filling machines compared to dosator-nozzle machines.

RATES OF COMPRESSION AND EJECTION

The initial and final powder bulk density achieved are important for a low coefficient of fill weight variability, but the rate with which the powder is densified has also been identified as a major factor in successful capsule filling and plug formation.[112] In order to compare rates of compression and ejection between tabletting and capsule-filling machines, it is necessary to compare force–time profiles obtained on these different machines and to parameterize them.

Figure 9.1a shows a schematic drawing of a force–time profile that would be obtained on an eccentric tablet press. In order to draw this graph, it was assumed that the tablet press would run at a tabletting speed of 43.6 rpm, as then numerical data published by Konkel and Mielck[66] could be used to construct the graph in line with the shape of a general force–time profile as described by Jones.[113] The consolidation time (distance between points A and B) is defined as the time for the force to rise almost linearly with time, whereby the punch speed remains fairly constant.[67,114] The beginning of the slowdown of the punch movement can be detected by the stronger bend of the curve just before point B. Upper and lower punch are at their closest distance at point C; that is, the force has already dropped to a slightly lower value when the maximum upper punch displacement has been reached. This time shift was first reported by David and Augsburger[115] and has been attributed to the viscoelastic behavior of tablet formulations.[116] The time span between points B and C is classed as the dwell time.[67] Other authors prefer the determination of the time difference between the maximum force value and the maximum upper punch displacement.[66] The contact time is the time where the upper punch is in contact with the powder and/or formed compact (points A to D). At point E, the tablet is ejected and the ejection force can be measured if the lower punch is instrumented, and at point F, the tablet has been removed from the die table. For the rate of compression, the velocity of the upper punch between points A and B is determined. For example, on a Manesty F 3 eccentric tablet press running at 60 rpm, this is approximately 100 mm s^{-1},[67] and the corresponding contact time is approximately 100 ms.[114]

Figure 9.1b shows a schematic drawing of a force–time profile that would be obtained at the upper punch of a rotary machine. It was constructed from data obtained using pregelatinized starch compressed on a Fette P 2 rotary machine.[117] Again, there is an initial steep rise in force with time (point A to point B), followed by a dwell time (point B to point C) and a gradual decrease in force until there is no further contact between the compact and the upper punch (point C to point D). The length of the dwell time depends on various machine-related and powder-related parameters,[117,118] whereas the decompression phase is very much a function of the elastic properties of the formed compact.[119] Compression rates of approximately 20–70 mm s^{-1} and 40 mm s^{-1} have been reported;[67,117] that is, the compression rate on a rotary tablet machine is slower despite a much higher production output.

In an intermittent dosator-nozzle machine (e.g., Zanasi AZ 20; LZ 64; Macofar), the nozzle and plunger are pushed in a vertical direction into the powder bed. In a continuous dosator-nozzle machine, the movement of the nozzle is controlled by the cam tracks of the machine as the nozzles rotate, similar to a rotary tablet machine. A schematic drawing of the force–time profile that would be obtained on an intermittent dosator-nozzle capsule-filling machine is shown in Figure 9.1c. The drawing is based on reports by Small and Augsburger[35] and Mehta and Augsburger[83] who recorded such traces for lubricated microcrystalline cellulose, anhydrous lactose, and pregelatinized starch. When the dosing tube starts to dip into the powder bed, forces are only recorded once the powder bed height and the piston inside the dosing tube are at the same level (point A), and any further downward travel of the dosing tube results in pre-compression of the powder. The maximum precompression force is reached at point B. After a lag time of approximately 100 ms, at point C, the piston starts to compress the powder and consequently there is a further increase in force up to the maximum compression force, which is reached at point D and coincides with the maximum displacement of the piston. For some powders and compression settings, there is also a short and finite dwell time,[35] and as with eccentric tablet presses, the maximum force recorded and the maximum piston displacement can be shifted, and in this respect, values of about 40 ms have been observed.[83] The force then drops, depending on the elastic properties of the powder, more or less rapidly back to zero (points D to E) before an ejection force (not shown) is applied to push the powder plug out of the dosing tube into the capsule body. Due to the quasi-linear movement of the piston, compression rates are higher compared to tabletting machines, and values of 120–160 mm s^{-1} (Zanasi AZ 20) and 220–505 mm s^{-1} (Macofar MT 13/2) have been recorded.[120] The pre-compression rates are even higher, that is, 242–350 mm s[-1] and 301–600 mm s[-1] for Zanasi AZ 20 and Macofar MT 13/2 machines, respectively.[120] On a continuous dosator-nozzle machine (e.g., mG2), the force–time profiles recorded[36] appear similar, but there is a lack of accurate time scales to allow exact comparisons. Values for rates achieved on these machines are not available.

Finally, Figure 9.1d shows a schematic drawing of the force–time profile obtained on a single tamping head. The drawing is based on numeric data obtained using a pneumatic tamping head installed at tamping station 3 with pregelatinized starch,[38] but the trace has been smoothed similar to traces observed using strain gauges.[68] Again, there is a rapid rise of the tamping force (point A to point B) followed by a short dwell time (point B to point C, approximately 10–20 ms, depending on the tamping station and powder), followed by a drop in force owing to the deflection of the overload spring (point C to point D), a second dwell time (point D to point E, approximately 40–50 ms), and then the final drop of the tamping force to zero owing to the retraction of the tamping pin (point E to point F).[38] On a GKF 330 tamp-filling machine, depending on the pin penetration setting, Cropp et al.[68] found times to peak force between 54 and 117 ms, which is similar to compression rates of 9 to 74 mm s[-1].

A special situation is found when using compaction simulators. While these can, in theory, reproduce any force–time and force–displacement profile recorded on eccentric or rotary tablet machines, they are usually used in the so-called "saw-tooth" profile mode; that is, the force is applied linearly with displacement, which results also in a linear compaction rate up to a point where the moving punch has to slow down and come to a standstill in order for the travel to be reversed (unloading phase). Using the saw-tooth profile, compaction simulators can achieve speeds up to 3000 mm s[-1],[121] but in capsule-filling studies, only compaction rates between 10 and 100 mm s[-1] have been used[39,97] to mimic more closely the compaction rates achieved in such machinery.

To date, ejection rates have only be reported for dosator-nozzle machines and range from 453 to 653 mm s[-1] and from 272 to 834 mm s[-1] for Zanasi AZ 20 and Macofar MT 13/2 machines, respectively.[120] On a rotary tablet machine, the full ejection force is applied within less than 50 ms.[100] Using a physical testing instrument, Anuar and Briscoe[122] achieved a tablet ejection rate of 167 µm s[-1].

MECHANICAL STRENGTH

The determination of the mechanical strength of tablets forms an essential test procedure in development and production, in-process, and quality control. The USP 38/NF33,[123] method 1217 "Tablet Breaking Force" describes the mechanical testing of tablets in great depth and is very thorough in providing exact requirements for the design of tester to be used, load cell requirements, test speed and loading configurations, and the development of an adequate test procedure for a given product. To date, the shape of tablets is no longer simply round and cylindrical, requiring different test configurations, which have been reviewed recently.[124] For the time being, the USP restricts the recommended test configurations to two, namely, the diametral compression test[125–127] and a flexural bending test,[128,129] and the USP also encourages researchers to calculate a value of tensile strength rather than simply to record failure loads. For the tensile strength of standard tablets, an optimum value of 1.5–2.5 MPa has been suggested as a rule of thumb.[27]

In capsule filling, the mechanical strength of the powder plugs is important for their transfer from the die into the capsule body. Poor mechanical plug strength has been identified as one major reason for underfilling of hard capsules, and it was observed that plugs made from powders are generally weaker than those formed from granules.[130] Empirically, plugs are visually inspected for their integrity and lightly handled with, for example, a tamping pin to see whether they crumble easily, or whether they are firm enough to break into two halves.[131] This is illustrated in Figure 9.2.

Mehta and Augsburger[84] reported the development of equipment sensitive enough to subject powder plugs to a flexural bending test in order to determine their mechanical strength, similar to the three-point bending test reported for tablets.[129] They modified a commercially available benchtop tensile-strength tester. The powder plugs were collected directly from an intermittent dosator-nozzle

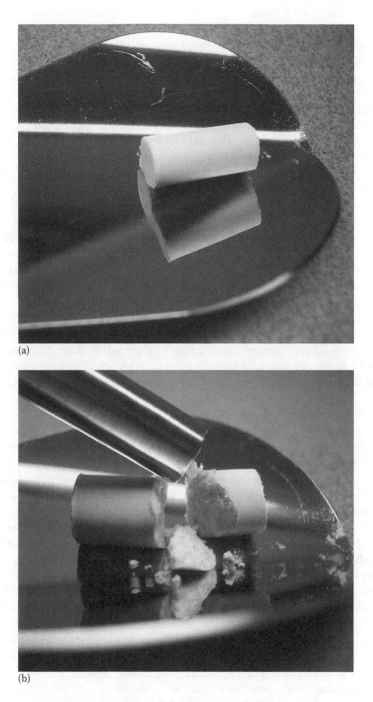

FIGURE 9.2 Empirical testing of the mechanical strength of powder plugs produced under defined conditions. (a) Plug after ejection from the die. (b) Plug with sufficient mechanical strength. (Courtesy of Robert Bosch Inc., Utah, USA.)

machine by removing the capsule bodies from the bushings and were placed into the tester on two supports, mounted 8 mm apart. A blunt stainless steel edge (25 × 0.9 mm) was suspended from a load cell and lowered very slowly onto the powder plug at a rate of 4.4 μm s⁻¹. On contact, the blunt edge's further downward movement caused the plug to bend, and the breaking force was reported. However, there was no indication as to the mode of failure. They found that when filling capsules with a lubricated microcrystalline cellulose-based drug formulation (1% and 2% magnesium stearate) at a compression force of 213 N, the powder plugs were too weak to be tested for their mechanical strength despite filling well into the capsules. Varying the magnesium stearate concentration between 0.05% and 0.75% significantly decreased the mechanical strength of the plugs from 824 to 18 mN. Between 0.05% and 0.1%, the strength reduction was only about 10%, but a further increase in lubricant concentration to 0.2% decreased the plug strength by a further 45%, and the resistance to bending became negligible for 0.5% and 0.75%. With anhydrous lactose, the mechanical strength of the powder plugs was low (170–125 mN), but an increase in magnesium stearate concentration from 0.05% to 0.75% only reduced the values by less than 30%.

Augsburger's research group improved the bending tester so that it had a greater measurement range and higher precision.[40] When using a tamp-filling machine, they found that an increase in tamping force resulted in an increase in plug strength, with the fill weight remaining constant. The mechanical strength of individual segments did not increase further when an additional segment was compressed over them using the same tamping force. They showed that with microcrystalline cellulose, the addition of 0.1% magnesium stearate was the optimum concentration for both fill weight and mechanical strength of the plugs, whereby the mechanical strength of the plugs varied from approximately 2 to 26 mN, depending on the compression forces applied.

Guo et al.[71] measured the breaking force of size 1 powder plugs of 12 mm length made on a compaction simulator at a saw-tooth speed of 50 mm s[-1] and an approximate force of 250 N. Similarly to tabletting,[132] the use of a compaction simulator enabled the recording of the "work of plug formation" (i.e., area under the force–displacement curve).[71] Pregelatinized starch did not form plugs of measurable mechanical strength and anhydrous lactose plugs were found to have a mechanical strength of 160 mN, whereas various microcrystalline and silicified microcrystalline cellulose batches formed plugs of mechanical strengths between 240 and 820 mN. The work of plug formation was similar for pregelatinized starch, anhydrous lactose, and silicified microcrystalline cellulose with a median particle size of 50 μm, yet the mechanical strength of the plugs of the latter material was significantly greater than that for anhydrous lactose. Equally, the work recorded for microcrystalline cellulose, median particle size of 90 μm, was approximately the same as that recorded for the equivalent high-density silicified microcrystalline cellulose, but the mechanical strength was only about half that for the plugs made from the silicified powder. As in tabletting, the work put into plug formation not only is translated into interparticulate adhesion but also reflects losses attributed to interparticulate and particle-die wall friction as well as loss attributed to emission of heat.[133] As silicification changes the surface topography of microcrystalline cellulose,[134] one reason for the increase in plug strength might be an increase in interparticulate forces and a reduction in interparticulate and particle-die wall friction owing to the silicon dioxide particles that are mainly located on the surface of the microcrystalline cellulose particles.[135] Another explanation could be the higher density of the silicified powders and the formation of less porous plugs.[71] The difference in surface topography and its effect on friction could also explain the differences in the mechanical properties observed for pregelatinized starch compared to anhydrous lactose plugs, but differences in particle density and plug porosity achieved are equally likely. Presumably, both mechanisms will contribute to these findings, but to a varying degree depending on the powders tested.

Heda et al.[72] reported values for the mechanical strength of plugs made from binary powder mixtures. They presented plug breaking force as a function of the ratio between the two mixture components, that is, for mixtures of anhydrous lactose and pregelatinized starch, anhydrous lactose and coarse-grade microcrystalline cellulose, and direct-compression ascorbic acid and coarse-grade microcrystalline cellulose. The breaking force–mixture ratio profiles showed a remarkable similarity to those obtained in tabletting when compressing mixtures of brittle lactose monohydrate and ductile sodium chloride;[136] that is, the development of the plug strength is neither synergistic nor additive for the three types of mixtures studied. Fell[136] attributed the non-synergistic, non-additive behavior of binary mixtures to the differences in particle deformation under load; the increase in the number of lactose monohydrate particles in the binary mixture attributed to brittle fragmentation was stated as the reason for the drop in mechanical strength when lactose monohydrate was used in higher proportions than the ductile sodium chloride. However, the powder plugs were made with a compression force of only 200 N,[72] which should not cause significant particle deformation other than from the elastic type and hence the reasoning proposed by Fell[136] does not apply here. Heda et al.[72] unfortunately did not comment further on their findings.

Guo and Augsburger[85] compared the maximum breaking force of plugs made with a dosator-nozzle machine at 50 and 100 N. They found that when doubling the compression force, the maximum breaking force of a variety of microcrystalline and silicified microcrystalline cellulose powders trebled or even quadrupled, but no explanation was provided for this effect.

In the articles cited above published by Augsburger's research group, the breaking forces were determined with an in-house apparatus. It appears equally possible to use dynamic mechanical analysis (DMA). DMA equipment is very versatile, and one of the attachments is a three-point bending rig. DMA can test the samples using a defined stress or strain ratio and can apply forces in a constant and increasing fashion until the sample fails, similar to the equipment used by Augsburger's group. However, DMA also allows the use of dynamic nondestructive test methods; it can measure creep and relaxation and can provide temperature–time and frequency scans.[137] For purposes of research, DMA has been used as a nondestructive test alternative in investigations of the mechanical strength of tablets[138,139] and hence could provide useful information about the structure and mechanical behavior of powder plugs.

LOW-PRESSURE COMPRESSION

MODELING OF LOW-FORCE COMPRESSION

In 1999, Heda et al.[97] proposed that classical compression physics routinely used in the development and optimization of tablet formulations should be extended to the development of powder/granule-filled hard capsule formulations by adapting the models to the much lower pressures used in both dosator-nozzle and tamp-filling machines. This approach has since been called "low-force compression physics." In adapting standard tabletting models for this purpose, Heda et al.[97] employed a compaction simulator equipped with a die that was much longer than usual tabletting dies to facilitate the formation of the comparatively long powder plugs used for capsule filling. The use of this simulator is a scientific approach that allows the precise control of applied stresses and strains as well as their rates, which can affect the outcome of such studies. Unfortunately, compaction simulators are rather expensive and not generally accessible. In 1988, Jones[25] reported the use of a powder plug simulator, a low-cost benchtop equipment to study plug formation as a function of applied pressure and/or achieved plug length. In 1998, Jones[6] reported that after 10 years of experience with this equipment, the results obtained had demonstrated that this simulator could be successfully used to assess the filling performance of formulations for both tamp-filling and dosator-nozzle machines. In this paper, he demonstrated how this equipment could be used to optimize formulations in terms of excipients used, optimum lubricant concentration, and mixing time. By then, he had developed a fully digitized prototype of the powder plug simulator, which was used as a template for the development of the commercially available Bosch capsule plug simulator (Figure 9.3). This apparatus can be used in a similar way to the compaction simulator, but it relies more on the skill of the operator to ensure an even stress or strain rate.

Low-force compression physics is based on the parameterization of the relationship between plug properties such as length, volume, and density, and the force or pressure applied. The model parameters obtained have to be interpreted in line with solid-state physics principles, which can be problematic. As discussed by Lüdde and Kawakita,[140] low-force compression can be applied to a powder by means of a compaction machine (e.g., tablet press, compaction simulator, and powder plug simulator) or by tapping the powder in a jolting volumeter. Models for the parameterization of the low-force

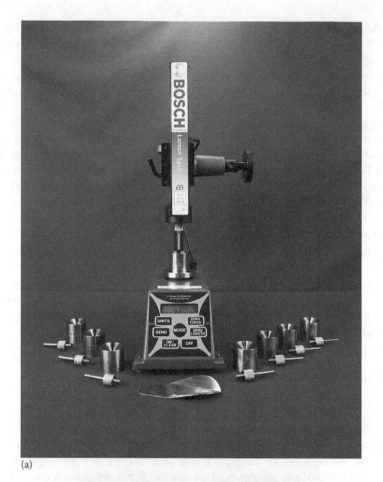

(a)

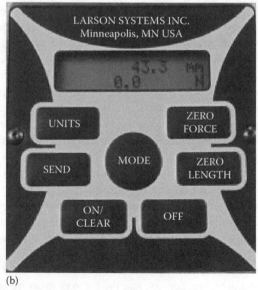

(b)

FIGURE 9.3 Digital powder plug tester (Robert Bosch Inc). (a) Digital powder plug tester. (b) Electronic control panel of the digital powder plug tester.

compression profiles can hence be resourced from the literature on powder compaction and flow. In the following sections, several of these models will be studied for their power and meaningfulness when used to parameterize low-force compression profiles related to capsule filling.

The work on parameterization of low-force compression profiles has mainly been conducted by three research groups, that is, Augsburger's at Maryland University in Baltimore, Sonnergaard's at the Royal Danish School of Pharmacy, and Podczeck's at University College, London. They favored different models and also used different types of equipment, which makes an objective comparison of their work difficult. Hence, a small study was undertaken to obtain low-force compression profiles for a set of powders and granules of different particle sizes. Basic information of the powders and granules used is collated in Table 9.1, and the low-force compression profiles are shown in Figure 9.4.

TABLE 9.1
Information about Powders Used in Low-Force Compression Experiments

Powder	Manufacturer	Median Particle Size (µm)	Material Density (g cm⁻³)	Plug Weight (mg)	Plug Formation
MCC 105	FMC, Little Island, Cork, Ireland	19	1.52	200	Firm
MCC 101	FMC, Little Island, Cork, Ireland	50	1.52	180	Firm
MCC 102	FMC, Little Island, Cork, Ireland	90	1.52	180	Firm
LM fine	Borculo Whey, Saltney, UK	6	1.54	330	Firm, sticky
LM Medium	Borculo Whey, Saltney, UK	43	1.54	330	Firm
LM Coarse	Borculo Whey, Saltney, UK	101	1.54	330	Crumbling
Sorbitol[a]	Merck, Darmstadt, Germany	375	1.49	240	Firm
Sorbitol[b]	Merck, Darmstadt, Germany	980	1.49	215	Firm

Note: LM, lactose monohydrate; MCC, microcrystalline cellulose.

[a] Sorbitol Instant 300–500 µm.

[b] 710–1400 µm.

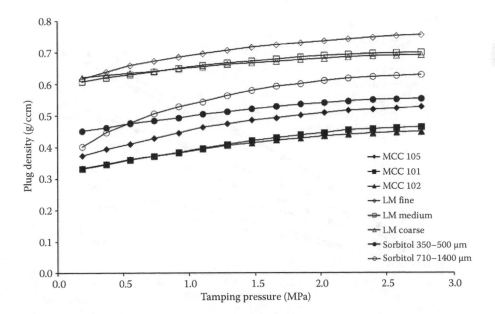

FIGURE 9.4 Plug density as a function of tamping pressure for a series of pharmaceutical excipients, obtained using the digital powder plug tester first described by Jones.[6]

The low-force compression models are in fact pressure relationships; the force values, which ranged from 10 to 150 N, were converted into pressures. Plugs were formed with size 0 tooling.

The models are studied in the order of (1) models taken from powder flow studies using tapping devices, (2) models that have been applied to both tap and compression data, and (3) models that require powder compression in a punch and die system. Within these categories, the models are investigated in the order of the year of their first recorded use.

Angle of Internal Flow[61]

Varthalis and Pilpel[61] studied powder flow using a jolting volumeter. They plotted a term, K ($K = E^2 n/(1 - E)$, with E being the porosity of the powder bed after n taps), as a function of the number of taps n and found that for a number of powders and powder mixtures, this resulted in a straight line of the form $K = bn + K_0$. They ignored the intercept K_0 and only used the slope b, from which they obtained the angle of internal flow θ ($\theta = \tan^{-1} b$). For use in low-force compression, the number of taps has to be replaced by the compression pressure P, that is,

$$\frac{E^2 P}{1 - E} = bP + c. \tag{9.4}$$

The application of Equation 9.4 to the data introduced in Figure 9.4 is illustrated in Figure 9.5. The model does not provide a set of straight lines for low-force compression using the powder plug simulator. Instead, there is an initial nonlinear phase, followed by a linear part, which starts approximately at 1.29 MPa. The relationships have been treated statistically using linear regression analysis, including only data between 1.29 and 2.76 MPa. The results are summarized in Table 9.2. For the powders, the angle of internal flow θ increases with particle size, while for the granules, it decreases. As values for this model have not been reported for low-force compression in the literature, a direct comparison is not possible. According to Varthalis and Pilpel,[61] the value of θ is an indirect measure of interparticulate friction during powder flow. In terms of low-force compression, this would mean that the value represents interparticulate friction during particle rearrangement

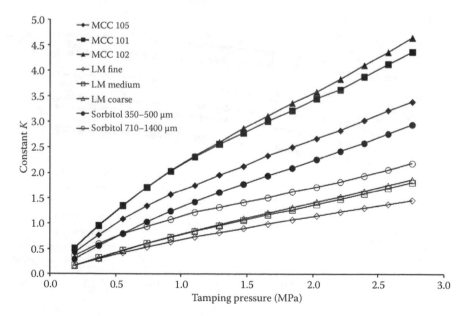

FIGURE 9.5 Parameterization of the data presented in Figure 9.4 using Equation 9.4, that is, a modification of the model described by Varthalis and Pilpel.[61]

TABLE 9.2

Results of the Parameterization of Low-Force Compression Profiles Shown in Figure 9.4 Using the Modified Varthalis–Pilpel Model[61] (Equation 9.4)

Powder	K_0 (MPa)	tan θ	θ (°)	R^2	RMS
MCC 105	0.704	0.974	44.2	0.999	1.39
MCC 101	0.979	1.220	50.7	0.999	1.74
MCC 102	0.821	1.377	54.0	0.999	1.96
LM fine	0.268	0.435	23.5	1.000	0.62
LM medium	0.214	0.577	30.0	1.000	0.82
LM coarse	0.207	0.600	31.0	1.000	0.86
Sorbitol[a]	0.452	0.897	41.9	0.999	1.28
Sorbitol[b]	0.546	0.586	30.4	0.997	0.84

Note: LM, lactose monohydrate; MCC, microcrystalline cellulose; R^2, linear determinant; RMS, root–mean–square deviation (residual analysis).

[a] Sorbitol Instant 300–500 μm.

[b] 710–1400 μm.

enforced by the applied pressure. The values (Table 9.2) imply that there is more interparticulate friction between microcrystalline cellulose particles than between lactose monohydrate particles, which could be explained by differences in their surface morphology, with microcrystalline cellulose particles being much rougher than those of lactose monohydrate. This can be inferred from scanning electron micrographs for microcrystalline cellulose[141] and lactose monohydrate.[142] Equally, Sorbitol granules have a fairly rough surface structure, which could explain their comparatively higher values of θ, but here, the relationship with particle size is inverted. The difference in particle size is almost three times and might have resulted in very large differences in initial powder porosity, which might be easier to densify with a low force than an already densely packed powder bed with no room for free movement.

When determining the angle of internal flow from powder packing studies, Newton and Bader[143] found a decrease in its value with increasing particle size of lactose monohydrate and acetylsalicylic acid, but the values had similar magnitudes ranging from about 20° to 50°. They reported linear relationships between the angle of internal flow and capsule fill weight and drug dissolution time when filling acetylsalicylic acid alone using a tamp-filling machine simulator. The fill weight decreased and the drug dissolution time increased with an increase in the value of θ. Similarly, there was a linear relationship between the angle of internal flow and capsule fill weight for mixtures of the drug with lactose monohydrate, but the relationship with the drug dissolution time was no longer present. When using an instrumented mG2 dosator-nozzle machine simulator, no relationships between particle size and the values of θ were found.[112] Nikolakakis et al.[144] also did not observe any significant relationships between θ values obtained with tapping experiments and the coefficient of fill weight variability when filling powders on a dosator-nozzle machine. When filling herbal powders, Podczeck et al.[69] found that the coefficient of fill weight variability was directly related to the angle of internal flow when using a tamp-filling machine and inversely related when using a dosator-nozzle machine. Tan and Newton[112] defined a powder having an angle of internal flow of 45° as "relatively free flowing," while powders with values higher than 50° were classed as "cohesive." When using low-force compression, such interpretation is less straightforward. Microcrystalline cellulose type 102 is free flowing, as are coarse lactose monohydrate and Sorbitol granules, yet the values for θ range between 54° and 30.4°, and the non-free-flowing powders have values in between this range. Similar powders except for fine and medium lactose monohydrate and microcrystalline cellulose type 105 could be successfully filled into hard capsules using a tamp-filling machine without addition of a lubricant.[55,60] The relevance of the angle of internal flow determined from low-force compression values for the filling of powders and granules into two-piece hard capsules hence requires further investigation.

Compaction Constant T according to Mohammadi and Harnby[145]

When determining the minimum bulk density of a powder using the standard measuring cylinder method, it is very difficult to derive at an exact value and success depends on the skills of the operator. Mohammadi and Harnby[145] suggested overcoming this problem by fitting tap density data obtained with a jolting volumeter to a model equation describing the relationship between volume reduction and number of taps. By exchanging the number of taps with the pressure applied, the following model equation can be obtained:

$$d_\mathrm{P} = d_{\mathrm{P}\infty} - (d_{\mathrm{P}\infty} - d_0)\exp^{-P/T}. \tag{9.5}$$

Here, d_P is the plug density at pressure P, d_0 is the theoretical powder (plug) density at zero pressure, and $d_{\mathrm{P}\infty}$ is the plug density at the maximum pressure applied, and T is the compaction constant. In order to obtain the model constants, nonlinear regression analysis is required. The results obtained from the low-force compression profiles shown in Figure 9.4 are listed in Table 9.3. The values for $d_{\mathrm{P}\infty}$ are equivalent to the maximum pressure of 2.76 MPa applied. The start values for the nonlinear regression analysis were 0.4, 0.6, and 5 for d_0, $d_{\mathrm{P}\infty}$, and T, respectively, and for fine and medium lactose monohydrate as well as size fraction 300–500 μm of the Sorbitol granules, a constraint model with d_0 and $d_{\mathrm{P}\infty}$ set to ≥0 had to be used. For microcrystalline cellulose and lactose monohydrate, maximum values for T are observed for the medium particle size grades, and in general, the values are very small. When using tap density data, the values for T reported were in the range of 5–40[60] and 12–21[43] for powders, 75–136 for granules,[55] and 18–135 for powdered herbs.[69,146] As expected, when applying an axial pressure to powders in a die, densification is much more rapid than when using a tap volumeter. Aling and Podczeck[146] filled herbal leaf powders into size 1 hard capsules using a tamp-filling machine and found that a larger fill weight could be achieved for powders with smaller values of T, whereby T was determined from parameterization of powder plug

TABLE 9.3
Results of the Parameterization of Low-Force Compression Profiles Shown in Figure 9.4 Using the Compaction Constant T as Described by Mohammadi and Harnby[145] (Equation 9.5)

Powder	T	d_0 (g cm^{-3})	$d_{\mathrm{P}\infty}$ (g cm^{-3})	R^2	RMS
MCC 105	1.425	0.345	0.560	0.998	1.06
MCC 101	2.107	0.312	0.525	0.997	0.93
MCC 102	1.728	0.315	0.486	0.998	0.91
LM fine	1.340	0.595	0.777	0.999	1.58
LM medium	4.995	0.607	0.846	0.999	1.49
LM coarse	2.328	0.610	0.731	0.997	1.48
Sorbitol[a]	4.997	0.447	0.719	0.982	1.15
Sorbitol[b]	1.060	0.357	0.653	0.999	1.25

Note: LM, lactose monohydrate; MCC, microcrystalline cellulose; R^2, linear determinant; RMS, root–mean–square deviation (residual analysis).

[a] Sorbitol Instant 300–500 μm.

[b] 710–1400 μm.

density–pressure profiles according to Equation 9.5. The T value was also predictive of the coefficient of fill weight variability at higher compression settings. This is, however, the only report on the use of Equation 9.5 to parameterize low-force compression data to date.

Two-Phase Densification Model according to Hauer et al.[81,109]

Hauer et al.[81] described the densification process, when powders are subjected to tapping, as a two-phase process similar to a first-order chain reaction. The powder is initially transferred from the state of minimum bulk density "A" by a rapid first-order densification process (rate constant k_1) to a state of densification "B," and from here onward, the densification process is slower, described by the first-order rate constant k_2, until the final maximum bulk density "C" has been reached. For lactose powders of various particle sizes, these authors found that the rate of densification k_1 was up to 100 times that of the rate k_2, but the difference became less, as the median particle size increased. They used the value of k_1 to optimize the lubricant concentration, assuming that larger values of k_1 are an indication of better lubrication.[109] Podczeck and Newton[60] found that there was an inverse relationship between the adhesion of powders to the tamping pins and the plug density achieved, and the rate constant k_1, when filling various powders into size 1 hard capsules on a tamp-filling machine. To be able to use this model for low-force compression, the equation has to be adapted, so that

$$d_P = a + b\,P\,\exp^{-k_1} + c\,P\,\exp^{-k_2}, \tag{9.6}$$

where d_P is the plug density at pressure P, k_1 and k_2 are the densification rates, and a, b, and c are constants. The results for the low-force profiles shown in Figure 9.4 are listed in Table 9.4. The data were processed with constraint nonlinear regression analysis and values of 0.5, 0.4, and 0.1 as start values for the constants a, b, and c, respectively, and $k_1 > 0$ (0.1) and $k_2 > 0$ (0.01). The rate constants as such are not very different between powders, and for microcrystalline cellulose, the model identifies unexpectedly large k_2 values. This could potentially be a sign of elastic particle deformation overlaying the densification process by particle rearrangement, as this powder is soft and elastic. Interestingly, when filling microcrystalline cellulose powders on a tamp-filling machine, it was observed that at higher cumulative tamping distances, the increase in capsule fill weight was more

---

TABLE 9.4

Results of the Parameterization of Low-Force Compression Profiles Shown in Figure 9.4 Using the Two-Phase Densification Model Described by Hauer et al.[81,109] (Equation 9.6)

Powder	k_1[a]	k_2[a]	a	b	c	R^2	RMS
MCC 105	0.364	0.443	0.385	0.090	0.006	0.940	0.82
MCC 101	0.412	0.612	0.334	0.034	0.055	0.968	0.72
MCC 102	0.401	0.594	0.339	0.030	0.045	0.956	0.70
LM fine	0.328	0.185	0.631	0.187	0.101	0.938	1.22
LM medium	0.337	0.191	0.614	0.180	0.112	0.947	1.15
LM coarse	0.337	0.189	0.621	0.175	0.117	0.973	1.15
Sorbitol[b]	0.351	0.286	0.455	0.142	0.079	0.959	0.89
Sorbitol[c]	0.360	0.302	0.436	0.168	0.048	0.903	0.97

Note: LM, lactose monohydrate; MCC, microcrystalline cellulose; R^2, linear determinant; RMS, root–mean–square deviation (residual analysis).

[a] k_1 and k_2 are rate constants with g cm^{-3} MPa^{-1} as unit.

[b] Sorbitol Instant 300–500 µm.

[c] 710–1400 µm.

pronounced than at lower cumulative tamping distances.[60] Lactose monohydrate has the largest differences in the rate values of the two phases, which could be the result of these particles being non-deformable at low compaction pressures. In tamp-filling, lactose monohydrate had a limited response to an increase in tamping force/cumulative tamping distance.[60] For the fine grade of microcrystalline cellulose, the first densification phase appears very long, compared to the second phase ($b \gg c$), whereas for the medium and coarse grades, the second phase was slightly longer than the first phase, indicating the possibility of elastic particle deformation. For all lactose monohydrate grades and the smaller granule fraction, the first phase takes about two-thirds of the complete densification process. In conclusion, the use of Equation 9.6 appears to be promising for the modeling of low-force pressure data in relation to capsule-filling performance.

Parameterization Using the Kawakita Equation[140,147]

The Kawakita equation[140,147] is one of the most used models in powder technology. These authors published two versions of this equation: one for uniaxial powder compression and one for powder tap density data. From this, its applicability to low-force compression is obvious. The relationship

$$C = \frac{V_0 - V_P}{V_0} = \frac{abP}{1+bP} \tag{9.7a}$$

is usually applied in its linearized form:

$$\frac{P}{C} = \frac{1}{ab} + \frac{1}{aP}, \tag{9.7b}$$

where P is the applied pressure, V_0 and V_P are the zero-pressure and at-pressure volumes of the powder, respectively, and a and b are constants.

In tabletting studies, it is usually assumed that the value of V_0 is equal to the maximum bulk volume of the powder. However, Hüttenrauch and Roos[148] have shown that this assumption does not hold and that the density of a powder after filling into a die is usually greater than the minimum bulk density; that is, the volume occupied will be less than the maximum bulk volume. The "working bulk volume" V_w has hence to be obtained if correct model data are sought. This can be achieved if instead of the commonly used linear regression analysis on basis of Equation 9.7b the following equation[146] is adopted and solved by nonlinear regression analysis:

$$V_P = V_w - \frac{V_w abP}{1+bP}. \tag{9.8}$$

For the powders listed in Table 9.1, the low-force compression profiles shown in Figure 9.4 have been processed using Equation 9.8 and start values of 0.3, 0.1, and 3 for a, b, and V_w, respectively, using nonlinear regression analysis. The results are shown in Table 9.5. The values of the Kawakita constants depend on the pressure range adopted.[149] The constant a describes the maximum volume reduction under the given loading conditions and is usually listed in percent. When using tapping as the mode of loading, theoretically this constant should be equal to Carr's compressibility index.[140] To have a comparison between the Kawakita constant a and Carr's compressibility index,[58] the latter was determined for all powders and listed in Table 9.5. When comparing tapping and low-force compression, Podczeck and Lee-Amies[150] found that, on average, the constant a obtained from low-force compression (in the range of 0.7–7.3 kPa) was approximately 5% higher than Carr's compressibility index and a is obtained using a high-speed (250 taps min⁻¹) low-lift (2 mm) jolting volumeter.[123,151] The relationship was not perfectly linear, and the greater

TABLE 9.5

Results of the Parameterization of Low-Force Compression Profiles Shown in Figure 9.4 Using the Kawakita Equation[140,147] (Equation 9.8)

Powder	a (%)	b (MPa^{-1})	$1/b$ (MPa)	V_w (cm^{-3} g^{-1})	R^2	RMS	Carr's[a] (%)
MCC 105	48.3	0.975	1.026	2.901	0.997	4.83	30.2
MCC 101	53.6	0.593	1.686	3.188	0.997	5.53	24.3
MCC 102	46.0	0.771	1.297	3.171	0.997	5.59	20.3
LM fine	30.5	0.953	1.049	1.700	1.000	3.19	38.0
LM medium	25.1	0.628	1.592	1.692	0.996	3.37	28.4
LM coarse	24.5	0.357	2.801	1.639	0.997	3.38	13.6
Sorbitol[b]	36.2	0.571	1.751	2.303	0.996	4.38	10.1
Sorbitol[c]	54.3	1.956	0.511	2.903	0.999	4.13	12.8

Note: LM, lactose monohydrate; MCC, microcrystalline cellulose; R^2, linear determinant; RMS, root–mean–square deviation (residual analysis).

[a] Carr's index[56] obtained using a slow-speed (30 taps min^{-1}) high-lift (2.54 cm) jolting volumeter (Jencons Scientific Equipment, Radon Ind. Electronics, Worthing, UK).

[b] Sorbitol Instant 300–500 μm.

[c] 710–1400 μm.

the constant a, the smaller the increase attributed to low-force compression. The values for a and Carr's index in Table 9.5 do not support this and rather indicate that the difference between values from low-force compression and tapping experiments is material dependent, bearing in mind that the pressure range was between 0.2 and 2.8 MPa, that is, four times that of Podczeck and Lee-Amies,[150] and that a slow-speed (30 taps min^{-1}) high-lift (2.54 cm) jolting volumeter had been used. For example, for the two Sorbitol granule fractions, Carr's indices are 10.1% and 12.8%, whereas the values for a are 36.2% and 54.3%, respectively (see Table 9.5), that is, more than just 5% above the values observed by tapping the powder. Podczeck et al.[55] reported Carr's indices of 4.8% and 5.3% for similar granules, using a USP/Ph Eur-jolting volumeter,[123,151] which indicates that the choice of the tapping equipment is also of importance. On the other hand, for a variety of microcrystalline cellulose products, values for Carr's index between 24% and 30% were reported[60] and are close to those reported in Table 9.5. The differences to the values for a are hence not as big as those for the Sorbitol granules. The differences are even smaller for the lactose monohydrate batches. This confirms that the differences between a obtained from low-force compression data and Carr's compressibility index or a obtained from powder tap density measurements are material dependent, being largest for granules and smallest for hard crystalline powders. The large difference observed for the Sorbitol granules might indicate granule fragmentation under the low loads applied with the powder plug simulator.

Yamashiro et al.[152] defined the value of $1/b$ as a measure for the cohesiveness between powder particles, and Adams and McKeown[153] related this term to the failure stress of the individual particle agglomerates, which might be interesting when studying granules under low-force compression conditions. Lüdde and Kawakita[140] defined b as a constant related to the ease with which powder particles can slide along each other during packing, and larger values for b were found for powders with poor fluidity. Adams et al.[154] reported that b was inversely proportional to the shear strength of powder agglomerates. From Table 9.5, it can be observed that the values of b decrease with an increase in particle size except for Sorbitol, where the opposite is the case. Following the theory presented by Adams et al.,[154] the shear strength of the Sorbitol granules would be $0.7/b$, that is, 1.23 and 0.36 MPa for 300–500 μm and 710–1400 μm granule size, respectively. Adams and McKeown[153] had found that the agglomerate tensile strength of individual granules was similar to the value of $1/b$, and this would mean that Sorbitol granules of 300–500 μm and 710–1400 μm will fragment at tensile loads of about 1.7 and 0.5 MPa, respectively. However, it has to be pointed out that these two relationships are only valid for granules, not for individual crystals.

Heda et al.[97] used a compaction simulator with speeds of 1 and 100 mm s[-1] and a plug length of 12 mm. They also found excellent fit of their data to the Kawakita equation. Microcrystalline cellulose type 102 was found to be more compressible than anhydrous lactose (a about 60% and 40%, respectively), and anhydrous lactose was strain rate sensitive in this respect, that is, the value of a was significantly smaller at the higher compaction speed. Pregelatinized starch was similar to anhydrous lactose in terms of both value and strain rate sensitivity. This similarity is somewhat surprising, considering that anhydrous lactose particles are comparatively hard crystals, whereas pregelatinized starch particles are soft and deformable. The ranking of the materials on the basis of the constant b was anhydrous lactose > pregelatinized starch > microcrystalline cellulose. This would mean that anhydrous lactose is least cohesive and thus should reduce its volume more readily than the other two powders, which is what Heda et al.[97] found.

Kopleman et al.[73] reported that for dry herbal extracts, the value of the constant a decreased significantly with an increase in plug length. They interpreted this as a sign for greater densification and packing of the powders with an increase in the die cavity depth. They also found that the value of b decreased with an increase in plug length, that is, increasing resistance to densification.

Guo et al.[71] found for several grades of microcrystalline and silicified microcrystalline cellulose, anhydrous lactose, and pregelatinized starch that regardless of punch speed or plug length, the value of a remained fairly consistent, that is, could be interpreted as a material-specific constant. They also observed that the value of b decreased with an increase in compaction speed from 1 to 50 mm s[-1]. This was interpreted as increase in resistance to packing and densification and a reflection of interparticulate friction. Anhydrous lactose and pregelatinized starch exhibited much larger values for b than the cellulose products.

Low-Force Compression Model Proposed by Chowhan and Chow[155]

Chowhan and Chow[155,156] applied small loads to powders filled into a measuring cylinder by dead-weight loading. They used different cylinder widths (2.5, 3.5, and 4.5 cm) and different powder bed heights (9.5, 18, and 27 cm) and derived powder consolidation ratios. Their test conditions are different to powder columns confined into the space of a dosator-nozzle or dosing bore of a tamping disc, but these authors had related their consolidation ratio to the coefficient of fill weight variability,[156,157] which hence warrants the inclusion of this model into this section:

$$\ln \frac{V_0 - V_P}{V_P} = K \ln \left(\frac{P}{P_0} \right) + C. \tag{9.9}$$

Here, V_0 and V_P are the powder volumes at zero pressure and at pressure P, and P_0 is set arbitrarily to 1 mPa in order to get to a dimensionally homogeneous equation. K and C are constants, whereby C is termed the "consolidation rate" and is the intercept of the linear equation. Figure 9.6 shows the outcome using the data presented in Figure 9.4. As can be seen, initially, that is, below a pressure of 1 MPa, the relationship is linear, but above this threshold, linearity is not maintained. It is noteworthy that Chowhan and Chow[155] used much lower pressures, resulting in $\ln(P/P_0)$ values between 2.5 and 5 only, which could explain the discrepancies with respect to linear/nonlinear behavior. One could argue that it could be possible to calculate the intercept of the equations using the data below 1 MPa only, but this would be based on four points only,

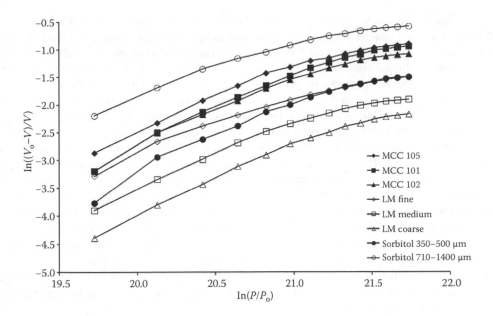

FIGURE 9.6 Parameterization of the data presented in Figure 9.4 using Equation 9.9 described by Chowhan and Chow.[155]

which is dubious. It can be seen from Figure 9.6, however, that for lactose monohydrate and microcrystalline cellulose, the intercept values would decrease in the order coarse > medium > fine powder, but for the Sorbitol granules, the opposite trend would apply. The differences in the overall profiles are marginal for the microcrystalline cellulose powders, whereas they are distinct for the other two materials. Smaller consolidation ratios were associated with larger coefficients of fill weight variation.[156,157]

Heckel Equation[158,159]

Heckel[158] considered the compaction process of powders as a first-order process analogous to a chemical reaction, the pores of the powders being the "reactant." The process could therefore be described as proportionality between pore fraction and change in powder density with applied pressure. After differentiation, the following expression was obtained:

$$\ln\left(\frac{1}{1-D}\right) = KP + \ln\left(\frac{1}{1-D_0}\right). \tag{9.10}$$

Here, D and D_0 are the relative density of the powder at pressure P and at zero pressure, and the term $1 - D$ defines the pore fraction of the powder, that is, powder porosity. The reciprocal value of K, that is, of the slope of the linear portion of the Heckel plot is termed "yield pressure"[160] and is related to the ability of a powder to deform under load.[159] The logarithmic term on the right hand in parenthesis in Equation 9.10 is usually replaced by a constant A. When using linear regression analysis and extrapolating the value of A as the intercept, it is found that its value is typically somewhat larger than $\ln(1/(1 - D_0))$.[158] The value of A supposedly represents powder densification owing to filling of the die and the degree of packing achieved at low pressures as a result of particle rearrangement attributed to particles slipping over one another[159] and depends mainly on particle size and shape but also on the hardness of the particles. A series of intrinsic factors, for example, the way of filling the dies, compaction speed, consolidation time, dimensions of the compacts, method of determining the compact height (see below), and sample preparation all affect the shape of the function and the slop of the linear portion, and comparisons can hence only be made by keeping all experimental conditions constant.[161–163] Heckel[158] defined two principal *modes of operandi* for the determination of the data; at zero-pressure and at-pressure measurements. In the former method, each compact is removed from the die and the dimensions are measured afterward, whereas in the latter method, the dimensions of the compact are determined under load, which requires calibration of punch deformations and displacement and is best undertaken with a compaction simulator. Values obtained at-pressure are affected by the degree of elastic deformation and hence are more difficult to interpret.[164] The Heckel model is strictly only valid for materials that undergo plastic deformation under load,[158,159] but deviations from linearity are often interpreted as a sign of brittle fragmentation.[165] Carstensen and Hou[166] reported that nonlinearity of the Heckel plot observed for direct-compression tricalcium phosphate could have been avoided by substituting the material density used to determine the relative densities of the compacts with the mercury intrusion density. The yield pressure resulting from this approach (265 MPa) was very similar to values reported for direct-compression inorganic phosphates[165] when manipulating nonlinear Heckel plots.

A number of further relationships were suggested to describe the ratio between densification owing to die filling and particle rearrangement (obtained from constant A) and the yield strength of the powder (from constant K).[159]

Adams et al.[154] suggested that the Heckel equation was not very useful when compacting particle agglomerates rather than powders, because the stress developing in a bed of granules when subjected to uniaxial loading is not homogeneously distributed; it is transmitted through a network of "backbone granules," while other granules remain unstressed. Hassanpour and Ghadiri[167] questioned the validity of the Heckel model as such. They used the distinct element method to simulate the behavior of particles as part of a powder bulk under load and found that the results from Heckel analysis are dependent on the ratio of Young's modulus of the material to the yield stress of the particles, and that in some situations, the yield stress derived from the slope of the Heckel plot substantially exceeded the true yield stress of the particles. They suggested caution when using the Heckel function.

Heda et al.,[97] using a compaction simulator, suggested that the Heckel function could be used to parameterize low-force compression profiles. They used compression pressures up to 14 MPa and found that for microcrystalline cellulose, anhydrous lactose, and pregelatinized starch, the Heckel plot became linear at around 4–6 MPa. It is hence not surprising that when using the data presented in Figure 9.4, no linear relationship could be found and Heckel analysis could not be undertaken (see Figure 9.7). The applicability of this model clearly depends on the applied pressure range.

Heda et al.[97] pointed out that the pressure range used did in fact fall into the range of the expected particle rearrangement phase. They were able to derive yield pressures from the linear portions of their plots, but in acknowledging the low pressures used, they termed these values "apparent" yield pressures. This was defined as the resistance of the powder to volume reduction, not to yielding. The apparent yield pressures increased with compression speed except for anhydrous lactose, which seemed unaffected unless the highest speed of 100 mm s^{-1} was used. They explained this by the reduction in time for particle rearrangement at higher speeds and thus greater resistance to volume reduction. The apparent yield pressure also increased with an increase in plug length. For various dry extracts of *H. perforatum*, Kopleman et al.[73] reported that the apparent yield strength increased systematically with an increase in compaction speed (compaction simulator), but that there was no relationship with plug length. Guo et al.[71] studied the apparent yield pressure of a series of microcrystalline and silicified microcrystalline cellulose brands in comparison to anhydrous lactose and pregelatinized starch, also using a compaction simulator. Again, an increase in the apparent yield pressure with compaction speed was found, but to a different degree. They interpreted the increase in the values as a response to interparticulate and die wall friction as well as resistance to general volume reduction. They found that die wall lubrication effects observed at higher compaction speeds were not reflected in the apparent yield pressure values.

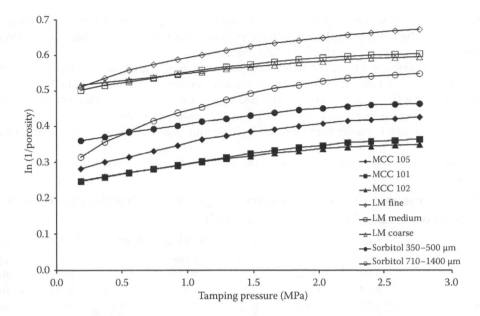

FIGURE 9.7 Parameterization of the data presented in Figure 9.4 using the Heckel function (Equation 9.10).[158]

Cooper–Eaton Relationship

Cooper and Eaton[168] studied the compression of ceramic powders. They described the densification process as two distributed processes, which are the filling of the voids in the powder bed that are larger or of the same size as the particles, and the filling of the voids in the powder bed that are smaller than the particles. The first process is similar to powder particle rearrangement attributed to slippage and rearrangement, overcoming interparticulate friction, and the second process involves particle deformation such as elastic deformation, plastic flow, and fragmentation. As there is a distribution of different void sizes for each process, there will be a range of pressures required to fill the voids during each process, and the processes might also overlap. In Equation 9.11, V_0, V_P, and V_∞ are the powder volume at zero pressure, at pressure P, and at infinite pressure; a_1 and a_2 are dimensionless constants; and k_1 and k_2 are constants with units of pressure:

$$\frac{V_0 - V_P}{V_0 - V_\infty} = a_1 \exp^{-k_1/P} + a_2 \exp^{-k_2/P}. \tag{9.11}$$

The dimensionless constants indicate the two densification processes. Their sum $(a_1 + a_2)$ equals unity when the compaction can be completely described by these two processes. A sum of less than unity indicates that other processes are active before complete densification has been achieved. In principle, the sum could also become larger than unity, which would indicate that zero porosity could be achieved by the two densification mechanisms at a lower than infinite pressure. The values of the constants k_1 and k_2 are indicative of the pressures at which the two related densification processes might occur with greatest probability.

If Equation 9.11 is to be used for low-force compression data, a redefinition of the processes that are observed has to be undertaken. Under conditions of low-force compression, the first phase might represent filling of voids larger than the powder particles and is characterized by smooth particle slippage along one another without greater interparticulate friction. The second phase would represent filling of voids larger than or equal to and maybe slightly smaller than the powder particles, but under the assumption that larger degrees of interparticulate friction have to be overcome, plus some degree of elastic deformation might also occur.

The data presented in Figure 9.4 have been processed applying Equation 9.11, and the results are listed in Table 9.6. Constraint nonlinear regression analysis was employed, and the start values used were $a_1 > 0 = 0.2$, $a_2 > 0 = 0.8$, $k_1 = 0.5$, and $k_2 = 2$. Figure 9.8 shows that indeed the powder densification process is biphasic, even under low-force compression conditions. The values of the constant a_1 are all much smaller than those for a_2, indicating that frictionless particle rearrangement

TABLE 9.6
Results of the Parameterization of Low-Force Compression Profiles Shown in Figure 9.4 Using the Cooper–Eaton Equation[168] (Equation 9.11)

Powder	a_1	a_2	$a_1 + a_2$	k_1 (MPa)	k_2 (MPa)	R^2	RMS
MCC 105	0.187	0.495	0.682	0.085	0.935	0.999	0.80
MCC 101	0.174	0.502	0.676	0.133	1.293	0.999	0.69
MCC 102	0.171	0.431	0.602	0.133	1.203	0.999	0.64
LM fine	0.334	0.386	0.720	0.207	1.465	1.000	0.80
LM medium	0.136	0.400	0.536	0.121	1.234	0.999	0.56
LM coarse	0.102	0.378	0.480	0.153	1.605	0.999	0.42
Sorbitol[a]	0.133	0.415	0.548	0.125	1.283	0.998	0.55
Sorbitol[b]	0.431	0.386	0.817	0.127	0.828	0.999	1.12

Note: LM, lactose monohydrate; MCC, microcrystalline cellulose; R^2, linear determinant; RMS, root mean square deviation (residual analysis).

[a] Sorbitol Instant 300–500 μm.

[b] 710–1400 μm.

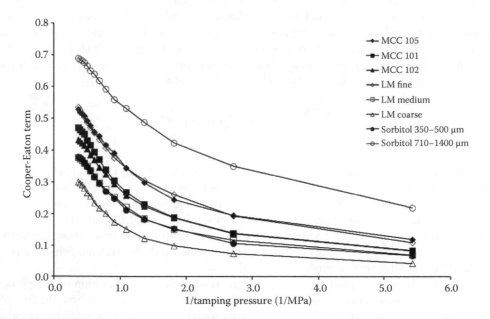

FIGURE 9.8 Parameterization of the data presented in Figure 9.4 using the Cooper–Eaton equation (Equation 9.11).[168]

occurs, but to a far lesser degree than particle rearrangement overcoming interparticulate friction. In no case was the densification process complete, which is not surprising, as there was not enough pressure to cause permanent particle deformation. Considerable interparticulate friction appears to set in at pressures of about 1.2–1.6 MPa (compare constant k_2), except for microcrystalline cellulose type 105 and the larger Sorbitol granule fraction, where this happens already at pressures below 1 MPa. Microcrystalline cellulose type 105 is a fine, fibrous powder with a rough surface structure,[141] which also has a comparatively higher bulk density than the other grades, which could explain the earlier onset of considerable interparticulate friction. For the larger Sorbitol granule fraction, it was concluded from the Kawakita constant $1/b$ that the agglomerates probably start to fragment into smaller agglomerates or individual particles at a pressure of 0.5 MPa. This would mean that, here, the second phase of the densification process is related to agglomerate fragmentation and filling of voids smaller than the original granule size. The k_2 value of about 0.8 MPa fits well with this assumption and indicates that the majority of Sorbitol granules will crumble at this pressure value.

Other Approaches That Could Be Used to Model Low-Force Compression

Walker[169] compressed powders with static loads up to 40 and dynamic loads up to 3 MPa (impact speed, 1.7–4.9 m s^{-1}). He plotted the relative volume of the powders ($V_{rel} = V/\rho_p$; V = observed powder volume; ρ_p = material density) as a function of the resistance to compression ($\ln_{10} R_C$) and extrapolated values for the resistance to static loading R_p and impact loading R_i from these graphs. He defined the resistance ratio R_C as R_i/R_p and found that the value of R_C reflected the viscoelastic properties of the powders. Using compaction simulation at defined speeds instead of impact loading, it should be possible to adapt this relationship to study the viscoelastic behavior of powders during capsule filling.

Sonnergaard developed the so-called "log-exp-model"[170] and applied it to low-force compression.[171] His model assumes that two compaction processes proceed simultaneously, one of which can be described with a logarithmic, the other with an exponential function:

$$V_{rel} = V_1 - w \ln(P) + V_0 \exp^{P/P_m}. \tag{9.12}$$

Here, V_{rel} is the relative volume of the powder as defined above, V_0 and V_1 are the relative volume of the powder at zero load and when compressed at $P = 1$ MPa, respectively, and w and P_m (average pressure to cause agglomerate fragmentation) are constants. Sonnergaard[170] established the validity of this model for compaction pressures above 1 MPa but was unable to apply it to the area below 1 MPa.[171] This seems unsurprising, considering that the logarithmic part of the model is thought to describe particle or agglomerate fragmentation and the exponential part is thought to describe irreversible plastic deformation. In order to check the validity of the model above 1 MPa, the data shown in Figure 9.4, using the values above 1 MPa only, were processed with nonlinear regression analysis. However, it was found that this model could not be fitted successfully. This might be attributed to the pressure being applied manually using the powder plug simulator. A final conclusion should only be made once the model has been tested using a compaction simulator, and after establishing that the model constants are indicative of capsule-filling performance.

As in tabletting, it should be possible to investigate the use of force–displacement,[132,172] force–time,[66] and 3D-models,[173,174] as long as it is possible to record the force or pressure applied as a function of the punch displacement and/or compaction time with high accuracy. Heda et al.[97] recorded force–displacement profiles using a compaction simulator. They found an apparent increase in the applied force with compaction speed and explained this with the reduced time for particle rearrangement at higher speeds. Anhydrous lactose formed an exception in that it was not affected by speed owing to its relatively higher packing density after die filling. The authors also determined the work of compression ("network") by integrating the force–displacement curves. The network decreased from microcrystalline cellulose > pregelatinized starch > anhydrous lactose. Force–displacement curves were also recorded by Cropp et al.[68] using an instrumented tamp-filling machine. They also found that the network for microcrystalline cellulose was much larger than that of anhydrous lactose, plus the values increased with pin penetration setting (i.e., tamping force) and spring constant.

Densification Simulations Using DEM

During powder densification, complex stress states are involved, and on a macroscopic level, that is, treating the powder as a continuum and employing the models discussed above, the densification process depends on discrete particle interactions affected by material properties such as particle hardness, surface roughness, and surface free energy. However, the microscopic particle interactions are equally important for a full understanding of the response of a powder bulk to compaction. For this, DEM simulations are useful. The compaction process of interest in low-force compression during capsule filling is phase one,[175] that is, densification mainly by particle rearrangement. According to Martin et al.,[176] particle rearrangement induces a higher average coordination number together with a lower average contact area and, as a result, does not change the pressure response of the powder greatly (pressure response $\propto$ coordination number $\times$ contact area). Contact orientation owing to elongated or irregular particle shape has a more pronounced influence on the pressure response during phase one.[175] Rotation of the particles is as important in phase one as particle rearrangement by slippage.[177] Rotations by up to 15° occur in the absence of larger amounts of interparticulate friction, but the increase in particle-particle friction attributed to densification reduces the amount and degree of rotation.[178]

STABLE ARCH FORMATION AND ITS SIGNIFICANCE IN CAPSULE FILLING

The filling of powders and granules into two-piece capsules using a dosator-nozzle system requires an accurate amount of powder to be picked up and retained within the cylindrical dosing tube during plug transfer. Similarly to hoppers, which can block because powder is supported by the hopper walls due to transfer of stress, powders could be retained in dosator tubes. Retention may be improved by applying sufficient pre-compression or compression to form a mechanically stronger plug. Jolliffe et al.[179] applied theories derived from mass flow hoppers[180,181] to this problem and is based on two assumptions: First, the maximum nozzle diameter across which arching can occur is limited by the maximum of shear developed at the nozzle walls, and second, the strength present in the powder for arching to occur is the unconfined yield strength. This approach showed that the angle of powder–wall friction is important for the determination of the stress distribution of the powder within the nozzle and that there is an optimum value for this angle, for which the compressive force required to ensure arching is at a minimum. Both the properties of the dosator-nozzle wall and the particles will affect this optimum value. Jolliffe and Newton[182] studied changes in powder–wall friction in relation to the powder built up on the walls of a dosator-nozzle using eight different size fractions of lactose monohydrate. They observed that the angle of powder–wall friction increased asymptotically because of increasing amounts of powder sticking to the wall until 15–20 plugs had been formed. At the same time, the plug weights decreased, reaching a constant value at about 20 capsules. They postulated that the increase in powder–wall friction made movement of the powder at the nozzle wall, as it packed under compression, more difficult. This was thought to have a buffering effect on the piston, gradually slowing it down. The loss of energy, which occurred in this way, resulted in less compressive stress available for transmission to lower parts of the plug. There was hence less frictional support available to the lower part of the forming plug and consequently the powder was less firmly held inside the nozzle. Plugs were easier to eject. The reduced ability to retain the plug was thought to be a possible reason for the observed decrease in plug capsule fill weight.

Using six different grades of microcrystalline cellulose, Faulhammer et al.[183] found that the mean volume diameter of these comparably soft powders did not influence the angle of powder–wall friction except for the coarse, agglomerated[141] Avicel PH-200, where the angle of powder–wall friction was almost twice the value of the other grades. Jolliffe and Newton[184] studied eight different size fractions of lactose monohydrate within a mean size range of 15.6–155.2 μm. While the effective angle of internal friction, determined using a linear shear cell, was independent of particle size, the angles of powder–wall friction, determined on face ground and turned stainless steel surfaces, decreased with an increase in mean particle size up to 40 μm, above which they also became constant. Jolliffe and Newton[184] furthermore reported that the rougher turned plate gave consistently higher values of the angle of powder–wall friction than the smoother face ground plate. Good powder retention by a dosator-nozzle, tested at a range of powder bulk densities, was only possible for the powders up to the mean particle size of 40 μm. Using the developed arching theory[182] it was possible to show that the strength required within the powders to ensure arching also increased with increasing particle size up to 40 μm, above which it became constant. Calculations confirmed that, as powders became freer flowing, a larger compressive stress was necessary and that the angle of powder–wall friction should be low to ensure stress is transmitted to the arching zone at the nozzle opening. Jolliffe and Newton[185] used spark erosion and lapping with abrasive paste to resurface dosator-nozzles used in an mG2 simulator and they also produced surfaces for a linear shear cell of matching surface roughness. In this way, they were able to study the influence of the surface roughness of the dosator-nozzle walls on plug retention applying the theory developed earlier. They found that very rough surfaces had similar values for the angle of powder–wall friction owing to domination of powder–powder over powder–wall friction. Surfaces produced by different techniques resulted in different values for the powder–wall friction coefficient despite similar surface roughness values, presumably as a result of different lay structures, which are not accounted for in surface profilometry. The original nozzle had the roughest surface and produced capsules with the lowest weight and largest coefficient of fill weight variation. With resurfaced nozzles, there was an increase in fill weight and reduction in coefficient of fill weight variation owing to better powder retention. One of the lapped nozzles slightly exceeded the others in improving filling performance, supporting the concept of an optimum angle of powder–wall friction for powder retention and thus reduced coefficient of fill weight variation.

Jolliffe and Newton[80] used an instrumented mG2 capsule-filling machine simulator to study the effect of the amount of compression, defined by the compression ratio,[18] on capsule fill weight uniformity, compression, and ejection forces, using four size fractions of lactose monohydrate (mean particle size, 15.6, 17.8, 37.5, and 155.2 μm). The range of compression ratios over which they could achieve uniform fill weights accompanied by a minimum stress in the dosing tubes depended on particle size. The fine particle size fractions produced uniform fill weights over a wide range of compression settings (0–0.65 and 0–0.53), but for the 37.5-μm powder, this ratio was reduced to 0.18–0.3, and for the coarse powder fractions, satisfactory filling was only achieved at a compression ratio of 0.3. The lower limits of the ranges of compression settings were defined by the ability of the powder to arch, whereas the upper limits were set by the ability of the powders to compact. Since fine powders are able to undergo greater volume reduction than coarse powders, the upper limit decreased with an increase in mean particle size. The same powders were then filled on an mG2 dosator-nozzle machine at a turret speed of 40 rpm.[186] The results showed that capsule fill weights obtained using the two fine fractions were relatively insensitive to the compression settings applied by the piston, and uniform fill weight was again achieved over a wide range of compression settings. As before, the coarse, free-flowing powder required a minimum compression setting and fill weight uniformity was only obtained for small increases in compression above this minimum setting. It was observed that attempts to compact the powders, regardless of their size, further than what can be achieved by simple particle rearrangement resulted in poor fill weight uniformity. As coarser powders were less compressible, this was seen already for lower compression setting when filling the larger particle sizes. All modified nozzles had improved filling ability, confirming that surface roughness will affect powder arching and, similar to Jolliffe and Newton,[185] that there exists an optimum surface roughness for good capsule-filling performance.

Jolliffe and Newton[187] extended their theory on the influence of powder–wall friction on arching and proposed using a nozzle, where the main part has a low value for the angle of powder–wall friction, but the wall near the outlet of the nozzle has a high value. They predicted that such a nozzle modification would result in effective stress transmission to its outlet with minimum losses in powder–wall friction. Hence, arching would be promoted by the rougher surface of the dosator-nozzle wall at the nozzle outlet, which reduces the amount of stress required for arching to occur and hence will improve powder retention. Unfortunately, no experimental evidence was provided.

Tan and Newton[188] calculated the theoretical compressive stress requirements for arch formation and powder retention in a dosator-nozzle for a variety of powders and their size fractions. They found that, in general, higher values of the required vertical stress in the arching zone also required higher values of compressive stress at the top of the powder bed. The magnitude of these stresses depended on material properties and particle size. The highest required stress values were determined for the calcium carbonate powder fractions with hard individual crystals, whereas the lowest stresses were determined for microcrystalline cellulose powder fractions. The stress requirements increased with particle size for all powders, but to a different degree, again depending on crystal hardness. However, these calculated stress values were found not to be the main controlling feature for capsule-filling performance. The authors found that all powders showed good ability to arch without the need for piston compression during filling, but it has to be borne in mind that the size fractions used all had mean particle sizes below 40 μm. Tan and Newton[79] filled pregelatinized starch and microcrystalline cellulose size fractions with mean particle size of less than 40 μm also using dosator tubes with modified surface texture. They found that differences in surface roughness did not affect capsule fill weight variability significantly. This is in contrast to findings on lactose monohydrate.[185] The findings imply that powders with little affinity to adhere to the dosator-nozzle wall hence do not form a coating and wall texture only marginally influences the capsule-filling performance. Tan and Newton,[189] using similar sets of fine powder fractions, confirmed that, in most cases, fill weight variation was lowest at a compression setting of zero (i.e., densification by precompression only). For the finest particle size fractions of pregelatinized starch and maize starch, however, powder retention had to be increased by applying a small amount of compression. For particle size fractions approaching 40 μm mean particle size, however, it was observed that higher compression settings resulted in jamming of the piston and failure to fill the capsules. The degree of nozzle wall coating increased with a decrease in particle size and an increase in powder compression. Calcium carbonate was found to produce the greatest amount of nozzle wall coating, and together with pregelatinized starch, it also produced the highest losses of powder behind the piston. With the exception of lactose monohydrate, filling powders with a coated nozzle gave comparable results to those obtained with a clean one. Capsule fill weights were less than predicted from the bulk density of the powder bed from which the samples were taken. The origins for these discrepancies were not identified.

PARTICLE DEFORMATION DURING CAPSULE FILLING

In tabletting, once the value of the compaction pressure has exceeded the yield strength of the powder particles, it will result in permanent particle deformation owing to plastic flow and/or fragmentation. Elastic particle deformation can occur during stages two and three of compaction, that is, as soon as volume reduction can no longer be achieved solely by particle rearrangement and rotation.[175] In capsule filling, volume reduction is achieved mainly by particle rearrangement and rotation, but rearrangement processes as well as deformation processes are governed by statistical laws and hence overlap to some degree. Adams and McKeown[153] have shown using single agglomerate strength tests that particle agglomerates and granules can fragment at loads as low as 0.2 MPa. This is well in the range of loads applied during capsule filling and hence a potential densification process for granulated powders during capsule filling. The use of the Cooper–Eaton model (see above) provided some experimental evidence for this.

Britten et al.[37] had already observed that elastic deformation plays a part in plug formation for soft powders such as pregelatinized starch. Shah et al.[40] reported for anhydrous lactose and dicalcium phosphate that the density of each plug segment formed during successive tamping remains constant, whereas Podczeck[74] found for microcrystalline cellulose and pregelatinized starch that each successive tamp further increased the density of the already formed plug segments. While lactose monohydrate is unlikely to deform by fragmentation or elastic flow under the low forces generated in a tamp-filling machine, both pregelatinized starch and microcrystalline cellulose are soft and pliable, which could have resulted in at least elastic deformation and thus consecutive plug densification. Heda et al.[97] suggested that the high values for the apparent yield pressure observed for microcrystalline cellulose and pregelatinized starch were an indication that more than just particle rearrangement had occurred despite the low forces applied. Again, this is most likely elastic deformation, which is known to overlay Heckel data.[133]

CONCLUSION

It is clear from the information presented that while there are some similarities in the production process of tablets and powder-filled hard capsules, there are also substantial differences between the two processes. The use of different forces results in distinctive different powder behavior during compression. Thus, the formulations should not be identical; they must account for these differences to achieve successful products.

ACKNOWLEDGMENT

The author wishes to thank Shashi Gupta (School of Pharmacy, University of London) for experimental work undertaken (Figure 9.4) and Robert Bosch Inc. for permission to use copies of pictures from their plug simulator manual.

LIST OF SYMBOLS

a	constant
a_1	constant
a_2	constant
A	Heckel constant
A_a	apparent area of compact-die contact
A_L	lateral surface area of a cylinder
A_O	total surface area of a cylinder
b	constant
c	constant
C	constant
$C(\%)$	compression ratio
d	powder column/plug diameter
d_0	theoretical powder/plug density at zero pressure
d_P	plug density at pressure P
$d_{P\infty}$	plug density at maximum applied pressure
D	diameter of the base of a cylinder; relative density of powder at pressure P (Heckel model)
D_0	relative density of the powder at zero pressure
DEM	Discrete Element Method
E	porosity
F_d	axial force lost to the die wall
F_e	maximum ejection force

F_L maximum force at the lower punch
F_U maximum force at the upper punch
h cylinder height; height of the powder bed after compression ("plug length")
h_0 original powder bed/powder column height
H height of the powder bed
k_1 rate constant (powder densification); constant with the units of pressure
k_2 rate constant (powder densification); constant with the units of pressure
K porosity-related term in powder packing; slope (Heckel model)
K_0 intercept of linear regression line (powder packing)
K_m material constant
L length of the dosing tube from its opening to the piston
n power law constant; number of taps (powder packing)
P compression pressure
P_0 pressure arbitrarily set to 1 mPa
P_e maximum ejection pressure
P_L maximum pressure at the lower punch
P_m average pressure to cause agglomerate fragmentation
P_M mean compaction pressure
P_r pre-compression ratio
P_U maximum pressure at the upper punch
r radius of the circular base of a cylinder
R axial force transmission ratio
R_C resistance to compression ratio
R_i resistance to impact loading
R_p resistance to static loading
T compaction constant
V volume of a cylinder; powder volume
V_0 powder volume at zero pressure
V_1 powder volume at a pressure of 1 MPa
V_P powder volume at pressure P
V_{rel} relative powder volume
V_w working bulk volume
V_∞ powder volume at infinite pressure
w constant
x distance
α correction factor
ρ_p material density
ρ_r powder densification ratio
θ angle of internal flow
μ_d die wall friction coefficient

REFERENCES

1. Cole GC. Powder characteristics for capsule filling. In: Ridgway K, ed. *Hard Capsules*, 1st edn. London: Pharmaceutical Press, 1987: 80–6.
2. Jones BE. Capsules, hard. In: Swarbrick J, Boylan JC, eds. *Encyclopaedia of Pharmaceutical Technology*, 2nd edn, Vol. 1. London: Informa Healthcare, 1997: 302–16.
3. Jones BE. The filling of powders into two-piece hard capsules. *Int J Pharm* 2001; 227: 5–26.
4. Podczeck F. Powder, granule and pellet properties for filling of two-piece hard capsules. In: Podczeck F, Jones BE, eds. *Pharmaceutical Capsules*, 2nd edn. London: Pharmaceutical Press, 2004: 101–18.
5. Lai SMH. *Expert System for Formulation Support of Hard Gelatin Capsules*. PhD Thesis, University of London, 1996: 144–5.

6. Jones BE. New thoughts on capsule filling. *STP Pharm Sci* 1998; 8: 277–83.

7. Small LE, Augsburger LL. Aspects of the lubrication requirements for an automatic capsule filling machine. *Drug Dev Ind Pharm* 1978; 4: 345–72.

8. Botzolakis JE, Augsburger LL. Disintegrating agents in hard gelatin capsules. Part I: Mechanism of action. *Drug Dev Ind Pharm* 1988; 14: 29–41.

9. Botzolakis JE, Augsburger LL. Disintegrating agents in hard gelatin capsules. Part II: Swelling efficiency. *Drug Dev Ind Pharm* 1988; 14: 1235–48.

10. Botzolakis JE, Small LE, Augsburger LL. Effect of disintegrants on drug dissolution from capsules filled on a dosator-type automatic capsule-filling machine. *Int J Pharm* 1982; 12: 341–9.

11. Newton JM. Drug release from capsules. In: Podczeck F, Jones BE, eds. *Pharmaceutical Capsules*, 2nd edn. London: Pharmaceutical Press, 2004: 213–37.

12. Brockedon W. Shaping of pills, lozenges and Black Lead by pressure in a die. English Patent Number 9977, London: 1843.

13. Lehuby JC. Mes enveloppes médicamenteuses. French Patent Number 4435, Paris: 1946.

14. Harris JW, Stocker H. *Handbook of Mathematics and Computational Science*. New York: Springer, 1998: 103.

15. Reier G, Cohn R, Rock S, Wagenblast F. Evaluation of factors affecting the encapsulation of powders in hard gelatin capsules I. Semi-automatic capsule machines. *J Pharm Sci* 1968; 57: 660–6.

16. Eskander F, Lejeune M, Edge S. Low powder mass filling of dry powder inhalation formulations. *Drug Dev Ind Pharm* 2011; 37: 24–32.

17. Crowder TM. Precision powder metering utilizing fundamental powder flow characteristics. *Powder Technol* 2007; 173: 217–23.

18. Tagaki K, Sugihara M, Kimura S. Studies on filling properties in automatic filling machines (in Japanese). *Yakuzaigaku* 1969; 29: 245–9.

19. Clement H, Marquardt HG. Experiences with automatic filling of hard gelatin capsules (in German). *Pharm Ind* 1970; 32: 169–76.

20. Kurihara K, Ichikawa I. Effect of flowability on capsule-filling-weight-variation. *Chem Pharm Bull* 1978; 26: 1250–6.

21. *Martindale: The Extra Pharmacopoeia*, 23rd edn. London: Pharmaceutical Press, 1952: 1284–9.

22. *Martindale: The Extra Pharmacopoeia*, 26th edn. London: Pharmaceutical Press, 1972: 2164–5.

23. Gunsel WC, Swartz CJ, Kanig JL. Tablets. In: Lachman L, Lieberman HA, Kanig JL, eds. *The Theory and Practice of Industrial Pharmacy*. Philadelphia: Lea & Febiger, 1970: 305–45.

24. Jones BE. Hard gelatin capsules. *Manuf Chem Aerosol News* 1969; 40(2): 25–9.

25. Jones BE. Powder formulations for capsule filling. *Manuf Chem* 1988; 59(7): 28–33.

26. Newton JM, Podczeck F, Lai S, Daumesnil R. The design of an expert system to aid the development of capsule formulations (in Japanese). In: Hashida M, ed. *Formulation Design of Oral Dosage Forms* (in Japanese). Tokyo: Yakugyo Jiho, 1998: 236–44.

27. Stricker H. *Physical Pharmacy* (in German). Stuttgart: Wissenschaftliche Verlagsgesellschaft, 1987: 506–8.

28. Stamm A, Boymond C, Mathis C. Some aspects of the formulation of hard gelatin capsules. *Drug Dev Ind Pharm* 1984; 10: 355–80.

29. Newton JM, Rowley G. *Drug Formulations*. US Patent 3,859,431, granted 7 January 1975.

30. Seth PL, Münzel K. Comparative investigation into the properties of tablets prepared on eccentric and rotary tablet machines (in German). *Pharm Ind* 1960; 22: 392–5.

31. MacLeod HM, Marshall K. The determination of density distributions in ceramic compacts using autoradiography. *Powder Technol* 1977; 16: 107–22.

32. Kandeil A, de Malherbe CM. The use of hardness in the study of compaction behaviour and die loading. *Powder Technol* 1977; 17: 253–7.

33. Charlton B, Newton JM. Application of gamma–ray attenuation to the determination of density distributions within compacted powders. *Powder Technol* 1985; 41: 123–34.

34. Nebgen G, Gross D, Lehmann V, Müller F. ^{1}H–NMR microscopy of tablets. *J Pharm Sci* 1995; 84: 283–91.

35. Small LE, Augsburger LL. Instrumentation of an automatic capsule-filling machine. *J Pharm Sci* 1977; 66: 504–9.

36. Jolliffe IG, Newton JM, Cooper D. The design and use of an instrumented mG2 capsule filling machine simulator. *J Pharm Pharmacol* 1982; 34: 230–5.

37. Britten JR, Barnet, MI, Armstrong NA. Studies on powder plug formation using a simulated capsule filling machine. *J Pharm Pharmacol* 1996; 48: 249–54.

38. Podczeck F. The development of an instrumented tamp-filling capsule machine I Instrumentation of a Bosch GKF 400S machine and feasibility study. *Eur J Pharm Sci* 2000; 10: 267–74.
39. Davar N, Shah R, Pope DG, Augsburger LL. The selection of a dosing disk on a Höfliger–Karg capsule-filling machine. *Pharm Technol* 1997; 21(2): 32–48.
40. Shah KB, Augsburger LL, Marshall, K. An investigation of some factors influencing plug formation and fill weight in a dosing disk-type automatic capsule-filling machine. *J Pharm Sci* 1986; 75: 291–6.
41. Shah KB, Augsburger LL, Marshall K. Multiple tamping effects on drug dissolution from capsules filled on a dosing disk-type automatic capsule–filling machine. *J Pharm Sci* 1987; 76: 639–45.
42. Felton LA, Garcia DI, Farmer R. Weight and weight uniformity of hard gelatin capsules filled with micro-crystalline cellulose and silicified microcrystalline cellulose. *Drug Dev Ind Pharm* 2002; 28: 467–72.
43. Gohil UC, Podczeck F, Turnbul, N. Investigations into the use of pregelatinised starch to develop powder-filled hard capsules. *Int J Pharm* 2004; 285: 51–63.
44. Nair R, Vemuri M, Agrawala P, Kim S. Investigation of various factors affecting encapsulation on the In-Cap automatic capsule-filling machine. *AAPS Pharm Sci Tech* 2004; 5(4): article 57.
45. Woodhead PJ, Hardy JG, Newton JM. Determination of porosity variations in powder beds. *J Pharm Pharmacol* 1982; 34: 352–8.
46. Wang Z, Afacan A, Nandakumar K, Chuang KT. Porosity distribution in random packed columns by gamma ray tomography. *Chem Engng Process* 2001; 40: 209–19.
47. Mueller GE. Radial porosity in packed beds of spheres. *Powder Technol* 2010; 203: 626–33.
48. Woodhead PJ, Newton JM. The influence of deposition method on the packing uniformity of powder beds. *J Pharm Pharmacol* 1983; 35: 133–7.
49. Woodhead PJ, Newton JM. The effect of sinusoidal vibration on the uniformity of packing of powder beds. *J Pharm Pharmacol* 1984; 36: 573–7.
50. Woodhead PJ, Chapman SR, Newton JM. The vibratory consolidation of particle size fractions of powders. *J Pharm Pharmacol* 1983; 35: 621–6.
51. Woodhead PJ. *The Influence of Powder Bed Porosity Variations on the Filling of Hard Gelatin Capsules by a Dosator System*. PhD Thesis: University of London, 1980: 271–83.
52. Llusa M, Faulhammer E, Biserni S et al. The effect of capsule-filling machine vibration on average fill weight. *Int J Pharm* 2013; 454: 381–387.
53. Besenhard M, Faulhammer E, Fathollahi S et al. Accuracy of micro powder dosing via a vibratory sieve-chute system. *Eur J Pharm Biopharm* 2015; 94: 264–72.
54. Guo Y, Kafui KD, Thornton C. Numerical analysis of density-induced segregation during die filling. *Powder Technol* 2009; 197: 111–19.
55. Podczeck F, Blackwell S, Gold M, Newton JM. The filling of granules into hard gelatine capsules. *Int J Pharm* 1999; 188: 59–69.
56. Miyake Y, Shinoda A, Nasu T et al. Packing properties of pharmaceutical powders into hard gelatine capsules (in Japanese). *Yakuzaigaku* 1974; 34: 32–7.
57. Newton JM, Bader F. The prediction of the bulk densities of powder mixtures, and its relationship to the filling of hard gelatin capsules. *J Pharm Pharmacol* 1981; 33: 621–6.
58. Carr JR. Evaluating flow properties of solids. *Chem Eng* 1965; 72: 163–8.
59. Podczeck F, Newton JM. Powder and capsule filling properties of lubricated granulated cellulose powder. *Eur J Pharm Biopharm* 2000; 50: 373–7.
60. Podczeck F, Newton JM. Powder filling into hard gelatine capsules on a tamp filling machine. *Int J Pharm* 1999; 185: 237–54.
61. Varthalis S, Pilpel N. Anomalies in some properties of powder mixtures. *J Pharm Pharmacol* 1976; 28: 415–19.
62. Schmidt PC, Tenter U, Hocke J. Force and displacement characteristics of rotary tabletting machines. 1. Instrumentation of a single punch for force measurements (in German). *Pharm Ind* 1986; 48: 1546–53.
63. Hardy IJ, Fitzpatrick S, Booth SW. Rational design of powder formulations for tamp filling processes. *J Pharm Pharmacol* 2003; 55: 1593–9.
64. Jovanović MD, Samardzaić ZJ, Djurić ZR, Sekulović DV. The effect of fillers, disintegrants and compression force on antacid activity of magnesium trisilicate tablets. *Pharm Ind* 1988; 50: 1090–2.
65. Hauer B, Mosimann P, Posanski U et al. Solid oral dosage forms. 1. Powders, granules, pellets, tablets and cores (in German). In: Sucker H, Fuchs P, Speiser P, eds. *Pharmaceutical Technology (in German)*, 2nd edn. Stuttgart: Georg Thieme, 1991: 244–318.
66. Konkel P, Mielck JB. Associations of parameters characterizing the time course of the tabletting process on a reciprocating and on a rotary tabletting machine for high-speed production. *Eur J Pharm Biopharm* 1998; 45: 137–48.

67. Armstrong NA. Time-dependent factors involved in powder compression and tablet manufacture. *Int J Pharm* 1989; 49: 1–13.
68. Cropp JW, Augsburger LL, Marshall K. Simultaneous monitoring of tamping force and pin displacement (F–D) on an Höfliger Karg capsule filling machine. *Int J Pharm* 1991; 71: 127–36.
69. Podczeck F, Claes L, Newton JM. Filling powdered herbs into gelatine capsules. *Manuf Chem* 1999; 70(2): 29–33.
70. Ashraf M, Iuorno VL, Coffin-Beach D et al. A novel nuclear magnetic resonance (NMR) imaging method for measuring the water front penetration rate in hydrophilic polymer matrix capsule plugs and its role in drug release. *Pharm Res* 1994; 11: 733–7.
71. Guo M, Muller FX, Augsburger LL. Evaluation of the plug formation process of silicified microcrystalline cellulose. *Int J Pharm* 2002; 233: 99–109.
72. Heda PK, Muteba K, Augsburger LL. Comparison of the formulation requirements of dosator and dosing disc automatic capsule filling machines. *AAPS Pharm Sci* 2002; 4(3): article 17.
73. Kopleman SH, Augsburger LL, NguyenPho A et al. Selected physical and chemical properties of commercial *Hypericum perforatum* extracts relevant for formulated product quality and performance. *AAPS Pharm Sci* 2001; 3(4): article 26.
74. Podczeck F. The development of an instrumented tamp-filling capsule machine II. Investigations of plug development and tamping pressure at different filling stations. *Eur J Pharm Sci* 2001; 12: 515–21.
75. Podczeck F, Jones BE. The in vitro dissolution of theophylline from different types of hard shell capsules. *Drug Dev Ind Pharm* 2002; 28: 1163–9.
76. Wilson WI, Peng Y, Augsburger LL. Generalization of a prototype intelligent hybrid system for hard gelatin capsule formulation development. *AAPS Pharm Sci Tech* 2005; 6(3): article 56.
77. Armstrong NA. Instrumented capsule-filling machines and simulators. In: Podczeck F, Jones BE, eds. *Pharmaceutical Capsules*, 2nd edn. London: Pharmaceutical Press, 2004: 139–55.
78. Tattawasart A, Armstrong NA. The formation of lactose plugs for hard shell capsule fills. *Pharm Dev Technol* 1997; 2: 335–43.
79. Tan SB, Newton JM. Capsule filling performance of powders with dosator nozzles of different wall texture. *Int J Pharm* 1990; 66: 207–11.
80. Jolliffe IG, Newton JM. An investigation of the relationship between particle size and compression during capsule filling with an instrumented mG2 simulator. *J Pharm Pharmacol* 1982; 34: 415–19.
81. Hauer B, Remmele T, Züger O, Sucker H. The rational development and optimization of capsule formulations with an instrumented dosator capsule filling machine I. Instrumentation and influence of the filling material and the machine parameters (in German). *Pharm Ind* 1993; 55: 509–15.
82. Cole GC, May G. The instrumentation of a Zanasi LZ/64 capsule filling machine. *J Pharm Pharmacol* 1975; 27: 353–8.
83. Mehta AM, Augsburger LL. Simultaneous measurement of force and displacement in an automatic capsule filling machine. *Int J Pharm* 1980; 4: 347–51.
84. Mehta AM, Augsburger LL. A preliminary study of the effect of slug hardness on drug dissolution from hard gelatin capsules filled on an automatic capsule-filling machine. *Int J Pharm* 1981; 7: 327–34.
85. Guo M, Augsburger LL. Potential application of silicified microcrystalline cellulose in direct-fill formulations for automatic capsule-filling machines. *Pharm Dev Technol* 2003; 8: 47–59.
86. Nelson E, Naqvi SM, Busse LW, Higuchi T. The physics of tablet compression. IV. Relationship of ejection, and upper and lower punch forces during compressional process: application of measurements to comparison of tablet lubricants. *J Am Pharm Assoc Sci Ed (J Pharm Sci)* 1954; 43: 596–602.
87. Sheinhartz I, McCullough HM, Zambrow JL. Method described for evaluation of lubricants in powder metallurgy. *J Metals* 1954; 6: 515–18.
88. Toor HL, Eagleton SD. Plug flow and lubrication of polymer particles. *Ind Eng Chem* 1956; 48: 1825–30.
89. Hölzer AW, Sjögren J. Comparison of methods for evaluation of friction during tableting. *Drug Dev Ind Pharm* 1977; 3: 23–37.
90. Lewis CJ, Shotton E. Some studies of friction and lubrication using an instrumented tablet machine. *J Pharm Pharmacol* 1965; 17(S1): 71S–81S.
91. Hölzer AW, Sjögren J. Influence of tablet thickness on measurements of friction during tableting. *Acta Pharm Suec* 1978; 15: 59–66.
92. Strickland Jr WA, Nelson E, Busse LW, Higuchi T. The physics of tablet compression. IX. Fundamental aspects of tablet lubrication. *J Am Pharm Assoc Sci Ed (J Pharm Sci)* 1956; 45: 51–5.
93. Wolff JE, de Kay HG, Jenkins GL. Lubricants in compressed tablet manufacture. *J Am Pharm Assoc Sci Ed (J Pharm Sci)* 1947; 36: 407–10.

94. Strickland Jr WA, Higuchi T, Busse LW. The physics of tablet compression. X. Mechanism of action and evaluation of tablet lubricants. *J Am Pharm Assoc Sci Ed (J Pharm Sci)* 1960; 49: 35–40.

95. Bowden FP, Tabor D. *The Friction and Lubrication of Solids.* Oxford: Clarendon Press, 1958: 176–96.

96. Lewis CJ, Shotton E. A comparison of tablet lubricant efficiencies for a sucrose granulation using an instrumented tablet machine. *J Pharm Pharmacol* 1965; 17(S1): 82S–86S.

97. Heda PK, Muller FX, Augsburger LL. Capsule filling machine simulation. I. Low-force powder compression physics relevant to plug formation. *Pharm Dev Technol* 1999; 4: 209–19.

98. Shaxby JH, Evans JC. On the properties of powders. The variation of pressure with depth in columns of powders. *Trans Faraday Soc* 1923; 19: 60–72.

99. Spencer RS, Gilmore GD, Wiley RM. Behavior of granulated polymers under pressure. *J Appl Phys* 1950; 21: 527–31.

100. Schmidt PC, Tenter U. Force and displacement characteristics of rotary tabletting machines. 5. Measurement and interpretation of ejection forces (in German). *Pharm Ind* 1989; 51: 183–7.

101. Mitrevej KT, Augsburger LL. Adhesion of tablets in a rotary tablet press. II. Effects of blending time, running time, and lubricant concentration. *Drug Dev Ind Pharm* 1982; 8: 237–82.

102. Train D. An investigation into the compaction of powders. *J Pharm Pharmacol* 1956; 8: 745–60.

103. Salpekar AM, Augsburger LL. Magnesium lauryl sulfate in tableting: Effect on ejection force and compressibility. *J Pharm Sci* 1974; 63: 289–93.

104. Flipot AJ, Gilissen R, Smolders A. Importance of stearates in fabrication of UO_2 and $(U,PU)O_2$ pellets. *Powder Metall* 1971; 14: 93–109.

105. Juslin MJ, Krogerus VE. Studies on tablet lubricants. I. Effectiveness of lubricants of some fatty acids, alcohols, and hydrocarbons measured as the relationship of the forces on the lower and upper punches of an eccentric tablet machine (in Finnish). *Farm Aikak* 1970; 79: 191–202.

106. Juslin MJ, Krogerus VE. Studies on tablet lubricants. II. On effectiveness of some fatty acids, alcohols, and hydrocarbons as lubricant in tablet compression judged from the amount of ejection force (in Finnish). *Farm Aikak* 1971; 80: 255–62.

107. Cole GC, May G. The instrumentation of a Zanasi LZ/64 capsule filling machine. *J Pharm Pharmacol* 1975; 27: 353–8.

108. Shah KB, Augsburger LL, Small LE, Polli GP. Instrumentation of a dosing disk automatic capsule filling machine. *Pharm Technol* 1983; 7(4): 42–54.

109. Hauer B, Remmele T, Sucker H. The rational development and optimization of capsule formulations with an instrumented dosator capsule filling machine II. Fundamentals of the optimization strategy (in German). *Pharm Ind* 1993; 55: 780–6.

110. Ullah I, Wiley GJ, Agharkar SN. Analysis and simulation of capsule dissolution problem encountered during product scale-up. *Drug Dev Ind Pharm* 1992; 18: 895–910.

111. Desai DS, Rubitski BA, Varia SA, Newman AW. Physical interactions of magnesium stearate with starch-derived disintegrants and their effects on capsule and tablet dissolution. *Int J Pharm* 1993; 91: 217–26.

112. Tan SB, Newton JM. Powder flowability as an indication of capsule filling performance. *Int J Pharm* 1990; 61: 145–55.

113. Jones TM. Physico-technical properties of starting materials used in tablet formulation. *Int J Pharm Tech Prod Manuf* 1981; 2: 17–24.

114. Charlton B, Newton JM. Theoretical estimation of punch velocities and displacements of single-punch and rotary tablet machines. *J Pharm Pharmacol* 1984; 36: 645–51.

115. David ST, Augsburger LL. Plastic flow during compression of directly compressible fillers and its effect on tablet strength. *J Pharm Sci* 1977; 66: 155–9.

116. Müller F. Viscoelastic models. In: Alderborn G, Nyström C, eds. *Pharmaceutical Powder Compaction Technology.* New York: Marcel Dekker, 1995: 99–132.

117. Schmidt PC, Tenter U. Force and displacement characteristics of rotary tabletting machines. 2. Comparison of the machines Fette P 2, Fette P 1000, Kilian LX 28 and Korsch PH 343 (in German). *Pharm Ind* 1987; 49: 637–42.

118. Schmidt PC, Tenter U. Force and displacement characteristics of rotary tabletting machines. 3. Comparison of different materials (in German). *Pharm Ind* 1988; 50: 376–81.

119. Schmidt PC, Koch H. The evaluation of force–time profiles (in German). *Eur J Pharm Biopharm,* 1991; 37: 7–13.

120. Britten JR, Barnett MI, Armstrong NA. Construction of an intermittent-motion capsule filling machine simulator. *Pharm Res* 1995; 12: 196–200.

121. Bourland ME, Mullarney MP. Compaction simulation. In: Augsburger LL, Hoag SW, eds. *Pharmaceutical Dosage Forms: Tablets*, 3rd edn. Vol. 1. New York: Informa Healthcare: 519–53.

122. Anuar MS, Briscoe BJ. The elastic relaxation of starch tablets during ejection. *Powder Technol* 2009; 195: 96–104.

123. United States Pharmacopoeia/National Formulary (USP38/NF33). Rockville, Maryland: The United States Pharmacopoeial Convention: 2015.

124. Podczeck F. Methods for the practical determination of the mechanical strength of tablets—From empiricism to science. *Int J Pharm* 2012; 436: 214–32.

125. Barcellos A. Tensile strength of concrete—Correlation between tensile and compressive concrete strength. *RILEM Bull* 1953; 15: 109–13.

126. Carneiro FLL. Tensile strength of concrete—A new method for determining the tensile strength of concretes. *RILEM Bull* 1953; 13: 103–7.

127. Fell JT, Newton JM. The tensile strength of lactose tablets. *J Pharm Pharmacol* 1968; 20: 657–8.

128. Münzel K, Kägi W. Test for the mechanical resistance of tablets (in German). *Pharm Acta Helv* 1957; 32: 305–21.

129. David ST, Augsburger LL. Flexure test for determination of tablet tensile strength. *J Pharm Sci* 1974; 63: 933–6.

130. Pfeifer W, Marquardt G. Investigations of the frequency and causes of dosage deviations during filling of hard gelatin capsules. 1. Dosage deviations during filling of powders and granules into hard gelatin capsules (in German). *Pharm Ind* 1984; 8: 860–3.

131. Bosch Inc. *Digital Slug Tester; Instruction Manual*, 2nd edn. Utah: Robert Bosch Inc., 2010: 5–6.

132. de Blaey CJ, Polderman J. Compression of pharmaceuticals. II: Registration and determination of force–displacement curves, using a small digital computer. *Pharm Weekbl* 1971; 106: 57–65.

133. Ragnarsson G. Force–displacement and network measurements. In: Alderborn G, Nyström C, eds. *Pharmaceutical Powder Compaction Technology*. New York: Marcel Dekker, 1995: 77–97.

134. Tobyn MJ, McCarthy GP, Staniforth JN, Edge S. Physicochemical comparison between microcrystalline cellulose and silicified microcrystalline cellulose. *Int J Pharm* 1998; 169: 183–94.

135. Edge S, Steele DF, Chen A et al. The mechanical properties of compacts of microcrystalline cellulose and silicified microcrystalline cellulose. *Int J Pharm* 2000; 200: 67–72.

136. Fell JT. Compaction properties of binary mixtures. In: Alderborn G, Nyström C, eds. *Pharmaceutical Powder Compaction Technology*. New York: Marcel Dekker, 1995: 501–15.

137. Menard KP. *Dynamic Mechanical Analysis. A Practical Introduction*. Boca Raton: CRC Press, 1999: 2–16.

138. Radebaugh GW, Babu SR, Bondi JN. Characterization of the viscoelastic properties of compacted pharmaceutical powders by a novel non-destructive technique. *Int J Pharm* 1989; 57: 95–105.

139. Hancock BC, Dalton CR, Clas S-D. Micro-scale measurement of the mechanical properties of compressed pharmaceutical powders. 2: The dynamic moduli of microcrystalline cellulose. *Int J Pharm* 2001; 228: 139–45.

140. Lüdde K-H, Kawakita K. Review: Powder compression (in German). *Pharmazie* 1966; 21: 393–403.

141. Sun CC. Cellulose, microcrystalline. In: Rowe RC, Sheskey PJ, Cook WG, Fenton M, eds. *Handbook of Pharmaceutical Excipients*, 7th edn. London: Pharmaceutical Press, 2012: 140–4.

142. Edge S, Kibbe AH, Shur J. Lactose monohydrate. In: Rowe RC, Sheskey PJ, Cook WG, Fenton M, eds. *Handbook of Pharmaceutical Excipients*, 7th edn. London: Pharmaceutical Press, 2012: 415–20.

143. Newton JM, Bader F. The angle of internal flow as an indicator of filling and drug release properties of capsule formulations. *J Pharm Pharmacol* 1987; 39: 164–8.

144. Nikolakakis I, Ballesteros Aragon O, Malamataris S. Resistance to densification, tensile strength and capsule-filling performance of some pharmaceutical diluents. *J Pharm Pharmacol* 1998; 50: 713–21.

145. Mohammadi MS, Harnby N. Bulk density modelling as a means of typifying the microstructure and flow characteristics of cohesive powders. *Powder Technol* 1997; 92: 1–8.

146. Aling J, Podczeck F. The filling of powdered herbs into two-piece hard capsules using hydrogenated cotton seed oil as lubricant. *Eur J Pharm Sci* 2012; 47: 739–51.

147. Kawakita K, Lüdde K-H. Some considerations on powder compression equations. *Powder Technol* 1970/71; 4: 61–8.

148. Hüttenrauch R, Roos W. Influence of density on dosage accuracy of powder mixtures—Introduction of a working density (in German). *Pharmazie* 1970; 25: 259–9.

149. Lordi NG, Cocolas H, Yamasaki H. Analytical interpretation of powder compaction during the loading phase. *Powder Technol* 1997; 90: 173–8.

150. Podczeck F, Lee-Amies G. The bulk volume changes of powders by granulation and compression with respect to capsule filling. *Int J Pharm* 1996; 142: 97–102.

151. European Pharmacopocia (8.5), 8th edn. Strasbourg: European Directorate for the Quality of Medicines and HealthCare, 2015.

152. Yamashiro M, Yuasa Y, Kawakita K. An experimental study on the relationships between compressibility, fluidity and cohesion of powder solids at small tapping numbers. *Powder Technol* 1983; 34: 225–31.

153. Adams MJ, McKeown R. Micromechanical analyses of the pressure–volume relationships for powders under confined uniaxial compression. *Powder Technol* 1996; 88: 155–63.

154. Adams MJ, Mullier MA, Seville JPK. Agglomerate strength measurement using a uniaxial confined compression test. *Powder Technol* 1994; 78: 5–13.

155. Chowhan ZT, Chow YP. Powder flow studies I. Powder consolidation ratio and its relationship to capsule-filling-weight variation. *Int J Pharm* 1980; 4: 317–26.

156. Chowhan ZT, Chow YP. Powder flow studies II. Powder compactibility factor and its relationship to powder flow. *Drug Dev Ind Pharm* 1980; 6: 1–13.

157. Chowhan ZT, Yang I-C. Powder flow studies III. Tensile strength, consolidation ratio, flow rate, and capsule-filling-weight variation relationships. *J Pharm Sci* 1981; 70: 927–30.

158. Heckel RW. Density–pressure relationships in powder compaction. *Trans Metal Soc AIME* 1961; 221: 671–5.

159. Heckel RW. An analysis of powder compaction phenomena. *Trans Metal Soc AIME* 1961; 221: 1001–8.

160. Hersey JA, Rees JE. Deformation of particles during briquetting. *Nature* 1971; 230: 96.

161. Rue J, Rees JE. Limitations of the Heckel relation for predicting powder compaction mechanisms. *J Pharm Pharmacol* 1978; 30: 642–3.

162. York P. A consideration of experimental variables in the analysis of powder compaction behaviour. *J Pharm Pharmacol* 1979; 31: 244–6.

163. Humbert-Dróz P, Gurny R, Mordier D, Doelker E. A quick method for determining compression behaviour in reformulation studies (in French). *Pharm Acta Helv* 1982; 57: 136–43.

164. Paronen P. Using the Heckel equation in the compression studies of pharmaceuticals. *Proc Fourth Int Conf Pharm Technol* 1986; Paris: 301–7.

165. Duberg M, Nyström C. Studies on direct compression of tablets. VI. Evaluation of methods for the estimation of particle fragmentation during compaction. *Acta Pharm Suec* 1982; 19: 421–36.

166. Carstensen JT, Hou X-P. The Athy–Heckel equation applied to granular agglomerates of basic tricalcium phosphate [$3(Ca_3PO_4)_2 \cdot Ca(OH)_2$]. *Powder Technol* 1985; 42: 153–7.

167. Hassanpour A, Ghadiri M. Distinct element analysis and experimental evaluation of the Heckel analysis of bulk powder compression. *Powder Technol* 2004; 141: 251–61.

168. Cooper AR, Eaton LE. Compaction behavior of several ceramic powders. *J Am Ceram Soc* 1962; 45: 97–101.

169. Walker EE. The properties of powders. VI. The compressibility of powders. *Trans Faraday Soc* 1923; 19: 73–82.

170. Sonnergaard JM. Investigation of a new mathematical model for compression of pharmaceutical powders. *Eur J Pharm Sci* 2001; 14: 149–57.

171. Sørensen AH, Sonnergaard JM, Hovgaard L. Bulk characterization of pharmaceutical powders by low-pressure compression. *Pharm Dev Technol* 2005; 10: 197–209.

172. Schmidt PC, Ebel S, Koch H et al. Force and displacement characteristics of rotary tabletting machines. 4. Quantitative evaluation of force–time profiles (in German). *Pharm Ind* 1988; 50: 1409–12.

173. Picker KM. The 3D model: Explaining densification and deformation mechanisms by using 3D parameter plots. *Drug Dev Ind Pharm* 2004; 30: 413–25.

174. Picker-Freyer KM. The 3D–model: Experimental testing of the parameters d, e and ω and validation of the analysis. *J Pharm Sci* 2007; 96: 408–17.

175. Zhu HP, Zhou ZY, Yang RY, Yu AB. Discrete particle simulation of particulate systems: A review of major applications and findings. *Chem Eng Sci* 2008; 63: 5728–70.

176. Martin CL, Bouvard D, Shima S. Study of particle rearrangement during powder compaction by discrete element method. *J Mech Phys Solids* 2003; 51: 667–93.

177. Zavaliangos A. A numerical study of the development of tensile principal stresses during die compression. *Particulate Sci Technol* 2003; 21: 105–15.

178. Procopio AT, Zavaliangos A. Simulation of multi-axial compaction of granular media from loose to high relative densities. *J Mechn Phys Solids* 2005; 53: 1523–51.

179. Jolliffe IG, Newton JM, Walters JK. Theoretical considerations of the filling of pharmaceutical hard gelatin capsules. *Powder Technol* 1980; 27: 189–95.
180. Walker DM. An approximate theory for pressures and arching in hoppers. *Chem Eng Sci* 1966; 21: 975–97.
181. Walters JK. A theoretical analysis of stresses in silos with vertical walls. *Chem Eng Sci* 1973; 28: 13–21.
182. Jolliffe IG, Newton JM. The effect of powder coating on capsule filling with a dosator nozzle. *Acta Pharm Technol* 1980; 26: 324–6.
183. Faulhammer E, Llusa M, Radeke C et al. The effects of material attributes on capsule fill weight and weight variability in dosator nozzle machines. *Int J Pharm* 2014; 471: 332–8.
184. Jolliffe IG, Newton JM. Practical implications of theoretical consideration of capsule filling by the dosator nozzle system. *J Pharm Pharmacol* 1982; 34: 293–8.
185. Jolliffe IG, Newton JM. The effect of dosator nozzle wall texture on capsule filling with the mG2 simulator. *J Pharm Pharmacol* 1983; 35: 7–11.
186. Jolliffe IG, Newton JM. Capsule filling studies using an mG2 production machine. *J Pharm Pharmacol* 1983; 35: 74–8.
187. Jolliffe IG, Newton JM. Extension theoretical considerations of the filling of pharmaceutical hard gelatin capsules to the design of dosator nozzles. *Powder Technol* 1983; 35: 151–7.
188. Tan SB, Newton JM. Minimum compression stress requirements for arching and powder retention within a dosator nozzle during capsule filling. *Int J Pharm* 1990; 63: 275–80.
189. Tan SB, Newton JM. Influence of compression setting ratio on capsule fill weight and weight variability. *Int J Pharm* 1990; 66: 273–82.

10 Modeling Powder Filling during Encapsulation

Ammar Khawam

CONTENTS

INTRODUCTION

Much work has been done to study encapsulation, including machine instrumentation,[1–5] compression analysis,[6–9] formulation requirements,[10–14] powder densification predictions,[15,16] and application of artificial intelligence.[17–20] However, more knowledge about encapsulation is needed, especially in establishing prediction tools that can reduce empiricism in the development of capsule dosage forms. For example, it is often required to estimate fill weights in different capsule sizes, which involves experimental evaluation that is not always possible because of scarcity of active ingredients; especially in early development stages, this gap can be filled by *in silico* prediction tools. Additionally, there is much empiricism in setting parameters during machine operation that can be improved if prediction tools were used. If a Zanasi 40E machine is considered as an example, there are more than 20,000 possible setting combinations for a single powder; prediction tools will narrow the number of settings needed to achieve the desired fill weight, which would reduce resources during machine operation and refine setting selection during a DoE study.[21]

ENCAPSULATION METHODS AND PRINCIPLES

Encapsulation methods can be generally classified into manual, semiautomatic, and automatic.[22,23]

MANUAL AND SEMIAUTOMATIC METHODS

Manual methods involve manually dispensing powder on a dosing tray containing capsule bodies housed within wells, and powder filling occurs volumetrically by spreading powder over capsules. Encapsulation fill weight is controlled by the amount of powder added into the tray and the extent of tapping performed. Semiautomatic methods resemble manual ones except that powder is delivered by vibration or by a rotating auger to a filling ring containing empty capsules, and the rate of powder flow and ring speed control the encapsulation fill weight.[22]

AUTOMATIC METHODS

Unlike manual filled capsules, automatic machines usually produce compacts (i.e., plugs or slugs) rather than loose fills (Figure 10.1). Automatic machines have two dosing principles, dosing disc and dosator. Dosing disc-based machines, also called tamping machines, include Bosch GKF, Höfliger-Karg, and Harro-Höfliger KFM encapsulation machines. The dosing disc is a perforated circular

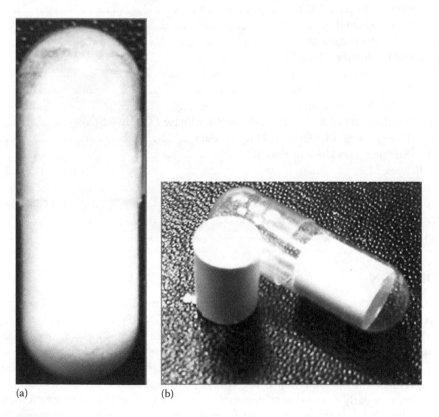

(a)   (b)

FIGURE 10.1   Capsules produced from two encapsulation methods: (a) manual filling (loose powder); (b) automatic machine (plug).

disc that rotates over a brass support ring.[1] A constant powder level is maintained above the dosing disc; the dosing disc consists of three to five tamping stations and a single ejection station. Tamping stations consist of cavities formed between the dosing disc and the brass support ring similar to a die cavity on a tablet press. The powder in the dosing disc fills the cavity, and a spring-controlled piston compresses the powder into plugs. These topics have been discussed in more detail in Chapter 6.

Machines having five tamping stations (Bosch GKF and Höfliger-Karg machines) compress the powder once at each station while those containing three tamping stations (Harro-Höfliger KFM machines) compress the powder twice at each station. After tamping, the dosing disc moves to the ejection station and a piston ejects the powder plug into an empty capsule body.[22,23]

Dosator-based machines, which are represented by the Zanasi and MG2, use a dosator for dosing powders. A dosator is a hollow cylinder containing a spring-controlled moving piston. Filling occurs when a dosator is immersed into a uniform powder bed, and a plug is then formed when the powder is densified by the piston. Plugs are then ejected into capsule bodies.

MODELING/POWDER FILL ESTIMATION DURING ENCAPSULATION

It is important to predict the amount of powder that can be filled into a capsule or the maximum fill a certain capsule size can hold. This information will affect capsule size selection, number of capsules to be administered per dose, and the processing method to be pursued.

ESTIMATIONS IN MANUAL CAPSULE FILLING

Traditionally, encapsulation fill weight is estimated according to Equation 10.1:

$$W = V \times \rho, \qquad (10.1)$$

where W is the fill weight, V is the capsule body volume, and ρ is the powder density.

Capsule volumes and dimensions are provided by capsule vendors for different capsule sizes[24] and are discussed in more detail in Chapter 2. The density term in Equation 10.1 could be either the bulk or the tapped density, but the tapped density is often used since the maximum fill weight of a capsule is usually targeted. Equation 10.1 is helpful in predicting fill weights of manually filled capsules and, to some extent, capsules filled by tamping (i.e., dosing disc).

Predictions do not necessarily correlate to dosator-based filling machines, because powders pack differently in dosators compared to capsule bodies. Therefore, a separate equation is required to make predictions in dosator-based machines. Failure of Equation 10.1 in making accurate predictions in dosator-based machines is further depicted in the case study below.

The Need for a Dosator-Based Model—A Case Study

BI 671800 ED is an investigational new pulmonary drug developed as a 100-mg capsule dosage form (200 mg fill weight) that was hand-filled into size 1 capsules. A 200-mg strength (400 mg fill weight) of the same common blend was to be developed using a capsule no larger than size "0EL." Both strengths were needed for Phase II clinical studies and were to be manufactured by a dosator-based encapsulation machine. The key challenge for the higher-strength development was that the fill weight was to be doubled without doubling the capsule volume (capsule body volume = 0.50 mL and 0.78 mL for size 1 and 0EL capsules, respectively).

The bulk and tapped powder densities of the BI 671800 ED powder blend (0.37 and 0.61 g/mL, respectively) were used according to Equation 10.1 to estimate fill weights in different sized capsules. According to these estimates (Table 10.1), encapsulating 400 mg of the powder blend (200 mg strength) in a size 0EL capsule was feasible since up to 476 mg of powder can be filled in a size 0EL capsule.

TABLE 10.1

Predicted Encapsulation Weights of BI 671800 ED Powder Using Equation 10.1

Capsule Size	Capsule Body Volume (mL)[a]	Predicted Fill Weight (mg) Based On	
		$\rho_{(Bulk)}$	$\rho_{(Tap)}$
00EL	1.02	377	622
00	0.91	337	555
0EL	0.78	289	476
0	0.68	252	415
1 EL	0.54	200	329
1	0.50	185	305
2 EL	0.41	152	250
2	0.37	137	226
3	0.30	111	183
4	0.21	78	128
5	0.13	48	79

[a] Based on Capsugel Coni-Snap capsules.

Hand-filling experiments confirmed the estimates and demonstrated that 400 mg of the BI 671800 ED powder blend could be hand-filled into a size 0EL capsule after tapping. Encapsulation attempts using a dosator-based automatic filling machine (Zanasi 6F) were successful for the 100-mg strength (200 mg fill weight) in size 1 capsules, but not the 200-mg strength (400 mg fill weight), which could not be encapsulated in a capsule smaller than size "00." The maximum fill weight that could be encapsulated in a size 0EL capsule using the Zanasi 6F was 380 mg, which is significantly different from the 476-mg fill weight predicted by Equation 10.1 (Table 10.1). This shows that Equation 10.1 is not an accurate predictor of fill weight in dosator-based machines and that a separate equation or model is needed for such machines.

ESTIMATIONS IN DOSATOR-BASED CAPSULE MACHINES

Many dosator-based machines have the same dosing principle but differ in some of the operational details. This section will describe dosator machines based on a Zanasi-type machine; differences between the Zanasi and other encapsulation machines are further described in the "Machine Differences" section.

A dosator is a hollow cylinder (i.e., dosing tube) containing a spring-controlled moving piston (Figure 10.2). In dosator-based machines, dosing occurs through three sequential stages: First, the powder bowl is filled and uniformly leveled to form a powder bed; then, the target dose is filled into the dosator and densified into a plug. Finally, the plug is ejected from the dosator into the capsule body; these steps are discussed in more detail in Chapter 6. Powder densification within a dosator is necessary to achieve a powder arch strong enough to support the powder's weight and keep it in the dosator during transfer between dosing and ejection stations. Unlike dosing discs that involve multiple steps, filling and densification in dosator-based machines occur in a single step.

Starting from Equation 10.1, the volume and density terms are modified to account for a cylindrical body (i.e., dosator) as follows:

$$W = \left(\left(\frac{D_{piston}}{2} \right)^2 \pi \times H_{dosator} \right) \times \left(\rho_{bulk} \times f_1(\rho) \right), \qquad (10.2)$$

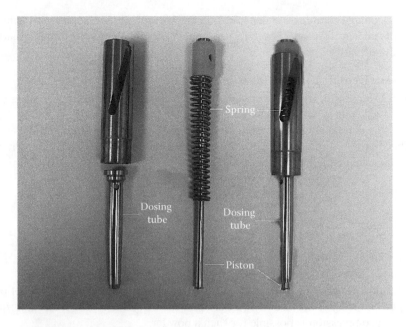

FIGURE 10.2 Composition of a dosator.

where W is the dosator fill weight, D_{piston} is the piston diameter, $H_{dosator}$ is the powder height in dosator, ρ_{bulk} is the bulk powder density, and $f_1(\rho)$ is the precompression densification factor.

The first term in Equation 10.2 represents the volume of a cylinder. Piston widths vary for each capsule size; they can be directly measured or provided by machine vendors. Powder height in a dosator ($H_{dosator}$) is the minimum value of either the powder bed height (H_{powder}) or the piston height (H_{piston}) as shown in Equation 10.3:

$$H_{dosator} = Min(H_{piston}, H_{powder})\qquad(10.3)$$

where H_{powder} is the powder bed height and H_{piston} is the piston height in the dosator tube.

The second term in Equation 10.2 is related to powder density inside the dosator. This density is defined by the bulk powder density (bulk density of powder in the bowl) multiplied by a factor representing the extent of densification a powder is subjected to as a result of dosator immersion. This is one of two types of powder densifications achieved in a dosator.

Powder Densification inside a Dosator

Powder densification within a dosator is required for two reasons: first, densification helps form arches that support the powder's weight and keep it in the dosator.[25] Densification is also needed to fit a plug into the capsule body. There are two types of densification within a dosator: precompression and compression. The powder density within a dosator ($\rho_{dosator}$) is a cumulative value from both types as shown in Equation 10.4:

$$\rho_{dosator} = \rho_{bulk} \times f_1(\rho) \times f_2(\rho),\qquad(10.4)$$

where $\rho_{dosator}$ is the powder density within the dosator, ρ_{bulk} is the bulk powder density, $f_1(\rho)$ is the precompression densification factor, and $f_2(\rho)$ is the compression densification factor.

Precompression and compression densification factors are unitless factors with values ≥ 1, where unity represents no densification. If both factors equal unity, the density within a dosator reduces to the bulk powder density.

Precompression Densification Factor ($f_1(\rho)$)

The precompression densification factor reflects densification that occurs during dosator insertion into the powder bed when the powder height is more than the piston height ($H_{powder} > H_{piston}$). The extent of precompression densification is determined by the powder-to-piston height ratio and powder flow behavior. The more fluid the powder, the less the precompression densification. Precompression densification factor is defined by Equation 10.5:

$$f_1(\rho) = \left((1-F) \ln \frac{H_{powder}}{H_{piston}} \right) + 1 , \tag{10.5}$$

where $f_1(\rho)$ is the precompression densification factor, F is the powder flow factor, H_{powder} is the powder height in the powder bowl, and H_{piston} is the piston height.

The powder flow factor (F) in Equation 10.5 is a unitless factor that is indicative of powder flow; it has an upper boundary limit of unity. A fluid powder will have a flow factor and $f_1(\rho)$ of unity, indicating no precompression is possible for such a powder.

Compression Densification Factor ($f_2(\rho)$)

Compression densification occurs from piston displacement against the powder after the dosator is immersed in the powder bed. This factor is defined by Equation 10.6:

$$f_2(\rho) = \frac{H_{dosator}}{H_{plug}} , \tag{10.6}$$

where $f_2(\rho)$ is the compression densification factor, $H_{dosator}$ is the powder height in the dosator (Equation 10.3), and H_{plug} is the plug height.

The plug height represents the powder height reached within the dosator as a result of piston displacement (ΔH):

$$H_{plug} = H_{dosator} - \Delta H , \tag{10.7}$$

where $H_{dosator}$ is the powder height in the dosator (Equation 10.3) and ΔH is the piston displacement against powder (i.e., distance a piston moves against powder).

The actual plug heights are expected to be slightly larger than those predicted by Equation 10.7 because of plug expansion after ejection. The plug height (H_{plug}) is an important parameter to control during encapsulation; it should be equal to or less than the effective capsule body length (h_{Caps}; Figure 10.3), which can be calculated using Equation 10.8:

$$h_{Caps} = h_0 + (h_1 - h_2), \tag{10.8}$$

where h_{Caps} is the effective capsule body length, h_0 is the length of the cylindrical portion of the capsule body, h_1 is the length of the spherical portion of the capsule body, and h_2 is the length of dead space.

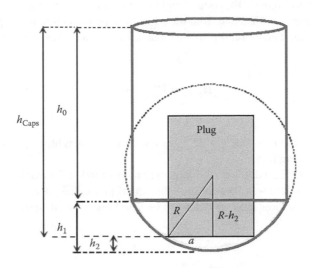

FIGURE 10.3   Schematic presentation of a plug inside the capsule body.

The effective capsule body length is higher than the cylindrical capsule body length because plugs have a smaller diameter than capsule bodies; therefore, the plug sinks in the spherical portion of the capsule body as shown in Figure 10.3. The effective capsule body length (h_{Caps}) would equal the cylindrical length of the capsule body (h_0) if the plug and capsule body widths were equal. The length of the dead space within a capsule is calculated using Equation 10.9:

$$h_2 = R - \sqrt{R^2 - a^2},\tag{10.9}$$

where R is the cup radius (i.e., radius of the spherical segment) and a is the plug radius.

The dead space represents the space where no fill is present. Values for h_0, h_1, and R are obtained from capsule specifications provided by capsule vendors.

PISTON MOVEMENT WITHIN A DOSATOR

Piston movement within a dosator is affected by two constraints: the spring and the powder.

The Spring Factor

At the maximum piston height, the spring within the dosator is at the most relaxed position; lowering the piston height in the dosator tube will involve spring compression. The actual height achieved is different from that set depending on the spring factor (k) as shown below:

$$k = \frac{\Delta H_0}{H_{com}},\tag{10.10}$$

where k is the spring factor, H_{com} is the set piston displacement, and ΔH_0 is the achieved piston displacement in an empty bowl.

The spring factor is a unitless number that is unique to that spring. If $k = 1$, then both set and achieved displacement values would be equal ($\Delta H_0 = H_{com}$).

According to Figure 10.4, piston height (distance from the open end of a dosator to the piston tip) and its displacement (distance from the maximum piston height to the piston tip) are determined by the same spring, Therefore, the actual distance a piston moves is given by

$$H_{\text{piston}} = H_{\text{piston}}^{\text{max}} - \left(k \left(H_{\text{piston}}^{\text{max}} - H_{\text{piston}}^{\text{set}} \right) \right), \tag{10.11}$$

where H_{piston} is the piston height, $H_{\text{piston}}^{\text{set}}$ is the set piston height, $H_{\text{piston}}^{\text{max}}$ is the maximum piston height, and k is the spring factor.

For example, for a dosator with a spring factor of 0.9 and a maximum piston height of 26 mm, if the set piston height was 16 mm, then the actual piston height would be 17 mm. This is important because it affects how much powder can be filled inside the dosator according to Equation 10.2.

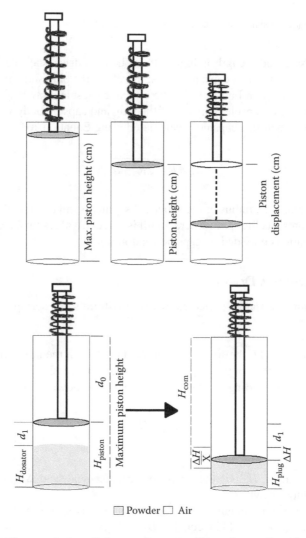

FIGURE 10.4   Schematic presentation of piston movement within a dosator (based on Zanasi machines).

Powder Compressibility

In addition to spring properties, the actual displacement achieved for a set value will depend on the compression resistance exhibited by the powder being compressed. Different powders have different compression properties; thus, achieved piston displacements will differ accordingly.

In the presence of powder, the actual distance traveled by the piston (i.e., piston displacement against powder) is related to the set value through the powder compression factor (X) as shown in Equation 10.12:

$$X = \frac{\Delta H}{H_{com}}, \tag{10.12}$$

where X is the powder compression factor, H_{com} is the set piston displacement, and ΔH is the achieved piston displacement against powder.

The powder compression factor is a unitless factor that is similar to the spring factor derived in Equation 10.10, except that it is measured in the presence of powder when the piston and powder heights are set to the maximum value $\left(H_{powder} = H_{piston} = H_{piston}^{max} \right)$.[25]

The powder compression factor (X) $\leq$ spring factor (k) because it accounts for the cumulative resistance to piston movement from both the spring and powder.

Equation 10.12 can be rearranged as

$$\Delta H = H_{com} X. \tag{10.13}$$

The more compressible the powder (i.e., higher X), the higher the actual piston displacement will be for a set compression. Equation 10.13 is a special case $\left(H_{powder} = H_{piston} = H_{piston}^{max} \right)$ of a general equation (Equation 10.14):

$$\Delta H = \left[H_{com} - (d_0 + d_1) \right] X, \tag{10.14}$$

where H_{com} is the set piston displacement, d_0 is the starting point of displacement, d_1 is the piston displacement against air, and X is the powder compression factor.

If the piston height and piston displacement settings are opposite settings controlled by the same spring (Figure 10.4), then the starting point of displacement (d_0) represents the value below which no piston displacement occurs. The value of d_0 depends on the difference between the maximum achievable piston height and set piston height according to Equation 10.15:

$$d_0 = \left(H_{piston}^{max} - H_{piston} \right), \tag{10.15}$$

where H_{piston}^{max} is the maximum piston height and H_{piston} is the piston height determined from Equation 10.11.

Piston displacement against air (d_1) represents the distance a piston moves within the dosator before contacting the powder (Figure 10.4); this occurs when the piston height is more than the powder height ($H_{piston} > H_{powder}$) as shown in Equation 10.16:

$$d_1 = \frac{(H_{piston} - H_{powder})}{k}, \tag{10.16}$$

where H_{piston} is the piston height determined from Equation 10.11, H_{powder} is the powder height in the powder bowl, and k is the spring factor.

For any densification to occur from piston displacement, the piston displacement setting (H_{com}) should exceed $d_0 + d_1$.

Equation 10.14 is important as it relates the set piston displacement (H_{com}) to that achieved against powder (ΔH), which is needed to calculate the plug height (i.e., plug length) according to Equation 10.7.

SUMMARY OF MODEL PARAMETERS

Equations 10.2 and 10.7 are the equations needed to predict the two measurable outcomes of encapsulation: fill weight (Equation 10.2) and plug length (Equation 10.7). Parameters in these equations can be classified as

1. Machine-programmable: H_{powder}, H_{piston}, H_{com}
2. Machine-specific: k, D_{piston}, H_{piston}^{max}
3. Powder-specific: ρ_{bulk}, F, X

Machine-programmable parameters consist of the three parameters that control encapsulation outcomes in dosator-based machines; these parameters are set by the operator during encapsulation. Machine-specific parameters are dependent on the machine and/or desired capsule size to be used during encapsulation. These parameters need to be determined for the specific machine before encapsulation. Table 10.2 lists some parameters for two common machines made by MG2 and IMA; these parameters are usually shared among different machines produced by the same manufacturer. Finally, powder-specific parameters are powder dependent and need to be determined for each powder before encapsulation.

EXPERIMENTAL EVALUATION OF THE MODEL

The model was experimentally evaluated using two formulations.[26] Comparisons of predicted and experimentally achieved results for both powders showed a high correlation for both the fill weight

TABLE 10.2

Machine-Specific Parameters of the IMA Zanasi 40E and MG2 Futura Encapsulation Machines

	Piston Diameter, D_{piston} (mm)	
Capsule Size	IMA Zanasi 40E	MG2 Futura
000	–	8.55
00 and 00EL	7.2	7.15
0 and 0EL	6.4	6.15
1 and 1 EL	5.7	5.55
2 and 2 EL	5.2	5.05
3	4.7	4.55
4	4.3	3.85
5	3.9	3.55
H_{piston} (mm)	3a–26	2–35
H_{powder} (mm)	15–50	8–55

a   Minimum piston height depends on spring factor (k) and set piston height value according to Equation 10.11. For a spring factor of 0.9 and a piston height set at the minimum value, the actual achieved piston height is 3 mm.

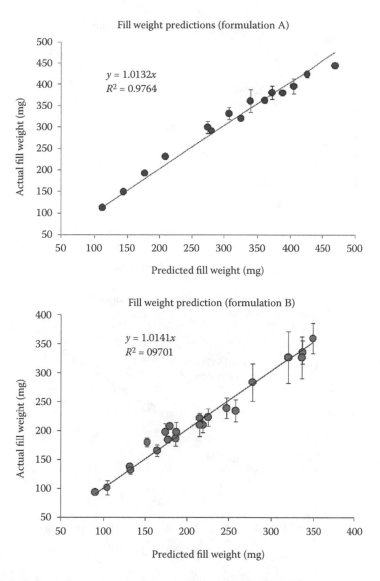

FIGURE 10.5 Comparison of experimentally achieved and model predicted fill weights for two powder formulations. (Data in this figure combined compression and precompression densification results shown in Figures 5 and 6 of Reference 26.)

(Figure 10.5) and plug height (Figure 10.6). This correlation suggests that the model successfully predicted encapsulation outcomes for both powders.

Machine Differences

The model discussed above was developed based on the IMA Zanasi 6F encapsulation machine. There are two main suppliers of dosator-based machines: IMA and MG2 (although Harro-Höfliger recently introduced a dosator-based machine in their production line). Machines produced by these companies share the same dosing principle; however, there are operational differences that could affect the encapsulation model for each machine.

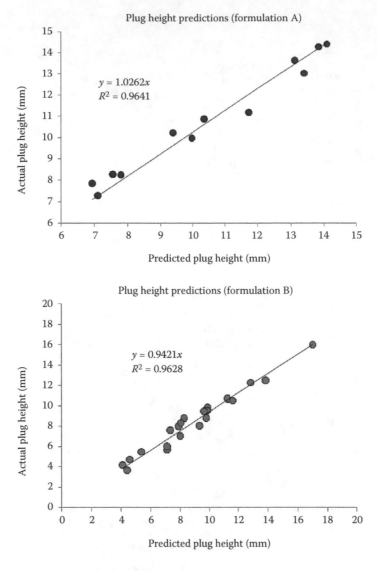

FIGURE 10.6 Comparison of experimentally achieved and model predicted plug lengths for two powder formulations. (Data in this figure combined compression and precompression densification results shown in Figures 7 and 8 of Reference 26.)

Figure 10.7 shows the dosing steps in two machines: IMA Zanasi (Figure 10.7a) and MG2 (Figure 10.7b). For the Zanasi machine, the piston height is adjusted from its maximum value (steps I and II; Figure 10.7a), after which the dosator is immersed into the powder bed (step III; Figure 10.7a) followed by powder compression (step IV; Figure 10.7a).

For MG2 machines, the piston is moved within the dosator from its maximum height (step I; Figure 10.7b) to the tip of the dosator opening above the maximum powder height level of the bowl (step II; Figure 10.7b). The dosator tube but not the piston is then immersed into the powder bed by a lowering cam (Figure 10.8) until the set piston height is achieved (step III; Figure 10.7b); this movement resembles a syringe when the syringe barrel is moved while holding the plunger in place. After the piston height is reached, both the dosator and piston are lowered into the full bowl depth

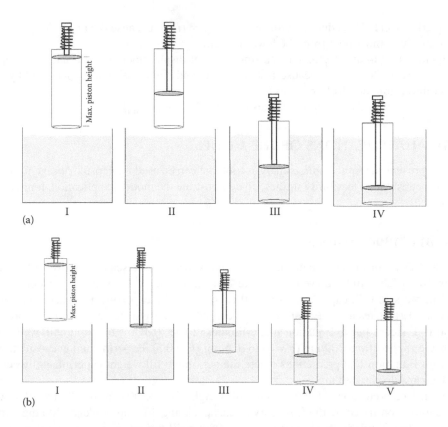

FIGURE 10.7   Powder dosing in two different dosator-type machines: (a) Zanasi; (b) MG2.

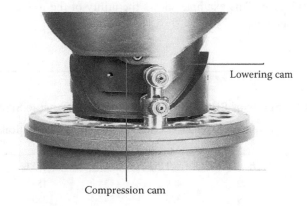

FIGURE 10.8   Lowering and compression cams used in an MG2 machine. (Courtesy of MG2 America.)

maintaining the piston height (step IV; Figure 10.7b). Finally, the powder is compressed within the dosator by piston movement (step V; Figure 10.7b) as a result of a compression cam (Figure 10.8). Consequently, the following equations are affected for MG2 machines:

- Equation 10.10: The spring factor (k) is no longer significant in determining piston displacement as it is related to the depth of the compression cam. Therefore, the spring factor reduces to unity.

- Equation 10.11: This equation reduces to $H_{piston} = H_{piston}^{set}$ because the piston height is set by dosator wall movement from the lowering cam.
- Equations 10.14 and 10.15: The starting point of displacement (d_0) in machines depicted by Figure 10.7b is zero because piston heights and compression are controlled by cams; therefore, Equation 10.14 reduces to $\Delta H = [H_{com} - d_1] X$.
- Equation 10.16: The equation reduces to $d_1 = (H_{piston} - H_{powder})$.

PRACTICAL APPLICATIONS OF THE MODEL

The model presents a useful *in silico* analysis tool that can be used for capsule dosage form development and encapsulation feasibility studies. To demonstrate the model's application, four case studies are discussed.

CASE I—BI 671800 DEVELOPMENT

BI 671800 ED is an investigational new pulmonary drug. As discussed above, estimates using Equation 10.1 (Table 10.1) showed that up to 476 mg of the BI 671800 ED powder blend could be filled into a size 0EL capsule; however, this could not be experimentally achieved on a dosator machine. Estimates using Equation 10.2 were substantially different from those predicted by Equation 10.1. According to Equation 10.2 estimates (Table 10.3), the maximum fill weight in a size 0EL capsule ranged from 309 mg ($F = 1$) to 376 mg ($F = 0.5$). Experimental encapsulation results agreed with Equation 10.2 predictions where the maximum fill weight experimentally achieved in a size 0EL capsule was 380 mg.

Equation 10.2 predictions of 392–476 mg fill weights in size 00 capsules (Table 10.3) were also experimentally confirmed by the feasibility of encapsulating 400 mg of blend (200 mg strength) in size 00 capsules. Similarly, predictions of 245–298 mg fill weights in size 1 capsules (Table 10.3) were confirmed experimentally by the feasibility of encapsulating 200 mg of powder blend (100 mg strength) in that capsule size. This example shows the utility of the model as a prediction tool in early formulation development.

TABLE 10.3

Fill Weight Estimates of BI 671800 ED in Different Capsule Sizes

Capsule Size[a]	Predicted Maximum Fill Weights[b,c] at Different Theoretical Flow Factors, $\rho_{Bulk} = 0.37$ g/mL (mg)				
	$F = 1$	$F = 0.9$	$F = 0.75$	$F = 0.6$	$F = 0.5$
00 and 00EL	392	409	434	459	476
0 and 0EL	309	323	343	363	376
1 and 1 EL	245	256	272	288	298
2 and 2 EL	204	213	226	240	248
3	167	174	185	196	203
4	140	146	155	164	170
5	115	120	127	135	140

[a] Based on Capsugel Coni-Snap capsules.

[b] Maximum fill weights were calculated according to Equation 10.2 using the maximum H_{piston} and H_{powder} values.

[c] Numbers represent the predicted powder weights within a dosator. Further densification of this powder might be needed to fit it into the capsule body.

TABLE 10.4

Fill Weight Estimates of a New Drug Product in Size 00 Capsules

	Predicted Fill Weight at Different Theoretical Flow Factors, ρ_{Bulk} = 0.25 g/mL (mg)									
	F = 1		F = 0.9		F = 0.75		F = 0.6		F = 0.5	
Machine	Min[a]	Max[b,c]	Min[a]	Max[b,c]	Min[a]	Max[b,c]	Min[a]	Max[b,c]	Min[a]	Max[b,c]
Zanasi 40E	31	265	35	282	43	308	50	334	55	351
MG2 Futura	20	351	23	367	27	391	31	415	34	431

[a] Minimum fill weights were calculated according to Equation 10.2 using the minimum H_{piston} and H_{powder} values.

[b] Maximum fill weights were calculated according to Equation 10.2 using the maximum H_{piston} and H_{powder} values.

[c] Numbers represent the predicted powder weights within a dosator. Further densification of this powder might be needed to fit it into the capsule body.

CASE II—DEVELOPMENT OF A NEW DRUG PRODUCT FOR PHASE I CLINICAL STUDIES

An active formulation of a new drug product was to be developed as a capsule dosage form to supply phase I clinical studies. An encapsulation feasibility assessment was needed to determine the minimum and maximum fill weights that can be encapsulated in a size 00 capsule on two available machines; MG2 Futura and Zanasi 40E. The required powder fill weight for the highest strength was 400 mg, and the bulk density of the final blend was 0.25 g/mL. Fill weights lower than 400 mg were needed to supply lower-strength capsules through a common blend approach. Using parameters in Table 10.2, fill weights were calculated using Equation 10.2 for the two encapsulation machines. Prediction results (Table 10.4) are shown for flow factors ranging from 0.5 (poor flow) to 1.0 (good flow).

a. For a freely flowing powder ($F = 1$): The minimum fill weight is estimated to be about 20 mg for an MG2 Futura and 31 mg for a Zanasi 40E; these weights increase to 34 and 55 for a poorly flowing powder ($F = 0.5$). Therefore, one-tenth the maximum strength (40 mg fill weight) can be filled on the MG2 machine and one-seventh (60 mg fill weight) of that can be filled on the Zanasi 40E.

b. A target fill weight of 400 mg could be achieved on the MG2, but only if the powder blend had poor flow characterized by a flow factor (F) less than 0.7; this would be a risk factor that needs to be considered if a capsule dosage form is to be developed.

Based on costs and risks involved, a decision was made to develop this drug product as a tablet dosage form rather than as a capsule dosage form.

CASE III—DEVELOPMENT OF A GENERIC DRUG PRODUCT

A generic drug product was to be developed as a capsule dosage form. Two strengths using a common blend having a bulk density of 0.61 g/mL were to be developed as follows:

a. 250 mg strength (300 mg fill weight) in a size 2 capsule

b. 500 mg strength (600 mg fill weight) in a size 0 capsule

An encapsulation feasibility study on the MG2 Futura was performed to assess the encapsulation process. Using parameters in Table 10.2, the fill weight was calculated using Equation 10.2 on the MG2 encapsulation machine. Results (Table 10.5) are shown for flow factors ranging from 0.5 (poor flow) to 1.0 (good flow).

TABLE 10.5
Fill Weight Estimates of a Generic Drug Product in Different Capsule Sizes

Capsule Size[a]	Predicted Maximum Fill Weights[b,c] at Different Theoretical Flow Factors $\rho_{Bulk} = 0.61$ g/mL (mg)				
	F = 1	F = 0.9	F = 0.75	F = 0.6	F = 0.5
00	857	896	954	1012	1051
0	634	663	706	749	778
1	517	540	575	610	633
2	428	447	476	505	524
3	347	363	386	410	426
4	249	260	277	293	305
5	211	221	235	250	259

[a] Based on Capsugel Coni-Snap capsules.
[b] Maximum fill weights were calculated according to Equation 10.2 using the maximum H_{piston} and H_{powder} values.
[c] Numbers represent the predicted powder weights within a dosator. Further densification of this powder might be needed to fit it into the capsule body.

Results show that both strengths can be encapsulated in the desired capsule size, even at the highest F factor. For example, the 500-mg strength with a target fill weight of 600 mg can be encapsulated in the size 0 capsule, which has a maximum predicted fill weight range of 634 mg ($F = 1.0$) to 778 mg ($F = 0.5$). Similarly, the 250-mg strength (target fill weight of 300 mg) can be encapsulated in the desired size 2 capsule, which has a maximum predicted fill weight range of 428 mg ($F = 1.0$) to 524 mg ($F = 0.5$). Predictions also showed that a size 3 capsule can be used to fill the 250-mg strength (300 mg fill weight) where the maximum predicted fill weight range at that size is 347 mg ($F = 1.0$) to 426 mg ($F = 0.5$). However, densification requirements of the bulk powder (Table 10.6)

TABLE 10.6
Powder Density and Minimum Densification Required to Fill Two Strengths of a Generic Drug Powder in Different-Sized Capsule Bodies

Capsule Size[a]	250 mg Strength (300 mg Fill Weight)		500 mg Strength (600 mg Fill Weight)	
	Powder Density[b] within Capsule Body (g/mL)	Minimum Powder Densification[c] Needed to Achieve Fill Weight (%)	Powder Density[b] within Capsule Body (g/mL)	Minimum Powder Densification[c] Needed to Achieve Fill Weight (%)
00	0.37	0	0.73	20
0	0.54	0	1.08	77
1	0.74	21	1.47	141
2	0.97	58	1.93	217
3	1.33	118	2.66	337
4	2.05	235	4.09	571
5	3.20	424	6.39	948

[a] Based on Capsugel Coni-Snap capsules.
[b] Powder density calculated according to effective capsule body length given by Equation 10.8.
[c] Values represent the densification required of the bulk powder with a bulk density of 0.61 g/mL and assuming a powder flow factor (F) = 0.75.

show that if the final blend is to be filled into a size 2 capsule, the powder density needs to be increased from 0.61 g/mL (i.e., bulk powder density) to 0.97 g/mL to fit in a size 2 capsule (equivalent to about 58% densification), and to a density of 1.33 g/mL (118% densification) to be filled in a size 3 capsule. This is a high densification that might not be reliably achieved on a capsule machine; as a result, a size 2 capsule was used for the 250-mg strength.

CASE IV—STICKING ONTO DOSATOR PINS

A new orally administered antitumor drug was developed as a capsule dosage form. A 600-mg powder (bulk powder density = 0.58 g/mL) was filled into a size 00 capsule.

Encapsulation runs on the Zanasi 48E showed significant powder sticking onto dosator pins.

Sticking was studied by simulating plug formation using a mechanical material tester (Instron Universal Tester) and measuring forces required to eject these plugs. In these experiments, plugs were formed from active powder formulations using an Instron material testing system with a 7-mm flat-faced punch at several compression forces ranging from 50 to 500 N at a 2-s dwell time. After compression, a second compression cycle was performed at a constant force of 50 N to eject the compact (i.e., plug) and the ejection force was recorded. The plug weight and length were measured after ejection and the plug density was calculated (Table 10.7). The normalized ejection force (i.e., ejection force divided by plug height) was plotted against plug density as shown in Figure 10.9. Results showed that a higher ejection force (i.e., higher sticking) was observed as a function of plug density. According to Figure 10.9, sticking could be reduced by reducing plug densification.

An investigation of encapsulation parameters showed that powder densification in the dosator ($\rho_{dosator}$) was about 0.98 g/mL and the plug length (H_{plug}) was 14.8 mm, which was significantly less than the effective capsule body length for that capsule size (18.2; Table 10.8). Two settings were proposed (Table 10.8) to decrease powder sticking. Experimentally, both settings showed a significant decrease in sticking tendency. However, the process change was not a permanent resolution to the sticking issue observed since new lots of API had significantly smaller particles and showed increased sticking, which was remedied by a formulation change.

TABLE 10.7
Plug Characteristics of a New Orally Administered Antitumor Drug Produced Using an Instron Mechanical Material Tester

| Compression Force (N) | Plug Dimensions[a] | | | | Ejection Force (N) | Normalized Ejection Force (N/mm) |
	Length (mm)	Weight (mg)	Volume (mL)	Density (g/mL)		
500	6.44	260	0.248	1.05	30	4.66
500	7.58	300.8	0.292	1.03	18.3	2.41
400	6.81	267	0.262	1.02	15	2.20
400	6.86	269	0.264	1.02	16	2.33
300	6.32	241.6	0.243	0.99	7.2	1.14
300	7.49	289.5	0.288	1.01	5.1	0.68
250	7.46	279.2	0.287	0.97	4.5	0.60
250	7.32	273.5	0.282	0.97	4.4	0.60

[a] Plugs produced at compression forces below 250 N were too soft to give reliable ejection force values.

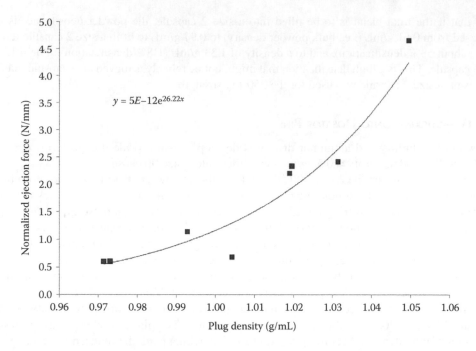

FIGURE 10.9 Normalized ejection forces of plugs of an active anticancer drug formulation as a function of plug density.

TABLE 10.8

Densification Parameters of an Orally Administered Antitumor Drug Using an IMA Zanasi 48E Encapsulation Machine

Parameter	Original Setting	Proposed Setting 1	Proposed Setting 2
$\rho_{dosator}$ (g/mL)	0.98	0.80	0.72
H_{plug} (mm)	14.8	18.2	20.2
Capsule size	00	00	00EL
Effective capsule body length, h_{Caps} (mm)[a]	18.2	18.2	20.2

[a] Calculated according to Equation 10.8 based on Capsugel Coni-Snap capsules.

MODEL CHALLENGES

The model is a useful tool during development and manufacturing of capsules; however, like any model, it is based on assumptions and has its application challenges. The main challenge is that powder-specific parameters such as powder flow (F) and compression (X) factors need to be experimentally measured for each powder for accurate predictions; the measurement process was discussed earlier[26] and involves experimental runs on the encapsulation machine. It would be beneficial if these parameters were deduced from other material properties (i.e., Carr index, flow functions, or Heckel compressibility parameters); extensive testing of several powder formulations would be required to show if such a relationship exists.

One of the main assumptions in the model involves the density term in Equation 10.2. It is assumed that the powder bed density and bulk powder density are equal. This is a reasonable assumption but deviations could be observed if the powder bed density changes during operation. These changes could be attributed to many factors including: machine type, speed effects, and encapsulation settings.

SPEED EFFECTS

Encapsulation speed can affect the powder density within the bowl if it causes significant vibrations that compact the powder. In this case, Equation 10.2 will underpredict the fill weight because the actual powder density within the powder bed is higher than the bulk powder density. This was observed on the Zanasi 6F machine where the intermittent motion at higher speeds caused significant tapping of the powder inside the powder bed. Figure 10.10 shows the encapsulation fill weight of a placebo formulation (Formulation A[26]) encapsulated at two speeds (30 and 100 capsules per hour) using the settings in Table 10.9. Results (Figure 10.10) show that fill weights were higher at high speeds for all tested settings. Fill weight predictions from Equation 10.2 were closer to weights obtained at lower speeds (30 CPH) compared to those at higher speeds (100 CPH). Further experiments conducted at different speeds for a single setting (Setting 6; Table 10.9) confirmed this trend as shown in Figure 10.11.

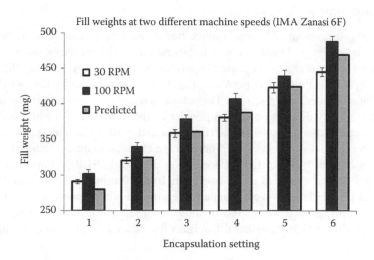

FIGURE 10.10 Predicted and actual fill weights of a placebo formulation at two different encapsulation speeds.

TABLE 10.9
Encapsulation Settings Used to Encapsulate a Placebo Formulation at Two Different Speeds

Setting	H_{powder} (mm)	H_{piston}^{set} (mm)	H_{com} (mm)
1	15.5	17	23
2	18	18	18
3	20	20	18
4	21.5	22	18
5	23.5	25	19.5
6	26	26	18

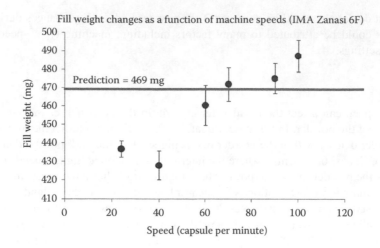

FIGURE 10.11   Fill weight variation of a placebo formulation as a function of encapsulation speed.

INDUCED DENSIFICATION OF POWDER BED

Powder bed height adjustment order can induce bed densification if heights are set from higher to lower values; the extent of densification will depend on the difference between the two powder height values. Densification occurs because the leveled powder already forming the powder bed is not emptied or replenished with new powder but is further compacted by the powder leveler as a response to the new powder height setting. This causes a temporary increase in the fill weight. The fill weight will gradually decrease once the powder in the bowl is replenished with new powder throughout the encapsulation process. In such cases, Equation 10.2 will underpredict the fill weight.

This issue can be avoided if powder bed heights are changed in an ascending manner. Induced densification was observed during the encapsulation of Avicel PH-105 (Formulation B[26]) where the powder height setting was reduced in two cases from 20 mm to 12 mm and 15 mm, respectively (piston and powder heights were equated to eliminate precompression effects). Fill weights achieved at these settings were compared to those achieved at the same settings but with fresh powder. Results (Figure 10.12) show that fill weights for induced densification settings were higher

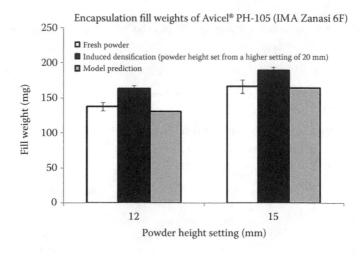

FIGURE 10.12   Effect of induced powder bed densification on encapsulation fill weights of Avicel PH-105 using the IMA Zanasi 6F.

than those predicted and experimentally achieved when a fresh powder was used. Predictions were closer to results obtained using the fresh powder as shown in Figure 10.12. Therefore, powder height settings should be changed in an ascending manner during encapsulation.

POWDER BED AERATION WITH TIME

Powder aeration is a case where fill weights would deviate from those predicted by Equation 10.2 because the powder bed density decreases with time owing to the air entrapment. This was observed during the encapsulation of the BI 671800 ED on the IMA Zanasi 6F where fill weights were decreasing with time (Figure 10.13a). This was only observed for poorly flowing formulations.

An investigation attributed this to the powder plowing mechanism of the Zanasi 6F where different plowing blades would disturb the powder bed. These blades are needed to break (i.e., plow) cavities formed within the powder bed from dosator insertion (Figure 10.14). If these blades were removed, empty capsules would be produced as the dosator is immersed into the same position within the powder bed. Zanasi bowls are equipped with vacuum suction to densify

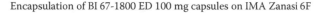

Encapsulation of BI 67-1800 ED 100 mg capsules on IMA Zanasi 6F

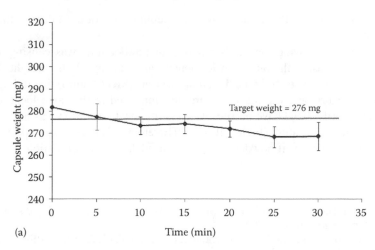

(a)

Encapsulation of BI 671800 ED 100 mg capsules on MG2 Futura

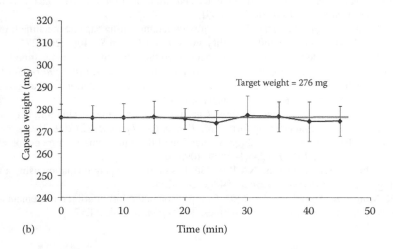

(b)

FIGURE 10.13   Encapsulation of BI 671800 ED 100-mg capsules: (a) IMA Zanasi 6F; (b) MG2 Futura.

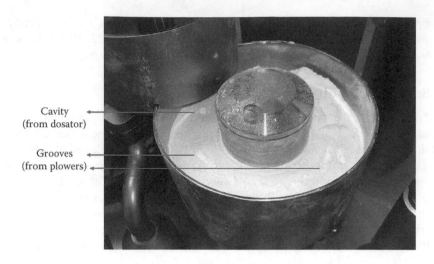

FIGURE 10.14   Powder bed disturbance during encapsulation (Zanasi 6F machine).

the powder bed and improve this issue; however, vacuum was not used during these encapsulation experiments.

The combination of plowing mechanism and poor powder flow was causing aeration of the powder bed, thus decreasing the bulk powder density and the capsule fill weight. To resolve this issue, the powder was encapsulated on a different machine (MG2 Futura) that did not have powder plowers/blades. Dosators on these machines are not immersed in the same location until several revolutions of the powder bowl have passed. As a result, powder aeration was not observed during encapsulation on the MG2 Futura (Figure 10.13b). Therefore, it is necessary to design formulations with improved flow properties if powder plowers are used during encapsulation.

REFERENCES

1. Shah K, Augsburger LL, Small LE, Polli GP 1983. Instrumentation of a dosing disc automatic capsule filling machine. *Pharm Technol* 7(4):42–54.
2. Small LE, Augsburger LL 1977. Instrumentation of an Automatic Capsule-Filling Machine. *J Pharm Sci* 66(4):504–509.
3. Mehta AM, Augsburger LL 1980. Simultaneous measurement of force and displacement in an automatic capsule filling machine. *Int J Pharm* 4:347–351.
4. Podczeck F 2000. The development of an instrumented tamp-filling capsule machine I. Instrumentation of a Bosch GKF 400S machine and feasibility study. *Eur J Pharm Sci* 10(4):267–274.
5. Podczeck F 2001. The development of an instrumented tamp-filling capsule machine II. Investigations of plug development and tamping pressure at different filling stations. *Eur J Pharm Sci* 12(4):515–521.
6. Chowhan ZT, Chow YP 1980. Powder flow studies I. Powder consolidation ratio and its relationship to capsule-filling—Weight variation. *Int J Pharm* 4:317–326.
7. Heda PK, Muller FX, Augsburger LL 1999. Capsule filling machine simulation. I. Low-force powder compression physics relevant to plug formation. *Pharm Dev Technol* 4(2):209–219.
8. Guo M, Muller FX, Augsburger LL 2002. Evaluation of the plug formation process of silicified microcrystalline cellulose. *Int J Pharm* 233(1–2):99–109.
9. Britten JR, Barnett MI, Armstrong NA 1996. Studies on powder plug formation using a simulated capsule filling machine. *J Pharm Pharmacol* 48(3):249–254.
10. Heda PK, Muteba K, Augsburger LL 2002. Comparison of the formulation requirements of dosator and dosing disc automatic capsule filling machines. *AAPS pharmSci* 4(3):E17.

11. Irwin GM, Dodson GJ, Ravin LJ 1970. Encapsulation of clomacran phosphate [2-chloro-9[3-(dimethylamino) propyl]acridan phosphate] I. Effect of flowability of powder blends, lot-to-lot variability, and concentration of active ingredient on weight variation of capsules filled on an automatic capsule-filling machine. *J Pharm Sci* 59(4):547–550.

12. Small LE, Augsburger LL 1978. Aspects of the lubrication requirements for an automatic capsule-filling machine. *Drug Dev Ind Pharm* 4(4):345–372.

13. Podczeck F, Newton JM 2000. Powder and capsule filling properties of lubricated granulated cellulose powder. *Eur J Pharm Biopharm* 50(3):373–377.

14. Guo M, Augsburger LL 2003. Potential application of silicified microcrystalline cellulose in direct-fill formulations for automatic capsule-filling machines. *Pharm Dev Technol* 8(1):47–59.

15. Miyake Y, Shimoda A, Jasu T, Furukawa M, Nesuji K, Hoshi K 1974. Packing properties of pharmaceutical powders into hard gelatin capsules. *Yakuzaigaku* 34(1):32–37.

16. Newton JM, Bader F 1981. The prediction of the bulk densities of powder mixtures, and its relationship to the filling of hard gelatin capsules. *J Pharm Pharmacol* 33(10):621–626.

17. Guo M, Karla G, Wilson W, Peng Y, Augsburger LL 2002. A prototype intelligent hybrid system for hard gelatin capsule formulation development. *Pharm Technol* 26:44–60.

18. Wilson WI, Peng Y, Augsburger LL 2005. Comparison of statistical analysis and Bayesian networks in the evaluation of dissolution performance of BCS Class II model drugs. *J Pharm Sci* 94(12):2764–2776.

19. Wilson WI, Peng Y, Augsburger LL 2005. Generalization of a prototype intelligent hybrid system for hard gelatin capsule formulation development. *AAPS PharmSciTech* 6(3):E449–457.

20. A. Ali MDM, York P, Rowe R 2011. *Prediction of Pellets Characteristics and Capsule Filling Performance Using Artificial Intelligence Technology*. AAPS, ed., Washington D.C.

21. Khawam A 2012. Reply to Filling hard gelatin capsules by the dosator nozzle system—Is it possible to predict where the powder goes? *Int J Pharm* 436(1–2):880–882.

22. Augsburger LL 2002. Hard and soft shell capsules. In Banker GS, Rohdes CT, editors. *Modern Pharmaceutics*, 4th ed. New York: Marcel Dekker, pp. 335–380.

23. Podczeck F 2004. Dry filling of hard capsules. In Podczeck F, Jones BE, editors. *Pharmaceutical Capsules*, 2nd ed. Pharmaceutical Press, pp. 119–138.

24. 2010. Common capsule sizes. *Tablets & Capsules* 8(8):40.

25. Khawam A 2011. Modeling powder encapsulation in dosator-based machines: I. Theory. *Int J Pharm* 421(2):203–209.

26. Khawam A, Schultz L 2011. Modeling powder encapsulation in dosator-based machines: II. Experimental evaluation. *Int J Pharm* 421(2):210–219.

11 Scale-Up and Transfer of Hard Shell Formulations across Machine Types

Larry L. Augsburger and Michael Levin

CONTENTS

INTRODUCTION

Scale-up of any physical process implies increasing the batch size or a procedure for applying the same process to different output volumes. Once you understand what makes these processes of different scales similar, you can eliminate many scale-up problems. A rational approach to scale-up has been used in physical sciences, viz., fluid dynamics and chemical engineering, for quite some time. This approach is based on process similarities between different scales and uses dimensional analysis that was developed a century ago and has since gained wide recognition in many industries, especially in chemical engineering.[1] This approach is warrantied when there is a geometric, kinematic, and dynamic similarity between processes of different scales.

In encapsulation, as well as in tableting unit operations, batch size enlargement does not mean a size increase of the processing volume. In both tableting and capsule-filling applications, the process scale-up involves production in what is essentially the same unit volume (die cavity or capsule size). However, unlike tableting, encapsulation scale-up is generally achieved by means of increasing the number of processing units rather than the speed of operation. Since the size of each unit volume is fixed, one of the conditions of the theory of models (similar geometric space) is partially met when using similar equipment. However, there are still kinematic and dynamic parameters that need to be investigated and matched for any scale-up or process transfer. Technology transfer to machines of a different type presents another difficulty as the procedures to maintain quality are mainly empirical. One way to eliminate potential scale-up or technology transfer problems is to develop formulations that are very robust with respect to processing conditions.

Scale-up problems may require post-approval changes that affect formulation composition, site change, and manufacturing process or equipment changes (by the way, from the regulatory standpoint, scale-up and scale-down are treated with the same degree of scrutiny). In a typical drug development cycle, once a set of clinical studies have been completed or NDA/ANDA (New Drug Application/Abbreviated New Drug Application) has been approved, it becomes very difficult to change the product or the process to accommodate specific production needs. Such needs may include changes in batch size and manufacturing equipment or process. Post-approval changes in the size of a batch from the pilot scale to larger or smaller production scales call for submission of additional information in the application, with a specific requirement that the new batches are to be produced using similar equipment and in full compliance with current good manufacturing practices (CGMPs) and the existing standard operating procedures (SOPs). Manufacturing changes may require new stability, dissolution, and *in vivo* bioequivalence testing. This is especially true for Level 2 equipment changes (change in equipment to a different design and different operating principles) and the process changes of Level 2 (process changes including changes such as mixing times and operating speeds within application/validation ranges) and Level 3 (change in the type of process used in the manufacture of the product, such as a change from wet granulation to direct compression of dry powder).

If the process is different after scale-up, the company has to demonstrate that the product produced by a modified process will be equivalent, stability studies and dissolution profiles. Of practical importance are the issues associated with a technology transfer in a global market. Equipment standardization inevitably will cause a variety of engineering and process optimization concerns that, generally speaking, can be classified as SUPAC (scale-up and post-approval changes). In what follows, we will address these issues in detail.

SCALING UP WITHIN THE SAME DESIGN AND OPERATING PRINCIPLE

REGULATORY MEANING OF SAME DESIGN AND OPERATING PRINCIPLE

The current (1999) guidance, "SUPAC-IR/MR: Immediate Release and Modified Release Solid Oral Dosage Forms Manufacturing Equipment Addendum"[2] applies to both immediate- and modified-release oral solid dosage forms. It was developed by the US Food and Drug Administration (FDA) with the assistance of the International Society of Pharmaceutical Engineering (ISPE) and is an update of earlier documents, SUPAC-IR (1995)[3] and SUPAC-MR (1997).[4] This guidance is organized in broad categories of unit operations (e.g., blending, drying, granulation, etc.). For each unit operation, a table is provided in which equipment is classified by class (operating principle) and subclass (design characteristic). Generally, equipment within the same class and subclass are considered to have the same design and operating principle under SUPAC-IR (1995) and SUPAC-MR (1997). A change from equipment in one class to equipment in a different class would usually be considered a change in design and operating principle.

The SUPAC Guidances classify changes according to their level. The documentation and reporting requirements also vary according to the level of changes. Scale up to and including a factor of 10 times the size of the pilot/bio-batch is considered a Level 1 change provided the equipment used to produce the test batch(es) is of the same design and operating principles, CGMPs are followed, and the same SOPs, controls, and formulation and manufacturing procedures are used. Level 1 changes are not likely to cause any detectable impact on formulation quality or performance and need only be reported in the annual report.

Scale-up beyond 10 times the pilot/bio-batch is a Level 2 change provided the equipment used to produce the test batch(es) is of the same design and operating principles and the same SOPs, controls, and formulation and manufacturing procedures are used. Level 2 changes are defined as those changes that could significantly affect formulation quality and performance and require the filing of "changes being effected supplement." Interestingly, neither case requires *in vivo* bioequivalence data to support the change of scale. The guidance should be consulted for a full description of the test documentation needed to be reported to FDA in these cases.

However, equipment changes to a different subclass within the same class should be carefully considered and evaluated on a case-by-case basis. By definition, *encapsulating*, or the "division of material into a hard gelatin capsule," is an *operating principle*. That is, all encapsulators should have in common rectification, separation of caps from bodies, dosing of fill material/formulation, rejoining of caps and bodies, and ejection of the filled capsules. Nevertheless, the various methods of dosing the formulation represent different design characteristics and are considered *subclasses*. Thus, a change from a dosator machine to a dosing disc machine would constitute a change in subclass, but not of operating principle.

According to a survey of industry practices, 64% of companies develop formulations using small-scale equipment of the same design and operating principles as the production equipment, whereas about 18% of the responding companies indicated that they use small-scale development equipment of a subclass different from the intended production equipment.[5] Preferences among the companies appeared about evenly divided between dosator and dosing disc machines, with about 18% using both machine types. In the following sections, we will address some of the issues involved in scaling up or transferring formulations within and between these subclasses.

SCALING UP WITHIN THE SAME SUBCLASS

Generally, there should be minimal problems when changing scale within the same subclass. Higher-output plug-forming machines of the same manufacturer's series typically do not make plugs any faster than the lower-output machines. Higher throughput is primarily achieved in these machines by increasing the number of dosing units. Nevertheless, there are factors that formulators should take into account when make making such scale changes. For example, the greater diameter and turning radius of the powder bowl of larger dosing disc machines may need to be considered. To minimize weight variation in such machines, there may be an optimal flow criterion that should be met, and that criterion may vary with the turning radius. Kurihara and Ichikawa[6] studied the relationship between the angle of repose, weight variation, and the degree of acceleration that takes place in disc movement, which, in turn, depends on dosing disc diameter and rotational speed. They reported a minimum point in the plot of the angle of repose versus coefficient of variation of filling weight for a dosing disc machine (Höfliger Karg GKF 1000). This observation indicates that powder is distributed over the dosing disc by the centrifugal action of the indexing rotation (baffles are provided to help maintain a uniform powder level). It means that powders with sufficiently high angles of repose may not have sufficient mobility to distribute well over the dosing disc via the intermittent indexing motion, whereas powders having angles of repose that are sufficiently low may be too fluid to maintain a uniform bed. Working with an instrumented GKF model 330, Shah et al.[7] observed that a uniform powder bed height was not maintained at the first tamping station because of its proximity to the scrape-off device adjacent to ejection. More recent workers have also pointed to the need to properly calibrate the flow properties of formulations for this type of filling machine. Heda et al.[8] studied several model formulations, each having different flow properties, on a GKF 400 machine. They proposed that Carr Compressibility Index (CI) values should be in the range of 18–30% to maintain low weight variation, which agrees well with Podczeck and Newton[9] who reported an optimum range of 15–30% based on a study of various materials filled on a GKF 400S machine. More poorly flowing powders (CI > 30%) were found by Heda et al. to dam up around the ejection station. Podczeck[10] reported that poor flowing powders display an "avalanching behavior" in front of the ejection station; that is, the powder mass alternatively builds up and collapses in the manner of an avalanche at certain intervals of time such that the powder mass over stations 1 and 2 can vary dramatically and cause increased capsule fill weight variation.

Nalluri et al.[11] found weight variability to correlate with the angle of internal friction and the avalanche energy of blends of acetaminophen and microcrystalline cellulose 102 filled on a Harro Höfliger KFM III-C dosing disc machine. Beyond about 75% of drug loading, variability increased and changed differently as a function of drug level. This threshold level was also predicted by percolation theory and is considered the point beyond which flowability becomes dominated by the drug.

The MG-2 series of continuous motion dosator machines also exhibit similar plug-forming parameters across machines with different production capacities. To illustrate this point, one can compare the 16-station (rated up to 48,000 capsules per hour [cph]) and 64-station machines (rated up to 200,000 cph). These two machines are reported to operate at the same revolutions per minute (RPM), have the same spacing between dosators, and have similar dosator penetration and withdrawal speeds, plug compression dwell times, and plug ejection speeds.[12] The powder bed into which dosators dip to form plugs is scraped off neatly to a specific bed height and is presented in an annular ring (the "powder trough") that rotates with the dosator turret (dosing head). Because the powder bed and dosing head rotate at slightly different speeds, a plug is not formed from the same location in the powder bed until approximately 8–10 revolutions have occurred when the bed is presumed to have been restored and stabilized.[12] Maintaining a uniform powder bed density is critical for dosators to pick up uniform weights of powder in all cases. Contributing to plug uniformity in MG2 machines is the fact that the dosators in these machines do not punch vertical holes through the bed. The difference in rotational speeds between the turret and the powder trough also causes the dosators to enter the powder bed at an angle. The axes of rotation of the annular powder bed and the dosing head are offset such that as the turret rotates, dosators alternatively pass over the annular powder trough where they form plugs and then over bushings bearing capsule bodies where they eject the plugs.

With the MG-2 Futura series of machines, formulations can be scaled up within the same machine by changing the number of dosators to yield outputs ranging from 6,000 to 96,000 cph. Since the turret and annular powder bed dimensions are unchanged, few problems should be expected when scaling up within this range. However, when fewer than the full complement of 16 dosators are installed, the dwell time of powder in the trough and feed mechanism will be longer compared to the fully tooled machine.

Differences in dwell time in the feed mechanism of MG-2 machines have been reported to affect dissolution and content uniformity. For instance, Desai et al.[13] found the dissolution rates of three drugs of varying solubility to slow after 30 or 45 min of running on an MG-2 machine fitted with four dosators. This slowdown, which was most apparent with the least-soluble drug, was attributed to increased coating of particles with hydrophobic magnesium stearate as a result of prolonged mixing by the propeller blade in the hopper. Desai et al. carried out a simulation in which the capsule machine was run for up to 60 min without filling capsules. During this time, the propeller blade continued to mix the formulation in the hopper. Capsules were hand filled (to eliminate possible confounding effects of plug compression) from the powder initially and at the end of a run. After 60 min, dissolution from capsules filled from the hopper was significantly reduced from that of capsules filled before the start of the run.

The positive results of additional studies carried out by Desai et al. supported various formulation changes that may ameliorate the problem, for example replacing magnesium stearate with more hydrophilic lubricants (Stear-O-Wet or sodium stearyl fumarate), reducing the level of magnesium stearate, and replacing pre-gelatinized starch (10% in the subject formula) with equal concentrations of a super disintegrant (Explotab or Primojel).[13]

In another example, Johansen et al.[14] reported both a segregation problem and an overmixing problem on an MG-2 model G36/4 machine during a trial production run of 25-mg indomethacin capsules. The formulation was mixed using a planetary mixer, with magnesium stearate being added separately and mixed for 5 min. Both drug content and dissolution were found to vary with time during the run. They concluded that the powder throughput was so slow at the mixing blade rotational velocity of 1 RPM that overmixing occurred. Removing the mixing blade and fitting the hopper with an insert to convert it to a mass flow hopper apparently solved both problems.

As a predictive stress test to determine the likelihood of encountering a dissolution problem on scale-up attributed to lubricant overmixing, Harding et al.[15] proposed the use of a Turbula high-intensity mixer. They reported a qualitative relationship between changes in the properties of a 500-g batch caused by mixing in a 2-L Turbula for 6 h and the effects of a 6-h run of a 10-kg batch of the same formulation in a Zanasi LZ-64 intermittent motion dosator machine.

Air compressors, vacuum pumps, and the drive motor all contribute to filling machine vibration and the greater vibration realized at higher running speeds may increase powder density and fill weight in dosator machines. Llusa et al.[16] fitted a laser Doppler vibrometer to a research MG2 machine (Labby). They found that machine vibrations were not significant at a running speed of 500 cph, and powder density was not measurably affected. At 3000 cph, vibration and powder bed densification were significant and fill weight was significantly increased. The study was limited to a single capsule size (#3) and the filling of several grades of microcrystalline cellulose. No lubricants (i.e., magnesium stearate) were included, which could have modified their findings owing to the ability of magnesium stearate often to enhance the initial packing density of powder blends and form denser plugs, including those formed from microcrystalline cellulose. For example, Shah et al.[7] found the bulk and tapped densities of microcrystalline cellulose (Avicel PH 101) to increase with the percent magnesium stearate within the concentration range of 0.1–0.5%. The weight and breaking strength of the plugs formed from these lubricated blends on an instrumented H&K 330 dosing disc machine were greater than were found with the unlubricated filler. The 0.1% level appeared optimal in that it resulted in maximum weight and plug breaking strength. At the 0.25% and 0.5% levels, breaking strength decreased with magnesium stearate concentration, but weight exhibited little change. The lubricant effects that contribute to plug breaking strength and those that tend to soften plugs appear competitive, with those contributing to softening dominating at the higher magnesium stearate levels. In another example using a tabletop plug-forming device, Jones[17] found that plug density increased with mixing time when 1% magnesium stearate was added to either microcrystalline cellulose (Avicel PH 102) or pre-gelatinized starch (Starch 1500). Such densified formulations may have limited ability to undergo further vibrational densification in the machine. Nevertheless, the direct observation of significantly increased vibratory consolidation of a powder bed at the high running speed is a significant finding for dosator machines for which powder bed density is a significant determinant of fill weight. However, the significance of this finding should not be limited to dosator machines since vibratory consolidation can occur in both dosator and dosing disc machines. Considering the operational characteristics of these machines, vertical vibration may be more important in dosing disc machines. Beyond effects on fill weight, increased vibration at higher speeds could also encourage segregation in susceptible formulations. The reader is referred to Lin et al.[18] for a useful analysis of the relationship between bulk powder properties and the segregation tendency of powder formulations from a Quality by Design perspective.

Differences in various parameters may be encountered when scaling up within the same subclass but across different manufacturers of the equipment, which have the potential to affect the success of the scale change. For example, using a filling machine simulator, Britten et al.[19] found that plug ejection speed had little effect on plug properties, but higher compression speeds led to reduced plug consolidation and lower weights. Machines of the same subclass produced by different manufactures may exhibit differences in powder handling, mixing mechanisms, and throughput rates that could cause formulations to perform differently.

TRANSFERRING BETWEEN DOSATOR AND DOSING DISC MACHINES

Few studies comparing the formulation requirements of machines in different subclasses (i.e., dosator and dosing disc machines) have been published. The substantial differences in the way these two types of machines handle the powder feed and form plugs could cause differences in plug bonding and densification and dissolution. Since plugs may be formed in one stroke (dosator machines) or multiple strokes (dosing disc machines), compression dwell times, consolidation, and uniformity of plug density are likely to differ substantially between the machines. The discussion that follows compares dosing disc and dosator machines on the basis of their formulation requirements, specifically flowability, densification, compactibility, and lubrication requirements. It is hoped that this discussion will help formulators design formulations that can be run on either type of machine or transfer formulations from one machine type to the other.

BULK POWDER PROPERTIES

Bulk Density and Densification

Since the multiple tamping principle of the dosing disc machine is more efficient at densification than the single stroke dosator machine (without vacuum densification), dosing disc machines may be able to accommodate a broader range in powder properties. Comparing the same model formulations on instrumented Zanasi LZ-64 and Höfliger-Karg (H&K) GKF-400 machines, Heda et al.[8] found that though similar fill weights could be attained on both machines, the dosator machine required a higher piston height setting (18 mm), compared to the disc height (15 mm) required for the dosing disc machine.

Compactibility

Early in the history of automatic capsule filling machines, Ridgway and Callow[20] recognized that dosator machines would require a higher degree of compactibility owing to the exposure of the unsupported plug from the open end of the dosator. In dosator machines, when plug compression is complete, the dosator bearing the plug is lifted out of the powder bed and positioned over an open capsule body where it is ejected by the piston. It is thus clear that a successful filling operation with these machines requires the powder within the dosator to be quantitatively retained during this transfer process. At least, a stable powder arch needs to be formed at the dosator outlet to prevent loss of material during the time that the open end of the dosator tube is exposed.[21,22] This stable arch is dependent on the angle of wall friction of the powder with the dosing tube and the degree of compression applied. It can be shown that there is an optimum angle of wall friction for which the compression force required to ensure a stable arch is a minimum.[22] Ideally, the plug should also remain reasonably intact during the ejection event to avoid or minimize material loss during transfer. Heda et al.[8] demonstrated with instrumented filling machines that certain model formulations produced greater weight variation when run on a Zanasi machine than when run on an H&K GKF machine and related that difference to a greater compactibility requirement of the dosator machine.

Flowability

The optimal flow criteria for dosing disc and dosator machines may overlap. Heda et al.[8] observed that a CI value of 20–30% appeared to be a suitable value for filling model formulations on both machines as judged by weight variation analysis. Highly free-flowing powders that tend to flood can cause filling problems in either type of machine. Since dosing disc machines build up plugs gradually through a multiple tamp process, they may be less sensitive than dosator machines to powder flow problems.[9,23] Further, some freely flowing powders that do not form plugs well enough to be transferred by a dosator may be able to be managed in dosing disc machines by increasing the powder bed height.[9]

LUBRICANT REQUIREMENTS

Ullah et al.[24] transferred a formulation developed on a dosator machine (Zanasi) to a dosing disc machine (H&K GKF 1500) and found that the drug dissolved more slowly from the capsules filled on the dosing disc machine. They proposed that the slower dissolution rate was caused by excessive coating of the formulation with the hydrophobic lubricant, magnesium stearate, owing to shearing of the laminar lubricant during the tamping step in the H&K machine. Based on a study using a laboratory-scale mixer/grinder to simulate the shearing action of the filling machine, they solved the problem by reducing the initial level of lubricant from 1% to 0.3%. They obtained satisfactory dissolution from 570- and 1100-kg (full production) size batches using this reduced level of lubricant.

Heda et al.[8] compared model formulations at equivalent magnesium stearate levels and compression forces and found that plug ejection forces were lower on the H&K GKF 400 machine than on the Zanasi LZ-64. The dosing disc machine appeared to require about half as much magnesium stearate for the materials and conditions studied to achieve similar ejection forces. In part, this observation may reflect greater shearing of magnesium stearate in the dosing disc machine, as proposed by Ullah et al.[24] However, Heda et al.[8] also found lower ejection forces on the dosing disc machine when unlubricated microcrystalline cellulose was run at the same compression force. This observation suggests that materials may recover differently in the two types of machines. Post-compression elastic recovery can reduce residual radial pressures in dosators and dosing disc cavities and likely lead to reduced adhesion to those confining surfaces. Heda et al.[8] hypothesized that the gradual buildup of plugs in segments may allow for more complete elastic recovery than would occur in the dosing disc machines where plugs are formed from a single stroke. Interestingly, the effect of differences in elastic recovery on plug ejection was observed by Britten et al.[19] who compared two materials, pre-gelatinized starch (Starch 1500) and lactose, that exhibit substantially different elastic nature using a Macofar dosator machine simulator. They found that pre-gelatinized starch exhibited considerable elastic recovery, substantially lower residual radial pressure, and undetectable ejection pressure. All other things being equal, the significance of any such difference in post-compression recovery between machines will depend on the ability of the formulation itself to recover.

DISSOLUTION OUTCOMES

The same formulation run on the two types of machines may exhibit different dissolution profiles owing to differences in the shearing of magnesium stearate, but, conceivably, other factors could also affect dissolution. Dissolution may be affected by differences in plug density/porosity owing to differences in such variables as compression force, dwell time, rates of compression, and the number of tamping or compression events involved in forming the plugs. Studies using a Macofar dosator machine simulator revealed that greater piston compression speed resulted in a less consolidated plug[19] and that plug porosity was inversely related to the piston compression force.[25] In dosing disc machines, the greater time under pressure that already-formed plug segments can experience at subsequent tamping stations may lead to further densification of ductile formulations.[26]

Multiple tamping in a dosing disc machine may affect dissolution. When dicalcium phosphate was the filler, Shah et al.[27] found slower dissolution of hydrochlorothiazide from capsules after two and again after three tamps at a particular tamping force compared to a single tamp at the same compression force. The effect was more apparent at a compression force of 200 N than at 100 N and more dramatic than was observed with the soluble filler lactose. These results may be reflecting changes in the plug density. The effect of multiple tamping on the mean pore diameter of plugs (dicalcium phosphate filler) produced with the same 100 N tamping force was measured by Hg intrusion. The mean pore diameter decreased from 12.8 μm after one tamp to 10.8 μm after two tamps, but no further decrease in men pore size was noted after a third tamp. For either filler, adding 4% of the super disintegrant croscarmellose to the formulation effectively eliminated the effects of multiple tamps or compression force (100 N vs. 200 N) on dissolution.

Heda et al.[8] compared the dissolution profiles of model formulations from capsules filled on Zanasi LZ-64 and H&K GKF 400 machines at 100 N and 200 N compression forces. Among a series of ascorbic acid model formulations, there were two instances where the f_2 value comparing the dissolution profiles was less than 50. This finding suggests that the dissolution profiles for those formulations are different when filled on the two machines with the same compression force. When the dissolution profiles of hydrochlorothiazide formulations were compared, the f_2 value was less than 50 for one formula at the compression force of 100 N. These dissolution differences indicated by the f_2 metric would suggest the need for a preapproval supplement, were they the result of a post-approval change in filling machines. According to the SUPAC guidance, a change from a dosator machine to a dosing disc machine would constitute a change in subclass, but not of operating principle. Although such a change likely would not require filing a preapproval supplement, provided certain conditions are met, the guidance notes that such changes should be carefully considered and evaluated on a case-by-case basis, and the burden is placed on the applicant to provide the supporting data and rationale at the time of change to determine whether or not a preapproval supplement is justified. Such data are reviewed by FDA at its discretion.

GRANULATIONS

According to a survey[5] of industry practices, approximately 46% of the firms sampled favor direct filling of powders as a first choice over granulation before filling capsules. Thirty-six percent of firms would allow formulators to decide whether to granulate at their own discretion and 18% of firms favor granulation of all formulations before encapsulation. Despite these preferences, it is interesting that half of the firms responding report that only 0–10% of their hard shell capsule products are actually direct-fill powder formulations. Moreover, only 27% of the firms reported that greater than half of their capsules were developed as direct-fill formulations. Some of these non–direct-fill formulations may well be modified-release formulations (e.g., bead products); however, formulation problems may account at least in part for this relatively small proportion of direct-fill formulations developed.

Conventional wet and dry methods are used to granulate powders. That same survey of industry practices revealed that 64% of the firms sampled favored wet granulation for capsule formulations and 18% favored dry granulation.[5] The remainder had "no policy." Formulators often granulate before encapsulation to increase the formulation density. This allows the weight that can be filled in a given size capsule to be increased or a smaller capsule size to be selected. However, granulation also can improve flowability and compression properties, reduce dustiness and adhesion to metal surfaces, improve robustness by reducing variability in raw material physical properties, and improve content uniformity by holding drug particles in granules that can allow handling without loss of blend quality. Wet granulation may also improve the wettability and dissolution of poorly soluble drugs through hydrophilization,[28,29] that is, the increased wettability that can occur from the deposition and spreading of hydrophilic binders over particle surfaces during granulation. The liquid phase in wet granulation also provides a convenient vehicle by which to introduce and uniformly disperse a very low dose drug. Newton and Rowley[30] showed that dissolution of a poorly soluble drug was enhanced by granulation owing to formation of more permeable plugs from granules, as opposed to powders.

With some qualification, the same principles that apply to filling powders should apply to filling granulations. Podczeck et al.[31] found that an acceptable filling performance was always achieved when different granule size fractions of Sorbitol instant were filled on both a dosing disc (Bosch GKF 400) machine and a dosator (Zanasi AZ 5) machine. However, the dosing disc machine operation, which depends less on forming firm plugs, seemed slightly better suited to the coarser granule size fractions than the dosator machine. This was particularly the case when a solid plug cannot be formed. Generally, the dosator machine produced plugs that were denser than the formulation maximum bulk density, suggesting that this dosing principle might be more useful for granulations where the dose is large or where smaller capsule size is desired. With the dosing disc machine, the maximum bulk density apparently could not be attained for the smaller granule sizes under the conditions of the study. These investigators suggested that the lower-density plugs that can be run on a dosing disc machine may disintegrate more easily and thus be preferred for low bioavailability formulations.

The results of a study with granulated powdered cellulose suggest that a compromise may have to be met in selecting the proper lubricant level for some granulations.[32] The relationship between dosing disc machine running characteristics (Bosch GKF 400S), bulk powder properties, and the percent magnesium stearate lubricant in the formulation was found to be complex. Increasing the magnesium stearate concentration up to 0.8% resulted in easier machine operation with reduced friction between moving parts but was not necessarily beneficial in reducing fill weight variation.

REFERENCES

1. Zlokarnik M. *Scale-Up in Chemical Engineering.* Weinheim: Wiley-VCH, 2006: 2–37.
2. Guidance for Industry, SUPAC-IR/MR—Manufacturing Equipment Addendum, FDA, CDER, January 1999; http://www.fda.gov/cder/guidance/1721fnl.pdf.
3. Guidance for industry, SUPAC IR: Immediate Release Oral Solid Dosage Forms: Scale-Up and Post Approval Changes: Manufacturing and Controls, In Vitro Dissolution Testing and In Vivo Bioequivalence Documentation, FDA, CDER, FDA, Nov. 1995; http://www.fda.gov/cder/guidance/cmc5.pdf.
4. Guidance for industry, SUPAC-MR: Modified Release Solid Oral Dosage Forms. Scale-Up and Postapproval Changes: Chemistry, Manufacturing, and Controls; In Vitro Dissolution Testing and In Vivo Bioequivalence Documentation. FDA, CDER, FDA, Sep. 1997; www.fda.gov/downloads/Drugs/GuidanceComplianceRegulatoryInformation/Guidances/UCM070640.pdf.
5. Heda PK. A comparative study of the formulation requirements of dosator and dosing disc encapsulators. Simulation of plug formation, and creation of rules for an expert system for formulation design. PhD Dissertation, University of Maryland, Baltimore, MD, 1998.
6. Kurihara K, Ichikawa I. Effect of powder flowability on capsule filling weight variation. *Chem Pharm Bull* 1978; 26: 1250–1256.
7. Shah KB, Augsburger LL, Marshall K. An investigation of some factors influencing plug formation and fill weight in a dosing disk-type automatic capsule-filling machine. *J Pharm Sci* 1986; 75(3): 291–296.
8. Heda PK, Muteba, K, Augsburger LL. Comparison of the formulation requirements of dosator and dosing disc automatic capsule filling machines. *AAPS Pharm Sci* 2002; 4(3) article 17.
9. Podczeck F, Newton JM. Powder filling into hard gelatine capsules on a tamp filling machine. *Int J Pharm* 1999; 185: 237–254.
10. Podczeck F. Powder, granule and pellet properties for filling of two-piece hard capsules, Chapter 5 in Podczeck F, Jones BE, eds. *Pharmaceutical Capsules*, 2nd ed. London: Pharmaceutical Press, 2004: 101–118.
11. Nalluri RV, Puchcov M, Kuentz M. Toward a better understanding of powder avalanching and shear cell parameters of drug-excipient blends to design minimal weight variability into pharmaceutical capsules. *Int J Pharm* 2013; 442: 49–56.
12. McKee J. MG America, Fairfield, NJ, Personal Communication, 2005.
13. Desai DS, Rubitska BA, Bergum JS et al. Physical interactions of magnesium stearate with starch-derived disintegrants and their effects on capsule and tablet dissolution. *Int J Pharm* 1993; 91: 217–226.
14. Johansen H, Anderson I, Leedgaard H. Segregation and continued mixing in an automatic capsule filling machine. *Drug Devel Ind Pharm* 1989; 15: 477–488.
15. Harding VD, Higginson SJ, Wells JJ. Predictive stress tests in the scale-up of capsule formulations. *Drug Devel Ind Pharm* 1989; 15: 2315–2338.
16. Llusa M, Faulhammer E, Biserni S et al. The effect of capsule-filling machine vibrations on average fill weight. *Int J Pharm* 2013; 454: 381–387.
17. Jones BE. New thoughts on capsule filling. *STP Pharma Sciences* 1998; 8(5): 277–283.
18. Lin X, Huiquan W, Meiyu S et al. Quality-by-design (QbD): Effects of testing parameters and formulation variables on the segregation tendency of pharmaceutical powder measured by the ASTM D 6940-04 segregation tester. *J Pharm Sci* 2008; 97(10): 4485–4497.
19. Britten JR, Barnett MI, Armstrong NA. Studies on powder plug formation using a simulated capsule filling machine. *J Pharm Pharmacol* 1996; 48: 249–254.
20. Ridgway K, Callow JAB. Capsule-filling machinery. *Pharm J* 1973; 212: 281–285.
21. Jolliffe IG, Newton, JM, Walters JK. Theoretical considerations of the filling of pharmaceutical hard gelatine capsules. *Powder Tech* 1980; 27: 189–195.
22. Jolliffe IG, Newton JM, Cooper D. The design and use of an instrumented mG2 capsule filling machine simulator. *J Pharm Pharmacol* 1982; 34: 230–235.
23. Felton LA, Garcia DI, Farmer R. Weight and weight uniformity of hard gelatin capsules filled with microcrystalline cellulose and silicified microcrystalline cellulose. *Drug Devel Ind Pharm* 2002; 28(4): 467–472.
24. Ullah I, Wiley GJ, Agharkar SN. Analysis and simulation of capsule dissolution problem encountered during product scale-up. *Drug Devel Ind Pharm* 1992; 18(8): 895–910.

25. Tattawasart A, Armstrong NA. The formation of lactose plugs for hard shell capsules. *Pharm Devel Tech* 1993; 2: 335–343.
26. Podczeck F. The development of an instrumented tamp-filling capsule machine II: Investigations of plug development and tamping pressure at different filling stations. *Eur J Pharm Sci* 2001; 12: 501–507.
27. Shah KB, Augsburger LL, Marshall K. Multiple tamping effects on drug dissolution from capsules filled on a dosing-disk type automatic capsule filling machine. *J Pharm Sci* 1987; 76: 639–645.
28. Lerk CF, Lagas M, Fell JT, Nauta P. Effect of hydrophilization of hydrophobic drugs on release rate from capsules. *J Pharm Sci* 1978; 67: 935–939.
29. Lerk CF, Lagas M, Lie-a-Huen L et al. In vitro and in vivo availability of hydrophilized phenytoin from capsules. *J Pharm Sci* 1979; 68: 634–637.
30. Newton JM, Rowley G. On the release of drug from hard gelatin capsules. *J Pharm Pharmacol* 1981; 33: 621–626.
31. Podczeck F, Blackwell S, Gold M, Newton JM. The filling of granules into hard gelatine capsules. *Int J Pharm* 1999; 188: 59–69.
32. Podczeck F, Newton JM. Powder and capsule filling properties of lubricated granulated cellulose powder. *Eur J Pharm Biopharm* 2000; 50: 373–377.

12 Modified-Release Delivery Systems
Extended-Release Capsule Platform

Reza Fassihi

CONTENTS

INTRODUCTION

Pharmaceutical drug delivery embraces a range of delivery carriers and constructs that have dimensions ranging from several nanometers (nanotechnology) to numerous millimeters (conventional dosage forms, i.e., pellets, tablets, and capsules). Such delivery systems spawn a whole array of assemblies for delivery of highly potent active drugs through different routes of administrations to numerous sites and targets in the human or animal body to treat disease conditions. Such delivery types and carrier systems, with their relative sizes together with some molecules and bacterial cells, are shown in Figure 12.1.

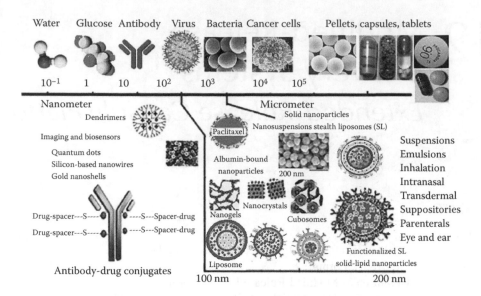

FIGURE 12.1   (See color insert.) Approximate size spectrum showing dimensions of typical molecules, carrier types, and drug delivery systems based on the published literature and some of the commercialized nanotechnology products, conventional dosage forms, modified-release technologies, and their combinations.

Typical pharmaceutical carriers, nanosized active agents, and delivery systems include dendrimers and nanoparticles with functionalized surface, antibody–drug conjugates, nanocrystals, nanoparticle albumin bound (nab) systems, lipid–polymer hybrid nanoparticles, liposomes, stealth liposomes, half-antibody functionalized ligand-targeted systems, micro-emulsions, nanosuspensions, emulsions, suspensions, oral-soluble strips, microcapsules, pellets, tablets, osmotic pumps, and encapsulated drug delivery systems in a capsule carrier. The latter seven delivery systems constitute greater than 80% of routinely used pharmaceuticals in current therapy.

According to the US Food and Drug Administration (FDA) and the US Pharmacopeia (USP), modified-release solid oral dosage forms encompass delayed/enteric-coated and extended-release drug products. Besides the delayed- and/or extended-release features, other newer types of oral modified-release products may include pulsatile-release, combination drugs (e.g., single dosage form containing immediate-release, enteric-coated, and/or extended-release components), targeted delivery (e.g., oral-mucosa, stomach, proximal intestine, distal intestine, and/or colon), or delivery systems that are based on the chronopharmacokinetics and interactions of drugs in the milieu of biologic rhythms from a clinical perspective and chronotherapeutics. These dosage forms can be designed to deliver drugs in a controlled and predictable manner over a prolonged time period or at a target location within the gastrointestinal (GI) tract to elicit the desired therapeutic effect. Moreover, development of such delivery systems having complicated features involved in their design has presented numerous challenges to the industry and regulatory authorities in ensuring pharmaceutical equivalence, bioequivalence, and therapeutic equivalence. Commonly used oral modified-release systems can be formulated as single-unit (e.g., tablet matrices, composites of layered tablets and compressed pellets) or multiple-unit dosage forms (e.g., based on encapsulation of pellets, spheres, granules, or multiparticulates). The relative merits of multiple unit dosage forms in terms of "release flexibility, increased bioavailability, predictable gastrointestinal transit time, less localized GI disturbances, more consistent blood levels, less intra or inter subject variability due to the food effects and greater product safety" over single-unit products are well established. In modified-release systems, the design of the dosage form allows for a specific drug delivery pattern so that the release rate becomes the rate-limiting step. This should be viewed in the context of existing parameters within the GI tract. For example, the two major rate-limiting factors to drug absorption are GI environment (e.g., pH, absorption site, and regional differences in drug permeability across GI mucosa, gut metabolism, and GI content) and transit rate of the dosage form. From a manufacturing point of view, irrespective of the type of the dosage form (single or multiple units), currently the utilization of hydrophilic matrices, mini-tablets, coated pellets or spheres, and osmotic systems is common and offers significant flexibility in pharmaceutical technology. In view of the many benefits offered by multiple-unit dosage forms, it is speculated that such systems are particularly useful in many chronic disease conditions and delivery of highly irritant and potent drugs for site-specific targeting within the GI tract and for delivery of non-steroidal anti-inflammatory drugs, colonic delivery of anticancer drugs, enzymes, peptides/proteins, and vaccines.

CAPSULES AS A CARRIER PLATFORM FOR ORAL EXTENDED-RELEASE DRUG DELIVERY

The purpose of this chapter is to highlight and describe potential uses of hard shell capsules as carriers for extended-release drug delivery systems that, by virtue of their design and popularity, satisfy features of an ideal technology platform for drug delivery and reliable pharmaceutical production. These features include the following:

a. Availability, types, and sizes of the capsule shells through different suppliers
b. Simplicity, flexibility and ease of production, low cost, and time efficient
c. Process familiarity and acquaintance with technology and equipment
d. Robust, manageable, quick changeover, transferability, suitable for worldwide manufacturing
e. Significant potential for innovation including multiple drug delivery options for modified release, targeted release, and delivery of drug combinations

The word *capsule* is derived from the Latin word *Capsula*, meaning "a small box or packet."[1,2] Therefore, hard shell capsules can be regarded as containers for delivery of formulated drug substances that are generally designed for oral administration, although non-oral products for rectal or vaginal administration are available. Capsules as a platform for delayed or controlled-release delivery offer numerous advantages and adaptabilities over tablets. They can readily accommodate a range of special excipients, formulations, and pre-fabricated systems to target specific regions of the GI tract including the following:

a. Powders, particulate systems, pellets, mini-tablets, coated particulates, or mixed coated beads with enteric coat or diffusion-controlled membrane
b. Multiple tablets, smaller hard or soft shell capsules, small drug wafers, or casted sheets containing drug
c. Enteric-coated systems with or without sustained release components
d. Various controlled-release forms
e. Drug combinations for targeting different regions of the GI tract for both local and systemic effects
f. Micronized or nanosized formulated drug(s) with pH-sensitive coatings for delivery to stomach, proximal intestine, distal intestine, or colon
g. Incompatible drugs where one drug in the form of a coated pellet, tablet, small soft shell capsule can be separated by placing it in a larger capsule before adding the second drug
h. Fixed-dose combinations

Hard shell capsule sizes range from number 5, the smallest, to number 000, which is the largest, except for veterinary sizes. However, size number 00 generally is the largest size acceptable to patients. Hard shell capsules consist of two parts, cap and body piece. Generally, there are unique grooves or indentations molded into the cap and body portion to provide firm closure when fully engaged or fitted, which helps prevent the unintended separation of the filled capsules during shipping and handling.[2] To assure strong closure, spot fusion "welding" of the cap and body piece together through direct thermal means, or application of ultrasonic energy, sealed banding, or liquid sealing can be applied. This further guarantees greater product stability by limiting oxygen and moisture penetration and also augments consumer safety by making the capsules tamper proof and difficult to open without producing noticeable damage to the dosage form and the shell's integrity.

Two-piece hard shell capsules are commercially available and are manufactured from gelatin (animal derived) or hypromellose (hydroxypropylmethylcellulose [HPMC], plant derived) via the thermal gelation process.[2,3] The HPMC capsules referred to as Vcaps Plus capsules or second-generation capsules are based on pure HPMC and generally dissolve similarly in different pH's or ionic strengths and have a lower moisture content (4% to 9% w/w) relative to gelatin capsules (13% to 16% w/w). Unlike gelatin shells, which can undergo cross-linking in the presence of aldehyde groups and cause dissolution problems, the HPMC shells are stable and are not affected by the presence of aldehyde groups.

MODIFIED-RELEASE DOSAGE FORMS

Modified-release drug delivery technologies, which include both enteric-coated systems and a variety of controlled-release solid dosage forms, including capsules, have evolved as a multidisciplinary science. For example, the extended-release Spansule capsule, containing a large number of coated and uncoated drug beads (i.e., coated spheres) to modify drug dissolution by controlling access of GI fluids to the drug through a coating barrier, was first introduced and patented in 1952, as shown in Figure 12.2.

A similar approach has been practiced since the 1950s, and today, there are dozens of modified-release capsule dosage forms using the same or similar principle that are commercially available. Some examples of modified-release hard shell capsules that have been FDA approved and

Spansule delivery system
Sustained release capsule containing about 600 tiny coated and uncoated pellets of antihistamine (chlorprophenpyradamine maleate) 12 mg.

Patent specification

715,305

Date of application and filing complete specification: Dec. 2, 1952.

No. 30552/52.

Application made in the United States of America on July 18, 1952.
Complete specification published: Sept. 8, 1954.

Index at acceptance:—Class 81(1), B11B(3:6).

We, Smith Kline and French International Co., a Corporation organised under the Laws of the State of Delaware, United States of America, of 1530, Spring Garden
5 Street, Philadelphia, Pennsylvania, United States of America, do hereby declare the invention, for which we pray that a patent may be granted to us, and the method by which it is to be performed, to be particu-
10 larly described in and by the following statement:—

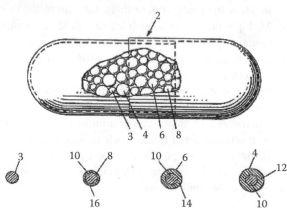

FIGURE 12.2 An issued patent in 1952 describing the Spansule capsule showing the hard shell gelatin capsule containing hundreds of coated and uncoated drug beads for extended release of an antihistamine.

are currently available in the marketplace are presented in Table 12.1. The list is not an exhaustive list of the available extended-release capsule products but rather an exemplary sample list that also includes fixed-dose combination products. Many of these products are marketed in different dose strengths for ease of clinical management of the disease conditions. For example, extended-release morphine sulfate (Kadian), listed in Table 12.1, has many different strengths with diversity in color(s), capsule size, and imprints in order to safely adjust the required dose for management of pain in patients having different pain thresholds and pain severity.

A brief but comprehensive history of modified-release delivery systems and significance of their performance through either manipulation of the drug molecule itself or delivery types with specific release configurations is presented elsewhere.[4] The groundbreaking theoretical developments of various scientists[5–9] and others whose contributions allowed for a more rational understanding and application of basic principles to the design and development of an array of more sophisticated and multifaceted controlled-release systems should not be overlooked. Extended-release capsules are produced in such a way as to deliver their content upon oral administration either in the stomach or different regions of the GI tract for absorption over a few hours to about 12 to 24 h. Figure 12.3

TABLE 12.1
Some Examples of FDA-Approved and Currently Marketed Modified-Release Capsule Dosage Forms

Brand Name	Generic Name	Therapeutic Class
Effexor-XR	Venlafaxine HCl	Antidepressants
Cardizem CD	Diltiazem HCl	Calcium channel blocker
Dilacor XR	Diltiazem HCl	Antihypertension
Pancrecarb	Pancrelipase	Pancreatic enzyme insufficiency
Dilantin Kapseals	ER phenytoin sodium	Prevention and treatment of seizures
Bontril SR	Phendimetrazine tartrate	Management of exogenous obesity
Oruvail	Ketoprofen	Nonsteroidal anti-inflammatory
Cartia XT	Diltiazem HCl	Calcium channel blocker
Metadate CD	Methylphenidate HCl	Attention deficit hyperactivity disorder
Carbatrol	Carbamazepine	Anticonvulsant drug
Kadian	Morphine sulfate	Management of pain
Cardene SR	Nicardipine HCl	Treatment of hypertension
Adderall XR	Amphetamine, dextroamphetamine mixed salts	Attention deficit hyperactivity disorder
Verelan PM	Verapamil HCl	Calcium channel blocker
Prozac Weekly	Fluoxetine HCl	Antidepressant
Nexium	Esomeprazole magnesium	Treatment of erosive esophagitis
Prilosec	Omeprazole	Treatment of duodenal ulcer
Delzicol	Mesalamine	Ulcerative colitis
Linzess	Linaclotide	Irritable bowel syndrome with constipation
Fixed-dose combinations		
Aggrenox	Aspirin/ER dipyridamole amlodipine	Reduce the risk of stroke
Lotrel	besylate and benazepril HCl	Treatment of hypertension

Modified-release capsules encompass both enteric and extended-release products.

Note: Four selected modified-release capsule delivery systems representing different release mechanisms will be discussed in more detail in this text: Dilacor XR (multiple tablet matrices in capsule); Carbatrol extended release (diverse coated and uncoated multiparticulates in capsule); Prilosec delayed-release/enteric-coated pellets in capsule; and Linzess capsule containing drug-coated beads of a polypeptide for delivery to the distal intestine for topical effect via receptor binding in the intestine and colon.

Gastric solution		Small intestine solution
Volume ~ 50 mL to 300 mL pH = 1–3 Water, Hcl, Na$^+$, K$^+$, PO$_4$$^{-3}$ SO$_4$$^{-2}$, HCO$_3$$^-$, mucus Pepsin, protein Residence time–variable 0.25 to > 5 h Surface tension < water Permeability low	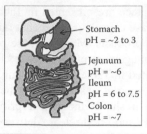 Stomach pH = ~2 to 3 Jejunum pH = ~6 Ileum pH = 6 to 7.5 Colon pH = ~7	Volume ~ 500 mL, pH ~ 4–7.5 HCO$_3$$^-$, Mucus, maltase-lactase- Sucrase-lipase-nuclease Carboxy and amino peptidase Fats-fatty acids, lecithin Bile salts, surface tension low Surface are ~ 200 m^2 Transit time ~ 3–4 h Permeability high

Complex colonic micro and macro environment
Permeability–drug dependent
Transit time 1 to > 24 h
Redox potential –400 mv
Bacteria(cfu/g), 1 × 10^{12}
pH ~ 7
Fluid ~ 187 mL(total), 13 mL(free)
Length = 1.66 m
Surface area = 3 m^2

FIGURE 12.3 Physiological constraints and variations in pH, transit time, permeability, and fluid compositions within the dynamic environment of the GI tract.

shows various physiological constraints and GI environments that a modified-release capsule dosage form encounters upon oral administration.

The GI constraints should be considered in conjunction with characteristics and limitations described by way of the Biopharmaceutics Classification System (BCS), implemented in 1995 as a new approach to better predict oral drug absorption and adopted by the FDA.[10,11] According to the BCS, drug substances are classified as follows:

Class I—High Permeability, High Solubility
Class II—High Permeability, Low Solubility
Class III—Low Permeability, High Solubility
Class IV—Low Permeability, Low Solubility

Furthermore, the class boundaries described above is based on the following premise:

1. A drug substance is considered highly soluble when the highest dose strength is soluble in <250 mL of water over a pH range of 1 to 7.5.
2. A drug substance is considered highly permeable when the extent of absorption in humans is determined to be >90% of an administered dose, based on mass balance or in comparison to an intravenous reference dose.
3. A drug product is considered to be rapidly dissolving when >85% of the labeled amount of drug substance dissolves within 30 min using USP apparatus I at 100 rpm or II at 50 rpm in a volume of ≤900 mL of buffer solutions.

The hard shell capsule itself, once in the desired GI environment/region, would dissolve fairly rapidly (10–30 min) and releases its content immediately (i.e., in the case of immediate release) for rapid absorption as opposed to modified-release systems such as controlled release or sustained release as shown in Figure 12.4.

When capsule dosage forms are designed for providing a particular release profile or sustained drug delivery, upon oral administration, it would deliver its content for further disintegration, dissolution, and release followed by absorption in various regions of the GI tract as shown in Figure 12.5.

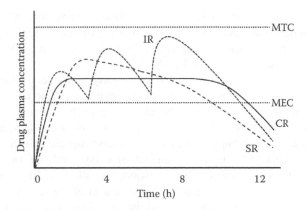

FIGURE 12.4 A graphical representation of the plasma concentration against time following the oral administration of an immediate-release (IR) capsule given every 4 h and a controlled-release (CR) and a sustained-release (SR) product given once a day. MTC, minimum toxic concentration; MEC, minimum effective concentration. CR maintains a constant therapeutic plasma concentration of drug; SR ensures prolonged duration of plasma levels of drug, and IR requires multiple administrations with peaks and troughs.

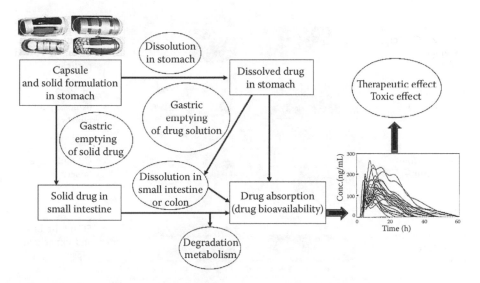

FIGURE 12.5 A simplified process of drug dissolution and absorption after oral administration of modified-release capsule dosage forms as it transits through various regions of the GI tract. Typical population plasma concentration–time profile for a small number of healthy human subjects is also shown.

TERMINOLOGY AND DEFINITION OF MODIFIED-RELEASE DOSAGE FORMS

FDA defines modified-release dosage forms as "dosage forms whose drug release characteristics of time course and/or location are chosen to accomplish therapeutic or convenience objectives not offered by conventional dosage forms, such as a solution or an immediate-release dosage form. Modified-release solid oral dosage forms include both delayed- and extended-release drug products."[12]

The USP recognizes several types of modified-release systems including extended release, delayed release, or targeted release. However, expressions such as "prolonged-action," "repeat-action," "controlled-release," "pulse-release," "modified-release," "ascending-release," and "sustained-release" have also been used to describe such dosage forms. Although many of these terms have been used interchangeably, the terms "extended-release" and "modified-release" are used for Pharmacopeial purposes, and requirements for drug release typically are specified in the individual monographs [see general release standard USP ⟨724⟩ and ⟨1088⟩].[13]

The platform is highly flexible and lends itself to a variety of delivery system designs that could be complementary with different biopharmaceutical properties of the drug in relation to physiological constraints imposed by the GI tract. Ideally, the extended-release delivery system should provide release rate and duration of release that would match the necessary amount of drug in the blood for a specific duration of therapy. The modified-release capsule delivery platform permits for constant release (zero-order), variable release (pulsatile), delayed release, or extended drug release and absorption over a prolonged period after ingestion. Capsules can be enteric coated, or coated pellets/granules that resist releasing in the acidic environment of the stomach can be encapsulated. Enteric coating delays release of medicament until the capsule or its contents have passed through the stomach. Potential modified-release capsule delivery systems and sophisticated release rates and patterns that can be realized from manufacturing of different controlled-release capsule delivery designs are shown in Figures 12.6 and 12.7a and b.

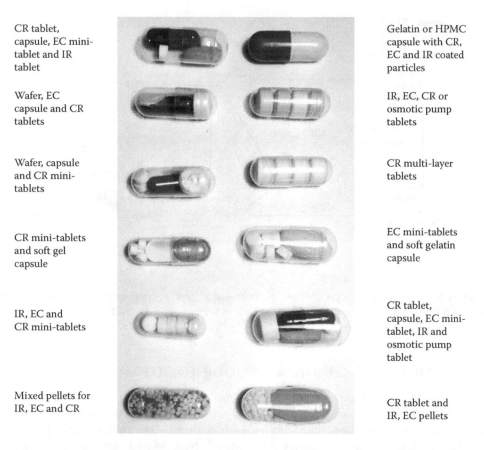

CR tablet, capsule, EC mini-tablet and IR tablet

Gelatin or HPMC capsule with CR, EC and IR coated particles

Wafer, EC capsule and CR tablets

IR, EC, CR or osmotic pump tablets

Wafer, capsule and CR mini-tablets

CR multi-layer tablets

CR mini-tablets and soft gel capsule

EC mini-tablets and soft gelatin capsule

IR, EC and CR mini-tablets

CR tablet, capsule, EC mini-tablet, IR and osmotic pump tablet

Mixed pellets for IR, EC and CR

CR tablet and IR, EC pellets

FIGURE 12.6   (See color insert.) Controlled-release capsule drug delivery systems with different types of dosages or encapsulated formulations (transparent shell is chosen to show the content). Some of these are commercially available; others are possible examples that can be for investigation. EC, enteric coated; CR, controlled release; IR, immediate release.

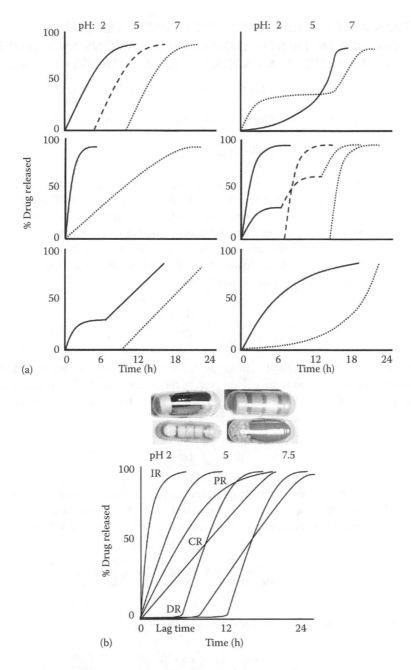

FIGURE 12.7 (See color insert.) (a) Typical modified-release capsule delivery system and potential drug release rates and duration of release during dissolution studies. Drug may be released in a pulsatile manner, one portion may provide for a bolus dose while another portion provides for delayed release, or maintenance dose either at constant rate, ascending rate, repeat action, or sustained release. System may allow for delivery of either one drug or drug combinations (i.e., fixed-dose combination). (b) Types of drug release from different modified-release capsule dosage forms containing multiple tablets, enteric or controlled-release coated pellets and tablets, coated mini-tablets, and enteric-coated small capsule placed in a larger capsule with different tablet combinations. Various release profiles from different combinations are possible for different time periods (i.e., 1- to 24-h duration). Systems may allow for either one drug or drug combinations. Type of release: immediate release (IR); prolonged release (PR, with or without a bolus dose); delayed release (DR): release after lapse of certain time in a desired pH environment; controlled release (CR) with zero-order kinetics.

DISSOLUTION RATE OF DRUG FROM DRUG PARTICLES, PELLETS, OR FROM VARIOUS MODIFIED-RELEASE FORMULATIONS AND DELIVERY SYSTEMS ENCAPSULATED IN A CAPSULE SHELL AS A DELIVERY CARRIER

There are two major classes of dosage forms or drug delivery systems for oral administration:

1. Immediate-release solid dosage forms (orally disintegrating and immediate-release tablets and capsules)
2. Modified-/controlled-/sustained-release dosage forms

Drug release in vitro or in vivo from a conventional capsule is very similar to an immediate-release tablet dosage form except for a small lag time of less than 30 min for the capsule shell to dissolve. Release and subsequent bio-absorption are controlled by the physicochemical properties of the drug, its formulation, and the physiological conditions and constraints imposed by the GI tract. The release of a drug from these delivery systems is rapid and involves factors of dissolution and diffusion. The earliest work describing diffusion was by Fick in 1855. Fick's first law of diffusion considers diffusion only under steady-state conditions.

$$J = -D \cdot \frac{dc}{dx},$$
(12.1)

where J is the diffusion current, D is the diffusion coefficient, and dc/dx is the concentration gradient assumed to be constant at steady state. However, as the concentration of drug changes with time, Fick's second law of diffusion is used; hence, it considers non-steady-state conditions.

$$\frac{dc}{dt} = D\left(\frac{d^2c}{dx^2}\right)$$
(12.2)

where dc/dt is the dissolution rate of the drug. Based on Fick's second law of diffusion, Noyes and Whitney[14] established a fundamental equation for dissolution. In its simplest form, the in vitro rate of solubility or dissolution rate of a drug substance is described by the Noyes–Whitney equation:

$$\frac{dC}{dt} = \left(\frac{D}{h} \times S\right) \times (C_s - C_t)$$
(12.3)

Under sink conditions, $C_s \gg C_t$, and Equation 12.3 becomes

$$\frac{dC}{dt} = \frac{(D \times S \times C_s)}{h},$$
(12.4)

where dC/dt is the dissolution rate at time t, D is the diffusion rate constant, h is the thickness of the stagnant layer, S is the surface area of the dissolving solid, C_s is the concentration of the drug in the stagnant layer, and C_t is the concentration of the drug at time t in the bulk solution. Note that if the concentration in bulk solution is ≤15% of saturation solubility, "sink condition" prevails.

In an *in vivo* situation after dissolution, drug molecules move across a distance into a membrane and its membrane permeability depends on the velocity with which it moves. Apart from the role of transporters, channels, and carriers, a simplified absorption is described by Fick's law of diffusion, which involves movement of the drug molecule from a region of high concentration to low

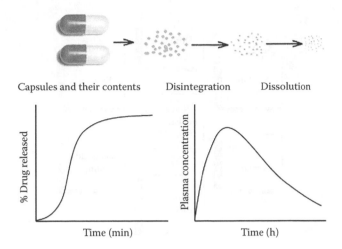

FIGURE 12.8 Disintegration, dissolution, and absorption of a drug after oral administration of an immediate-release capsule dosage form.

concentration. Thus, the drug tends to move toward a region that we may regard as sink, which is passage through the epithelial membrane into blood circulation in accordance with the following equation:

$$\frac{dC}{dt} = \frac{P_e \times A \times D \times (C_{GI} - C_{Blood})}{h},$$

(12.5)

where dC/dt is the rate of absorption, P_e is effective permeability, A is the surface area of the membrane, D is the diffusion coefficient of the drug molecule in water, $C_{GI} - C_{Blood}$ is concentration gradient across the GI membrane, and h is membrane thickness. In Equation 12.5, it is assumed that the unstirred aqueous boundary layer next to the membrane does not significantly affect the total transport process. Therefore, it is important to note that many factors influence the dissolution rate of a drug both in vivo and in vitro, including physicochemical (i.e., particle size, molecular size, hydrophilicity/hydrophobicity, and crystallinity), physiological (i.e., presence of surfactants, GI motility, viscosity and volume of GI fluid, and pH), and in vitro factors (i.e., surfactants, stirring rate and hydrodynamics, viscosity, pH, and volume of medium).

Typically when immediate-release capsule dosage forms are administered orally, the capsule shell disintegrates within a few minutes (i.e., <15 min) and its content dissolves, and the dissolved drug is absorbed as shown in Figure 12.8.

OPERATING RELEASE MECHANISMS ASSOCIATED WITH DIFFERENT ENCAPSULATED MODIFIED-RELEASE DOSAGE FORMS

Modified-release delivery from hard shell capsules may contain a variety of fabricated delivery systems. These include granules, powders, systems with different functional coatings such as enteric-coated, extended-, sustained-, controlled- (such as osmotic pump), and/or programmed-release systems including pulsatile or targeted-delivery systems and drug combinations, all of which can be placed in a capsule shell as a carrier for administration. It is also customary to coat hard shell capsules with polymers that prevent dissolution at low pH and can avert gastric degradation or release. Formulation methods vary and usually when needed allow for rapid release followed by slow release of the maintenance dose. All modified-release formulations employ a chemical, physical,

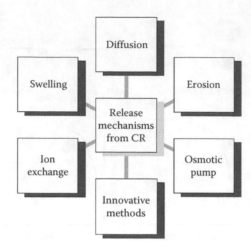

FIGURE 12.9 Various principles of operating release mechanisms associated with different encapsulated modified-release dosage forms. Such delivery systems, individually or in combination, can be placed in hard shell capsules to achieve specific goals of drug delivery.[15]

or electrical constraint to deliver sustained release of the drug dose. In general, they can be divided into two major groups:

1. Matrix based systems—pellets, mini-matrices, or small tablets
2. Membrane diffusion-controlled systems—coated pellets, tablets, and osmotic pumps

Production of modified-release delivery systems is based on numerous formulation approaches, methodologies, and innovative methods, and they each have their own specific operating release-controlling mechanisms as shown in Figure 12.9.

MATHEMATICAL MODELS TO DESCRIBE RELEASE KINETICS FROM EXTENDED-RELEASE CAPSULES CONTAINING FORMULATED DELIVERY SYSTEMS

Various mathematical models have been used to describe the rate of drug release from different types of encapsulated dosage forms and modified-release systems. For example, an analysis of drug diffusion from simple monolithic devices (i.e., cylinders or spheres representing small tablet matrix or an extruded and spheronized pellet type) designed for controlled release of drug has been described using exact solutions or reasonably accurate approximations.[16,17] From experimental work, it is evident that, from such monolithic systems, initial amount of drug released (i.e., early time) is in accordance with the square root of time while release in a later stage follows an exponential decay with time (i.e., late time). Equations shown in Table 12.2 predict such drug release from an infinite system, assuming that the edge or end effects are inconsequential.[17]

M_t is the amount released at time t, M_∞ is the total amount of drug, and D is the diffusion coefficient of the solute.

Besides, a more practical approach in evaluating drug release from matrix systems designed for controlled release using "insoluble waxes or hydrophilic and soluble/erodible polymers such as polyethylene oxide or hydroxypropylmethyl cellulose or hydroxypropyl cellulose" is described by the Higuchi approach:[5]

$$\frac{M_t}{M_\infty} = k\sqrt{t},$$

$$(12.6)$$

TABLE 12.2
Approximate Solutions for Diffusional Release from Cylinder and Spheres

Geometry	Early Time	Late Time
Cylinder	$\dfrac{M_t}{M_\infty} = 4\left(\dfrac{Dt}{\pi r^2}\right)^{1/2} - \dfrac{Dt}{r^2}$	$\dfrac{M_t}{M_\infty} = 1 - \dfrac{4}{(2.405)^2}\exp\left(\dfrac{-(2.405)^2 Dt}{r^2}\right)$
Sphere	$\dfrac{M_t}{M_\infty} = 6\left(\dfrac{Dt}{\pi r^2}\right)^{1/2} - 3\dfrac{Dt}{r^2}$	$\dfrac{M_t}{M_\infty} = 1 - \dfrac{6}{\pi^2}\exp\left(\dfrac{-\pi^2 Dt}{r^2}\right)$

where M_t/M_∞ indicates that the fraction of drug released is proportional to the square root of time. K is a constant reflecting formulation characteristics, which may include drug diffusion coefficient in matrix D, the solubility of drug in polymer/wax matrix C_s, the porosity ε, tortuosity of the capillary systems created within the matrix, and property of the matrix (i.e., homogeneous, granular, hydrophilic, erodible, or insoluble). The model assumes that in these matrices, drug dissolves from the exposed surface regions, and as it becomes exhausted of dissolved drug, a more gradual drug depletion of the deeper regions to the core is followed, as shown in Figures 12.10 and 12.11.

It is an important fact to note from Equation 12.6 that, in general, the relationship between M_t/M_∞ and square root of time is linear for both simple insoluble and hydrophilic granules, pellets, mini-tablets or matrices. A more general equation that can be applied to most types of drug delivery systems (excluding osmotic pump systems) to describe drug release rate is a modification of the above equation:

$$\frac{M_t}{M_\infty} = kt^n,$$

(12.7)

where exponent n has values between 0.45 and ≤ 0.85. The values around 0.5 or square root are generally associated with a burst effect (rapid initial drug release) followed by a tailing of release profiles beyond at least 60% drug release.[18,19]

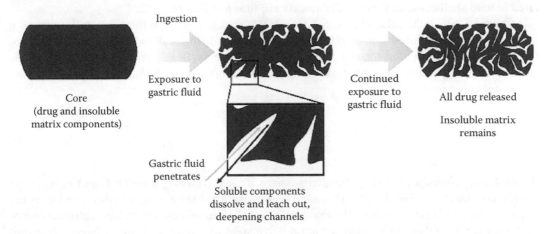

FIGURE 12.10 Release of drug from a granular insoluble matrix dosage form. Schematic shows the receding boundary as drug diffuses from the dosage form.

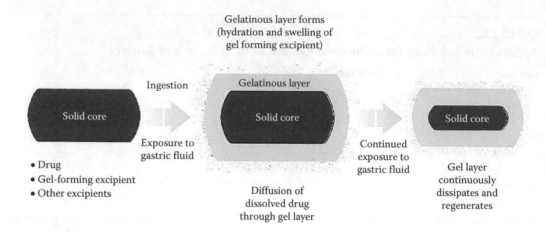

FIGURE 12.11 Release of drug from a hydrophilic matrix dosage form. Schematic shows the hydration, swelling, drug diffusion, and continuous erosion of the gel layer.

On the other hand, reservoir systems for extended release are characterized by a drug core surrounded by a particular polymeric membrane that determines rate of release from the system. The process of drug release is described by Fick's law of diffusion and, in its simplest form, it can be written as

$$J = \frac{M_t}{M_\infty} = \frac{DAK\Delta c}{L},$$

(12.8)

where J or M_t/M_∞ indicates that the fraction of drug released with time is proportional to the surface area A, the diffusion coefficient D, the distribution coefficient K of the permeant toward the polymer, and Δc is the concentration difference across the membrane having thickness L. Therefore, alteration of polymer in terms of type, molecular weight, and degree of crystallinity coupled with membrane thickness and drug properties can give rise to the desired drug release. Equations of similar form can be written for other geometries such as spheres, cylinders, or multi-laminates. Graphic representations for pellets or matrices with different properties that are routinely encapsulated in hard shell capsules for extended release are shown in Figure 12.12.

In systems where the value of n is in excess of 0.5, release rates tend to approach linearity as n increases and mechanisms of drug release depend on both diffusional and erosional properties of the system (i.e., hydrophilic matrix). This situation is more applicable when a polymer matrix is swellable and erodible at the same time. A well-known empirical model that describes these phenomena is given by[20,21]

$$\frac{M_t}{M_\infty} = k_1 t^m + k_2 t^{2m},$$

(12.9)

where M_t/M_∞ represents the drug fraction released in time t ($M_t/M_\infty \leq 60\%$); k_1 and k_2 represent kinetic constants associated with diffusional and relaxational release, respectively; and m is the purely Fickian diffusion exponent. For example, when small matrix tablets with potential for encapsulation were formulated using guar, a natural polymer, as its rate-controlling excipient, verapamil hydrochloride as a model drug, and glycine as a soluble release aid excipient, zero-order release of drug in pH 1–6 was achieved (see Figure 12.13). When such a matrix formulation is placed in a

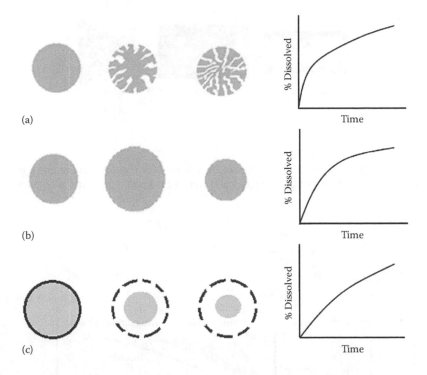

FIGURE 12.12 An illustration of cross section of pellets, matrix systems, or coated spheres and their corresponding drug release rate by diffusion through channels from an insoluble matrix (a), swelling and eroding matrix (b), and diffusion from the reservoir system (c).

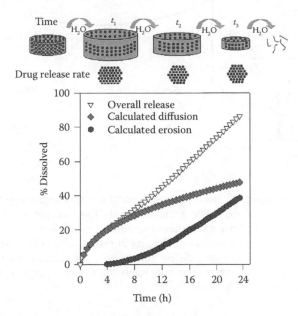

FIGURE 12.13 Verapamil release from guar matrix using USP apparatus-II, 1000 mL, buffer pH 1.5 at 50 rpm. Upper schematics show dynamics of changes in matrix dimensions in terms of swelling/erosion over time during dissolution. The sum of calculated curves using Equation 12.9 showing drug release based on the principle of diffusion and/or erosion results in an experimentally determined linear release rate shown with open triangles. Calculated diffusion and erosion contributions as part of release mechanisms associated with this hydrophilic matrix are also shown.[22,23]

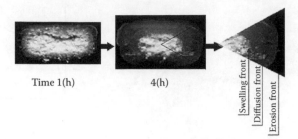

FIGURE 12.14 Changes in physical appearance of the matrix showing the swelling and eroding nature of matrix during dissolution. Matrices were sectioned at different time points and various fronts identified.[24]

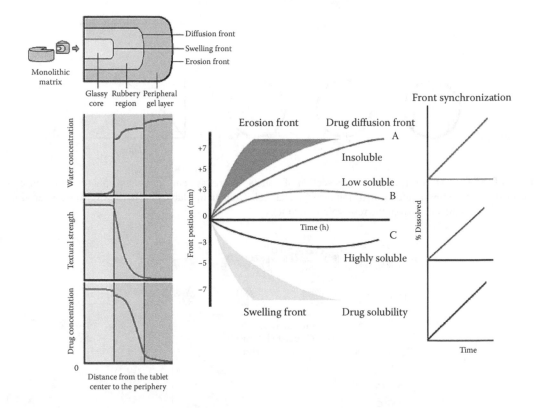

FIGURE 12.15 **(See color insert.)** Graphic representation of a matrix undergoing hydration and swelling. Depending on the properties of polymer(s), drug, and excipients. Exact release is influenced by synchronization of various fronts as shown. Left panel illustrates hydration of matrix from periphery to the center of the matrix showing different fronts and dynamics of changes in matrix from tablet center to the erosion front. Middle panel shows synchronization of drug diffusion front within a hydrating matrix dominated by either swelling aspect or erosion aspect contingent upon drug solubility. The right panel shows achievement of zero-order drug release owing to front synchronization.[25,26]

capsule shell, it is assumed that the capsule shell will dissolve within 15–30 min, and drug release would follow and release mechanism can be best described by Equation 12.9.

Accordingly, the degree and exactness of control over the rate of drug release from modified-release delivery systems differ according to the system design and associated mechanism(s) by which drug release is accomplished. Thus, the rate of drug release from the designed delivery systems may result in an input rate for absorption, which would match the desired concentration in the blood to elicit the preferred clinical outcome and potentially allow for establishment of level A *in vitro–in vivo correlation (IVIVC)*.[19]

For example, control over the rate of drug release from matrix-type systems that are based on hydrophilic/swelling and eroding polymers is exemplified for drugs of different solubility by analyzing dynamics of changes that occur during dissolution testing, leading to desired release as shown in Figures 12.14 and 12.15.

Multiple small matrices using swelling and eroding principles or different populations of multiparticulates, such as coated and uncoated pellets or multiple small coated pellets that release the drug by generation of osmotic pressure within the core, can be placed in a single hard shell capsule to provide for different release patterns, including zero order, delayed release, delayed and extended release, ascending, and/or pulse drug release, which are commercially available.

TYPES OF BLOOD LEVELS FOR DIFFERENT THERAPEUTIC EFFECTS

Typically, zero-order release or bolus and zero-order release may include profiles in which rapid attainment of a therapeutic level followed by either a constant maintenance level or prolonged duration of blood levels is the objective (Figure 12.16). Other delivery alternatives include repeat-action, delayed-release, extended-release, and ascending-release delivery systems, as shown in Figures 12.17 and 12.18.

EXAMPLES OF COMMERCIALLY AVAILABLE HARD SHELL EXTENDED-RELEASE CAPSULE DELIVERY SYSTEMS

ENCAPSULATED MATRIX TABLETS FOR EXTENDED DRUG RELEASE

Representative and commercially available modified-release capsule dosage forms containing four individual tablet matrices each containing 60 mg diltiazem hydrochloride designed for 24-h zero-order release is shown in Figure 12.19. In this delivery system, each tablet has three layers. Two external layers act as a barrier to release from the middle layer, which contains a highly soluble drug. The system is hydrophilic and will hydrate and swell, allowing drug diffusion. Diffusion of drug occurs laterally as barrier layers remain on both side of the middle matrix layer. The delivery

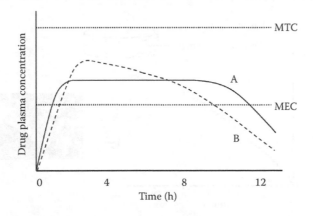

FIGURE 12.16 A graphical representation of the plasma concentration against time following the oral administration of controlled (A) and sustained (B) release products. MTC, minimum toxic concentration; MEC, minimum effective concentration. A maintains constant therapeutic plasma concentration of drug; B ensures prolonged duration of plasma levels of drug.

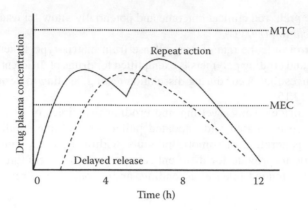

FIGURE 12.17 A graphical representation of the plasma concentration against time following the oral administration of a repeat action dosage form or a delayed release product. MTC, minimum toxic concentration; MEC, minimum effective concentration.

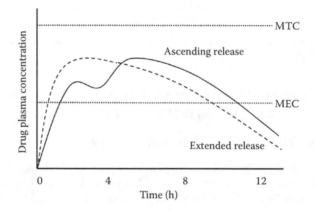

FIGURE 12.18 A graphical representation of the plasma concentration against time profiles following the oral administration of an ascending-release product and an extended-release dosage form. MTC, minimum toxic concentration; MEC, minimum effective concentration. Ascending-release dosage form provides for disease conditions in which chronopharmacological interactions prevail. An extended-release dosage form ensures prolonged duration of plasma levels of drug and more desirable therapeutic effect.

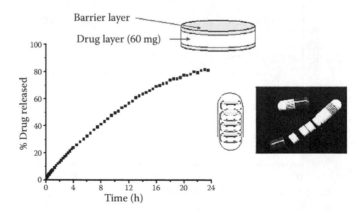

FIGURE 12.19 Near-zero-order delivery of highly soluble drug diltiazem hydrochloride (240 mg) from hard shell capsule containing 4 three-layer tablets each with 60 mg diltiazem sandwiched between two barrier layers. Dissolution was performed using USP-26, apparatus-II, in 900 mL of phosphate buffer (pH 6.8) at 37°C, with a paddle rotation of 100 rpm.

system provides 240 mg of diltiazem release in a near-zero-order manner. The principle mechanism of drug release is based on surface restriction, matrix swelling, drug diffusion, and system erosion as illustrated in the earlier discussion (see Figures 12.14 and 12.15).

ENCAPSULATED COATED AND UNCOATED PELLETS FOR EXTENDED DRUG RELEASE

Many marketed extended-release capsule dosage forms containing different populations of pellets, mini-tables, granules, or multiparticulates with varying polymer types and functionality to sequentially release their drug content in different pH's and regions of GI tract for prolonged absorption are commercially available. For example, in one US patent, specific formulation strategies to provide rapid, delayed, and extended release with enhanced solubility features for extended release of carbamazepine base especially in a more alkaline portion of the distal intestine are shown in Figure 12.20. In pellet C, one of the excipients used in the core is citric or tartaric acid. Since carbamazepine base has low solubility and limited dissolution in the more alkaline pH environment of distal intestine, the addition of acidic excipient in the pellet core once dissolved will create a low-pH microenvironment with increased osmotic pressure, thus enhancing diffusion and dissolution rate of carbamazepine. A similar approach has also been adopted in matrix systems to control dynamics of hydrations and dissolution rates of highly soluble compounds.[27]

The main mechanism of drug release from these three pellet types is based on immediate release and dissolution of pellet A, followed by delayed release from pellet B, and a more extended release that is based on enhanced solubility of the drug within the coated pellet C followed by diffusion from inside to outside of the permeable membrane as a result of both osmotic pressure and concentration gradient across the coating barrier. These release principles are discussed under the section "Dissolution Rate of Drug from Drug Particles, Pellets, or from Various Modified-Release Formulations and Delivery Systems Encapsulated in a Capsule Shell as a Delivery Carrier."

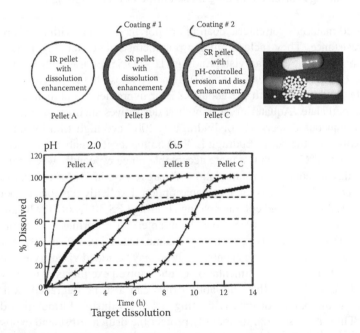

FIGURE 12.20 Extended-release carbamazepine capsule (200 mg) containing three different bead types, each with their own formulation and rate controlling membrane, combined in exact proportions to provide sustained release of drug in different pH environment within the GI tract. Each pellet type is designed to release drug in different pH's at different rates. Summation of all release portions from each pellet type after dissolution testing is also shown. (For more details, see US patent 5326570.)

ENCAPSULATED ENTERIC-COATED PELLETS AND ENTERIC-COATED MINI-TABLETS FOR DELAYED RELEASE AND/OR DELAYED EXTENDED RELEASE

The coating of solid substrates in the form of pellets or tablets is one of the most commonly used operation in the pharmaceutical industry for purposes of taste masking, esthetic and trade marking matters, stability improvement, or generating functionalized coatings such as enteric or controlled-release coatings. The functional coating option allows formulators to develop pH-dependent dosage forms of the drug that can resist gastric dissolution or to induce delayed release kinetics as part of modified-release drug delivery systems. A variety of dissolution kinetics can be addressed in this way, together with GI targeting of drug via pulsatile release or slow release through permeable or semipermeable coating having one or more orifices. Coating is accomplished by applying a uniform coat on a substrate in a drum/pan coater or fluidized bed system by means of liquid spraying, immersion into a liquid, or powder deposition by electrostatic forces.[28,29]

Enteric coating is typically and successfully employed when

1. Drug substance is destroyed by gastric acid or enzymes and should be protected.
2. Drug causes irritation to the gastric mucosa and thus improving tolerability is achieved by release in the small intestine.
3. Absorption and bioavailability is substantially enhanced in the intestine via temporal and pH-dependent dissolution and release.
4. It is desirable to deliver the drug after a time delay (i.e., controlled onset delivery) particularly as part of controlled-release drug delivery.
5. Targeting in the GI tract is desirable, especially in delivery to the colon, for topical effect or systemic absorption. For example, delayed release in pH ≥7.0 (ileum and colon) for distal GI delivery is particularly advantageous in the treatment of ulcerative colitis and Crohn's disease (i.e., dosage forms containing mesalamine or budesonide).[30]

Frequently used materials for enteric coating are polymeric acids with free carboxyl groups that confer gastric resistance. They include anionic polymethacrylates (copolymerisate of methacrylic acid: methylmethacrylate or ethyl acrylate, Eudragit L 30 D-55, Eudragit FS 30 D, or Eudragit-L100, with a pH value of aqueous dispersion of ~3.05) and cellulose-based polymers (i.e., hypromellose acetate succinate [HPMCAS], with pH about 3.85) or hypromellose phthalate (HPMCP), aqueous cellulose acetate phthalate (Aquateric), or polyvinyl derivatives such as polyvinyl acetate phthalate (Coateric). Since aqueous dispersions of Eudragit L 100 have high film-forming temperatures of about 85°C, mixing with the softer Eudragit L 30 D 55 makes it possible to reduce the film-forming temperature to about 40°C, which is a more acceptable range especially when hard gelatin capsules and HPMC capsules are coated. For modulation of drug release in pH 5.5 to 7.0, further mixing with Eudragit NE 30 D and FS 30 D is an acceptable option. Explicitly aqueous dispersions for enteric coating (Eudragit L 30 D-55) and colonic coating (Eudragit FS 30 D) of HPMC and hard shell gelatin capsules have been investigated.[31,32] Apart from enteric film formers, other enteric film coating components include plasticizers (i.e., diethyl phthalate, triacetin), anti-adhesion agents, colorants, pigments, solubilizers, and dispersing agents. To these may be added viscosity-enhancing suspension stabilizers designed to retard the sedimentation of undissolved excipients or dispersed film formers.

Mention must be made that the acid-labile drugs can also be degraded as a consequence of contact with the acidic nature of enteric coating polymers during formulation development and manufacturing. Thus, it is essential to not only protect the drug against acid exposure in the acidic environment of the stomach and prevent its degradation but also have protective measures during formulation development to prevent degradation and also enhance drug storage stability for predictive bioavailability and therapeutic efficacy after oral administration.[33,34] Figure 12.21 shows a typical pellet with an acid-labile drug omeprazole that is layered onto a sugar sphere and protected with a layer of neutral barrier before the application of acidic enteric coating solution.

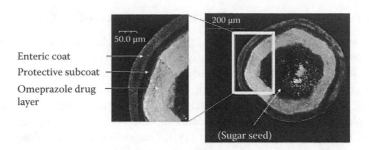

FIGURE 12.21 Fluorescence image of a fractured omeprazole pellet, where a spherical nonpareil seed was coated with the omeprazole drug layer followed by application of an inert barrier layer and further coating with an acidic polymer enteric layer on top of the subcoat for the enhancement of drug stability during manufacturing and shelf life storage stability.[35]

Two frequently used techniques to produce pellets that contain drugs include drug layering onto spherical substrates or direct pelletization via wet extrusion of drug and excipient mixture followed by spheronization and drying.[36] Pellets can be directly enteric coated with pH-sensitive polymers or coated for the controlled-release delivery of drug over a prolonged period. The coating process can be accomplished by using an air suspension coating approach where the solution of the polymers or suspension of drug in polymer solution is sprayed via nozzle(s) atomization onto the pellets in a fluid bed apparatus under the controlled conditions of air pressure and temperature to achieve percent target weight gain (i.e., desired coat thickness) for specific delivery rate or release location in the GI tract. The core materials could also be a formulated mini-tablet or a filled capsule, where both fluidization or the pan coating approach are used.[37,38] Typical examples of encapsulated enteric-coated pellets of omeprazole, a proton pump inhibitor, and delayed extended-release coated mini-tablets of 5-amino salicylic acid, an anti-inflammatory drug, for delivery to the proximal and distal intestine (i.e., ileum and colon) with their respective dissolution profiles are shown in Figure 12.22.

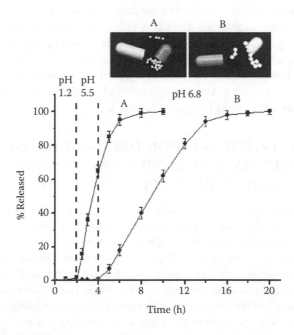

FIGURE 12.22 Dissolution profiles for encapsulated enteric-coated omeprazole pellets and delayed extended-release 5-amino salicylic acid mini-tablets, using USP 26, apparatus-II at 100 rpm, 900 mL of buffers with different pH's.

ENCAPSULATED BEADS OF A POLYPEPTIDE LINACLOTIDE FOR ONCE-A-DAY ORAL ADMINISTRATION

Linaclotide is a 14-amino acid peptide agonist of guanylate cyclase-C (GCC). Both linaclotide and its active metabolite bind to GCC and act locally on the luminal surface of the intestinal epithelium that is intended for the treatment of chronic idiopathic constipation and irritable bowel syndrome constipation in adults. It reduces activation of colonic sensory neurons, which reduces pain, and activates colonic motor neurons, which increases smooth muscle contraction and thus promotes bowel movements. The product is a hard gelatin capsule (145 and 290 μg strengths) containing linaclotide drug substance coated onto microcrystalline cellulose beads along with HPMC and stabilizing agents such as calcium chloride dihydrate and L-lucine for once-a-day administration. The molecular formula of linaclotide is $C_{59}H_{79}N_{15}O_{21}S_6$, and its molecular weight is 1526.8. It is a 14-amino acid synthetic peptide with three disulfide bridges. All amino acids are of L-configuration with the following sequence: L-tyrosine, L-cysteinyl–L-cysteinyl–L alpha-glutamyl–L-tyrosyl–L-cysteinyl–L-cysteinyl–L-asparaginyl–L-prolyl–L-alanyl–L-cysteinyl–L-threonylglycyl–L-cysteinyl-, cyclic (1↔6),(2 ↔10),(5 ↔13)-tris(disulfide).

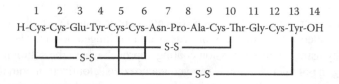

It is an amorphous, white powder with no x-ray powder diffraction patterns, soluble in water; pH (2.4 mg/mL) = 3.4; isoelectric point (IP) = 4.0; specific optical rotation = −235° to −261° (589 nm, c = 0.1 in 1% acetic acid). Linaclotide is minimally absorbed with low systemic availability following oral administration (i.e., plasma levels are below the limit of quantitation after oral doses of 145 μg or 290 μg). Its solubility in aqueous solution over a pH range 1.0 to 7.5 is >100 μg/mL. Therefore, it is considered to be a BCS Class 3 (high solubility, low permeability) compound. The hard shell capsule appears to be an ideal carrier for this compound. Being a polypeptide, if subjected to compression forces used in tableting, it is likely to lose its structural features owing to mechanical shearing followed by loss of its therapeutic value. It is known that mechanical perturbation and shearing forces of impaction and compression during tableting consolidation are high enough to kill bacterial cells and mold spores.[39] Consequently, if proteins and polypeptides are subjected to similar conditions, they may not maintain their molecular stability and folded state and result in conformational changes with loss of biological function.

ENCAPSULATED DRUG FORMULATION FOR TIME-DELAYED AND TARGETED DELIVERY DURING DRUG DEVELOPMENT PHASES AND RESEARCH TO ASSESS DRUG ABSORPTION

Multiple delivery systems with potential use in chronotherapeutics in concord with the circadian rhythms of the disease have been developed with specific time-dependent "trigger" mechanisms for delivery of drug at a particular rate to a specific region of the GI tract. One such delivery system is Pulsincap,[40,41] which consists of an insoluble and impermeable capsule body and a water-soluble cap with possibility for pH-sensitive coating as graphically shown in Figure 12.23. The capsule cap is soluble in water or a desired pH environment while the capsule body is impermeable to water. Drug and swelling polymer can be used as part of drug formulation together or independent of each other and filled into the body of the capsule. A swelling and eroding hydrogel plug or an eroding compressed tablet is used to seal the content. Upon oral administration, the cap will dissolve in the specific pH environment followed by gradual but controlled hydration, swelling, and erosion of the plug. Compositionally, the plug is made of a swellable, erodible (e.g., HPMC, soluble

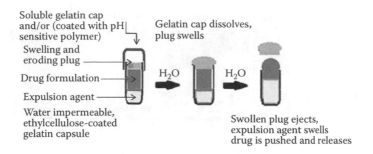

FIGURE 12.23 Pulsincap delivery system with time-delayed release using an erodible plug or erodible compressed tablet as a time trigger inciting drug release.

polymethacrylate, polyvinyl alcohol), or congealed melted excipient (e.g., glyceryl monooleate), or an enzymatically degradable polysaccharide like pectin. Once the plug is dissolved, fluid gradually enters the capsule body from the open end. For rapid release of insoluble drugs, a disintegrant or an effervescent agent may be added to the formulation. The expulsion agent also swells and expands and the drug formulation is expelled for complete dissolution. The second-generation Pulsincap has been further optimized for a more predictable and accurate plug ejection and composition of the expulsion agent to rapidly and completely expel the contents. The system has been used in several human studies demonstrating that the system was well tolerated in the volunteers as well as in the clinic, and its performance and location within the GI tract are monitored using scintigraphy studies.

Port System

Another system that has been investigated in research include the Port System, which is a compartmentalized semipermeable gelatin or HPMC capsule body divided into multiple compartments and is capable of drug delivery in accordance with zero order, pulse release, or their combinations especially for release in the lower ileum or colon.[42,43] The mechanism of drug release is based on water diffusion into the capsule body. Dissolved drug and excipients will generate an osmotic pressure gradient across the slidable separator and between the inside and outside of the capsule body pushing the separator and the dissolved drug into the GI tract.

Egalet

This particular system, which is also based on delayed release to achieve temporal or spatial targeted delivery of actives to the distal intestine, involves Egalet technology.[44] The system consists of an impermeable shell with two eroding lag plugs enclosing a formulation plug in the middle of the unit. Release mechanism is mainly based on swelling and erosion of the plugs and formulation. Other variants of the Egalet system allowing for burst release followed by extended or pulsatile release have also been investigated.

Electronic Capsule Devices for Site-Specific Determination of the Drug Absorption

Over the last 30 years, a number of electronic capsule devices with sizes generally equivalent to standard capsule size of "0" or "00" have been developed and investigated in humans to determine the drug absorption in various regions of the GI tract in a noninvasive manner.[45–47]

The primary emphasis of these electronic capsule devices has focused on control of time and the location of drug release via external activation of the capsule device after oral administration.[48]

One of the more advanced capsule shape devices in this category is called the Enterion capsule.

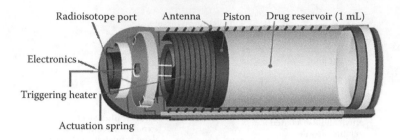

Radioisotope port   Antenna   Piston   Drug reservoir (1 mL)

Electronics

Triggering heater

Actuation spring

FIGURE 12.24 **(See color insert.)** The Enterion capsule can be used to assess absorption of drug from modified-release formulation during product development in different clinical phases. (Courtesy of Quotient Clinical, UK.)

The Enterion capsule shown in Figure 12.24 is designed and patented by Quotient Clinical to assess targeted delivery of a wide range of modified-release drug formulations. It is a remote-controlled device that is capable of precisely delivering drug formulations (both liquid and solid) to specific sites within the GI tract. It is a round-ended capsule with a drug chamber of about 1 mL in volume and can be loaded with either liquid dispersions, pellets, mini-tablets, or particulate matters, through an opening of 9 mm in diameter, which is then sealed by inserting a push-on cap fitted with a silicone O-ring. The base of the drug reservoir chamber is the piston face, which is held back against a compressed spring by a high-tensile strength polymer filament. The filament can be melted or ruptured wirelessly, pushing the drug formulation out of its chamber into the region of interest within the GI tract. The drug released may provide local and topical effect or it may be absorbed. A gamma-emitting marker may be placed inside a separate sealed tracer port to allow real-time visualization and transit location of the capsule in the GI tract after oral administration via scintigraphy.

The technology has potential for targeted delivery of highly potent drugs in specific regions of the GI tract especially when high localization of drug within a narrow segment of intestine for topical effect is needed. Such an application may include delivery of peptides, proteins, and anticancer drugs in colon cancer within any part of the colonic environment.[49]

INTELLICAP DEVICE

Medimetrics' IntelliCap is a wirelessly controlled, electronic capsule system that delivers drug to the region of interest in the GI tract for regional absorption studies. The 11 mm × 26 mm (approximately "000" size capsule) is composed of a microprocessor, battery, pH sensor, temperature sensor, wireless transceiver, fluid pump, and drug reservoir capable of storing up to 275 μL of test compound (see Figure 12.25). It communicates via its wireless transceiver to an external control unit worn by the subject.

Radiolabeling and scintigraphic monitoring of IntelliCap allow one to determine its position within the GI tract (Figure 12.26). This assures that the drug is released at the desired site, thus increasing its value in animal and clinical studies during product development phases.

The IntelliCap system allows for more predictable drug release within the target region. At the same time, transit time from stomach to colon can be easily monitored via a wireless pH sensor. Figure 12.27 shows representative data collected from an IntelliCap study in a dog. The capsule was programmed to release atenolol at a constant rate for 6 h starting at arrival in the duodenum. The zero-order release strategy allowed examining the entire intestinal tract with a single experiment. Regional transit and location are clearly described along with the pH data, drug release duration, and concurrent plasma concentration of the drug. An additional application of IntelliCap device for quantifying regional drug delivery and absorption in humans in bioequivalency studies using diltiazem as model drug is presented elsewhere.[50]

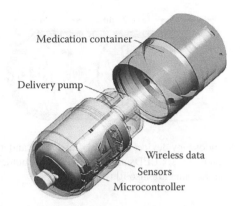

FIGURE 12.25 **(See color insert.)** "IntelliCap" system and its components. (Courtesy of Medimetrics.)

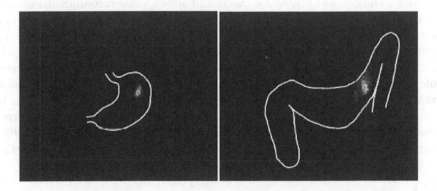

FIGURE 12.26 **(See color insert.)** A scintigraphic study showing the location of IntelliCap device after oral administration. (Courtesy of Medimetrics and Bio-Images Research partnership.)

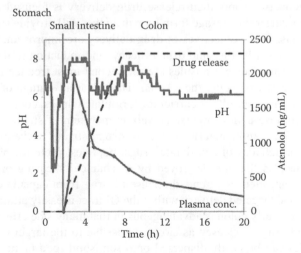

FIGURE 12.27 Concurrent determination of drug release, transit time, pH values, and drug plasma concentration; data collected from an IntelliCap study in a dog. (Courtesy of Medimetrics.)

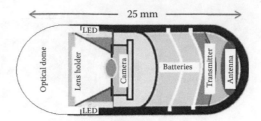

FIGURE 12.28 Typical capsule endoscopy device; its actual dimensions and its components are shown. The middle picture shows the capsule end with six LEDs and a camera. Lens holder, locations of LEDs, camera, batteries, electronic transmitter, and antenna are also illustrated.

ENDOSCOPY CAMERA CAPSULES

Wireless capsule endoscopy is a new and noninvasive tool to examine all or specifically parts of the GI tract (i.e., the middle portion of the small intestine) that cannot be seen with other types of endoscopy. The technique was invented in Japan and allows video recording and imaging of the digestive tract for use in medicine. The capsule dimensions and its features are generally equivalent to capsule size "00," and its general components are shown in Figure 12.28. Common reasons for doing capsule endoscopy is to diagnose GI tract problems such as internal bleeding, abdominal pain, detection of polyps, ulcers, tumors, and inflammatory bowel disease such as Crohn's disease. The capsule endoscope is a wireless and disposable device able to capture images and transmit these images to electrodes attached to the patient's body, permitting data storage. The capsule is capable of transmitting at a rate of 2 images per second, about 50,000 images within 8 h. There are four different manufacturers of capsule endoscopes: Endo Capsule (Olympus America), PillCam SB2 (Given Imaging), MiroCam (IntroMedic), and OMOM (Jinshan Science and Technology).

SUMMARY

Because of space limitations, complete coverage of all types of mechanisms and delivery innovations related to modified-release capsules as drug delivery was not possible. However, an attempt has been made to comprehensively elucidate and cover the major and more commonly used extended-release capsules that are FDA approved and currently marketed. The development of hard shell capsule products for modified-release drug delivery is focused on the choice and/or construction of the most desirable dosage form for a drug that will provide safe and effective drug delivery to treat patients. Other objectives of drug delivery are improvement in patient compliance, enhancement of bioavailability and drug efficacy, and reduction in dosing frequency with improved therapeutic performance. Capsules are the second most frequently used dosage forms for oral drug delivery (e.g., first being the tablets). The major advantage of capsules as delivery systems is that the shell can be used as a carrier for formulated drugs, coated pellets, mini-tablets, multiparticulates, fixed-dose combinations, as well as inclusion of smaller capsules or delivery systems. The capsule shell can be enteric coated for drug delivery to the proximal and/or distal intestine, especially for delivery of acid-labile drugs, peptides, proteins, biotechnology-derived drugs, and macromolecules that are destroyed by mechanical shearing or manufacturing processes. Additionally, controlled or extended release of drug from capsule delivery system with potential for pulsatile and targeted delivery within the GI tract is easily attainable. Drug targeting of the GI tract and specifically colon is advantageous in that many side effects are reduced, lower drug dose is used, and drug is released as close as possible to the target region. In some cases, the content of capsules can be easily dispersed onto semisolid food or liquids for patients who cannot swallow the dosage form. Furthermore, a variety of innovations in design of new capsule shells (i.e., microbiologically triggered systems, biodegradable, rupturable, or pressure-sensitive shells) and delivery types for targeting various regions of the GI tract are under investigation and development. Extended-release capsule delivery systems offer many opportunities and challenges not only in delivering drug in a controlled manner to the target area within GI tract but also in developing bio-relevant and appropriate in vitro dissolution methods simulating the in vivo conditions. The future of modified-release and extended-release capsules as drug delivery systems is limited only by the inventiveness of research scientists involved in the field.

REFERENCES

1. Jones, B.E. (2004) The history of the medicinal capsules. In: *Pharmaceutical Capsules*, 2nd edition, Chapter 1. Pharmaceutical Press: London, UK.
2. Augsburger, L.A. (1995) Hard and soft gelatin capsules. In: Banker, G.S., Rhodes, C.T. (Eds.), *Modern Pharmaceutics*. Marcel Dekker: New York, pp. 395–440.
3. Stegemann, S. (2000) Capsules as a delivery system for modified-release products. In: Dressman, J.B., Lennernäs, H. (Eds.), *Oral Drug Absorption*, Chapter 14. Marcel Dekker: New York.
4. Florence A.T. (2001) A short history of controlled drug release and an introduction. In: Wilson, C.G., Crowley, P.J. (Eds.), *Controlled Release in Oral Drug Delivery*, Chapter 1, Advances in Delivery Science and Technology, DOI 10.1007/978-1-4614-1004-1_1, Controlled Release Society.
5. Higuchi, T. (1963) Mechanism of sustained-action medication: Theoretical analysis of rate of release of solid drugs dispersed in solid matrices. *J Pharm Sci* 52:1145–1149.
6. Higuchi, W.I. (1967) Diffusional models useful in biopharmaceutics: Drug release rate processes. *J Pharm Sci* 56:315–324.
7. Ritschel, W.A. (1973) *Angewandte Biopharmazie*, Chapter 12, pp. 181–198; Wissenschaftliche Verlagsgesellschaft MBH, Stuttgart.
8. Langer, R. (1980) Polymeric delivery systems for controlled drug release. *Chem Eng Commun* 6:1–48.
9. Peppas, N. (1984) Mathematical modelling of diffusion processes in drug delivery polymeric systems. In: Smolen, V.F., Ball, L. (Eds.), *Controlled Drug Bioavailability*, Vol. 1. Wiley: New York, pp. 203–237.
10. Guidance for industry (2000) Waiver of *in vivo* bioavailability and bioequivalence studies for immediate release solid oral dosage forms based on a Biopharmaceutics Classification System. US Department of Health and Human Services Food and Drug Administration Center for Drug Evaluation and Research (CDER), Silver Spring, MD.
11. Amidon, G.L., Lennernäs, H., Shah, V.P., Crison, J.R. (1995) A theoretical basis for a biopharmaceutic drug classification: The correlation of in vitro drug product dissolution and in vivo bioavailability. *Pharm Res* 1995;12:413–420.
12. U.S. Department of Health and Human Services, Food and Drug Administration Center for Drug Evaluation and Research (CDER), Guidance for Industry, SUPAC-MR: Modified Release Solid Oral Dosage Forms. September 1997, p. 34, CMC8.
13. United States Pharmacopeia 23/National Formulary 18, USPC, Inc., Rockville, MD, 1995.
14. Noyes, A., Whitney, W. (1897) The rate of solution of solid substances in their own solutions. *J Am Chem Soc* 19: 930.
15. Jamzad, S. (2006) Analysis and application of bio-erodible swelling polymers in development of controlled release matrix systems for low dose BCS class-II drugs. Doctoral dissertation, submitted and approved; Temple University, School of Pharmacy.
16. Crank, J. (1975) *The Mathematics of Diffusion*, 2nd edition, Clarendon Press: Oxford, UK.
17. Wood, D.A. (1984) Polymeric materials used in drug delivery systems. In: Florence, A.T. (Ed.), *Materials Used in Pharmaceutical Formulation*. Society of Chemical Industry: London, UK, pp. 71–123.
18. Harland, R.S., Gazzaniga, A., Edvige Sangalli, M., Colombo, P., Peppas, N.A. (1988) Drug/polymer matrix swelling and dissolution. *Pharm Res* 5:488–494.
19. Fassihi, R., Ritschel, W.A. (1993) Multiple-layer, direct-compression, controlled-release system: In vitro and in vivo evaluation. *J Pharm Sci* 82(7):750–754.
20. Peppas, N.A., Sahlin, J.J. (1989) A simple equation for the description of solute release. III. Coupling of diffusion and relaxation. *Int J Pharm* 57:169–172.
21. Reynolds, T.D., Gehrke, S.H., Hussain, A.S., Shenouda, L.S. (1998) Polymer erosion and drug release characterization of hydroxypropyl methylcellulose matrices. *J Pharm Sci* 87:1115–1123.
22. Durig, T., Fassihi, R. (2002) Guar-based monolithic matrix systems: Effect of ionizable and non-ionizable substances and excipients on gel dynamics and release kinetics. *J Controlled Release* 80:45–56.

23. Pillay, V., Fassihi, R. (2000) A novel approach for constant rate delivery of highly soluble bioactives from a simple monolithic system. *J Controlled Release* 67:67–78.
24. Jamzad, S., Tutunji, L., Fassihi, R. (2005) Analysis of macromolecular changes and drug release from hydrophilic matrix systems. *Int J Pharm* 292:75–85.
25. Jamzad, S, Fassihi, R. (2006) Development of a controlled release low dose class-II drug glipizide. *Int J Pharm* 312:24–32.
26. Kim, H., Fassihi. R. (1997) Application of a binary polymer system in drug release rate modulation 1. Characterization of release mechanism. *J Pharm Sci* 86(3):316–322.
27. Pillay, V., Fassihi, R. (2000) A novel approach for constant rate delivery of highly soluble bioactives from a simple monolithic system. *J Controlled Release* 67:67–78.
28. Munday, D.L., Fassihi, A.R., De Villiers, C. (1991) Bioavailability study of a theophylline oral controlled release capsule containing film coated mini-tablets in beagle dogs. *Int J Pharm* 69:123–127.
29. Munday, D.L., Fassihi, A.R. (1991) Changes in drug release rate: Effect of stress storage conditions on film coated mini-tablets. *Drug Dev Ind Pharm* 17:2135–2143.
30. Kolte, B.P., Tele, K.V., Mundhe, V.S., Lahoti, S.S. (2012) Colon targeted drug delivery system—A novel perspective. *Asian J Biomed Pharm Sci* 2:21–28.
31. Thoma, K., Bechtold, K. (2000) Enteric coated hard gelatin capsules, BAS 145 E 2000, Capsugel Library, pp. 1–17.
32. Cole, E.T., Scott, R.A., Connor, A.L., Wilding, I.R., Petereit, H.U., Schminke, C., Beckert, T., Cade, D. (2002) Enteric coated HPMC capsules designed to achieve intestinal targeting. *Int J Pharm* 231:83–95.
33. Mathew, M., Das Gupta, V., Bailey, R.E. (1995) Stability of omeprazole solutions at various pH values as determined by HPLC. *Drug Dev Ind Pharm* 21:965–971.
34. Sharma, V.D., Akocak, S., Ilies, M.A., Fassihi, R. (2015) Solid-state interactions at the core–coat interface: Physicochemical characterization of enteric-coated omeprazole pellets without a protective subcoat. *AAPS PharmSciTech* 16:934–943.
35. Missaghi S. (2006) Formulation design and approaches to enteric coating delivery via compression coating or encapsulation of acid-labile compounds using omeprazole as a model drug. PhD dissertation, Chapter 4, Temple University, School of Pharmacy, Philadelphia.
36. Jantzen, G.M., Robinson, G.R. (2002) Sustained-and controlled-release drug-delivery systems. In: Banker, G.S., Rhodes, C.T. (Eds.), *Modern Pharmaceutics*, 4th edition. Marcel Dekker: New York, pp. 501–528.
37. Porter, S.C. (2000) Coating of pharmaceutical dosage forms. In: Gennaro, A.R. (Ed.), *Remington, the Science and Practice of Pharmacy*, 20th edition: Lippincott Williams and Wilkins: Philadelphia, PA, pp. 894–902.
38. Munday, D.L., Fassihi, A.R. (1989) Controlled release delivery: Effect of coating composition on release characteristics of mini-tablets. *Int J Pharm* 52:109–114.
39. Fassihi, R., Parker, M.S. (1987) Inimical effects of compaction speed on microorganisms in powder systems with dissimilar compaction mechanisms. *J Pharm Sci* 76(6):466–470.
40. McNeil, M.E., Rashid, A., Stephens, H.N.E. (1993) Drug Dispensing Device. GB Patent 2230442.
41. Stephens, H.N.E., Rashid, A., Bakhshaee, M. (1995) Drug Dispensing Device. US Patent 5474784.
42. Amidon, G.L., Lessman, G.D. (1993) Pulsatile Drug Delivery System. US Patent 5229131.
43. Amidon, G.L., Lessman, G.D., Sherman, L.B. (1995) Multi-Stage Delivery System. US Patent 5387421.
44. Lee, W.W., Mahony, B.O., Bar-Schalom, D., Slot, L., Wilson, C.G., Blackshaw, P.E., Perkins, A.C. (2000) Scintigraphic characterization of a novel injection molded dosage form. *Proc Int Symp Control Rel Bioact Mater* 27:1288–1289.
45. Gardner, D., Casper, R., Leith, F., Wilding I.R. (1997) The InteliSite capsule: A new easy to use approach for assessing regional drug absorption from the gastrointestinal tract. *Pharm Technol* 21:82–89.
46. Prior, V.D., Connor, L.A., Wilding, I.R. (2003) Modified release drug delivery technology. In: Rathbone M.J., Hadgraft. J., Roberts, M.S. (Eds.), *The Enterion Capsule*. Marcel Dekker: New York, pp. 273–288.
47. Wilding, I.R., Hirst, P.H., Connor, A.L. (2000) Development of a new engineering based capsule for human drug absorption studies. *Pharm Sci Technol Today* 3:385–392.
48. Casper, R.A., McCartney, L.M., Jochem, W.J., Parr, A.F. (1992) Medical Capsule Device Activated by Radiofrequency (RF) Signal. US Patent 5170801.
49. McCaffrey, C., Chevalerias, O., O'Mathuna, C., Twomey, K. (2008) Swallowable capsule technology. *Pervasive Computing* January–March: 23–29 (www.computer.org/pervasive).
50. Becker, D., Zhang, J., Heimbach, T., Penland, R.C., Wanke, C., Shimizu, J., Kulmatycki, K. (2014) Novel orally swallowable IntelliCap® device to quantify regional drug absorption in human GI tract using diltiazem as model drug. *AAPS PharmSciTech* 15(6):1490–1497.

13 Analytical Testing and Evaluation of Capsules

Stuart L. Cantor and Asish K. Dutta

CONTENTS

INTRODUCTION

Capsules are a diverse dosage form prepared using different polymeric materials and using different methods. Two main types are commonly used, and they are classified according to the nature and flexibility of the capsule shell. While soft gelatin capsules are composed of a liquid or semisolid fill, hard capsules typically can contain either powder or beads. Other important differences include the fact that soft gelatin capsules contain between 20% and 30% w/w of plasticizers (i.e., glycerin, sorbitol, propylene glycol [PG]) while hard capsules do not. The equilibrium moisture content of hard gelatin capsules is between 13% and 16%, but the level in soft gelatin capsules is lower at between 6% and 10% [1].

In general, the conditions that can cause brittleness to be observed in gelatin shells range between 0% and 20% relative humidity (RH) and between 7.6% and 10.0% moisture. Acceptable conditions lie within a broader range at between 20.0% and 58.0% RH and between 10.0% and 17.8% moisture. The gelatin shell will begin to soften when the moisture level goes above approximately 18.0% (Figure 13.1) [2].

Another issue pertinent to gelatin capsules is cross-linking reactions from aldehydes. The presence of even low levels of aldehydes inherent in the excipients and drug or produced via decomposition during storage can cause an unexpected delay in drug release as well as stability problems [3–5]. In addition to the presence of aldehydes, the other main contributory factors toward cross-linking were found to be storage stresses (i.e., high temperatures, high humidity, and excessive light exposure) [4].

However, sometimes this reaction can be beneficial. Gelatin, like the majority of protein-based films, has a limited barrier to water vapor transmission. Increasing cross-linking by reacting gelatin

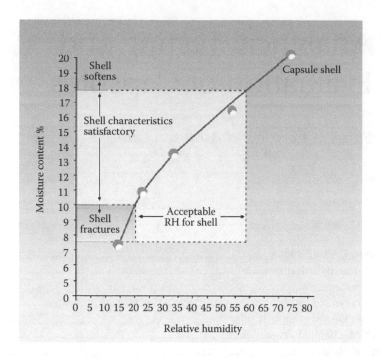

FIGURE 13.1 Equilibrium moisture content of empty gelatin capsule shells stored at different relative humidities for 2 weeks at 20°C. (Reprinted from *Adv Drug Del Rev*, 60, Cole ET, Cade D, Benameur H, Challenges and opportunities in the encapsulation of liquid and semi-solid formulations into capsules for oral administration, 747–756, Copyright 2008, with permission from Elsevier.)

films with formaldehyde not only can improve gelatin's mechanical properties but also can provide gastro-resistance [6,7]. It has also been reported by Kuijpers et al. [8] that chemical cross-linking via the carboxylic acid groups on gelatin can increase the resistance of the gels against thermal degradation.

Pina et al. [9] studied seven drugs with different solubilities in gastric juice. These drugs were then encapsulated and the gelatin capsules were coated with different formaldehyde concentration solutions ranging from 3.0 to 20.0% w/w. The results allowed for the establishment of a relation between the drug's solubility in gastric juice (S), and formaldehyde concentration in coating solution (C). It is given by

$$C = 248.556 \cdot S + 2.101 \quad (r = 0.999),$$ (13.1)

where C is the formaldehyde concentration and S is the drug's solubility in gastric juice.

The capsule wall may comprise gelatin or another suitable polymer such as hypromellose also called hydroxypropylmethylcellulose (HPMC). The equilibrium moisture content of HPMC capsules is lower and ranges from 2% to 6%. These capsules are also not susceptible to cross-linking reactions with aldehydes as this polymer does not contain chemically reactive groups. The choice of whether to use a hard or soft capsule will depend on several factors, including the nature of the formulation components, the compatibility of the excipients with the shell polymer, the best storage stability conditions, and the drug release characteristics.

The physicochemical properties of both HPMC and gelatin capsules are presented in Table 13.1 [10,11]. The largest difference between the two shell materials is in their moisture contents, which is between 2% and 6% for HPMC capsules and 13% and 16% for gelatin capsules. The relationship between the moisture content of the capsule shells and the resultant brittleness has previously

TABLE 13.1
Physicochemical Properties of HPMC and Gelatin Capsules

Property	HPMC	Gelatin
Moisture content	2–6%	13–16%
Glass transition temperature	170–180°C	50–60°C
Water vapor permeability	Low	Higher
Substrate for protease	No	Yes
Maillard reaction with drug fill	No	Yes
Deformation by heat	>80°C	>60°C
Water dissolution at room temperature	Soluble	Insoluble
Static	Low	High
Light degradation	No	Possible

Source: Honkanen O. Biopharmaceutical Evaluation of Orally and Rectally Administered Hard Hydroxypropyl Methylcellulose Capsules. Dissertation submitted to the Faculty of Pharmacy, University of Helsinki, 2004; Rowe RC, Sheskey PJ, Cook WG, Fenton ME (Eds.). *Handbook of Pharmaceutical Excipients*, 7th edition, 2012. Pharmaceutical Press, Philadelphia, PA.

been demonstrated using a hardness tester [12]. HPMC and gelatin capsules were filled with acetylsalicylic acid and stored at 60°C for 2 weeks. While drug potency was maintained above 95% for HPMC capsules, it decreased to 85% of its initial concentration when stored in gelatin capsules, apparently as a result of hydrolysis. Moreover, the percentage of broken gelatin capsules increased to almost 100% as the moisture content of the capsule shells decreased below 10%. In contrast, HPMC capsules remained undamaged even at moisture levels of only 2%. These data suggest that HPMC capsules could be more appropriate for actives that are either hygroscopic or prone to hydrolysis.

Another polymer that has received GRAS (generally recognized as safe) status from the Food and Drug Administration (FDA) in 2002 is pullulan. This polymer has already been approved in Japan for more than 20 years and is currently being evaluated for use as a food additive in Europe. These capsules are made from a pullulan polymer naturally fermented from tapioca starch [13–15]. Pullulan films display excellent oxygen barrier properties and the capsules have a crystal-clear transparency and a high degree of luster, ideal for marketing in the natural products industry. The other marketing advantages for these capsules are that they are Kosher, allergen-free, and manufactured from non-genetically modified organisms.

Capsules may also be enteric coated in order to prevent the premature release of their contents in the stomach, where the low-pH conditions can damage those active ingredients susceptible to acid hydrolysis [7,8,16]. An added benefit is that the capsule coating helps mask any unpleasant ingredient odor or taste. These capsules would be ideal for acid-sensitive active ingredients such as resveratrol, clopidogrel (Plavix), and 5-hydroxytryptophan (5-HTP) and also for items such as garlic.

Each of the different polymers used in the manufacture of capsules have different physicochemical and mechanical properties that will affect the release rate and stability of the drug product. There are a number of analytical methodologies that can yield important information regarding the capsule dosage form itself during manufacturing and storage, and these include the polymer's glass transition temperature (T_g) and level of moisture loss. The amount of moisture loss can affect the brittleness of the capsule shell during storage and also affect the *in vivo* drug release.

These analytical techniques include differential scanning calorimetry (DSC), dissolution, and high-performance liquid chromatography (HPLC). DSC can be used to yield a true picture of what is occurring on a micro-scale with the polymeric film before physical changes (e.g., capsule shrinkage, deformation, and/or brittleness) are observed. Moreover, these techniques can also be used with other complementary spectroscopic techniques (i.e., Fourier transform infrared spectroscopy,

Raman spectroscopy, or near-infrared spectroscopy [NIRS]) in order to identify potential impurity profiles and to confirm the identity of certain HPLC peaks of interest.

POLYMERS USED IN CAPSULES

GELATIN

Gelatin is a product obtained by the partial hydrolysis of collagen derived from the skin, connective tissue, and bones of animals. Gelatin is an amphoteric material. When derived from an acid-treated precursor, it is known as Type A; when derived from an alkali-treated precursor, it is known as Type B. Gelatin may be colored with certified colors, may contain no more than 0.15% of sulfur dioxide, and may also contain a suitable concentration of sodium lauryl sulfate (SLS) and suitable antimicrobial agents. The pharmacopeial specifications for gelatin are presented in Table 13.2.

A standard test to measure the gelling ability of various gelatins is termed the bloom strength and is measured in grams. This test is described under USP General Chapter gel strength of gelatin <1081> [17]. This test measures the force required to depress the surface of a 6.67% w/w gel, matured at

TABLE 13.2
Pharmacopeial Specifications for Gelatin

Test	JP XV	PhEur 7.4	USP35-NF30
Identification	+	+	+
Characters	+	+	−
Microbial contamination	−	+	+
Aerobic bacteria	−	≤10^3 CFU/g	≤10^3 CFU/g
Fungi	−	≤10^2 CFU/g	−
Residue on ignition	≤2.0%	−	≤2.0%
Loss on drying	≤15.0%	≤15.0%	−
Odor and water-insoluble substances	+	−	+
Isoelectric point	+	+	−
Type A	7.0–9.0	6.0–9.5	−
Type B	4.5–5.0	4.7–5.6	−
Conductivity	−	≤1 mS/cm	−
Sulfur dioxide	−	≤50 ppm	≤0.15%
Sulfite	+	−	−
Arsenic	≤1 ppm	−	≤0.8 ppm
Iron	−	≤30 ppm	−
Chromium	−	≤10 ppm	−
Zinc	−	≤30 ppm	−
Heavy metals	≤50 ppm[a]	−	≤50 ppm
pH	−	3.8–7.6	−
Mercury	≤0.1 ppm	−	−
Peroxides	−	≤10 ppm	−
Gel strength	−	+	−

Source: Reprinted with the permission of the American Pharmacists Association (Washington, DC) from Rowe RC, Sheskey PJ, Cook WG, Fenton ME (Eds.). *Handbook of Pharmaceutical Excipients*, 7th edition, 2012. Pharmaceutical Press, Philadelphia, PA.

[a] ≤20 ppm for purified gelatin.

10°C for 16–18 h in a standard bottle, adjusted for a depression of 4 mm using a 12.7-mm-diameter flat-bottomed plunger.

The physical properties of bloom strength and viscosity vary with the moisture content of the dry gelatin, and it is commonplace to correct these values to a standard moisture content of 11.5%. The bloom strength can vary depending on the source of the gelatin and whether it is used for soft or hard shell manufacture. For example, the bloom strength of Type B, fish-derived, and Type A gelatins used for soft capsules ranges from 150 to 175, from 160 to 210, and from 180 to 210, respectively. However, the bloom strength of Type B and Type A (from bone) ranges from 200 to 220 and from 245 to 270, respectively [1].

Stability Issues: Cross-Linking

Gelatin is mixed with a plasticizer, such as glycerin, to produce soft gelatin capsules. For hard gelatin capsules, the residual water acts as a plasticizer. While it can also be treated with formaldehyde to produce gastro-resistance, there are toxicity issues with this compound [18]. Analytical methods are available for the identification and quantification of aldehydes. While Li et al. [19] described a headspace gas chromatographic method, del Barrio et al. [20] utilized a gas chromatographic–mass spectroscopy (GC-MS) method and claimed that the detection limit for formaldehyde was 0.2 parts per million (ppm) (range, 0.2–10,000 ppm). However, another simple and sensitive method using HPLC can also be utilized for those labs without GC-MS capability [21].

A pivotal study by Meyer et al. [22] compared cross-linked (stressed) hard and soft gelatin capsules of acetaminophen with their unstressed controls. The authors found that the *in vitro* rate of dissolution dramatically decreased when the degree of cross-linking increased. Additionally, capsules stressed to the greatest extent were not bioequivalent to the unstressed control capsules.

This study resulted in the adoption of a USP two-tier procedure for dissolution testing of gelatin capsules that allowed the use of enzymes such as pepsin and pancreatin in the dissolution media when pellicle formation (i.e., a thick skin or film formed on a liquid) causes a delay in drug dissolution [4,23]. The USP states that pepsin and pancreatin can be added to dissolution media containing either simulated gastric fluid (SGF) or simulated intestinal fluid (SIF), respectively, depending on the dissolution media specified for the product and the drug's solubility. This revised procedure using enzymes enables an improved ability to distinguish whether gelatin capsules are bioequivalent to each other. Only in cases where the enzymes have been added and the test still shows poor dissolution rate should a negative effect attributed to cross-linking be assumed.

Details on the types and amounts of enzymes to be used can be found in the USP General Chapter <711> Dissolution. Where water or a medium with a pH of less than 6.8 is used, purified pepsin can be added to the medium in an amount that results in an activity of 750,000 U or less per 1000 mL. For media with a pH of 6.8 or greater, pancreatin can be added to produce not more than 1750 U of protease activity per 1000 mL. The pancreatin or pepsin to be used should meet the USP monograph requirements [24].

Marchais et al. [23] designed studies to determine whether the use of both enzyme and surfactant in the dissolution medium changes the *in vitro* drug release from cross-linked hard gelatin capsules containing the water-insoluble drug carbamazepine. Hard gelatin capsules were cross-linked by a controlled exposure to formaldehyde, resulting in different stressed capsules. *In vitro* dissolution studies were conducted with enzymes and using SGF containing pepsin and SIF containing pancreatin. SLS was also added in the dissolution medium at a concentration of 2% w/v in both SGF and SIF.

The percentage of carbamazepine dissolved was reduced by increasing the degree of gelatin cross-linking. For unstressed hard gelatin capsules, 36% of the carbamazepine was released after 1 h. However, this was greatly lowered to 5% for highly stressed hard gelatin capsules in the SGF. A similar effect was also observed with SIF. In the case of moderately stressed hard gelatin capsules, addition of enzyme in the dissolution medium enhanced the percentage of carbamazepine dissolved. The dissolution level increased from 12% to 39% in SGF with pepsin for hard gelatin capsules cross-linked with 1500 ppm formaldehyde. On the contrary, the use of enzyme in the dissolution medium did not increase the dissolution of carbamazepine from highly stressed hard gelatin capsules. Surprisingly, the addition of SLS in either medium did not allow the release of the carbamazepine. The results of this study demonstrate that the use of enzymes in the dissolution medium is justified for moderately cross-linked hard gelatin capsules. However, the action of a surfactant added in the medium containing enzymes remains unclear.

The selection of the formulation excipients is important because of their potential interaction with the capsule shells and their negative impact on both long-term stability and drug dissolution rate. Pellicle formation can be dependent on the excipients present in the gelatin shell. For example, Chang et al. [25] observed that after 12 weeks of storage at 40°C/75% RH, gelatin capsules containing lactose-based granules had reduced dissolution rates owing to pellicle formation inside capsule shells, while capsules containing mannitol-based granules showed faster dissolution profiles without noticeable pellicle formation.

There is some concern that a number of excipients for liquid-filled capsule formulations such as fats, polyethylene glycols (PEGs), aliphatic alcohols, phenols, polyoxylenated glycerides, and esters of unsaturated fatty acids can undergo auto-oxidation to form aldehydes [26]. It has previously been found that lactose can be incompatible with gelatin capsules owing to the presence of a preservative, hexamethylenetetramine, which decomposes into formaldehyde and causes cross-linking reactions with gelatin [4]. However, while this additive is approved in the European Union, it is not approved for use in the United States, Australia, or New Zealand.

When glycine and citric acid were incorporated together into a triamterene/hydrochlorithiazide formulation, cross-linking was completely prevented. Dissolution profiles remained the same throughout a 3-month accelerated stability program at 50°C. These results were confirmed using gemfibrozil and piroxicam as model drugs and showed that pellicle formation during dissolution was prevented [27]. The cross-linking susceptibility of capsules under ambient conditions was compared by Ku et al. [28] using lactose spiked with 25 ppm formaldehyde. After 1 week of storage at room temperature, the dissolution of acetaminophen from the HPMC shell (Vcaps Plus, containing no gelling agent) remains unchanged while the gelatin shell showed a significant decrease in the drug release (Figure 13.2).

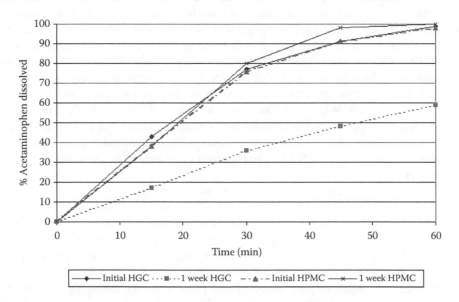

FIGURE 13.2 Dissolution of acetaminophen in hard gelatin capsules (HGC) and HPMC capsule shells after 1-week exposure to lactose spiked with formaldehyde. (Reprinted from *Int J Pharm*, 386, Ku SM, Li W, Dulin W, Donahue F, Cade D, Benameur H, Hutchison K. Performance qualification of a new hypromellose capsule: Part I. Comparative evaluation of physical, mechanical and processability quality attributes of Vcaps Plus, Quali-V and gelatin capsules, 30–41, Copyright 2010, with permission from Elsevier.)

Attenuated total reflection Fourier transform infrared spectroscopy (FTIR) has been used by Tengroth et al. [29] to study cross-linking reactions in hard gelatin capsules induced by exposure to formaldehyde, acetaldehyde, and propionaldehyde. These aldehydes are known to cause cross-linking between the amino acid chains of gelatin. Using FTIR spectroscopy, it is possible to analyze the cross-linking mechanisms by studying changes in the vibrational bands of the gelatin spectrum. The FTIR spectrum changes over time when the capsules are left in an aldehyde-rich environment. Analysis of the spectra shows that the early observed spectral changes conform to reaction intermediates proposed in previous work based on nuclear magnetic resonance experiments, specifically the formation of an amine methyl alcohol. Thus, the aldehydes combine with the primary amine groups from the arginine and lysine residues and this is followed by the formation of cross-links.

Further spectral changes appear to be mostly from unreacted aldehydes absorbed to the gelatin, although a minor shift of the amide II peak is attributed to cross-link formation. Another quality issue affecting the stability of capsule shells is moisture transfer. While it has been known that brittleness in hard gelatin capsules is a function of moisture content, a minimum quantity of sorbed moisture is necessary to act as a plasticizer and maintain the capsules in a pliable state. Kontny and Mulski [30] showed that the brittleness of both empty gelatin capsules and formulation-filled capsules becomes prevalent at RH values of less than 40%. The initial moisture contents and masses of all components are important in establishing the final equilibrium RH in a given capsule system.

Variation in moisture content of the capsule shells due to either the change of storage conditions or the moisture transfer between the capsule shell and its contents may lead to undesired physical properties, such as capsule brittleness and stickiness. Chang et al. [31] used Sorption–Desorption Moisture Transfer model fitting to study the effects of using a very hygroscopic drug encapsulated in hard gelatin shells and to predict the equilibrium RH in their system. The neat drug (moisture level, 1.7%) was compared to a formulation where the active was pre-moistened to a moisture content of 7%. Both samples were stored under various stability conditions for a period of 1 year. The authors found that by adding an adequate amount of water to the drug substance, moisture transfer issues and gelatin brittleness on storage can be reduced or eliminated.

Gold et al. [32] used NIRS to predict the degree of cross-linking from formaldehyde-stressed hard gelatin capsules. Capsules were filled with amoxicillin and then exposed to a 150 ppb (parts per billion) atmosphere of formaldehyde vapor for 2.3, 4.6, 9.4, 16, and 24 h. Dissolution profiles were obtained and then principal component regression (PCR) was used to analyze the data. The dissolution of amoxicillin was found to decrease with increasing exposure time to the formaldehyde atmosphere. The authors found that a good correlation ($R^2 = 0.963$) was established when principal components were regressed against amoxicillin percentage dissolved at 45 min. Furthermore, the water content of the capsules was the largest determinant in the variation between the capsule's spectra at each exposure time. The NIRS absorbance of the capsules at 1450 and 1949 nm decreased with the increased exposure time to formaldehyde.

Hydroxypropylmethylcellulose

Gelatin capsules may not provide sufficient protection against moisture for some active pharmaceutical ingredients (APIs) and the gelatin shells can also become brittle over time leading to capsule breakage [33–35]. Furthermore, while some consumers prefer that their medicines be free of animal-derived ingredients such as gelatin because of issues such as bovine spongiform encephalopathy, vegetarian capsules manufactured using hypromellose or HPMC have been on the market since 1998 [10].

Traditionally, hard gelatin capsule manufacturing is performed using dip molding where stainless steel pins at ambient temperature are dipped into a heated solution of liquid gelatin. The preparation of HPMC capsules is the opposite. The stainless steel molding pins are heated and subsequently dipped into an HPMC solution at ambient temperature. However, previously, HPMC required secondary gelling agents such as kappa-carrageenan or gellan gum as well as ionic promoters (i.e., potassium or sodium ions, respectively), in order to form a quick setting film on the molding pins. The issue with the use of secondary gelling systems is that they can interact with the dissolution media and cause an unexpected delay in drug release [36].

Differences have been shown in the *in vitro* dissolution rate between gelatin and HPMC capsules [37]. However, the bioavailability of ibuprofen, a BCS Class II drug, delivered from the two capsule types was not statistically different when AUC and C_{max} values were compared using pharmacoscintigraphic evaluation. Recent advances made in HPMC capsule manufacturing technology have resulted in the achievement of similar *in vitro* dissolution rates as compared with gelatin capsules.

Ku et al. [28] described the qualification of a new high-performance hypromellose capsule shell that contains no gelling agent and is dissolution friendly. Comparisons to gelatin and HPMC capsules containing carrageenan showed that the new HPMC capsules without any gelling agent are superior in terms of mechanical strength, hygroscopicity, and compatibility with a wide range of drugs. Specifically, the new HPMC capsules demonstrated improved weight variation, machineability, and powder leakage than the HPMC capsules containing carrageenan. The new capsule also demonstrated a broader applicability than gelatin capsule for new drug development because of its inertness and compatibility for a wide range of excipients including those used for liquid fill formulations. On the basis of the superior dissolution performance and other quality attributes, the new HPMC capsule is satisfactorily qualified and has since been used successfully for nearly 20 investigational new drug compounds.

The HPMC capsule was studied further by Ku et al. [38]. This new capsule does not contain any gelling agent and is manufactured by a thermal gelation process. Rupture time of the carrageenan-containing capsule (HPMC Shell 1) and HPMC Shell 2 (containing no gelling agent), as measured by an improved real-time detection method, showed only slight differences that did not manifest *in vivo*. The absence of a gelling agent appeared to give HPMC Shell 2 advantages in dissolution in acidic media and in buffers containing potassium ions. Slow drug release of HPMC Shell 1 in 0.1 M HCl was attributed to the interaction of carrageenan with drug compounds, whereas the presence of potassium ions, a gelling promoter for carrageenan, caused a delay in capsule opening and a larger capsule-to-capsule variation. Disintegration and dissolution performances of both hypromellose capsules are comparable in other dissolution media tested.

Ku et al. [38] showed that the HPMC shell containing carrageenan tended to open up somewhat faster than the pure HPMC shell material (Figure 13.3). The authors believed that the carrageenan helped to facilitate the dissolution of the HPMC polymer. The average capsule rupture time in the various media is in the range of 2.7–4.3 min for HPMC Shell 1 and 6.1–8.1 min for HPMC Shell 2. The differences (<4 min) in capsule opening/rupture times between the two HPMC capsules are not expected to have a significant impact on their *in vivo* performance. Other studies have shown that the *in vitro* rupture time or disintegration time of HPMC Shell 1 is generally slower than that of hard gelatin capsules in dissolution media at 37°C [39,40]. Additionally, it has also been shown that there is no significant difference in the *in vivo* capsule disintegration and dissolution times and, thus, no impact on the pharmacokinetic parameters [41].

The effect of elevated temperature and time was compared between hypromellose and gelatin capsules and studied by Missaghi and Fassihi [42]. The results showed that the longer exposure to elevated temperatures resulted in a larger moisture loss for gelatin shells as compared with hypromellose shells (i.e., 21.99% vs. 3.62% at 72 h, respectively). The authors believed that this extended period was responsible for reducing the plasticity of the gelatin capsules, thus resulting in their increased brittleness in Table 13.3. There are four different grades of HPMC, with the major differences being the levels of methoxy and hydroxypropoxy groups. The pharmacopeial specifications for hypromellose are presented in Table 13.4.

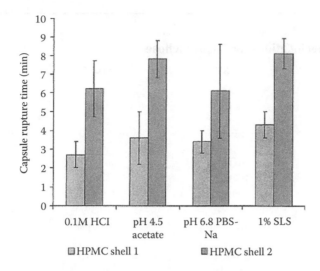

FIGURE 13.3 Disintegration/rupture time of HPMC Shell 1 (Quali-V) and HPMC Shell 2 (VCaps Plus) in four dissolution media, 0.1 M HCl, pH 4.5 acetate buffer, pH 6.8 phosphate (sodium salt), and 1% SLS in water. The error bars represent standard deviation of six capsules. (Reprinted from *Int J Pharm*, 416, Ku M, Lu Q, Li W, Chen Y. Performance qualification of a new hypromellose capsule: Part II. Disintegration and dissolution comparison between two types of hypromellose capsules, 16–24, Copyright 2011, with permission from Elsevier.)

TABLE 13.3

Extent of Weight Reduction for Empty Shells of Hypromellose and Gelatin, Compared to Their Initial Weight and after Storage at 45°C for Different Periods

	Weight Reduction(%)	
Exposure Time to 45°C (h)	Hypromellose Capsules	Gelatin Capsules
1	2.80 ± 0.22	5.92 ± 0.47
24	2.97 ± 0.27	7.55 ± 0.85
72	3.62 ± 0.32	21.99 ± 2.97

Source: Adapted from Missaghi S and Fassihi R. Evaluation and comparison of physicomechanical characteristics of gelatin and hypromellose capsules. *Drug Dev Ind Pharm* 2006; 32: 829–838. Reproduced with permission of Taylor & Francis via Copyright Clearance Center.

Note: Data are reported as mean value and standard deviation ($n = 20$).

PULLULAN

Pullulan is a linear, neutral exopolysaccharide produced by the fungus *Aureobasidium pullulans*. This polymer consists of maltotriose repeating units joined by α-1,6 linkages. The internal glucose units within maltotriose are connected by α-1,4-glycosidic bonds. The molecular weight for pullulan ranges from 4.5×10^4 to 6.0×10^5 daltons and depends on the growth conditions of the organism. Pullulan is non-hygroscopic and non-reducing, is soluble in hot and cold water but generally insoluble in organic solvents, and has a glass transition temperature of over 150°C [16]. Its unique linkage pattern grants pullulan films several distinctive physical properties such as mucoadhesive

TABLE 13.4
Pharmacopeial Specifications for Hypromellose

Test	JP XV	PhEur 7.4	USP35-NF30
Identification	+	+	+
Characters	–	+	–
Appearance of solution	–	+	–
pH (2% w/w solution)	5.0–8.0	5.0–8.0	5.0–8.0
Apparent viscosity	+	+[a]	+
<600 mPa s	80–120%	80–120%	80–120%
≥600 mPa s	75–140%	75–140%	75–140%
Loss on drying	≤5.0%	≤5.0%	≤5.0%
Residue on ignition	≤1.5%	≤1.5%	≤1.5%
Heavy metals[b]	≤20 ppm	≤20 ppm	≤20 ppm
Methoxy content			
Type 1828	16.5–20.0%	16.5–20.0%	16.5–20.0%
Type 2208	19.0–24.0%	19.0–24.0%	19.0–24.0%
Type 2906	27.0–30.0%	27.0–30.0%	27.0–30.0%
Type 2910	28.0–30.0%	28.0–30.0%	28.0–30.0%
Hydroxypropoxy content	+	+[a]	+
Type 1828	23.0–32.0%	23.0–32.0%	23.0–32.0%
Type 2208	4.0–12.0%	4.0–12.0%	4.0–12.0%
Type 2906	4.0–7.5%	4.0–7.5%	4.0–7.5%
Type 2910	7.0–12.0%	7.0–12.0%	7.0–12.0%

Source: Reprinted with the permission of the American Pharmacists Association (Washington, DC) from Rowe RC, Sheskey PJ, Cook WG, Fenton ME (Eds.). *Handbook of Pharmaceutical Excipients*, 7th edition, 2012. Pharmaceutical Press, Philadelphia, PA.

[a] May be a functionality-related characteristic.

[b] This test has not been fully harmonized at the time of publication.

TABLE 13.5
Pharmacopeial Specifications for Pullulan

Test	JP XV	USP35-NF30
Identification	+	+
Viscosity (kinematic)	100–180 mm^2 s^{-1}	100–180 mm^2 s^{-1}
Microbial limits		
Bacteria	–	<100 CFU/g
Yeasts and molds	–	<100 CFU/g
pH	4.5–6.5	4.5–6.5
Loss on drying	≤6.0%	≤6.0%
Residue on ignition	≤0.3%	≤0.3%
Heavy metals	≤5 ppm	≤5 μg/g
Content of monosaccharide, disaccharide, and oligosaccharides	≤10.0%	≤10.0%
Nitrogen content	≤0.05%	≤0.05%

Source: Reprinted with the permission of the American Pharmacists Association (Washington, DC) from Rowe RC, Sheskey PJ, Cook WG, Fenton ME (Eds.). *Handbook of Pharmaceutical Excipients*, 7th edition, 2012. Pharmaceutical Press, Philadelphia, PA.

ability, the capacity to form fibers and thin biodegradeable films, which are transparent and imper-meable to oxygen [43].

The mechanical strength of hard gelatin capsules depends on the RH both inside and outside the capsule. Sakata and Otsuka [44] studied the relationship between moisture content and the mechanical strength of both hard pullulan capsules filled with potato starch and solvent-cast pul-lulan films (15% w/w) using thermomechanical analysis and FTIR spectroscopy. They observed that the mechanical strength of the capsules decreased along with the water activity in the cap-sule wall during storage, and that this led to a contraction of the capsule length. Further study of the films using FTIR and PCR showed that the film contraction and water content could be adequately predicted using a calibration model. Moreover, the main peaks for the regression vector (the spectrum pattern comprising the loading vectors of the first two principal compo-nents) of the water content were observed to be similar to those for the pullulan film contraction. Thus, the results suggested that the calibration model for the film contraction could be predicted based on the model used for the water content. The compendia specifications for pullulan are similar between Japan and the United States. The pharmacopeial specifications for pullulan are presented in Table 13.5.

THERMAL ANALYSIS

Changes in temperature and humidity have a significant impact on the quality as well as the physical properties (i.e., brittleness) of the gelatin capsules as water is known to migrate between the powdered excipients or the liquid fill and the gelatin shell. Modulated differential scanning calorimetry (MDSC) or conventional DSC can be used to detect imperceptible changes in the gelatin shells attributed to either external factors or formulation ingredients long before they can be confirmed using visual observation. For improved accuracy, Coleman and Craig [45] advised that at least six modulations in MDSC should be observed throughout the duration of each ther-mal event.

The shift in the reversible heat flow determined using MDSC is used to measure the glass tran-sition temperature (T_g) of gelatin. During this transition, the heat capacity of the polymer is also decreased. Nazzal and Wang [46] studied various model formulations of Cremophor EL (polyoxyl castor oil) with water, alcohol, and PG for soft gelatin capsules (SGCs) and noted that such thermal events are correlated with the hardness data. The authors observed that there was a good correlation between the shift of gelatin's T_m (unfolding or melting temperature) toward lower temperatures and the hardness loss for SGCs containing water and PG as part of the fill formulation. It has also been shown by Fitzpatrick and Saklatvala [47] that moisture uptake by an excipient sample and, there-fore, moisture loss from the gelatin shell will result in an increase in the glass transition temperature of gelatin.

D'Cruz and Bell [48] studied those polyols that had a plasticizing effect on gelatin, as dem-onstrated by the lowering of the T_g values below that of anhydrous gelatin (157°C) (Table 13.6). Polyols with a lower glass transition temperature (e.g., glycerol) plasticized gelatin more efficiently than polyols with a higher T_g (i.e., trehalose). The glass transition temperature values of the gela-tin mixtures also decreased as the polyol concentrations increased. The plasticizing effect of the polyols promotes increased molecular mobility and also changes the gelatin's thermal properties. Moreover, the polyols also promoted a lowering of the gelatin's T_m value. This destabilizing effect also depended on the polyol type and concentration level. The T_m values decreased with decreasing polyol T_g and with increasing polyol concentration. Thus, the polyols promote a reduction in the thermal stability of gelatin, as indicated by lower T_m values.

With the glass transition temperature of gelatin films in the range of 50–60°C [49], aging of these films is expected even at room temperature. The process of physical aging is manifested by changes in a film's thermal and mechanical properties such as enthalpy and tensile modulus, and is an important phenomenon to consider during storage stability of capsule shells. When a polymer

TABLE 13.6

Effect of Polyol Type and Concentration on the Glass Transition Temperature (T_g) of the System and Unfolding Temperature (T_m) of Gelatin for Gelatin–Polyol Samples

Polyol (T_g)	Concentration (%)	Onset T_g^a (°C)	T_m^a (°C)
Glycerol (−92°C)	10	85 ± 9	117 ± 5
	20	51 ± 1	84 ± 1
	30	ND[b]	69 ± 2
Xylitol (−18.5°C)	10	101 ± 3	133 ± 3
	20	74 ± 3	111 ± 1
	30	53 ± 3	88 ± 2
Sorbitol (−2°C)	10	108 ± 5	131 ± 1
	20	80 ± 4	116 ± 1
	30	58 ± 6	98 ± 1
Sucrose (74°C)	10	109 ± 7	142 ± 6
	20	100 ± 5	132 ± 7
	30	86 ± 8	125 ± 4
Trehalose (115°C)	10	131 ± 1	161 ± 1
	20	119 ± 6	145 ± 1
	30	101 ± 5	139 ± 1

Source: D'Cruz NM and Bell LN: Thermal unfolding of gelatin in solids as affected by the glass transition. *J Food Sci.* 2005. 70(2). E64–E68. Copyright Wiley-VCH Verlag GmbH & Co. KGaA. Reproduced with permission via Copyright Clearance Center.

[a] Average ± standard deviation.

[b] Not determined.

---

is cooled and reheated near its T_g, a hysteresis in the transition's enthalpy is observed. The enthalpy of the polymer glass decreases toward its equilibrium value as it is aged below its T_g. During aging, there is a change in the polymer's heat capacity, and the T_g peak is classically overshot. The area underneath the endothermic peak at the T_g can be used to quantify the extent of the enthalpic relaxation [50].

By adjusting the temperature and humidity storage conditions, Dai and Liu [50] prepared gelatin films having different levels of structural gelatin content (i.e., crystallinity) as measured by $\Delta H_{crystal}$ and aging enthalpy as measured by ΔH_{age}. Gelatin films of ~15 μm thickness were dried under temperatures between 20°C and 50°C and 50%RH. The values for $\Delta H_{crystal}$ and ΔH_{age} ranged from 0 to 16 J/g and from 0 to 5 J/g, respectively. As shown in Figure 13.4a, the DSC thermogram for the gelatin film dried at 50°C and 50% RH for 12 h shows that the gelatin is completely amorphous with a T_g around 60°C. With increasing drying time at the same humidity and temperature, a T_g overshooting peak is observed to indicate an increase in aging enthalpy during the drying process. However, for gelatin films dried at a lower temperature of 35°C and 50% RH for 12 h, the DSC scan indicated that some structural order in gelatin with a melting temperature (T_m) of around 95°C exists, as shown in Figure 13.4b. Similarly, with increasing drying time, an aging enthalpy peak around its T_g grows with drying time.

For gelatin films with even higher crystallinity, the gelatin films were dried at lower temperatures of 30°C and 20°C with their respective DSC thermograms shown in Figure 13.4c and 13.4d. The authors observed that gelatin films with crystallinity values less than 5 J/g failed predominantly by brittle cracking fracture regardless of their aging enthalpy, while for films with the largest crystallinity (>15 J/g), deformation was caused predominantly by shear yielding irrespective of the aging enthalpy. The authors also noted that the ductility of the gelatin films increased with increasing

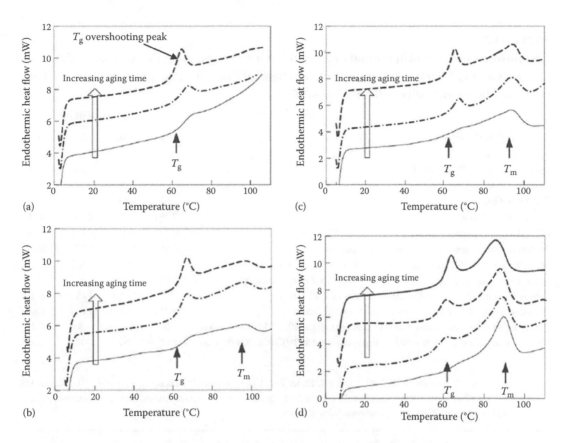

FIGURE 13.4 DSC thermograms of gelatin films prepared and dried under different conditions at (a) 50°C and 50% RH, (b) 35°C and 50% RH, (c) 30°C and 50% RH, and (d) 20°C and 50% RH. (Reprinted from *Mat Sci Eng A*, 423, Dai C-A, Liu M-W. The effect of crystallinity and aging enthalpy on the mechanical properties of gelatin films, 121–127, Copyright 2006, with permission from Elsevier.)

crystallinity and decreased with increasing enthalpy. This change in mechanical properties owing to physical aging has been known for many synthetic glassy amorphous polymers when they have been annealed below their T_g values [50].

Chen et al. [51] investigated the effects of lipophilic components on the compatibility of lipid-based drug formulations containing PG and/or Capmul MCM (glyceryl monocaprylate) and Cremophor EL (polyoxyl castor oil). The four liquid-fill HGC formulations are presented in Table 13.7. The presence of Capmul MCM significantly affected the activity of PG in the fills and the equilibrium of PG between the capsule shells and fills. These changes in activity and equilibrium of PG were furthermore correlated to the mechanical and thermal properties of the liquid-filled capsules and subsequently linked to the shelf life (i.e., capsule deformation) of the capsules placed on stability. The authors also demonstrated that headspace gas chromatography (GC) to measure PG activity can be utilized as a time-efficient method to assess capsule-fill compatibility.

Figure 13.5 shows the DSC thermograms of the liquid-filled HGC formulations analyzed at both 1 and 7 weeks under 40°C/75% RH storage. While there was a 10°C increase in the T_g as compared to the control at the 1 week time point, the formulations exhibited a progressive decrease in their T_g values following 7 weeks' storage. At the end of the 7-week storage period, the final water content decreased to ~7–8% w/w. While the authors expected these capsules to be brittle, they found that a significant migration of PG from the fill into the HGC shells had occurred and that this compensated for and eventually overrode the effect of the water loss from the capsule shells.

TABLE 13.7
Composition of Liquid-Fill Formulations and Their Corresponding PG Activity/Activity Coefficient, PG Migration, Thermal and Mechanical Property Change of the Liquid-Filled HGC and Incompatibility with HGC at 40°C

	Fill Formulations			
Compositions (% w/w)	IIa	IIb	IIc	IId
Propylene glycol	10	10	10	10
Model lipophilic API (log P 6.1)	–	–	30	30
Capmul MCM	–	7	–	7
Cremophor EL	90	83	60	53
PG activity in fill (α_{PG})	0.294	0.275	0.337	0.313
PG activity coefficient (γ_{PG}) without considering FM content	0.374	0.405	0.525	0.552
PG activity coefficient (γ_{PG}) considering FM content	0.666	0.661	0.777	0.769
PG migrated into HGC at 7 weeks (% of total recovered from whole capsule)	17.0	14.2	25.9	29.9
Lowest glass transition onset temperature of HGC shell after 7 weeks (°C)	55	59	40	40
Tensile breaking force of HGC shell after 7 weeks at 40°C (N)	287.9	292.4	146.7	141.3
Elastic modulus of HGC shell after 7 weeks at 40°C (N/mm)	160.2	161.3	112.8	109.9
First event of deformation observed for capsules stored at 40°C/75% RH (weeks)	8	7	3	4
First event of deformation observed for capsules stored at 25°C/60% RH (weeks)	>2 years	>2 years	32	33–71

Source: Reprinted from *J Pharm Sci*, 99, Chen F-J, Etzler FM, Ubben J, Birch A, Zhong L, Schwabe R, Dudhedia MS. Effects of lipophilic components on the compatibility of lipid-based formulations with hard gelatin capsules, 128–141, Copyright 2010, with permission from Elsevier.

DISSOLUTION AND DISINTEGRATION TESTING

The presence of certain functional groups, such as aldehydes, has the potential to cross-link the gelatin polymer. Some of the excipients used in the liquid-fill formulations for capsules may contain, or generate during storage, low levels of aldehydes. These aldehydes can subsequently alter the solubility of gelatin and result in a delay in the drug dissolution rate.

Schamp et al. [52] demonstrated that a semisolid formulation of a BCS Class II drug in hard gelatin capsules resulted in better dissolution, stability, and bioavailability than a formulation manufactured using just a lactose powder blend. The semisolid formulation consisted of a mixture of Gelucire 44/14 and polyvinylpyrrolidone (PVP) as a solubilizing agent. Another benefit of this formulation is that the drug is retained in solution after release in the duodenum.

The dissolution testing of both hard and soft gelatin capsules had been the focus of interest of an FDA-Industry Working Group. With the aid of gamma scintigraphy [35], researchers were able to show that cross-linked hard gelatin capsules exhibit the same *in vivo* disintegration properties in the stomach as unstressed control capsules. In a further study [22], it was demonstrated that hard and soft gelatin cross-linked capsules were bioequivalent to unstressed capsules. The findings in the latter study resulted in a modified USP monograph for dissolution testing of gelatin capsules that permits the use of enzymes in the dissolution media when pellicle formation is deemed to cause a delay in the dissolution rate of the drug.

Cole et al. [37] studied the dissolution rates of acetaminophen from both gelatin and HPMC-gellan capsules (Figure 13.6) [53]. The gelatin capsules released the drug much faster than the HPMC capsules, irrespective of the media used. The slowest release profile was using HPMC-gellan capsules in 0.1 N HCl, pH 1.2, because the capsules failed to rupture. Moreover, the release delay was lessened when sodium ions were present instead of potassium in phosphate buffer at pH 7.2 or in acetate buffer at pH 4.5.

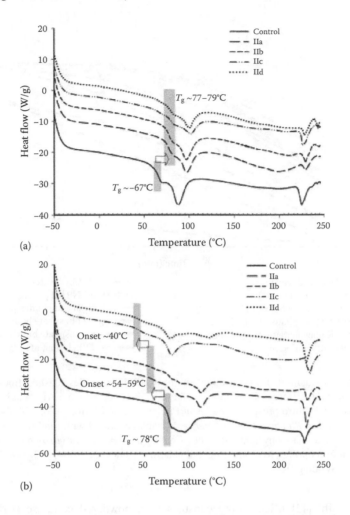

FIGURE 13.5 Thermograms of liquid-filled hard gelatin capsules at (a) 1-week and (b) 7-week time points by conventional differential scanning calorimetry. (Reprinted from *J Pharm Sci*, 99, Chen F-J, Etzler FM, Ubben J, Birch A, Zhong L, Schwabe R, Dudhedia MS. Effects of lipophilic components on the compatibility of lipid-based formulations with hard gelatin capsules, 128–141, Copyright 2010, with permission from Elsevier.)

The authors explained the hindrance of the HPMC-gellan capsule dissolution in potassium phosphate buffer as caused by the monovalent cations binding to the surface of the individual helices of gellan, lowering their charge density and reducing the electrostatic barrier to aggregation, and thus, solubility is reduced. They proposed that sodium ions are not as efficient binders as potassium, and therefore, disruption will be faster. They also explained that unlike the sulfate groups in a carrageenan gelling system, the carboxyl groups of gellan gum have a much higher pK_a, resulting in uncharged (-COOH) groups forming at low pH. This elimination of electrostatic repulsion between helices makes gellan gum less soluble at pH 1.2. HPMC solubility, on the other hand, is independent of pH, as it is a neutral polymer. Cole et al. [37] found that in both fasted and fed states, *in vivo*, gelatin capsules disintegrated faster than HPMC capsules (gellan gum used as the gelling promoter) in formulations containing ibuprofen. It is possible that the poorer performance of the HPMC-gellan capsules in an acidic environment is attributed to the gellan gum.

Differences have been seen in dissolution time between filled capsules of hypromellose (Quali-V, Shionogi Qualicaps Co., Ltd.) and gelatin (Coni-Snap, Capsugel) in different dissolution media.

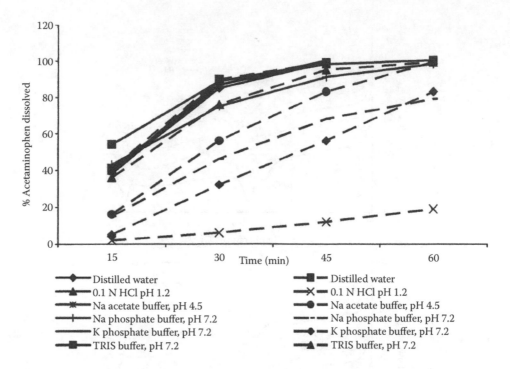

Distilled water

0.1 N HCl pH 1.2

Na acetate buffer, pH 4.5

Na phosphate buffer, pH 7.2

K phosphate buffer, pH 7.2

TRIS buffer, pH 7.2

Distilled water

0.1 N HCl pH 1.2

Na acetate buffer, pH 4.5

Na phosphate buffer, pH 7.2

K phosphate buffer, pH 7.2

TRIS buffer, pH 7.2

FIGURE 13.6 The dissolution of acetaminophen from HPMC capsules (dashed lines) and gelatin capsules (continuous lines) in different dissolution media ($n = 6$). (Adapted from Al-Tabakha MM. HPMC capsules: Current status and future prospects. *J Pharm Pharmaceut Sci* 2010; 13(3): 428–442, with permission from *Canadian Journal of Pharmaceutical Sciences*; Graph generated with kind permission from Springer Science+Business Media (via Copyright Clearance Center): *Pharm Res, In vitro* and *in vivo* pharmacoscintigraphic evaluation of ibuprofen hypromellose and gelatin capsules, 21, 2004, 793–798, Cole ET, Scott RA, Cade D, Connor Al, Wilding IR.)

Missaghi and Fassihi [42] filled empty capsules with powdered cellulose (Arbocel P290, JRS Pharma) and observed that in all immersion fluids tested, gelatin capsules showed a much faster disintegration as compared with hypromellose capsules. The authors attributed this to the fact that there are differences in water permeability of the capsules. In comparison to hypromellose, gelatin has been shown to be more water permeable, and this means that there will be a more rapid disintegration of the gelatin shell and its contents [54,55].

The disintegration time of gelatin capsules is the shortest in hydrochloric acid medium (pH 1.5), which may be attributed to the greater solubility of gelatin at such lower pH. On the other hand, the longest disintegration times for hypromellose capsules were observed in borate buffer, potassium phosphate monobasic buffer (K-PBS), and sodium phosphate monobasic buffer (Na-PBS), which was recorded as 288.3, 270.0, and 179.7 s, respectively. This is because potassium ions are present in the media; they are known to enhance the gel strength of carrageenan present in the hypromellose shells and thus delay capsule dissolution (Table 13.8).

The *in vitro* dissolution of theophylline in distilled water from two-piece hard shell capsules has been investigated using different types of capsule shells (gelatin, gelatin/PEG, and hypromellose). Analysis of variance confirmed that the formulation and the capsule shell materials were the most important factors influencing drug dissolution. The maximum extent of drug dissolution was significantly increased when HPMC capsules were used. The mean dissolution time (MDT) was significantly reduced, indicating a faster dissolution rate of the drug from HPMC capsules [55]. The use of the MDT is a model-independent approach. The MDT reflects the dissolution rate and is shorter the faster the dissolution process progresses [56].

TABLE 13.8

Disintegration Time (Seconds) for the Filled Capsules of Hypromellose and Gelatin in Selected Immersion Fluids

Disintegration Media	Hypromellose Capsules	Gelatin Capsules
Deionized water	154.0 ± 3.6	52.7 ± 2.5
Hydrochloric acid, pH 1.5	151.7 ± 16.8	34.0 ± 3.6
K-PBS, pH 6.8	270.0 ± 28.8	53.3 ± 6.6
Na-PBS, pH 6.8	179.7 ± 10.0	40.3 ± 4.5
Borate buffer, pH 10	288.3 ± 26.9	46.3 ± 5.0

Source: Adapted from Missaghi S and Fassihi R. Evaluation and comparison of physicomechanical characteristics of gelatin and hypromellose capsules. *Drug Dev Ind Pharm* 2006; 32: 829–838. Reproduced with permission of Taylor & Francis via Copyright Clearance Center.

Note: Data are reported as mean value and standard deviation ($n = 6$).

The addition of microfine cellulose (Vivacel A300) to the formulations as a filler reduced the MDT in all cases, whereas the addition of lactose monohydrate did not enhance drug dissolution. The study confirmed that a change from gelatin hard shell capsules to gelatin/PEG or HPMC hard shell capsules should not pose problems with respect to drug absorption or bioavailability. The authors also concluded that the use of HPMC capsule shells could be advantageous for low-solubility drugs [55].

Rossi et al. [57] developed and validated a dissolution procedure for ritonavir soft gelatin capsules (Norvir) based on *in vivo* data. The *in vivo* data were used to select the best dissolution test conditions based on an *in vitro–in vivo* correlation (IVIVC). The dissolution test was validated using an HPLC method. The best dissolution conditions used 900 mL of water containing 0.7% (w/v) of SLS and a paddle rotation speed of 25 rpm. Under these conditions, a significant linear relationship between the fraction of ritonavir absorbed and dissolved ($R^2 = 0.993$) and a level A IVIVC was established. The HPLC method showed RSDs for intraday and interday precision to be <1.6% and <1.4%, respectively. Accuracy was from 98.5% to 101.6% over the concentration range required for the dissolution test (4.0–124.0 µg/mL). Both the HPLC method and the dissolution test were validated and could be used to evaluate the dissolution profile of ritonavir soft gelatin capsules.

The release of high doses of APIs in a short amount of time or "dose dumping" is a potential safety and efficacy concern. Dose dumping is a particular concern for drugs used to manage pain such as Palladone, an opioid analgesic (hydromorphone HCl). Palladone extended-release capsules were withdrawn from the market in July 2005 because a clinical pharmacology study demonstrated that some patients who took Palladone with alcohol had six times the amount of drug in their blood as those who took Palladone with water (FDA, 2005) [58].

Smith et al. [59] conducted *in vitro* dissolution studies in various alcohol-containing media and found that, in 40% alcoholic media, 9 out of 10 capsules and 2 out of 17 tablets showed accelerated drug release. The authors noted that because the dose was released much quicker than expected, the extended-release product is performing more like an immediate-release formulation. Other modified-release drug products were also evaluated (i.e., anti-arrhythmic, calcium channel blocker, antidepressant, and anti-anginal) in 5% and 20% alcoholic media and in SGF (without enzymes) containing 20% alcohol. No tested capsules or tablets exhibited a significant increase in drug release in media containing only 5% alcohol within the first hour that was significantly different from the amount of drug released in purely aqueous media. The authors concluded that this study shows that *in vitro* dissolution may provide evidence regarding the ruggedness of formulations to ingested alcohol. An earlier study by Roberts et al. [60] reported an increase in drug release with an increase in alcohol concentration for aspirin tablets that were made using the excipient HPMC and when the testing was performed in 0%, 10%, 20%, 30%, and 40% ethanolic media.

Evaluation of Mechanical Properties

The mechanical properties of both gelatin and hypromellose capsule shells were studied by Missaghi and Fassihi [42] (Table 13.9). Based on its higher values of network of deformation and elastic modulus, gelatin appears to be a harder and tougher material than hypromellose. Thus, gelatin capsules are capable of absorbing more energy before their fracture. The authors stated that they believed that gelatin capsules may owe their improved mechanical properties to their reportedly higher water content, which makes this material more viscoelastic, as compared to hypromellose shells.

Nair et al. [61] used an In-Cap automatic capsule filling machine to compare filled capsules using both gelatin and HPMC (Quali-V) shells. The authors observed that the use of HPMC size #00 capsules resulted in a significant number of defective capsules. Some of the commonly observed defects included dimpled or dented bodies, split or chipped caps, and improperly closed caps. No such defects were observed for size #0 HPMC and gelatin capsules. The authors noted that the gelatin capsules did not show any dimple formation under identical filling conditions and concluded similar to Missaghi and Fassihi [42] that the HPMC capsules had a lower resistance to indentation load as compared with the gelatin capsules.

Kuentz and Rothlisberger [62] used texture analysis as a nondestructive test for HGC filled with liquid formulations to investigate the mechanical changes upon storage. Two different model formulations were prepared: (1) hydrophilic polymer mixtures containing water from 0% to 37.5%, PVP, and PEG; and (2) amphiphilic mixtures having high hydrophilicity–lipophilicity balance (HLB) values and containing water from 0% to 15%, colloidal silicon dioxide, and Labrasol (caprylocaproyl macrogol glycerides). The author's aim was to determine the most suitable amount of water present in the formulations to ensure maximum compatibility with the Licaps HGC, termed the balanced amount of water (BAW).

Kuentz and Rothlisberger [62] found that PVP did not show a great influence on the BAW in the range of 10–12% w/w for the first model mixture. However, capsules with the less hydrophilic Labrasol formulations retained their original stiffness after storage at 25°C/60% RH best with only half of that amount, that is, 5–6% w/w of water in the compositions. The authors stressed that while hydrophilic or amphiphilic liquid-fill formulations are often thought to be incompatible with gelatin capsules, there does exist an optimal water concentration (i.e., a BAW). The authors concluded by stating that texture profiling based on an experimental design can be used to determine hydrophilic or amphiphilic formulations that are compatible with gelatin capsules and that this

TABLE 13.9
Comparison of Compressive Properties of Empty Capsules Using a 10-mm Flat-Ended Probe

Compressive Properties (10-mm Probe)	Empty Capsules	
	Hypromellose	Gelatin
Work of compression (N/mm)	26.81 ± 2.31	42.62 ± 1.58
Work of recovery (N/mm)	4.77 ± 0.46	9.88 ± 0.23
Work of recovery/work of compression	0.18 ± 0.002	0.23 ± 0.003
Net work of deformation (N/mm)	22.04 ± 1.85	32.74 ± 1.35
Maximum force of deformation (N)	12.75 ± 0.99	18.47 ± 0.46
Elastic modulus (N/mm²)	4.70 ± 0.12	6.57 ± 0.20

Source: Adapted from Missaghi S and Fassihi R. Evaluation and comparison of physicomechanical characteristics of gelatin and hypromellose capsules. *Drug Dev Ind Pharm* 2006; 32: 829–838. Reproduced with permission of Taylor & Francis via Copyright Clearance Center.

Note: Data are reported as mean value and standard deviation ($n = 6$) at the Compression Depth of 4 mm.

information can be used to minimize the brittleness or softening issues that can occur in HGC owing to water migration during storage.

While hydrophilic solvents are incompatible with HGC, lipophilic materials such as monoglycerides, diglycerides, and triglycerides and other high-HLB surfactants with high molecular weight (e.g., Cremophors) do not seem to affect the mechanical properties of the capsules [2]. It was determined by Chen et al. [51] that ~26% and ~30% w/w of PG originally present in formulations IIc and IId, respectively, migrated into the HGC shells. Because PG functions as a plasticizer, this increase in PG content in the capsule shell provides a plausible explanation on the observed decrease in the T_g, tensile force, and elastic modulus of the capsule shells as shown in Figures 13.5b and 7b, respectively. Thus, the de-plasticization of the capsule shells attributed to water loss appears to be overcome by the migration of PG from the liquid-fills.

Empty capsules exhibited brittle fracture at a tensile force of 220.2 ± 8.2 N with an elastic modulus of 171.8 ± 1.6 N/mm. These values were found to be within the expected range for HGC with normal water content between 13% and 16% w/w [51]. Figure 13.7 shows the force–distance

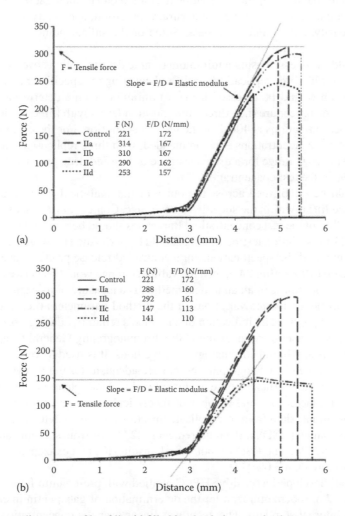

FIGURE 13.7 Force–distance profile of liquid filled hard gelatin capsules by texture analysis at (a) 1-week and (b) 7-week time points. (Reprinted from *J Pharm Sci*, 99, Chen F-J, Etzler FM, Ubben J, Birch A, Zhong L, Schwabe R, Dudhedia MS. Effects of lipophilic components on the compatibility of lipid-based formulations with hard gelatin capsules, 128–141, Copyright 2010, with permission from Elsevier.)

profiles for the plastic deformation (elongation) observed for the HGC formulations after 40°C/75% RH storage. It is evident from Figure 13.7b that after 7 weeks of storage, formulations IIc and IId exhibited lower elastic moduli and lower breaking force and were also observed to have greater softness and deformation as compared to formulations IIa and IIb (containing higher Cremophor EL levels). On the other hand, only ~17% and ~15% w/w of PG originally present in formulations IIa and IIb, respectively, migrated from the fills into the HGC shells. These PG levels that migrated from the fills into the shells appeared to compensate for the effect of water loss in the shells so that the mechanical properties of the capsules remained nearly identical to the controls.

ANALYTICAL METHOD VALIDATION

Analytical method development and validation go hand in hand with the determination of the drug release profile of capsule formulations during dissolution testing. Analytical method validation for compendia methods is described in detail under USP General Chapter <1225> [17] as well as FDA's *Guidance For Industry: Q2B Validation of Analytical Procedures: Methodology* [63], and is also part of the guidelines put forth by the International Council on Harmonization (ICH). Eight parameters are to be evaluated, and these include accuracy, precision, specificity, detection limit, quantitation limit, linearity, range, and robustness. Some of the salient points for these tests will be discussed below.

Accuracy should be assessed using a minimum of nine determinations over a minimum of three concentration levels with three replications each, and covering the specified range (i.e., 80%, 100%, and 120%). Precision should be assessed using a minimum of nine determinations covering the specified range for the procedure (i.e., three concentration levels with three replications each), or a minimum of six determinations at 100% of the test concentration. For the establishment of linearity, a minimum of five concentrations is recommended, with three replications performed per concentration level. The assay range for a drug substance or finished drug product should be evaluated from 80% to 120% of the test concentration.

Linearity should be established across the range of the analytical procedure, and all samples evaluated should be linear within the specified assay range. Content uniformity should cover a minimum of 70% to 130% of the test concentration. Impurities should be reported from 50% to 120% of the specification. For dissolution testing, testing should be performed between ±20% over the specified range; for example, if the specifications for a controlled-release product covered a region from 20% after 1 h, and up to 90% after 24 h, then the validated range would be between 0% and 110% of the label claim. The robustness of an analytical method is a measure of its capacity to remain unaffected despite small but deliberate variations in the method parameters (i.e., wavelength, column temperature, etc.) and provides an indication of a method's reliability during normal usage [63].

System suitability is discussed under the USP Chromatography General Chapter <621> and is an integral part of gas and liquid chromatographic methods. It is used to verify that the resolution and reproducibility of the chromatographic system are adequate for the analysis to be performed. Several measures of system efficiency are evaluated and include retention time, peak area, capacity factor (k'), tailing factor (T), and number of theoretical plates. Unless otherwise specified in the individual monograph, data from five replicate injections of the analyte are used to calculate the relative standard deviation (RSD), if the requirement is ≤2.0%, or from six replicate injections, if the RSD requirement is >2.0%. The RSD for both clindamycin HCl and oxazepam capsules is listed in the USP 35 as not more than 3.0% [17].

Ulu and Kel [64] developed a sensitive HPLC method with pre-column fluorescence derivatization using 4-fluoro-7-nitrobenzofurazan for the determination of gabapentin in capsules and using mexiletine as the internal standard. The assay was linear over the concentration range between 5 and 50 ng/mL. Moreover, the method was found to be sensitive with a low limit of detection (LOD; 0.85 ng/mL) and limit of quantitation (LOQ; 2.55 ng/mL). The results of the developed procedure for gabapentin content in capsules were compared with those by the official USP method. Statistical analysis by t and F tests showed no significant difference at the 95% confidence level between the two proposed methods.

However, Ciavarella et al. [65] had developed a novel method for the determination of gabapentin and its major degradation impurity in tablets and capsules without the need for a derivatization step. After this, Gupta et al. [66] developed and validated a simple, efficient, and selective reversed-phase HPLC method for the analysis of dissolution samples from five marketed gabapentin drug products. The standard calibration curve was prepared using eight concentration levels over the range of 0.05 to 0.65 mg/mL. While the two capsule products showed similar dissolution profiles with >90% dissolution within 10 min and >99% dissolution within 30 min, the three tablet samples exhibited more variability.

An HPLC method is described for the determination of duloxetine hydrochloride in capsules [67]. This method was also based on pre-column derivatization with 4-chloro-7-nitrobenzo-2-oxa-1,3-diazole using the fluorimetric detection technique. The linearity of the method was in the range of 10–600 ng/mL and the limits of detection and quantification were 0.51 and 1.53 ng/mL, respectively. The results were in good agreement with those obtained using the reference method of Prabu et al. [68]. Bonfilio et al. [69] reported on a reversed-phase HPLC method that was validated according to the ICH guidelines and showed accuracy, precision (intraday and interday RSD values were <2.0%), selectivity, robustness, and linearity ($r = 0.9998$) over a concentration range from 30 to 70 mg/L of losartan potassium. The limits of detection and quantification were 0.114 and 0.420 mg/L, respectively. The authors concluded that this validated method may be used to quantify losartan potassium in capsules and also to determine the drug's stability. Mohammadi et al. [70] reported on a stability-indicating HPLC method for orlistat capsules. The authors found that the method was linear over the concentration range of 0.02–0.75 mg/mL ($r = 0.9998$) and had limits of detection and quantitation of 0.006 and 0.02 mg/mL, respectively. Degradation products resulting from the stress studies did not interfere with the detection of orlistat, and the assay was thus found to be stability-indicating.

A validated method can be applied to the analysis of both innovator and generic products. Cyclosporin A (CyA) is a cornerstone immunosuppressant for the prophylaxis against allograft rejection after organ transplantation. Novartis is the innovator for the Neoral CyA formulation in soft gelatin capsules. A simple and reliable reversed-phase HPLC method was developed and validated by Bonifacio et al. [71] for the evaluation of four CyA degradation products and two related compounds aimed for the quality control of Neoral capsules and its generic formulations.

In a second step, the validated method was then compared to the USP assay method for CyA capsules, where some of the mentioned impurities were not adequately resolved from the CyA peak. Isocratic elution at a flow rate of 1.0 mL/min was employed using a C-18 analytical column (4 mm × 250 mm) maintained at 75°C with tetrahydrofuran:phosphoric acid (0.05 M) (44:56, v/v) as the mobile phase. The developed method was validated in terms of selectivity, linearity, precision, accuracy, LOD, and LOQ. The validated method was successfully applied to both innovator and generic Neoral capsules. Therefore, the proposed method was found to be suitable for the simultaneous determination of CyA as well as its major impurities in capsule formulations.

Two different methodologies were used to validate assays for capsules of fexofenadine HCl. A simple, accurate, and effective capillary electrophoresis (CE) method with ultraviolet absorbance detection was employed by Breier et al. [72]. The method was found to be linear ($r = 0.9999$) at concentrations ranging from 20 to 100 μg/mL, precise (RSD intra-assay and inter-assay = 1.5%), accurate (recovery = 98.1%), and specific. The limits of detection and quantitation were 0.69 and 2.09 μg/mL, respectively. This method was compared to the reversed-phase HPLC method developed previously by the authors for the same drug (Breier et al. [73]), and no significant differences were found between the two methods in fexofenadine HCl quantitation. In fact, the authors concluded that since the detection and quantitation limits were 0.341 and 1.033 μg/mL, respectively, these low values showed that the HPLC method possessed good sensitivity.

NUTRACEUTICALS

A wide variety of nutraceutical products are delivered to consumers using capsules; in fact, the HPMC capsules have grown to be very popular within the all-natural market. Many nutraceuticals have some type of antioxidant functionality and can be classified as phenolics, a category that comprises more than 4000 compounds divided into 12 subclasses. Currently, HPLC has become the analytical method of choice for phenolic compounds. Other techniques such as GC, CE, FTIR, and spectrophotometry have also been employed.

With HPLC, reversed-phase columns, particularly C18 with particle sizes of 5 µm, are most commonly used. In general terms, endcapped columns provide better separations as they have ultralow silanol activity and this eliminates unpredictable secondary interactions with analytes. Elution mobile phases are usually binary, with an aqueous acidified solvent (solvent A), that is, acetic acid, and an organic solvent, such as methanol or acetonitrile, generally acidified (solvent B). Trifluoroacetic acid in both solvents enhances the resolution and eliminates peak tailing of catechins [74].

In terms of detection systems, UV-visible with diode array detection is the standard method for detection of phenolic compounds [75]. Simple phenolic compounds present a single absorption band in the range of 240–290 nm, while more complex phenol compounds (flavonoids) present a second absorption band with a maximum in the 300–550 nm range [76].

Carotenoids are a class of more than 600 naturally occurring pigments synthesized by plants, algae, yeast, fungi, and photosynthetic bacteria. Fruits and vegetables provide most of the carotenoids in the human diet. Carotenoids can be broadly classified into two classes, carotenes (α-carotene, β-carotene, or lycopene) and xanthophylls (β-cryptoxanthin, lutein, or zeaxanthin). Lycopene, a bright red carotene pigment, was recently analyzed in nutritional supplements by an easier technique such as high-performance thin-layer chromatography (TLC) [77]. These authors analyzed four softgel samples, 300 µg, 3 mg, 5 mg, and 10 mg. The amount of lycopene in the tested samples ranged from 77.7% to 98.1% relative to the stated label claim. Accuracy was found to be within 1.90% of theoretical values for the 3-mg softgels and 1.10% of theoretical values for the 10-mg softgels. Precision was 1.44% and 2.39% RSD for the 10-mg and 3-mg softgels, respectively. For all analyses, polynomial regression produced r values ≥ 0.993. The LOQ of the method was equal to the weight of the lowest standard (294 ng), and the visual LOD was approximately 8 ng.

Other nutraceuticals have shown promise in the treatment of osteoarthritis. Chondroitin sulfate is a mucopolysaccharide that acts as an important structural component of cartilage, providing much of its resistance to compression. It has been determined in raw materials and formulations by CE-UV [78]. It has also been analyzed in dietary supplements using a specific and sensitive agarose-gel electrophoresis and strong anion-exchange HPLC method [79]. High-performance size-exclusion chromatography was subsequently used to determine the chondroitin sulfate molecular mass [80]. An HPLC-UV method was also developed and validated after enzymatic hydrolysis in order to quantify chondroitin sulfate in raw materials and dietary supplements at a range of about 5% to 100% (w/w) chondroitin sulfate. The precision %RSD for total chondroitin sulfate content was between 1.60% and 4.72%, and chondroitin sulfate recovery from the raw material negative control (e.g., heparin) was between 101% and 102% [81].

Two different CE approaches have been developed to determine levels of glucosamine, a compound shown to be effective in treating osteoarthritis pain and rehabilitating cartilage [82,83]. A simple capillary electrophoretic method was developed and validated more recently for the determination of glucosamine in capsules and tablets using in-capillary derivatization with o-phthalaldehyde [84]. The detector response was linear ($R^2 > 0.999$) in the concentration range 10–1000 µg/mL. The LOD was 1.3 mg/g. Spiked glucosamine recoveries at 50- and 100-mg/g levels were 95.1% and 104.3%, respectively. The concentrations of glucosamine from the commercial products were 109–705 mg/g, and the ratios of detected glucosamine content to the labeled value were 88.8%–124%. No significant bias was observed ($R^2 = 0.989$, $p < 0.01$), between the results obtained by the proposed CE method and the older colorimetric method of Rondle–Morgan [85].

In 2007, the USP added performance tests for the disintegration and dissolution of capsules under General Chapter <2040> for dietary supplements. Traditionally, the disintegration test was used for determining the disintegration time of all solid oral dosage forms. However, now, the rupture test for soft shell capsules has been added and it utilizes the dissolution test <711> with 500 mL of water as the immersion medium and Apparatus 2 (paddle) operated at 50 rpm. The test requirements are met if all capsules rupture within 15 min or if not more than 2 of the total of 18 capsules tested rupture in more than 15 min but not more than 30 min. For soft gelatin capsules that do not conform to the rupture test acceptance criteria, the test is repeated with the addition of purified pepsin to the medium that results in an activity of 750,000 U or less per 1000 mL [17]. Another difference is that for hard shell capsules, Chapter <2040> lists USP pH 4.5 buffer as the immersion medium while Chapter <701> lists water as the default medium if a monograph does not specify any other medium. A decision tree is presented in Figure 13.8.

There are limited scientific data comparing the performance of the rupture test with that of the disintegration test for soft shell capsules. Almukainzi et al. [86] recently conducted a study using five different soft shell capsule products: (1) amantadine (suspension), (2) flaxseed oil (oil base), (3) ginseng (oil base), (4) soybean oil (oil base), and (5) pseudoephedrine HCl (water-miscible solution). The study design compared capsules as received with capsules that were treated by coating them with the liquid contents of another capsule to simulate a production deficiency. The capsules were then incubated for 2 weeks at both ambient and 40°C and evaluated using both the rupture and disintegration tests. The results varied depending on the type of product. For example, while amantadine showed that the rupture test was not faster than the disintegration test, it was faster for the flaxseed oil capsules. Furthermore, for the soybean oil capsules, the disintegration test was able to differentiate between the storage conditions ($p = 0.0$). For this product, while the rupture test had the shortest test duration, the disintegration test was able to reveal the differences among the storage and the uncoated/coated conditions.

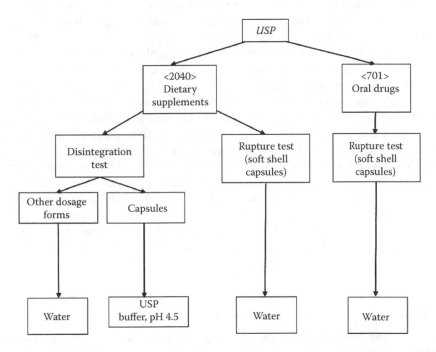

FIGURE 13.8 Schematic comparison of USP Chapters <2040> and <701>. (Adapted from Almukainzi M, Salehi M, Chacra NAB, Lobenberg R. Comparison of the rupture and disintegration tests for soft-shell capsules. *Dissolution Tech* Feb. 2011; 21–25, with permission from Dissolution Technologies, Hockessin, Delaware, USA.)

However, the authors concluded that the statistical analysis showed that there was no advantage of the rupture test over the disintegration test. On a product-by-product basis, both tests were sensitive to certain investigated parameters. They found that a noticeable difference between both tests was observed in most cases; the rupture test reached the defined endpoint faster than the disintegration test. The authors also stated that if the soft shell capsules were manufactured using a Quality-by-Design approach, they should be evaluated using both methods to determine which performance test is more sensitive to the specific product characteristics.

An international collaborative study involving 10 laboratories was conducted using an HPLC-UV method for the determination of coenzyme Q10 (Co-Q10, ubidecarenone) in raw materials and dietary supplements (softgels, hard gelatin capsules, and tablets). The method exhibited acceptable accuracy upon spiking at 50%, 100%, and 200% of the target Co-Q10 level. The average assay for all levels was 97.3%, with a %RSD of 0.5%. The repeatability %RSDs were about 2.2% for the raw material and about 5.0% for a softgel finished product dosage form. The LOD and LOQ for the method were determined to be 3 and 9 µg/mL, respectively. A 5-point calibration curve covering a range from 0.025 to 0.125 mg/mL Co-Q10 demonstrated that the method is linear over this range with a regression coefficient, R^2, of 0.9999 [87].

Standardized extracts of *Ginkgo biloba* leaves are considered a drug in many European countries and China while being listed as a top-selling dietary supplement in North America. The major active components of *G. biloba* extract are the flavonoids and terpene lactones. Ding et al. [88] developed a highly sensitive and specific fingerprint profile method using capillary HPLC–ion trap mass spectrometry (HPLC-MS) which could identify more than 70 components from *G. biloba*.

The authors obtained an LOD using standard compounds ranging from 8 to 25 ng/mL for flavonoids, while the LOD for terpene lactones ranged from 40 to 150 ng/mL. The overall sensitivity of this method was more than 10 times higher than normal bore HPLC-MS. Moreover, by re-processing the mass spectrometry data using tandem MS-MS, extracting ion current, and neutral loss information, considerably more information could be obtained to compare the similarity of *Ginkgo* extract originating from different countries. The authors concluded that this is a major advantage over HPLC-UV and other TLC methods, which are currently the main techniques used for fingerprinting analysis.

In a recent review article, Lockwood [89] summarized published reports of the quality of nutraceutical raw materials and finished products. His results have revealed wide variability, often as a result of a lack of clear regulatory definitions with respect to the size of polymeric entities and also the presence of glycosidic and salt forms. Published evaluations of more than 70 formulations of 25 different nutraceuticals from different countries revealed variable quality. No nutraceutical product examined showed consistent high quality, but a number revealed consistent low quality, thereby making the case for closer regulation of manufacturers. For example, overall, scientific studies have shown that the quality of chondroitin sulfate in commercially available products is often poor, as measured by the low percentage of products meeting an assay value between 95% and 105% of their label claim. Moreover, creatine products conformed poorly, as did polyunsaturated fatty acids (*n*-3-PUFAs), γ-linolenic acid, lutein, zeaxanthin, lycopene, and α-tocopherol. Complex materials such as soy and tea extracts were also found to have poor compliance. These highlighted points are important as they can contribute to side effects and drug interactions in patients in the future as nutraceutical usage becomes more widespread.

REFERENCES

1. Podczeck F and Jones BE (Eds.). *Pharmaceutical Capsules*, 2nd ed. 2004; Pharmaceutical Press, London.
2. Cole ET, Cade D, Benameur H. Challenges and opportunities in the encapsulation of liquid and semi-solid formulations into capsules for oral administration. *Adv Drug Del Rev* 2008; 60: 747–756.
3. Carstensen JT and Rhodes CT. Pellicle formation in gelatin capsules. *Drug Dev Ind Pharm* 1993; 19: 2709–2712.

4. Digenis GA, Gold TB, Shah VP. Cross-linking of gelatin capsules and its relevance to their *in vitro–in vivo* performance. *J Pharm Sci* 1994; 83: 915–921.
5. Singh S, Rao KVR, Venugopal K, Manikandan R. Alteration in dissolution characteristics of gelatin-containing formulations. A review of the problem, test methods, and solutions. *Pharm Technol* April 2002: 36–58.
6. de Carvalho RA and Grosso CRF. Properties of chemically modified gelatin films. *Braz J Chem Eng* 2006; 23(1): 45–53.
7. Pina M, Souza AT, Brojo AP. Enteric coating of hard gelatin capsules. Part 1: Application of hydroalcoholic solutions of formaldehyde in preparation of gastro-resistant capsules. *Int J Pharm* 1996; 133(1–2): 139–148.
8. Kuijpers AJ, Engbers GHM, Feijen J, de Smedt SC, Meyvis TKL, Demeester J, Krijhsveld J, Zaat SA, Dankert J. Characterization of the network structure of carbodiimide cross-linked gelatin gels. *Macromolecules* 1999; 32: 3325–3333.
9. Pina M, Souza AT, Brojo AP. Enteric coating of hard gelatin capsules. Part 2: Bioavailability of formaldehyde treated capsules. *Int J Pharm* 1997; 148: 73–84.
10. Honkanen O. Biopharmaceutical Evaluation of Orally and Rectally Administered Hard Hydroxypropyl Methylcellulose Capsules. Dissertation submitted to the Faculty of Pharmacy, University of Helsinki, 2004.
11. Rowe RC, Sheskey PJ, Cook WG, Fenton ME (Eds.). *Handbook of Pharmaceutical Excipients*, 7th edition, 2012. Pharmaceutical Press, Philadelphia, PA.
12. Ogura T, Furuya Y, Matsuura S. HPMC capsules—An alternative to gelatin. *Pharm Tech Eur* 1998; 11: 32–42.
13. Scott R, Cade D, He X. Pullulan Film Compositions. U.S. Patent #6,887,307 B1; May 3, 2005.
14. Scott R, Cade D, He X. Pullulan Film Compositions. U.S. Patent #7,267,718 B2; Sept. 11, 2007.
15. Martyn GP and St. John Coghlan D. Composition for Delivery of an Active Agent. U.S. Patent Application # 2009/0004275 A1, January 1, 2009.
16. Huyghebaert N, Vermeire A, Remon JP. Alternative method for enteric coating of HPMC capsules resulting in ready-to-use enteric-coated capsules. *Eur J Pharm Sci* 2004; 21: 617–623.
17. United States Pharmaceopeia (USP) 35/NF 20, 2012. United States Pharmaceopeial Convention, Inc., Rockville, MD.
18. Nishi C, Nakajima N, Ikada Y. In vitro evaluation of cytotoxicity of diepoxy compounds used for biomaterial modification. *J Biomed Mater Res* 1995; 29(7): 829–834.
19. Li Z, Jacobus LK, Wuelfing WP, Golden M, Martin GP, Reed RA. Detection and quantification of low-molecular-weight aldehydes in pharmaceutical excipients by headspace gas chromatography. *J Chromatogr A* 2006; 1104: 1–10.
20. del Barrio MA, Hu J, Zhou P, Cauchon N. Simultaneous determination of formic acid and formaldehyde in pharmaceutical excipients using headspace GC/MS. *J Pharm Biomed Anal* 2006; 41: 738–743.
21. Wu Y, Levons J, Narang AJ, Raghavan K, Rao VM. Reactive impurities in excipients: Profiling, identification and mitigation of drug–excipient incompatibility. *AAPS Pharm Sci Tech* 2011; 12(4): 1248–1263.
22. Meyer MC, Straughn AB, Mhatre RM, Hussain A, Shah VP, Bottom CB, Cole ET, Lesko LL, Mallinowski H, Williams RL. The effect of gelatin cross-linking on the bioequivalence of hard and soft gelatin acetaminophen capsules. *Pharm Res* 2000; 17: 962–966.
23. Marchais H, Cayzeele G, Legendre JY, Skiba M, Arnaud P. Cross-linking of hard gelatin carbamazepine capsules: Effect of dissolution conditions on in vitro drug release. *Eur J Pharm Sci* 2003; Jun; 19(2–3): 129–132.
24. USP, Physical Tests and Determinations, *Pharm Forum* 25, 7516 (1999).
25. Chang CK, Alvarez-Nunez FA, Rinella JV Jr, Magnusson LE, Sueda K. Roller compaction, granulation and capsule product dissolution of drug formulations containing a lactose or mannitol filler, starch, and talc. *AAPS Pharm Sci Tech* 2008; 9(2): 597–604.
26. Nassar MN, Nesarikar VN, Lozano R, Parker WL, Huang Y, Palaniswamy V, Xu W, Khaselev N. Influence of formaldehysde impurity in the polysorbates 80 and PEG-300 on the stability of a parenteral formulation of BMS0294352: Identification and control of the degradation product. *Pharm Dev Tech* 2004; 9: 189–195.
27. Adesunloye TA and Stach PE. Effect of glycine–citric acid on the dissolution stability of hard gelatin capsules. *Drug Dev Ind Pharm* 1998; 24(6): 493–500.
28. Ku SM, Li W, Dulin W, Donahue F, Cade D, Benameur H, Hutchison K. Performance qualification of a new hypromellose capsule: Part I. Comparative evaluation of physical, mechanical and processability quality attributes of Vcaps Plus, Quali-V and gelatin capsules. *Int J Pharm* 2010; 386(1–2): 30–41.

29. Tengroth C, Gasslander U, Andersson FO, Jacobsson SP. Cross-linking of gelatin capsules with formaldehyde and other aldehydes: An FTIR spectroscopy study. *Pharm Dev Technol* 2005; 10(3): 405–412.

30. Kontny MJ, Mulski CA. Gelatin capsule brittleness as a function of relative humidity at room temperature. *Int J Pharm* 1989; 54: 79–85.

31. Chang R-K, Raghavan KS, Hussain MA. A study on gelatin capsule brittleness: Moisture transfer between the capsule shell and its content. *J Pharm Sci* 1998; 87(5): 556–558.

32. Gold TB, Buice RG, Lodder RA, Digenis GA. Determination of extent of formaldehyde-induced crosslinking in hard gelatin capsules by near-infrared spectrophotometry. *Pharm Res* 1997; 14(8): 1046–1050.

33. Cole SK, Story MJ, Attwood D, Laudanski T, Robertson J, Barnwell SG. Studies using a non-ionic surfactant-containing drug delivery system designed for hard gelatin capsule compatibility. *Int J Pharm* 1992; 88: 211–220.

34. Liebowitz SM, Vadino WA, Ambrosio TJ. Determination of hard gelatin capsule brittleness using a motorized compression test stand. *Drug Dev Ind Pharm* 1990; 16: 995–1010.

35. Brown J, Madit N, Cole ET, Wilding IR, Cade D. The effects of cross-linking on the in vivo disintegration of hard gelatin capsules. *Pharm Res* 1998; 15(5): 1026–1030.

36. Cadé D. Vcaps® Plus Capsules. A New HPMC Capsule for Optimum Formulation of Pharmaceutical Dosage Forms. CAPSUGEL brochure BAS416; 2012.

37. Cole ET, Scott RA, Cade D, Connor Al, Wilding IR. *In vitro* and *in vivo* pharmacoscintigraphic evaluation of ibuprofen hypromellose and gelatin capsules. *Pharm Res* 2004; 21: 793–798.

38. Ku SM, Lu Q, Li W, Chen Y. Performance qualification of a new hypromellose capsule: Part II. Disintegration and dissolution comparison between two types of hypromellose capsules. *Int J Pharm* 2011; 416(1): 16–24.

39. Chiwele I, Jones BE, Podczeck F. The shell dissolution of various empty hard capsules. *Chem Pharm Bull* 2000; 48: 951–956.

40. El-Malah Y, Nazzal S. Hard gelatin and hypromellose (HPMC) capsules: Estimation of rupture time by real-time dissolution spectroscopy. *Drug Dev Ind Pharm* 2007; 33: 27–34.

41. Tuleu C, Khela MK, Evans DF, Jones BE, Nagata S, Basit AW. A scintigraphic investigation of the disintegration behavior of capsules in fasting subjects: A comparison of hypromellose capsules containing carrageenan as a gelling agent and standard gelatin capsules. *Eur J Pharm Sci* 2007; 30: 251–255.

42. Missaghi S and Fassihi R. Evaluation and comparison of physicomechanical characteristics of gelatin and hypromellose capsules. *Drug Dev Ind Pharm* 2006; 32: 829–838.

43. Cheng K-C, Demirci A, Catchmark JM. Pullulan: Biosynthesis, production, and applications. *Appl Microbiol Biotechnol* 2011; 92: 29–44.

44. Sakata Y and Otsuka M. Evaluation of relationship between molecular behavior and mechanical strength of pullulan films. *Int J Pharm* 2009; 374: 33–38.

45. Coleman NJ and Craig DQM. Modulated temperature differential scanning calorimetry: A novel approach to pharmaceutical thermal analysis. *Int J Pharm* 1996; 135: 13–29.

46. Nazzal S and Wang Y. Characterization of soft gelatin capsules by thermal analysis. *Int J Pharm* 2001; 230: 35–45.

47. Fitzpatrick S, Saklatvala R. Understanding the physical stability of freeze dried dosage forms from the glass transition temperature of the amorphous components. *J Pharm Sci* 92(12): 2495–2501.

48. D'Cruz NM and Bell LN. Thermal unfolding of gelatin in solids as affected by the glass transition. *J Food Sci* 2005; 70(2): E64–E68.

49. Coppola A, Djabourov M, Ferrand M. Phase diagram of gelatin plasticized by water and glycerol. *Macromol Symp* 2008; 273: 56–65.

50. Dai C-A, Liu M-W. The effect of crystallinity and aging enthalpy on the mechanical properties of gelatin films. *Mat Sci Eng A* 2006; 423: 121–127.

51. Chen F-J, Etzler FM, Ubben J, Birch A, Zhong L, Schwabe R, Dudhedia MS. Effects of lipophilic components on the compatibility of lipid-based formulations with hard gelatin capsules. *J Pharm Sci* 2010; 99(1): 128–141.

52. Schamp K, Schreder S-A, Dressman J. Development of an in vitro/in vivo correlation for lipid formulations of EMD 50733, a poorly soluble, lipophilic drug substance. *Eur J Pharm Biopharm* 2006; 62: 227–234.

53. Al-Tabakha MM. HPMC capsules: Current status and future prospects. *J Pharm Pharmaceut Sci* 2010; 13(3): 428–442.

54. Nagata S. Advantages to HPMC capsules: A new generation. *Drug Del Technol* 2002; 2(2): 34–39.

55. Podczeck F, Jones BE. The in vitro dissolution of theophylline from different types of hard shell capsules. *Drug Dev Ind Pharm* 2002; 9: 1163–1169.

56. Podczeck F. Comparison of in vitro dissolution profiles by Calculating Mean Dissolution Time (MDT) or Mean Residence Time (MRT). *Int J Pharm* 1993; 97: 93–100.

57. Rossi, RC, Cias CL, Donato EM, Martins LA, Bergold Am, Frohlich PE. Development and validation of dissolution test for ritonavir soft gelatin capsules based on in vivo data. *Int J Pharm* 2007; 338: 119–124.

58. FDA, 2005. Public Health Advisory: Suspended Marketing of Palladone (hydromorphone hydrochloride, extended-release capsules). [http://www.fda.gov/Drugs/DrugSafety/PostmarketDrugSafetyInformation forPatientsandProviders/DrugSafetyInformationforHeathcareProfessionals/PublicHealthAdvisories /ucm051743.htm; accessed online: December 30, 2012].

59. Smith AP, Moore TW, Westenberger BJ, Doub WH. In vitro dissolution of oral modified-release tablets and capsules in ethanolic media. *Int J Pharm* 2010; 398: 93–96.

60. Roberts M, Cespi M, Ford JL, Dyas AM, Downing J, Martini LG, Crowley PJ. Influence of ethanol on aspirin release from hypromellose matrices. *Int J Pharm* 2007; 332: 31–37.

61. Nair R, Vemuri M, Agrawala P, Kim S-I. Investigation of various factors affecting encapsulation on the In-Cap automatic capsule-filling machine. *AAPS Pharm Sci Tech* 2004; 5(4) Article 57.

62. Kuentz M, Rothlisberger D. Determination of the optimal amount of water in liquid-fill masses for hard gelatin capsules by means of texture analysis and experimental design. *Int J Pharm* 2002; 236: 145–152.

63. *FDA Guidance for Industry*: Q2B Validation of Analytical Procedures: Methodology. CDER & CBER (November, 1996).

64. Ulu ST, Kel E. Highly sensitive determination and validation of gabapentin in pharmaceutical preparations by HPLC with 4-fluoro-7-nitrobenzofurazan derivatization and fluorescence detection. *J Chromatogr Sci* 2011; 49(6): 417–421.

65. Ciavarella AB, Gupta A, Sayeed VA, Khan MA, Faustino PJ. Development and application of a validated HPLC method for the determination of gabapentin and its major degradation impurity in drug products. *J Pharm Biomed Anal* 2007; 43(5): 1647–1653.

66. Gupta A, Ciavarella AB, Sayeed VA, Khan MA, Faustino PJ. Development and application of a validated HPLC method for the analysis of dissolution samples of gabapentin drug products. *J Pharm Biomed Anal* 2008; 46: 181–186.

67. Tatar Ulu S. Determination and validation of duloxetine hydrochloride in capsules by HPLC with pre-column derivatization and fluorescence detection. *J Chromatogr Sci* 2012; 50(6): 494–498.

68. Prabu LS, Shahnawaz S, Kumar D, Shirwaikar A. Spectrofluorimetric method for determination of duloxetine hydrochloride in bulk and pharmaceutical dosage forms; *Ind J Pharm Sci* 2008; 70: 502–503.

69. Bonfilio R, Tarley CR, Pereira GR, Salgado HR, de Araújo MB. Multivariate optimization and validation of an analytical methodology by RP-HPLC for the determination of losartan potassium in capsules. *Talanta* 2009; 80(1): 236–241.

70. Mohammadi A, Haririan I, Rezanour N, Ghiasi L, Walker RB. A stability-indicating high performance liquid chromatographic assay for the determination of orlistat in capsules. *J Chromatogr A* 2006; 1116(1–2): 153–157.

71. Bonifacio FN, Giocanti M, Reynier JP, Lacarelle B, Nicolay A. Development and validation of HPLC method for the determination of Cyclosporin A and its impurities in Neoral capsules and its generic versions. *J Pharm Biomed Anal* 2009; 49(2): 540–546.

72. Breier AR, Garcia SS, Jablonski A, Steppe M, Schapoval EE. Capillary electrophoresis method for fexofenadine hydrochloride in capsules. *J AOAC Int* 2005; 88(4): 1059–1063.

73. Breier AR, Paim CS, Menegola J, Steppe M, Schapoval EE. Development and validation of a liquid chromatographic method for fexofenadine hydrochloride in capsules. *J AOAC Int* 2004; 87(5): 1093–1097.

74. Dalluge JJ, Nelson BC, Brown TJ, Sander LC. Selection of column and gradient elution system for the separation of catechins in green tea using high-performance liquid chromatography. *J Chromatogr A* 1998; 793: 265–274.

75. Hurst WJ. *Methods of Analysis for Functional Foods and Nutraceuticals*, 2002. CRC Press, Boca Raton, FL.

76. Andersen OM and Markham KR. *Flavonoids: Chemistry, Biochemistry, and Applications*, 2nd edition, 2007. CRC Press, Boca Raton, FL.

77. Vasta JD and Sherma J. Analysis of lycopene in nutritional supplements by silica gel high-performance thin-layer chromatography with visible-mode densitometry. *Acta Chromatographia* 2008; 20(4): 673–683.

78. Malavaki CJ, Asimakopoulou AP, Lamari FN, Theocharis AD, Tzanakakis GN, Karamanos NK. Capillary electrophoresis for the quality control of chondroitin sulfates in raw materials and formulations. *Anal Biochem* 2008; 374: 213–220.

79. Sim J-S, Im A-R, Cho SM, Jang HJ, Jo JH, Kim YS. Evaluation of chondroitin sulfate in shark cartilage powder as a dietary supplement: Raw materials and finished products. *Food Chem* 2007; 101: 532–539.

80. Volpi N and Maccari F. Quantitative and qualitative evaluation of chondroitin sulfate in dietary supplements. *Food Anal Methods* 2008; 1: 195–204.

81. JI D, Roman M, Zhou J, Hildreth J. Determination of chondroitin sulfate content in raw materials and dietary supplements by high-performance liquid chromatography with ultraviolet detection after enzymatic hydrolysis: Single-laboratory validation. *J AOAC Int* 2007; 90(3): 659–669.

82. Volpi N. Capillary electrophoresis determination of glucosamine in nutraceutical formulations after labeling with anthranilc acid and UV detection. *J Pharmaceut Biomed Anal* 2009; 49: 868–871.

83. Chen J-J, Lee YC, Cheng T-J, Hsiao H-Y, Chen RLC. Determination of glucosamine content in nutraceuticals by capillary electrophoresis using in-capillary OPA labeling techniques. *J Food Drug Anal* 2006; 14: 203–206.

84. Akamatsu S and Mitsuhashi T. Development of a simple capillary electrophoretic determination of glucosamine in nutritional supplements using in-capillary derivatisation with *o*-phthalaldehyde. *Food Chem* 2012; 130: 1137–1141.

85. Rondle CJM and Morgan WTJ. The determination of glucosamine and galactosamine. *Biochem J* 1955, 61(4): 586–589.

86. Almukainzi M, Salehi M, Chacra NAB, Lobenberg R. Comparison of the rupture and disintegration tests for soft-shell capsules. *Dissolution Tech* Feb. 2011; 21–25.

87. Lunetta S and Roman M. Determination of coenzyme Q10 content in raw materials and dietary supplements by high-performance liquid chromatography-UV: Collaborative study. *J AOAC Int* 2008; 91(4): 702–708.

88. Ding S, Dudley E, Plummer S, Tang J, Newton RP, Brenton AG. Fingerprint profile of *Ginkgo biloba* nutritional supplements by LC/ESI-MS/MS. *Phytochemistry* 2008; 69(7): 1555–1564.

89. Lockwood GB. The quality of commercially available nutraceutical supplements and food sources. *J Pharm Pharmacol* 2011; 63: 3–10.

14 Rheological Aspects of Capsule Shell Excipients and the Manufacture of Encapsulated Formulations

Lawrence H. Block

CONTENTS

INTRODUCTION

The invention of the capsule in the nineteenth century—and subsequent improvements to it in composition and manufacturing—focused on gelatin as the sole or principal film-forming component of the capsule shell. In time, other macromolecular excipients—for example, cellulosic polymers (e.g., HPMC alginates, ι- and κ-carrageenans, starch, and polyvinyl alcohol—have also been employed to form capsule shells, but to a much lesser extent. Nonetheless, all of these ingredients share a common characteristic [1]: the ability to form a gel or film rigid enough [in the case of hard shell capsules] or pliable enough [in the case of soft shell capsules] to serve as the envelope or container for a dose of a drug formulation. Gel formation is generally accomplished by a change in temperature: in general, for hard gelatin capsule shells, chilled capsule shell molds or pins are dipped into a heated solution of the gellant (usually gelatin at 45–55°C). In some instances, heated molds or pins are dipped into a chilled solution of the gellant (e.g., some cellulosic polymers). In either case, the coated pins are then slowly withdrawn from the coating solution. The viscosity of the coating solution determines the quantity of solution retained on the pins and the resultant thickness of the capsule shells. Gelation is also facilitated by the loss of solvent through evaporation and the concomitant increase in gellant concentration. The formed capsule shells are stripped from the pins and subsequently filled with the formulation matrix, typically by dosator or dosing disk methods. Injection molding processes have also been developed for the manufacture of hard shell capsules, for example, from starch [2,3] and other polymeric components [4]. As with dip coating processes, the formed shells are reserved for subsequent filling. Manufacturing of soft shell capsule products, on the other hand, involves a process wherein the capsule is formed *and* filled in tandem.

This chapter focuses on the rheological requirements for capsule shell excipients, rheological instruments, and procedures intended to test the suitability of the excipients for capsule shell production, and rheological considerations relevant to the filling of hard and soft capsules.

CAPSULE SHELL EXCIPIENT SOLUTION RHEOLOGY AND MEASUREMENT

SOLUTION SHEAR VISCOSITY

Gellant solution viscosity determinations are critical to the development of capsule shell manufacturing specifications, as the retention of the gel-forming solution on the capsule shell molds or pins during the shell formation process is primarily dependent on the solution's viscosity. As gellants are macromolecular or polymeric materials, solution viscosity is markedly affected by the gellant's concentration, its molecular weight distribution, and the applied hydrodynamic conditions, as well as by solution temperature, pH, electrolyte concentration, and additives such as plasticizers and co-solvents.

In *shear flow* of fluids, viscosity is a property defined by Newton's law:

$$\eta = \frac{\sigma}{\dot{\gamma}}, \tag{14.1}$$

where η is the Newtonian viscosity (mPa·s), σ is the shear stress (Pa), and $\dot{\gamma}$ is the rate of shear (s^{-1}). Newtonian fluids obey Equation 14.1; that is, there is a direct, time-independent, constant proportionality between σ and $\dot{\gamma}$, so that η is the same irrespective of σ or $\dot{\gamma}$. Macromolecular solutions, however, seldom exhibit true Newtonian behavior unless solution concentrations are very low. While non-Newtonian fluid rheology encompasses shear-thinning, shear-thickening, or plastic behavior, sometimes accompanied by time dependency (i.e., thixotropy or rheopexy) [5], most polymeric or macromolecular solutions exhibit shear-thinning behavior when sheared.

Huang and Sorensen [6] evaluated the shear rate dependence of viscosity of 3% w/w aqueous solutions of gelatin during the course of gelation. They found that although the apparent viscosity of the solutions was shear rate dependent (i.e., shear thinning), it was independent of the shear rate history of the solution.

The application of stress to polymeric materials often results in a change in the molecular weight distribution of the polymer [7]. Staudinger, in 1930, was apparently the first to observe shear-induced scission of polymers in solution [8]. Since then, numerous studies have confirmed the potentially deleterious effect of shear stress on the degradation of polymers in solution and the corresponding reduction in polydispersity as shear stress is increased [9]. It should be noted that reductions in polymer solution viscosity are not necessarily always attributed to depolymerization or degradation. Reduced viscosity could also result from deaggregation of macromolecular aggregates [9]. Conversely, there are reports in the literature of negligible effects of mechanical shear on polymer molecular weight. For example, Powell et al. [10] observed minimal degradation of hydroxyethyl cellulose under all but the most rigorous conditions (e.g., shear rates of ~1.9×10^6 s^{-1}). Given the unpredictable outcome when shear or stress is imposed on polymeric solutions—in the absence of prior experimental data—it would be advisable to estimate the shear stresses and rates of shear incurred in manufacturing or processing operations and then evaluate polymeric stability under those conditions, at relevant temperatures and concentrations, before any manufacturing proceeds. The spectrum of shear rates involved in capsule manufacturing operations ranges from those incurred in dip coating operations (10^{-1} to 10^2 s^{-1}) [11], precision pumping through dosator nozzles (10^0 to 10^3 s^{-1}) [12], to those encountered in soft gel capsule production that are orders of magnitude higher (10^4 to 10^5 s^{-1}).

Viscometers—instruments used to measure the viscosity of Newtonian fluids—are generally inappropriate for measuring the viscosity of non-Newtonian solutions as σ or $\dot{\gamma}$ cannot be varied accurately or precisely (e.g., sample geometry violates rheological principles). Furthermore, $\dot{\gamma}$ may vary substantially within the sample environment. The inability to control sample temperatures within a specific narrow range may also be problematic for some viscometers, given the temperature dependence of fluid or solution viscosity that often takes the form [13]

$$\left.\begin{aligned} \eta &= A \cdot e^{B/T} \\ &\text{or} \\ \ln \eta &= (B/T) + \ln A \end{aligned}\right\}, \tag{14.2}$$

where A and B are constants and T is absolute temperature (K).

Given the higher macromolecular concentrations that are used in gellant solutions (for dip coating, film forming, and injection molding processes) and the non-Newtonian behavior of the gellant solutions, the continued use of *single point* rheological methods intended for Newtonian fluids is potentially misleading and consequently unacceptable, especially for quality control/quality assurance (QA/QC) and quality-by-design (QbD) purposes, unless provisions can be made for varying the shear rate $\dot{\gamma}$ or shear stress σ. If that is done, an acceptable assessment of the gellant solution's rheological behavior can be made. Viscometers that are suitable for shear viscosity measurements of non-Newtonian fluids typically accommodate *multiple* shear rates so that data for shear stress σ as a function of shear rate $\dot{\gamma}$ can be obtained, thereby defining the rheological behavior of a test fluid. These instruments include pressure-driven capillary and microfluidic slit viscometers, drag flow (i.e., rotational) viscometers, and falling or rolling ball viscometers [5]. Instruments capable of precise measurements of deformation and flow in a geometrically defined space are often described as *rheometers*. In general, viscometers and rheometers and the corresponding methods employed with them are suitable for non-Newtonian fluids and are appropriate as a part of a QA/QC program for gellant characterization. These instruments and methodologies are described in detail elsewhere [5,11,14,15].

SOLUTION EXTENSIONAL VISCOSITY

While fluid flow and viscosity are often described in terms of steady shear of fluid laminae past one another, hard capsule manufacturing by a dip coating process necessitates consideration as well of the *elongational* or *extensional viscosity* of the film-forming solution occurring under non-shearing or "shear-free" conditions [16,17]. The thickness of the film coating the pins is a function of both the shear and extensional viscosities of the coating liquid, the rate of the pin's immersion in and withdrawal from the gellant solution, the surface tension of the gellant solution, and the angle at which the pin is immersed and withdrawn from the gellant solution [16,17]. As the coated pin is withdrawn from the gellant solution, a filament forms between the hemispherical end of the pin and the solution bath. The efficiency of the capsule manufacturing process is reflected in the time required for the filament to break [16]. Simulations of the stretching and breaking of the filament show the potentially substantial influence of the elongational viscosity of the gellant solution on the filament breakage time [17].

As shear flow of macromolecular solutions proceeds, the macromolecules orient in the direction of flow but undergo some rotation, owing to the differential velocity across the flow field, thereby reducing the stretching of the macromolecules. The velocity gradient in shear flow is at right angles to the direction of flow. However, extensional flow in macromolecular solutions—sometimes referred to as "shear-free" flow—involves less rotation than shear flow because of the absence of competing forces and correspondingly more stretching and elongation of the macromolecules. In addition, the velocity gradient is in the direction of flow [15]. In extensional flow, the extensional stress (i.e., tension) is σ_e and the rate of extension, or elongation (i.e., extensional strain rate) is $\dot{\gamma}_e$. For Newtonian fluids, *extensional viscosity,* η_e, in uniaxial flow, can be characterized in an analogous manner to *shear viscosity,* that is

$$\eta_e = \frac{\sigma_e}{\dot{\varepsilon}}. \tag{14.3}$$

For simple Newtonian or quasi-Newtonian fluids (at very low shear rates), $\eta_e = 3\eta$. This relationship between extensional and shear viscosities was first established in 1906 by Trouton [18]. However, for complex non-Newtonian fluids, extensional viscosities cannot be predicted readily on the basis of their shear flow behavior [19]. In such instances, experimentally determined extensional viscosities are best described as apparent extensional viscosities, that is, $\eta_{e,app}$. Just as the rheological behavior of macromolecular solutions can be described in terms of a power law relationship [5], the extensional rheological behavior of such solutions can be described in an analogous fashion. Thus, for extension-thinning fluids,

$$\eta_{e,app} = k|\dot{\varepsilon}|^{n-1}, \tag{14.4}$$

where k is a proportionality constant and n is the power law index.

Research on extensional viscous behavior of macromolecular solutions was not the subject of substantial research efforts until the 1980s mainly because of the difficulty in making the measurements [20–23]. Only recently has commercial instrumentation for extensional viscosity measurements—that is, CaBER, an acronym for **Ca**pillary **B**reakup **E**xtensional **R**heometer—become available[i] to supplant improvised in-house equipment.

CaBER instruments function by enabling the rapid separation (typically within 20–50 ms) of two discs between which a small volume of solution (generally <1 mL) has been placed. The instantaneous (user-selected) extensional strain rate imposed on the nearly cylindrical fluid sample by the rapid movement of the upper disc away from the lower stationary disc results in the formation of a uniform but unstable cylindrical filament of liquid that stretches between the discs. With the cessation of stretching, the fluid at the midpoint of the filament is subjected to an extensional strain rate and a corresponding drainage of fluid from the filament. The filament's midpoint diameter is monitored—as it thins—by a laser micrometer as a function of time. The apparent simplicity of the filament formation and monitoring processes tends to minimize or obscure consideration of the potential effects of pre-shear history on the extensional behavior of some fluids, although research to date implicates wormlike micelle solutions and immiscible polymer blends rather than polymer solutions [24]. A prudent approach to CaBER experimentation and use warrants attention to the pre-shear history of the fluid sample and an evaluation of the effect of changes in the rate and extent of the rapid elongation[ii] imposed on the nearly cylindrical fluid sample at the outset of the procedure.

---

[i] Thermo Haake, Karlsruhe, Germany.
[ii] These are the so-called "step-stretch" parameters.

For viscous Newtonian fluids undergoing capillary thinning, the breakup process proceeds linearly with time [25,26]. Thus, the mid-filament diameter (D_{mid}) decreases with time, t, in accordance with

$$D_{mid}(t) = \alpha \left(\frac{2\gamma}{\eta_s} \right) (t_b - t),$$ (14.5)

where α is a numerical coefficient, γ is the surface tension of the solution, η_s is solvent viscosity, and t_b is the time to breakup [26].

However, for non-Newtonian fluids, the breakup process is nonlinear. For viscoelastic fluids, the mid-filament diameter decreases exponentially [26]:

$$D_{mid}(t) \left(\frac{\eta_0 D_1^4}{2\bar{\lambda}\gamma} \right)^{1/3} \exp\left(-\frac{t}{3\bar{\lambda}} \right),$$ (14.6)

where $\eta_p = (\eta_0 - \eta_s)$ is the solution viscosity owing to the polymeric component, η_0 is the zero-shear rate viscosity of the solution, $\bar{\lambda}$ is the relaxation time of the viscoelastic filament, and D_1 is the mid-filament diameter after stretching has ceased.

Arnolds et al. [27] demonstrated the utility of a CaBER instrument for determining the extensional rheology of semi-dilute to concentrated aqueous solutions of polyethylene oxide. The authors noted that, in all instances, cylindrical filaments were formed that thinned down to a diameter of 5–10 μm before breaking. Filament breakage was immediately preceded by the formation of a beads-on-a-string structure that was apparently the result of flow-induced phase separation, with solvent predominating in the beads and the interbead filaments comprising highly extended polymer chains. This beads-on-a-string polymer solution behavior was consistent with the "blistering" phenomenon reported earlier by Sattler et al. [28] and further explicated by Sattler et al. in 2012 [29].

The extensional rheology of solutions of macromolecules that may be used as capsule shell excipients is, increasingly, the subject of ongoing research. Representative presentations and published reports that have focused on the extensional rheological behavior of biopolymer solutions include those on gelatin [30], ultrahigh-viscosity alginates [31], hydroxyethyl cellulose [32], methylhydroxyethyl celluloses [33], casein [34], and starches [34,35]. These citations provide further support for the use of extensional viscosity measurements of solutions of capsule shell excipients.[i]

Sol–Gel Transitions

Gel Formation

While many linear polymers undergo thermoreversible aggregation in dilute solution, most physical (non-covalent) gelation occurs in moderately concentrated polymer solutions as a result of the formation of supermolecular aggregates that extend continuously, as a network, throughout the system [36]. This description complements and extends the much earlier characterization—by P. H. Hermans [37]—of a gel as a "coherent system of at least two components, which exhibits mechanical

---

[i] An alternative device for measuring the apparent extensional viscosity of a fluid has recently become commercially available from RheoSense. It comprises a precision syringe pump that pushes fluid through a rectangular channel into a hyperbolic expansion/contraction zone. Fluid in the straight rectangular channel experiences shear flow, but as it enters the hyperbolic zone, it undergoes a uniform extension and a further pressure drop that is measured by embedded pressure sensors in the channel surface. The apparent extensional viscosity is calculated from the pressure drop, the flow rate, and the geometry of the contraction zone.

properties characteristic of a solid, where both the dispersed component and the dispersion medium extend themselves continuously throughout the whole system". Almdal *et al.* [38] reviewed the often ambiguous definitions and uses of the term *gel* in the literature and provided a further clarification based on the dynamic mechanical properties of these solid-like systems: Gels also exhibit a storage modulus G2, which exhibits a plateau extending to times at least of the order of seconds, and a loss modulus G3, which is considerably smaller than the storage modulus in the plateau region.

Non-covalent or physical gel network formation can be envisaged as resulting from macromolecular interactions as varied as van der Waals, dipole–dipole, Coulombic, charge transfer, and hydrophobic and hydrogen-bonding [39]. Data from rheological test measurements suggest that physical cross-links in gels move or break when a gel is stressed. Activation energies associated with cross-link breakage—estimated from the temperature dependence of viscoelastic parameters—range from 6 to 65 kcal/mol for gelatin and various polysaccharides [40].

Given the potential multiplicity of non-covalent interactions responsible for gel formation—particularly in systems with a substantial excess of solvent (typically water)—and limited information on pregel precursors, it is not surprising that the process of physical gelation is less completely understood than that of covalent gelation [41]. Nonetheless, Hermans [42] found that the cross-linking between N_0 hydrocolloid molecules—each having f identical groups ($f \gg 1$) capable of interacting with one group on another molecule—could be adequately described in terms of an equilibrium between the interactive surface sites. Hermans theorized that a fraction α of the f groups—distributed randomly over the macromolecules—has interacted to form intermolecular links and that the probability that any one group has interacted is independent of the number of groups on the same molecule that have interacted. Assuming the interactions comprise an equilibrium, the concentration of interacted groups is equal to a constant multiplied by the square of the concentration of the groups that have not interacted, that is,

$$\alpha f N_0 = K' \left[(1-\alpha) f N_0 \right]^2, \tag{14.7}$$

where K' is independent of molecular weight, that is, of f. When $\alpha \ll 1$, this reduces to

$$\alpha = K' f N_0 = K c, \tag{14.8}$$

where c is the concentration and K, as before, is independent of molecular weight. Thus, $\alpha \sim c$ for large values of f, and the fraction of the macromolecules in the gel phase, N_g, is related to α by

$$N_g - \left\{ 1 - \exp\left(-\alpha N_g / \alpha_c \right) \right\}, \tag{14.9}$$

where $\alpha_c = 1/f$. Since $N_g \geq 0$ only when $\alpha \geq \alpha_c$, then α_c is the degree of interaction of the functional groups at the point when a gel forms. Combining Equations 14.8 and 14.9, the gel point occurs at a concentration c_c inversely proportional to the length of the chain:

$$c_c = 1/Kf. \tag{14.10}$$

Thus, gelation occurs when one group on each macromolecule has interacted with another group on another macromolecule. Hermans posits that in cases of practical interest, α is of the same order of magnitude as α_c and that $\alpha \ll 1$. As Clark and Ross-Murphy [41] note, this leads to

$$\frac{\alpha}{\alpha_c} = \frac{c}{c_0}, \tag{14.11}$$

where $c_0 = M/Kf^2$ is the *critical* (gel) concentration, that is, the concentration below which no *macro*scopic gel is formed under the prevailing conditions for a macromolecular segment of molecular weight M.

The literature is sometimes unclear in differentiating the critical concentration c_0 from the *overlap* concentration c^*, the latter term defined as the macromolecular concentration at which molecular overlap and cross-link formation occur for a time-averaged volume of rotation. The generally accepted hypothesis for physical cross-link formation is that $c_0 < c^*$; that is, cross-link formation does not require the persistence of the macromolecules in each others' macromolecular space, except when the cross-link is formed [43]. Ferry [44] estimated that—given the average volume of solution pervaded by a polymer molecule with a molecular weight of $1-2 \times 10^5 \, Da$—molecular overlap occurs at concentrations as low as 2–5% and that higher concentrations involve considerable molecular overlap and entanglement. Ferry hypothesized that the resultant structure behaves as a network (i.e., gel) and that its response to stress will depend on the extent to which entanglement and disentanglement can occur for a given duration and magnitude of stress.

Gelation, the critical transition from the sol (molecularly dispersed) state to the gel (intermolecularly connected) state, is best appreciated in terms of the transition variable—connectivity—among the system components. In physical terms, connectivity refers to the physical bonds that link the fundamental units of a system. The transition from the sol to the gel state is evidenced by the development—at the gel point—of connectivity throughout the system. During gelation, the system changes from one in which connectivity exists only on a very short-range scale to one in which connectivity is ultimately evident at every scale throughout the sample [45]. The infinite cluster formed, that is, a network that extends throughout the system from one end of the sample to the other, can be described as an infinitely large macromolecule [46].

Various theories have been advanced over the years to characterize gel formation and gellant connectivity at the gel point. Classical models developed by Flory [47] and Stockmayer [48] characterized gelation as a random process of multimolecular interaction that was also consistent in a number of ways with a model for percolation in a three-dimensional lattice. Herrmann et al. [49] proposed an alternative, kinetic model of gelation that more effectively dealt with the complexity of the sol–gel transition.

Nonetheless, theories and models aside, practical concerns remain: (a) the determination of the gel point for a given gellant concentration and temperature, (b) the determination of the mechanical or physical nature (e.g., rigidity, brittleness) of the resultant gel, and (c) the concentration dependence of gel strength and gel time. As Ross-Murphy [43] has noted, most research in the past has been more concerned with the temperature dependence rather than the concentration dependence of gel parameters. This bias needs to be corrected, particularly as new excipients are developed for hard and soft shell capsule manufacture. Gelation characterization and gel point determinations are essential to the setting of appropriate formulation and manufacturing parameters, whether for hard or soft shell capsules; assessment of gel rigidity and brittleness is critical to ensuring capsule integrity during the encapsulation process and post-manufacture.

Gel Point Determination

Gel points are frequently estimated by measurements of the fluidity of a solution by a test-tube inverting method or by a ball-drop method [50] but are relatively inaccurate, particularly as gellant solutions become more viscous (e.g., in the vicinity of the gel point). As noted above, the determination of solution viscosity as a function of temperature and gellant concentration has often been relied upon to determine the gel point for a system. The relatively abrupt divergence of solution viscosity behavior as temperature or gellant concentration change is indicative of the gel point having been reached. Nonetheless, the viscous behavior of these fluids as gel formation proceeds is almost invariably accompanied by elasticity, that is, viscoelasticity. The time dependence and temperature dependence of the *viscoelastic* properties of physical gels at and near the gel point have been studied extensively and shown to follow a power law function [51,52]. Therefore, gel point determinations based on viscous flow behavior alone can be misleading. Accordingly, the viscoelastic nature of gels warrants the use of rheological methods suitable for characterizing such materials and the processes of gelation and melting [53]. These are described in "Gel and Film Characterization" section.

GEL AND FILM CHARACTERIZATION

In an early overview of the rheological properties of industrial materials, Scott Blair [54] set out 8 objective rheological criteria and 24 rheological methods that could be used to establish the quality of materials. For "Jellies"—the most relevant of the 31 categories of substances tabulated by Scott Blair—seven rheological parameters were suggested: viscosity, elastic modulus, hysteresis, shear-thinning, yield value, thixotropy, and tensile strength. In the more than 70 years that have elapsed since Scott Blair's critical review, rheological instrumentation has evolved dramatically—driven by marked improvements in engineering and computer hardware and software [55]—so that empirical tests [56] have increasingly given way to imitative tests that simulate the conditions to which material is subjected in use and to fundamental tests that measure well-defined physical properties.

Once a solution of a capsule shell excipient has gelled, rheological methods suitable for the rheological characterization of fluids are no longer practical or appropriate. The relationship between gel rigidity or elasticity and gellant concentration was recognized as far back as 1886 for gelatin gels [57,58]. But not until Ferry's work in the 1940s [59] was the correlation more firmly established—at least for gelatin gels—as a consequence of Ferry's use of gelatin samples of known average molecular weight and molecular size distribution.[i]

Deformation and penetrometer tests are among the oldest methods used to evaluate the potential gel strength afforded by capsule shell excipients. The Bloom gelometer test is one of the most widely employed empirical deformation procedures for evaluating the suitability of gellants (particularly gelatin) for capsule manufacture. It is rapid, is simple to perform, is suitable for routine quality control, and may correlate well with sensory test methods. Unfortunately, the Bloom test did not evolve from a fundamental understanding of gelation or gel rigidity, nor is its measurement convertible to fundamental physical parameters. Furthermore, as a one-point measurement, its replacement by quantitative fundamental and imitative rheological methods and instrumentation is warranted and long overdue.

Insofar as penetrometers are concerned, as Mitchell notes [40]: "rupture strength of a gel is not necessarily related to its elastic modulus and therefore single point measurements of 'gel strength' based on rupture [penetrometer] tests will not always rank a series of gels in the same order as tests which involve small deformations without rupture."

Dynamic oscillatory methods employ rotational rheometers to apply either a small or a large sinusoidally oscillating stress or strain at an angular frequency to a fluid or semisolid sample contained within concentric cylinder, parallel plate, or cone and plate geometries [5]. These cyclical variations of stress and strain comprise the most commonly employed methods for the characterization of viscoelastic materials, that is, materials that exhibit both viscous and elastic behavior. The time scale is defined by the frequency of oscillation, ω, or the cycle time (rad s^{-1}). By altering the time scales, one can establish the nature of the mechanisms underlying the material responses to the imposed strain.

The application of sinusoidal strain to a gel system can be represented by

$$\gamma = \gamma_0 \sin \omega t$$

and the *linear* response to low amplitudes of imposed strain, $\sim\gamma_0$, corresponds to

$$\sigma = \sigma_0 \sin (\omega t + \delta),$$

where δ is the phase shift or phase angle.

---

[i] Seventy years on, polymeric excipient specification by formulation scientists has still not routinely involved the characterization of the molecular weight distribution and compositional variation of such materials.

The stress response can also be represented as follows:

$$\sigma = \sigma_0 \cos\delta \sin\omega t + \sigma_0 \sin\delta \cos\omega t.$$

Quantifiable parameters of interest in this linear viscoelastic region[i] include, among others, the storage modulus, G', and the loss modulus, G'', the loss tangent or loss factor, tan δ, which corresponds to the tangent of the phase shift or phase angle[ii] δ or (G'/G''). The moduli can be defined as follows:

$$G' = \frac{\sigma_0 \cos\delta}{\gamma_0} = \frac{\text{in-phase stress amplitude}}{\text{strain amplitude}}$$

$$G'' = \frac{\sigma_0 \sin\delta}{\gamma_0} = \frac{\text{out-of-phase stress amplitude}}{\text{strain amplitude}}$$

An additional term, the complex viscosity, η^*, corresponds to (G^*/ω), wherein G^*—the complex shear modulus—is equal to

$$\sqrt{(G')^2 + (G'')^2}.$$

These various moduli—defined as ratios of stress and strain amplitudes—are the quantitative rheological parameters of gels most often evaluated [52]: the storage (elastic) modulus G', based on the amplitude of in-phase stress, is indicative of the amount of recoverable energy stored elastically; the loss (viscous) modulus G'', based on the amplitude of out-of-phase stress, corresponds to the amount of energy dissipated as heat during shear; and the complex modulus G^* defines the stiffness or rigidity of a sample.

Useful methods of representing the mechanical spectra of gellant solutions and characterizing the sol–gel transition include plotting tan δ, or both G' and G'', as a function of ω. The approximate[iii] gel point corresponds to tan $\delta = 1$, or when $G' = G''$ (the crossover point[iv]), that is, when the rheological behavior becomes predominantly solid-like, or elastic, rather than liquid-like [15]. Heuristically, the value of G' correlates with the cross-link density of the gel network.

Dynamic oscillatory measurements involving *small* amplitude oscillatory shear (SAOS) can provide substantial information on semisolids via so-called "sweep" methods conducted in the linear viscoelastic region [60]: (a) frequency sweeps, wherein G' and G'' are determined as a function of frequency ω at fixed temperatures; (b) temperature sweeps, in which G' and G'' are determined as a function of temperature at fixed ω; and (c) time sweeps, in which G' and G'' are determined as a function of time at fixed ω and temperature. Frequency sweep studies characterize the gel phase of a system wherein G' is higher than G'' throughout a frequency range, that is, when molecular rearrangements within the network over time are minimal. Temperature sweep data can establish the temperature dependence of gelation while time sweep data can establish the temporal change in gel strength and the length of time required for recovery of sample mechanical strength. For a given concentration of

---

[i] The linear viscoelastic region—determined experimentally—is defined as the region within which material properties do not depend on the rate of application of the strain, the magnitude of the strain, or the magnitude of the stress.

[ii] The phase angle—sometimes called the phase lag—ranges from 0°, for purely elastic (Hookean) materials, to 90°, for purely viscous (Newtonian) fluids.

[iii] The crossover point *per se* is not an exact indicator of the gel point since it has been observed to depend on the probing frequency. On the other hand, lines of tan $\delta(t)$ at several frequencies ($\omega_1, \omega_2, \omega_3 \ldots \omega_n$) decay gradually and intersect exactly at the gel point [61].

[iv] The crossover frequency, that is, the frequency at which G' and G'' intersect, is inversely proportional to the relaxation time, that is, the time required for a sample to relax (recover from) an imposed stress.

gellant, temperature and time sweep data provide important parameters for the capsule manufacturing process by establishing an appropriate temperature and time range for unit operations.

As noted above, the power law dependence of the moduli G'' and G' on frequency—in the linear viscoelastic region—characterizes the gel point at an intermediate state between a liquid and a solid:

$$G(t) = St^{-\Delta},$$

where S is the gel strength depending on the cross-linking density and the molecular chain flexibility; Δ is a network specific exponent ranging between 0 and 1. Precise gel point determinations were thus made for various biopolymers, including gelatin [51,52].

Other small strain rheological tests applied to viscoelastic solids include stress relaxation and creep methods. In stress relaxation tests, the gel is subjected to an instantaneous strain followed by measurement of stress as a function of time. The resultant curve provides an estimate of the relaxation time, that is, the time required for stress to decay to about 37% ($1/e$) of the initial value. Creep tests typically involve subjecting a gel to an instantaneous, constant stress followed by measurement of strain over time. Removal of the imposed load is accompanied by recovery of the elastic strain while viscous deformation remains. Many variants of stress relaxation and creep methods have been described in the literature to evaluate gel properties, especially in the food industry, and could be used to advantage in the characterization of gels encountered in capsule shell compositions [62,63].

Weak gel systems exposed to *large* amplitude oscillatory shear (LAOS) deformations are apt to behave as thixotropic systems as they undergo progressive structural breakdown of their networks into smaller clusters whereas strong gels undergo network rupture and flow discontinuity [64]. In 1993, Giacomin and Dealy [65] noted that although LAOS measurements are increasingly the focus of many rheological evaluations on nonlinear viscoelasticity, "no predominant test method has emerged amongst experimentalists." More recently, Ewoldt et al. [66,67] have introduced a comprehensive analytic framework for representing nonlinear responses to oscillatory shear deformation that can be considered a *"rheological fingerprint"* of complex fluids and soft solids. In this framework, the stress responses are resolved into their elastic and viscous components and plotted against the strain (γ) and strain rate $\left(\dot{\gamma}\right)$ input functions. The plots then are fitted to nth-order Chebyshev polynomials of the first kind, that is,

$$T_n(x) = 2xT_{n-1}(x) - T_{n-2}(x)$$

and the coefficients used to provide information about nonlinear rheological behavior.

An alternative to dynamic oscillatory measurements of gels, texture profile analysis (TPA) has gained substantial traction in the pharmaceutical industry in recent years although more than 50 years have passed since the patenting of a force-deformation measuring apparatus and its application to the rheological characterization of solids and semisolids [68]. As with SAOS and LAOS methods, instrumental limitations and the absence of software to facilitate data acquisition and analysis led to the relatively belated adoption of these objective tests of texture of foods and related materials. Over time, with the increasing sophistication of equipment and accessories and the provision of automatic data acquisition and software interpretation, these methodologies have become more widely used and relied upon by formulators and manufacturers. The widespread acceptance and use of instrumented TPA, in particular, must be tempered by proper selection of sampling and testing conditions in order to assure reasonable outcomes [69].

THE RHEOLOGICAL BEHAVIOR OF CAPSULE SHELL EXCIPIENTS

The rheological behavior of solutions and dispersions of capsule shell excipients varies with the concentration of the gellant, composition of the solution or dispersion, and process conditions to such an extent that no one rheological descriptor is adequate. At low gellant concentrations, solutions often behave as Newtonian fluids. At the higher solution concentrations often employed in the manufacture of hard and soft shell capsules, non-Newtonian behavior (especially viscoelasticity) is more frequently the rule rather than the exception. The diversity of rheological phenomena that these excipients give rise to and the influence of compositional and environmental factors on that rheological behavior underscore the need for the formulator to investigate solution or dispersion rheology for each individual formulation and excipient batch or lot to the fullest extent possible. Failure to do so could lead to process disruption, product loss, or product recalls with concomitant economic and regulatory consequences, at the least. Product failures could have dire medical outcomes as well.

In order to achieve a particular gel strength, capsule manufacturers often blend different batches or lots of gellants in order to achieve a particular gel strength based on one-point indicia such as the Bloom strength or number. The result of such co-mingling of batches is a macromolecular composition that is even more heterogeneous than before, batch-to-batch replicability that may be an even more elusive goal, and simplistic rheological tests that are misleading.

CAPSULE SHELL EXCIPIENT VARIABILITY AND ITS RHEOLOGICAL ASSESSMENT

More than 25 years ago, at a symposium on pharmaceutical excipient standards, G. E. Reier [70] spoke of excipient specifications that are developed to control the intrinsic properties of excipients. These intrinsic properties need to be controlled for excipients to be used. "Without specifications to control excipient properties," Reier said, "our products and our manufacturing operations would be uncontrolled." Unfortunately, as Shangraw noted in 1987 [71]: "While standards for drugs have, in the past, usually taken precedence over standards for excipients, history has provided numerous unfortunate lessons which have demonstrated the fallacy of this approach."

The advent of FDA's pharmaceutical cGMPs for the twenty-first century [72] and ICH Guidelines for QbD [73] has spurred efforts by pharmaceutical scientists to assess excipient variability. In 2005, the PQRI Excipient Working Group developed three surveys to gather responses from excipient manufacturers, excipient distributors, and drug product manufacturers about excipient quality control strategies: 70% or more of the respondents perform additional functionality or processability testing that is not part of any compendial monograph. Twenty-four percent of drug product manufacturers have products for which excipient variability is a problem despite extra-compendial testing [74].

Hard and soft capsule shell excipients are macromolecular materials that can exhibit considerable batch-to-batch, lot-to-lot, and manufacturer-to-manufacturer variations in their physical properties and functionality. This variability is exemplified by gelatin, the most common capsule shell excipient. Suppliers of commercial gelatins frequently offer low, medium, and high [gelling] grades characterized in terms of their respective Bloom strengths, numbers that correspond to the force required to depress the surface of a 6.67% w/w gelatin gel by 4 mm with a 12.7-mm-diameter flat-bottomed plunger. The corresponding Bloom strengths or numbers cited by various gelatin processors vary considerably from supplier to supplier: "low gelling strength" grades have been characterized by Bloom numbers of 50–125, 80–150, <120, and <150, respectively; "medium gelling strength" grades, 120–200, 150–220, and 175–225; and "high gelling strength" grades, >200, 220–280, and 225–325. Yet Bloom strength is widely accepted globally as a measure of quality even though gelatins are rarely used under conditions that even approximate those of the [Bloom] test procedure.[i]

---

[i] In hard capsule manufacture, for example, the gelatin gel coating the stainless steel pins is formed in a matter of seconds from an approximately 30% w/w solution on cooling from about 50°C to 25°C. In the manufacture of soft (gelatin) capsules, a concentrated gelatin solution is again rapidly gelled on a chilled drum, but in this case, the situation is complicated by the inclusion of a plasticizer, normally glycerol [75].

Efforts to characterize macromolecular excipient variability have employed a variety of analytical and instrumental technologies including spectroscopy (e.g., IR, NIR, Raman, or NMR), chromatography (e.g., SEC or GPC), and rheological procedures. Spectral or chromatographic procedures may well demonstrate inter-lot, inter-grade, or inter-manufacturer differences in excipients but such differences may not correlate with actual excipient performance in capsule shell manufacture. Additional testing is necessary in order to establish whether these *indirect* data correspond to *in-use* differences. On the other hand, rheological methods have the potential to *directly* reflect the functionality or performance of capsule shell excipients in the capsule shell-forming process [76,77].

As noted above, the subsequent transition of the gellant solution from the sol to the gel state—as a function of gellant concentration and solution temperature—is directly evident from rheological measurements such as small amplitude oscillatory measurements of a gellant solution's viscoelastic parameters [78].

Ultimately, the capsule manufacturer is concerned with the assessment and replicability of the hard or soft capsule shells formed. As mechanical properties (e.g., rigidity, elasticity, viscoelasticity, and tensile strength measurements) provide direct evidence of the suitability of the formed capsules, there is no need to resort to *indirect* test methods or procedures to validate the adequacy of capsule shell excipients or compositions.

In one report on the manufacture of alginate capsules, processing issues arose for ultrahigh-viscosity alginate solutions with the *same average molar mass* but *different molar mass distributions*. Unacceptable filament formation and uncontrolled back bouncing of drops during the dip-coating capsule molding process were problematic. Extensional flow measurements of these solutions of alginates—in contrast to steady-state shear flow or small-amplitude oscillatory measurements—were able to differentiate among the various alginate samples [31] and minimize the likelihood of thread formation during capsule shell manufacture.

RHEOLOGICAL ASPECTS OF HARD AND SOFT SHELL CAPSULE FILLING

SOLIDS

In the distant past, industrial-scale hard capsule filling operations for solids—in the form of powders, granules, or beads—began with the separation and loading of the capsule shells into holders or plates such that the capsule bases' openings were flush with the plate surface. The solid was then spread over the surface, allowed to flow into the capsule bases, and the excess then scraped away. This process was primarily dependent on gravity feed of the solids into the bases of the capsule shells. Over time, these empirical approaches to capsule filling gave way to more sophisticated analyses of the interrelationship between material properties and machine operating characteristics. Thus, Reier et al. [79], using stepwise regression analysis, characterized the relationship of machine speed, capsule size, powder specific volume, and *flowability*, in part, to mean capsule fill weight and weight variation. These gravity-feed methods have been supplanted, for the most part, by capsule filling processes based on the formation of a plug of powder via a progressive tamping process in a dosating disk or by the use of a dosating nozzle or tube. In either case, the compressive forces involved are relatively low (tens of newtons) compared to those involved in tabletting (tens of kilonewtons) [80].

Given the low compressive forces in capsule filling operations, particulate cohesion may be less problematic for capsule formulations than for tablet formulations but glidants and/or lubricants may still be necessary adjuncts to capsule formulation compositions in order to ensure uniform particulate flowability and fill. Given production rates of ca. 200,000 capsules per day with semiautomatic capsule filling equipment and 150,000 units per hour (or more) with automated equipment [81], particulate fluidity is no trifling matter. Heda et al. [82], comparing dosator and dosing disc capsule filling machines, concluded that an optimal degree of powder fluidity is required for successful encapsulation on either machine.

With increasing attention directed to powder rheology and rheometry [83–85], one can expect more effective characterization in the future of particulate flow *vis-à-vis* capsule filling operations. Problematic aspects of powder rheometry and rheology include the incomplete delineation of the geometry of the shear zone and the shear stresses therein [85]. Given the more complete understanding of bulk solids mechanics at present, Søgaard et al. [85] prefer shear testers, for example, shear cell methods [86], to powder rheometers to assess powder flowability characteristics. When drug quantities are limited (e.g., 250 mg), as in the early stages of drug product development, Guerin et al. [87] advocate the use of mercury porosimetry to obtain insight into the rheological properties of pharmaceutical solids.

Khawam [88], reviewing the theory of powder encapsulation in dosator-based capsule filling machines, acknowledges the importance of powder fluidity in achieving densification and successful production but does not link it to material properties of the powder—exemplified by the "Carr index, flow function, or Heckel compressibility parameters"—in the theoretical model proposed to predict encapsulation outcomes. Nonetheless, in a subsequent paper, the model successfully predicted encapsulation outcomes for two powder formulations with substantially different flow properties [89].

Further efforts to minimize empirical approaches to capsule filling processes need to proceed along the lines of Fung and Ng [90] who have presented a systematic procedure for developing a manufacturing process for tablet and capsule dosage forms based on chemical engineering principles and heuristic principles that can facilitate excipient selection and equipment choices. The prediction of particulate flow properties could be facilitated and, most likely improved, by extending Fung and Ng's work to include multiple descriptors of the size and shape distributions of the solids, as Yu et al. [91] demonstrated, rather than mean particle size.

Semisolids and Liquids

For solids, the paramount rheological concern regarding capsule filling is fluidity or ease of flow of the material. However, rheological concerns for capsule filling with liquids or semisolids, especially thermosetting semisolids or liquids, are often complicated by other parameters such as holding temperatures prior to filling and the stress and shear conditions encountered during the capsule filling process.[i] Potential problems with drug–excipient combinations may be uncovered by subjecting proposed formulations to cycling of both temperature and shear [92]. Mixing of these dispersions under vacuum minimizes the likelihood of air entrapment during the filling process and the need to incorporate a separate deaeration step [92,93]. Leakage from hard shell capsules can be minimized or avoided altogether by using thixotropic shear-thinning formulations at room temperature, where liquefaction is shear or stress induced or at moderately elevated temperatures during the filling process [12]. Alternatively, molten formulations that solidify rapidly after capsule filling minimize the likelihood of nonuniform distribution of drug in the capsule. An additional concern for filling capsules with liquid and thermosoftened formulations is ensuring a clean break (i.e., the avoidance of residue on the dosing nozzle or stringing) from fill to fill [94]. Screening formulations for stringiness or pituity could be readily accomplished via extensional viscosity measurements using instruments such as the CABER [95] [described above].

Walker et al. [96] described a liquid filling technique for the manufacture of hard gelatin capsules filled with water-soluble hot melt polymers such as polyethylene glycols or water-dispersible thixotropic systems comprising oils with thixotropic additives. The authors used a Zanasi LZ64 capsule filling machine adapted to fill liquids using a liquid filling pump. A review of liquid filling in hard gelatin capsules provides an extensive list of the excipients used therein, all of which are

---

[i] For example, Kattige and Rowley [93] estimated the shear rate, as material is drawn into the hopper of a Hibar capsule filler, at about 12 s^{-1}, and, during extrusion via the pump into the capsule, at about 340 s^{-1}.

either viscous liquids or low-melting point semisolids [97]. Polymeric excipients of the poloxamer type have also been evaluated for use in hard capsule dosage forms [92]. Obviously, rheological properties of these excipients and their formulations must be evaluated before any decisions are made regarding equipment and processing parameters.

McTaggart et al. [98] described a heated stainless steel reservoir and pneumatically operated liquid metering pump for use with a Zanasi LZ64 automatic, intermittent motion powder filling machine that enabled the manufacture of 4400 liquid-filled capsules per hour. The liquid metering pump was capable of delivering volumes of 0.05 to 1.5 mL at a rate of up to 150 doses per minute. Dosing volume was "infinitely variable" and temperature could be controlled over the range from ambient to 100°C; the reservoir and dosing nozzle were maintained above ambient temperature by heating tape and a heating block, respectively; thermostatic control was provided by thermistors. A variety of Newtonian and non-Newtonian filling materials was evaluated with nominal viscosities ranging from 108 to 270,000 mPa·s. Excellent fill weight uniformity was achieved irrespective of material viscosity and temperature [98].

High-viscosity pastes have been filled into hard gelatin capsules using a modified fully automated dosator production machine to form cylindrical plugs that are inserted into the capsule shells [99]. Bohne et al. [100] reported on a high-pressure process for filling capsules with highly viscous materials. Hawley et al. [101] determined that hard gelatin capsule filling could be accomplished satisfactorily for various thermosoftened excipients whose viscosities ranged from 0.1 to 24,000 mPa.s at 70°C. Cole et al. [94] suggest an appropriate viscosity range, at the temperature of filling, of 10 to 1000 mPa.s. Walters et al. [12] formulated thixotropic gels with various excipients that could be filled into hard gelatin capsules at or above room temperature. They eventually focused on combinations of several semisynthetic oils Miglyol 829[i] and Imwitor 780K[ii]—with colloidal silicon dioxide that they subsequently evaluated rheologically using a constant stress rheometer in conjunction with dynamic shear, creep, and SAOS techniques. They were able to characterize the rate of reformation of structure following thixotropic breakdown at 20°C in high shear under conditions comparable to those encountered in capsule filling.

Kattige and Rowley [93] described the liquid filling of thermosoftened systems of drug and poloxamers comprising either a molten liquid or a particulate dispersion. Not unexpectedly, they encountered difficulties with dispersions beyond a limiting concentration of the dispersed phase, depending on the particle size distribution of the solid and the poloxamer molecular weight. The limiting concentration is indicative of dense packing of the solid particles and insufficient fluid to facilitate the relative motion of the particles [102].

RHEOLOGICAL BEHAVIOR OF CAPSULE SHELLS AND OF FILLED CAPSULES

Capsule Shells

Texture analyses of empty capsule shells subjected to compressive force have been reported in the literature. Liebowitz et al. [103] and Scott et al. [104] applied force to capsule shells using a 1.5-inch-diameter circular platen and a 2-mm-diameter cylindrical probe, respectively, to determine capsule shell strength. Measurements of crushing force at capsule failure—a one-point measurement—was augmented in the latter's report by their estimation as well of the work of failure, where work of failure is the integration of applied force over the distance traveled by the probe. However, no significant advantage of work estimates over force estimates was evident [104].

---

[i] Caprylic, capric, and succinic triglycerides.
[ii] Isostearyl diglyceryl succinate.

Mei et al. [105] employed a texture analyzer to exert tensile force on capsule shells and evaluate the effect of hydrophilic solvent systems used in various formulations on the integrity of the capsule shells. The texture analyzer was equipped with a load cell to which two short (e.g., 3 mm diameter) rods or pins were attached, one above the other. An empty capsule shell section (body or cap) was mounted over the upper and lower pins and tensile force and then applied in the upward direction at a constant rate (e.g., 0.5 mm/s) until the capsule shell ruptured. Continuous recording of force as a function of time and distance provided estimates of the mechanical properties of the capsule shell, that is, elasticity (slope of the force–distance curve), tensile force at break, and elongation at break.

FILLED CAPSULES

Peleg and Rha [106] proposed a rheological model for liquid-filled capsules[i] wherein theoretical equations for capsule-pressure deflection, relaxation, and creep allow parametric fitting to experimental data. The experimental apparatus comprised an anvil and a pressure plate, with the capsule in between. Texture profile analysis has been employed as a nondestructive test for hard gelatin capsules to assess formulation compatibility with capsule shells [107].

CONCLUDING REMARKS

Rheological principles play a substantial role in every aspect of the manufacture of capsules—from the formulation and manufacture of capsule shells *per se* to the filling of hard or soft shell capsules. The sensitivity and utility of rheological test methods, irrespective of the chemical or molecular composition of the capsules or their contents, underscore the value of rheology for modern encapsulation techniques and processes. Finally, the advent of more sophisticated rheological instruments and software has put these methodologies within the reach of most formulators and technicians. They are no longer solely the province of rheologists.

REFERENCES

1. Podczeck F, Jones BE, eds. *Pharmaceutical Capsules*. 2nd ed., London: Pharmaceutical Press, 2004.
2. US 4,673,438. Wittwer F, Tomka I. Polymer composition for injection molding. Jan. 16, 1987.
3. Vilivalam VD, Illum L, Iqbal K. Starch capsules: An alternative system for oral drug delivery. *Pharm. Sci. Technol. Today* 2000; 3: 64–69.
4. US 7,842,308. McAllister SM, Raby Jr RK, Brown A, Clarke AJ. Pharmaceutical formulation. Nov. 30, 2010.
5. Block LH. Rheology, Chapter 37 in Allen Jr LV, ed., *Remington: The Science and Practice of Pharmacy*. 22nd ed., London: Pharmaceutical Press, 2012: 749–766.
6. Huang H, Sorensen CM. Shear effects during the gelation of aqueous gelatin. *Phys. Rev. E* 1996; 53: 5075–5078.
7. Cooper AR. Recent advances in molecular weight determination. *Polymer Eng. Sci.* 1989; 29: 2–12.
8. Ballauff M, Wolf BA. Thermodynamically induced shear degradation. *Adv. Polymer Sci.* 1988; 85: 1–31.
9. D'Almeida AR, Dias ML. Comparative study of shear degradation of carboxymethylcellulose and poly(ethylene oxide) in aqueous solution. *Polymer Degradation Stability* 1997; 56: 331–337.
10. Powell DR, Swarbrick J, Banker GS. Effects of shear processing and thermal exposure on the viscosity-stability of polymer solutions. *J. Pharm. Sci.* 1966; 55: 601–605.
11. Macosko CW. *Rheology Principles, Measurements, and Applications*. New York: Wiley-VCH, 1994.
12. Walters PA, Rowley G, Pearson JT, Taylor CJ. Formulation and physical properties of thixotropic gels for hard gelatin capsules. *Drug Dev. Ind. Pharm.* 1992; 18: 1613–1631.
13. Doolittle AK. Studies in Newtonian flow. I. The dependence of the viscosity of liquids on temperature. *J. Appl. Phys.* 1951; 22: 1031–1035.
14. Mezger TG. *The Rheology Handbook*. Hanover: Vincentz Network, 2011.

---

[i] The authors utilized caviar (Ossetra and Beluga) and capsules made from chitosan.

15. Steffe JF. *Rheological Methods in Food Process Engineering*. East Lansing, MI: Freeman Press, 1996.
16. Yasuda K, Koshiba T, Mori N. Effects of rheological property of coating liquid and withdrawal velocity on dip coating process in manufacturing of capsules. *Nihon Reoroji Gakkaishi* 2004; 32: 85–90.
17. Yamamoto T, Nojima N, Mori N. Numerical analysis of flow behavior in meniscus region of viscoelastic dip coating flows. *J. Text. Eng.* 2005; 51: 21–28.
18. Trouton FT. On the coefficient of viscous traction and its relation to that of viscosity. *Proc. Royal Soc.* 1906; 77: 426–440.
19. Jezek J, Rides M, Derham B, Moore J, Cerasoli E, Simler R, Perez-Ramirez B. Viscosity of concentrated therapeutic protein compositions. *Adv. Drug Del. Rev.* 2011; 63: 1107–1117.
20. James DF. Extensional viscosity, an elusive property of mobile liquids. Third European Rheology Conference and Golden Jubilee Meeting of the British Society of Rheology. Springer, 1990: 241–243.
21. Matta JE, Tytus RP. Liquid stretching using a falling cylinder. *J. Non-Newtonian Fluid Mech.* 1990; 35: 215–229.
22. Sridhar T, Tirtaatmadja V, Nguyen DA, Gupta RK. Measurement of extensional viscosity of polymer solutions. *J. Non-Newtonian Fluid Mech.* 1991; 40: 271–280.
23. Tirtaatmadja V, Sridhar T. A filament stretching device for measurement of extensional viscosity. *J. Rheol.* 1993; 37: 1081–1102.
24. Miller E, Clasen C, Rothstein JP. The effect of step-stretch parameters on capillary breakup extensional rheology (CaBER) measurements. *Rheol. Acta* 2009; 48: 625–639.
25. Entov VM, Hinch EJ. Effect of a spectrum of relaxation times on the capillary thinning of a filament of elastic liquid. *J. Non-Newtonian Fluid Mech.* 1997; 72: 31–53.
26. Anna SL, McKinley GH. Elasto-capillary thinning and breakup of model elastic fluids. *J. Rheol.* 2001; 45: 115–138.
27. Arnolds O, Buggisch H, Sachsenheimer D, Willenbacher N. Capillary breakup extensional rheometry (CaBER) on semi-dilute and concentrated polyethyleneoxide (PEO) solutions. *Rheol. Acta* 2010; 49: 1207–1217.
28. Sattler R, Wagner C, Eggers J. Blistering pattern and formation of nanofibers in capillary thinning of polymer solutions. *Phys. Rev. Lett.* 2008; 100: 164502-1–164502-4.
29. Sattler R, Gier S, Eggers J, Wagner C. The final stages of capillary break-up of polymer solutions. *Physics Fluids* 2012; 24: 023101.
30. Lubansky AS, Curtis DJ, Williams PR, Deganello D. Transient extensional rheology of an aqueous gelatin solution: Before and during gelation. AIP Conference Proceedings, July 7, 2008, Vol. 1027, Issue 1, p. 609.
31. Storz H, Zimmermann U, Zimmermann H, Kulicke W-M. Viscoelastic properties of ultra-high viscosity alginates. *Rheol. Acta* 2010; 49: 155–162.
32. Meadows J, Williams PA, Kennedy JC. Comparison of the extensional and shear viscosity characteristics of aqueous hydroxyethylcellulose solutions. *Macromol.* 1995; 28: 2683–2692.
33. Plog JP, Kulicke W-M, Clasen C. Influence of the molar mass distribution on the elongational behaviour of polymer solutions in capillary breakup. *Appl. Rheol.* 2005; 15: 28–37.
34. Chan PS-K, Chen J, Ettalaie R, Alevisopoulos S, Day E, Smith S. Filament stretchability of biopolymer fluids and controlling factors. *Food Hydrocoll.* 2009; 23: 1602–1609.
35. Xie F, Halley PJ, Avérous L. Rheology to understand and optimize processability, structures and properties of starch polymeric materials. *Progr. Polymer Sci.* 2012; 37: 595–623.
36. Te Nijenhuis K. Viscoelastic properties of thermoreversible gels. In Burchard W, Ross-Murphy SB, eds. *Physical Networks: Polymers and Gels*. London: Elsevier Applied Science, 1990.
37. Hermans PH. Gels. In Kruyt HR, ed. *Colloid Science*, Vol. II, Amsterdam: Elsevier, 1949: 483–651.
38. Almdal K, Dyre J, Hvidt S, Kramer O. Towards a phenomenological definition of the term 'gel'. *Polymer Gels Networks* 1993; 1: 5–17.
39. Ross-Murphy SB. Physical gelation of synthetic and biological macromolecules. In DeRossi D, Kajiwara K, Osada Y, Yamauchi A, eds. *Polymer Gels: Fundamentals and Biomedical Applications*. New York: Plenum Press, 1991: 21–39.
40. Mitchell JR. The rheology of gels. *J. Text. Stud.* 1980; 11: 315–337.
41. Clark AH, Ross-Murphy SB. The concentration dependence of biopolymer gel modulus. *British Polymer J.* 1985; 17: 164–168.
42. Hermans Jr J. Investigation of the elastic properties of the particle network in gelled solutions of hydrocolloids. I. Carboxymethyl cellulose. *J. Polymer Sci.* 1965; 3: 1859–1868; Investigation of the elastic properties of the particle network in gelled solutions of hydrocolloids. II. Cellulose microcrystals. *J. Appl. Polymer Sci.* 1965; 9: 1973–1980.

43. Ross-Murphy SB. Incipient behaviour of gelatin gels. *Rheol. Acta* 1991; 30: 401–411.

44. Ferry JD. Viscoelastic properties of polymer solutions. *J. Res. Nat. Bureau Std.* 1948; 41: 53–62.

45. Carnali JO. Gelation in physically associating biopolymer systems. *Rheol. Acta* 1992; 31: 399–412.

46. Stauffer D, Coniglio A, Adam M. Gelation and critical phenomena. *Adv. Polymer Sci.* 1982; 44: 103–158.

47. Flory PJ. Molecular size distribution in three dimensional polymers. I. Gelation. *J. Amer. Chem. Soc.* 1941; 63: 3083–3090.

48. Stockmayer WH. Theory of molecular size distribution and gel formation in branched-chain polymers. *J. Chem. Phys.* 1943; 11: 45–55.

49. Herrmann HJ, Landau DP, Stauffer D. New universality class for kinetic gelation. *Phys. Rev. Lett.* 1982; 49: 412–415.

50. Jeong B, Kim SW, Bae YH. Thermosensitive sol–gel reversible hydrogels. *Adv. Drug Delivery Rev.* 2002; 54: 37–51.

51. Cuvelier G, Launay B. Frequency dependence of viscoelastic properties of some physical gels near the gel point. *Makromol. Chem., Macromol. Symp.* 1990; 40: 23–31.

52. Michon C, Cuvelier G, Launay B. Concentration dependence of the critical viscoelastic properties of gelatin at the gel point. *Rheol. Acta* 1993; 32: 94–103.

53. Rao MA. *Rheology of Fluid and Semisolid Foods: Principles and Applications.* 2nd ed., New York: Springer, 2007.

54. Scott Blair GW. The measurement of the rheological properties of some industrial materials. *J. Sci. Instr.* 1940; 17: 169–177.

55. Barnes HA, Schimanski H, Bell D. 30 years of progress in viscometers and rheometers. *Appl. Rheol.* 1999; 9: 69–76.

56. Scott Blair GW. Rheology in food research. *Adv. Food Res.* 1958; 8: 1–61.

57. Leick A. Über künstliche Doppelbrechung und Elastizität von Gelatineplatten. *Ann. Physik.* 1904; 319: 139–152.

58. Sheppard SE, Sweet SS. The elastic properties of gelatin jellies. *J. Amer. Chem. Soc.* 1921; 43: 539–547.

59. Ferry JD. Mechanical properties of substances of high molecular weight. IV. Rigidities of gelatin gels; dependence on concentration, temperature and molecular weight. *J. Amer. Chem. Soc.* 1948; 70: 2244–2249.

60. da Silva JA, Rao MA. Rheological behavior of food gels. In Rao MA. *Rheology of Fluid and Semisolid Foods: Principles and Applications.* 2nd ed., New York: Springer, 2007: 339–401.

61. Winter HH, Mours M. Rheology of polymers near liquid-solid transition. *Adv. Polymer Sci.* 1997; 134: 1–70.

62. Bourne MC. *Food Texture and Viscosity: Concept and Measurement.* 2nd ed., San Diego: Academic Press, 2002.

63. Norton IT, Spyropoulos F, Cox P, eds. *Practical Food Rheology: An Interpretive Approach.* Chichester: Wiley-Blackwell, 2011.

64. Grassi M, Lapasin R, Pricl S. A study of the rheological behavior of scleroglucan weak gel systems. *Carb. Polymers* 1996; 29: 169–181.

65. Giacomin AJ, Dealy JM. Large-amplitude oscillatory shear. In Collyer AA, ed. *Techniques in Rheological Measurement.* Houten: Springer Netherlands, 1993.

66. Ewoldt RH, Hosoi AE, McKinley GH. Rheological fingerprinting of complex fluids using large amplitude oscillatory shear (LAOS) flow. *Ann. Trans. Nordic Rheol. Soc.* 2007; 15: 3–8.

67. Ewoldt RH, Hosoi AE, McKinley GH. New measures for characterizing nonlinear viscoelasticity in large amplitude oscillatory shear. *J. Rheol.* 2008; 52: 1427–1458.

68. MacAllister RV, Reichenwallner CJ. US 2,912,855. Force-Deformation Measuring Apparatus. 1959.

69. Pons M, Fiszman SM. Instrumental texture profile analysis with particular reference to gelled systems. *J. Texture Studies* 1996; 27: 597–624.

70. Reier GE. Excipient standardization: User's viewpoint. *Drug Dev. Ind. Pharm.* 1987; 13: 2389–2407.

71. Shangraw RF. Compendial standards for pharmaceutical excipients. *Drug Dev. Ind. Pharm.* 1987; 13: 2421–2439.

72. Food and Drug Administration. *Pharmaceutical CGMPs for the 21st Century—A Risk-Based Approach: Final Report.* Sept. 2004.

73. Food and Drug Administration. *Guidance for Industry: Q8(R2) Pharmaceutical Development.* Nov. 2009.

74. Larner G, Schoneker D, Sheehan C, Uppoor R, Walsh P, Wiens R. PQRI survey of pharmaceutical excipient testing and control strategies. *Pharm. Technol.* 2006; 30: 84, 86, 88, 90, 92, 94, 96.

75. Ridgway K, ed. *Hard Capsules: Development and Technology.* London: Pharm. Press, 1987.

76. Fu S, Thacker A, Sperger DM, Boni RL, Velankar S, Munson EJ, Block LH. Rheological evaluation of inter-grade and inter-batch variability of sodium alginate. *AAPS PharmSciTech* 2010; 11: 1662–1674.

77. Thacker A, Fu S, Boni RL, Block LH, Inter- and intra-manufacturer variability in pharmaceutical grades and lots of xanthan gum, *AAPS PharmSciTech* 2010; 11: 1619–1626.

78. Kavanagh GM, Ross-Murphy SB. Rheological characterization of polymer gels. *Progr. Polym. Sci.* 1998; 23: 533–562.

79. Reier GE, Cohn R, Rock S, Wagenblast F. Evaluation of factors affecting the encapsulation of powders in hard gelatin capsules. I. Semi-automatic capsule machines. *J. Pharm. Sci.* 1968; 57: 660–666.

80. Armstrong NA. The instrumentation of capsule-filling machinery. Chapter 10 in Ridgeway Watt P, Armstrong A, eds. *Tablet and Capsule Instrumentation.* London: Pharmaceutical Press, 2007: 207–222.

81. Rudnic EM, Schwartz JB. Oral solid dosage forms. In Troy DB, ed. *Remington: The Science and Practice of Pharmacy.* Philadelphia: Lippincott, Williams and Wilkins, 2005: 922.

82. Heda PK, Muteba K, Augsburger LL. Comparison of the formulation requirements of dosator and dosing disc automatic capsule filling machines. *AAPS PharmSci* 2002; 4(3) article 17.

83. Lindberg N-O, Pålsson M, Pihl A-C, Freeman R, Freeman T, Zetzener H, Enstad G. Flowability measurements of pharmaceutical powder mixtures with poor flow using five different techniques. *Drug Dev. Ind. Pharm.* 2004; 30: 785–791.

84. Navaneethan CV, Missaghi S, Fassihi R. Application of powder rheometer to determine powder flow properties and lubrication efficiency of pharmaceutical particulate systems. *AAPS PharmSciTech* 2005; 6: E359–E404.

85. Søgaard SV, Allesø M, Garnaes J, Baldursdottir S, Rantanen J. Development of a reproducible powder characterization method using a powder rheometer. *Ann. Trans. Nordic Rheol. Soc.* 2012; 20: 239–245.

86. Chapter <1174> Powder Flow, USP 36.

87. Guerin E, Tchoreloff P, Leclerc B, Tanguy D, Deleuil M, Couarraze G. Rheological characterization of pharmaceutical powders using tap testing, shear cell and mercury porosimeter. *Int. J. Pharm.* 1999; 189: 91–103.

88. Khawam A. Modeling powder encapsulation in dosator-based machines: I. Theory. *Int. J. Pharm.* 2011; 421: 203–209.

89. Khawam A, Schulz L. Modeling powder encapsulation in dosator-based machines: II. Experimental evaluation. *Int. J. Pharm.* 2011; 421: 210–219.

90. Fung KY, Ng KM. Product-centered processing: Pharmaceutical tablets and capsules. *AIChE J* 2003; 49: 1193–1215.

91. Yu W, Muteki K, Zhang L, Kim G. Prediction of bulk flow performance using comprehensive particle size and particle shape distributions. *J. Pharm. Sci.* 2011; 100: 284–293.

92. Kattige A, Rowley G. The effect of poloxamer viscosity on liquid-filling of solid dispersions in hard gelatin capsules. *Drug Dev. Ind. Pharm.* 2006; 32: 981–990.

93. Kattige A, Rowley G. Influence of rheological behaviour of particulate/polymer dispersions on liquid-filling characteristics for hard gelatin capsules. *Int. J. Pharm.* 2006; 316: 74–85.

94. Cole ET, Cadé D, Benameur H. Challenges and opportunities in the encapsulation of liquid and semi-solid formulations into capsules for oral administration. *Adv. Drug Delivery Rev.* 2008; 60: 747–756.

95. Tripathi A, Whittingstall P, McKinley GH. Using filament stretching rheometry to predict strand formation and "processability" in adhesives and other non-Newtonian fluids. *Rheol. Acta* 2000; 39: 321–337.

96. Walker SE, Ganley JA, Bedford K, Eaves T. The filling of molten and thixotropic formulations into hard gelatin capsules. *J. Pharm. Pharmacol.* 1980; 32: 389–393.

97. Vijaykumar N, Reddy RA. Liquid filling in hard gelatin capsules: A review. *J. Pharm.* 2013; online at <www.jponline.in>

98. McTaggart C, Wood R, Bedford K, Walker SE. The evaluation of an automatic system for filling liquids into hard gelatin capsules. *J. Pharm. Pharmacol.* 1984; 36: 119–121.

99. Strickrodt J. Verfahren zur vollautomatischen Abfüllung von hochviskosen Pasten in Hartgelatinekapseln. *Pharm. Ind.* 1990; 52: 1276–1279.

100. Bohne L, Dürr M, Gajdos B. Neues Verfahren zur Abfüllung von halbfesten Massen in Hartgelatinekapseln. Entwicklungs- und Produktionserfahrungen. *Pharm. Ind.* 1991; 53: 1127–1134.

101. Hawley AR, Rowley G, Lough WJ, Chatham S. Physical and chemical characterization of thermo-softened bases for molten filled hard gelatin capsule formulations. *Drug Dev. Ind. Pharm.* 1992; 18: 1719–1739.

102. Metzner AB. Rheology of suspensions in polymeric liquids. *J. Rheol.* 1985; 29: 739–775.

103. Liebowitz SM, Vadino WA, Ambrosio TJ. Determination of hard gelatin capsule brittleness using a motorized compression test stand. *Drug Develop. Ind. Pharm.* 1990; 16: 995–1010.

104. Scott DC, Shah RD, Augsburger LL. A comparative evaluation of the mechanical strength of sealed and unsealed hard gelatin capsules. *Int. J. Pharm.* 1992; 84: 49–58.
105. Mei X, Etzler FM, Wang Z. Use of texture analysis to study hydrophilic solvent effects on the mechanical properties of hard gelatin capsules. *Int. J. Pharm.* 2006; 324: 128–135.
106. Peleg K, Rha C. Rheology of liquid-filled capsules made of biomaterials. *J. Rheol.* 1988; 32: 367–385.
107. Kuentz M, Röthlisberger D. Determination of the optimal amount of water in liquid-fill masses for hard gelatin capsules by means of texture analysis and experimental design. *Int. J. Pharm.* 2002; 236: 145–152.

15 Quality-by-Design (QbD) for Capsule Formulation and Process Development

Regulatory Science Relevance, Scientific Case Studies, and Future Challenges[i]

Huiquan Wu, Lin Xie, Stephen W. Hoag, Larry L. Augsburger, and Mansoor Khan

CONTENTS

---

[i] The views and opinions are those of the authors and do not necessarily represent or reflect the official position and statement of the US FDA.

REGULATORY SCIENCE RELEVANCE ON PHARMACEUTICAL DEVELOPMENT

The manufacturing of pharmaceuticals suffers from the problem of drug development in general.[1] Many drug manufacturing processes are characterized by inefficiency, waste, and a slow adoption of modern process control technologies. Thus, the pharmaceutical manufacturing sector would benefit from incorporation of new science and technology. The US Food and Drug Administration (FDA) is spearheading these changes through its Pharmaceutical Quality for the 21st Century Initiative.[2] With the introduction and implementation of several key concepts such as Process Analytical Technology (PAT)[3] and Quality by Design (QbD),[4–6] the paradigm for pharmaceutical quality regulation has been shifting from a heavy reliance on end-product testing toward a greater focus on pharmaceutical development, process control,[7] and product and process understanding.[8] The Critical Path Initiative is FDA's national strategy for transforming the way FDA-regulated medical products are developed, evaluated, and manufactured.

As outlined in the ICH Guideline Q8(R2):[2] "The aim of pharmaceutical development is to design a quality product and its manufacturing process to consistently deliver the intended performance of the product. The information and knowledge gained from pharmaceutical development studies and manufacturing experience provide scientific understanding to support the establishment of the design space, specifications, and manufacturing controls. Information from pharmaceutical development studies can be a basis for quality risk management. It is important to recognize that quality cannot be tested into products, i.e., quality should be built in by design. Changes in formulation and manufacturing processes during development and lifecycle management should be looked upon as opportunities to gain additional knowledge and further support establishment of the design space. Similarly, inclusion of relevant knowledge gained from experiments giving unexpected results can also be useful." ICHQ8(R2) elaborated possible approaches to gain a more systematic, enhanced understanding of the product and process under development. Key elements of pharmaceutical development that utilizes the QbD concept[9] were suggested to include (i) quality target product profile (QTPP); (ii) critical quality attributes (CQAs); (iii) risk assessment: linking materials attributes and process parameters to drug product CQAs; (iv) design space; (v) control strategy; and (vi) product lifecycle management, process capability, and continuous improvement. As such, the following pharmaceutical development and related information are recommended to submit in Common Technical Document format: (i) quality risk management and product and process development, (ii) design space, (iii) control strategy, and (iv) drug substance-related information.

To implement this evolving science and risk-based regulatory science framework in the pharmaceutical sector, collaborative efforts among the regulated industry, the academia, and the regulatory agencies are needed such that best medical products are available to the public. We hope the QbD principles and scientific case studies discussed below would provide some examples on how robust process and consistent quality may be achieved by applying QbD principles to capsule formulation and process development. First, the general QbD principles applied to capsule formulation and process development will be introduced. Then, several scientific case studies that illustrate how QbD principles are applied to capsule-filling process control and product quality will be provided. Finally, the current challenges and future outlook on capsule fill QbD will be discussed.

QbD PRINCIPLES APPLIED FOR CAPSULE FORMULATION AND PROCESS DEVELOPMENT

When applying QbD principles as highlighted in relevant ICH quality guidelines[4–6] and ICH Guideline on the Common Technical Document[10] to capsule formulation and process development, the following vital technical and regulatory science aspects are to be considered: (i) variability understanding and management, (ii) risk assessment, (iii) formulation design considerations, (iv) process and equipment design considerations, (v) packaging design considerations, and (vi) control strategies for capsule-filling process. For each and every aspect, there are certain recognized tools, techniques, and methodologies that can be used: (i) design of experiments (DOE) and PAT tools for variability understanding and management; (ii) risk management tools listed in the ICH Q9 Guideline, such as flowcharts, Failure Mode Effects Analysis, Failure Mode, Effects and Criticality Analysis, Fault Tree Analysis, Hazard Analysis and Critical Control Points, Hazard Operability Analysis, Preliminary Hazard Analysis, supporting statistical tools, and so on; (iii) formulation design practices to improve powder flowability and minimize capsule plug weight variation, and so on; (iv) process design and equipment design integrations to achieve consistent capsule product quality; (v) packaging design considerations to maintain the stability of the capsule products; and (vi) established control strategies for capsule-filling process to maintain the process in a state of Statistical Process Control. Most of the tools and methodologies listed above are well established and have been adopted by other industrial sectors for process control, quality assurance, and risk assessment and management for many years.[11–13] Several relatively new concepts such as PAT real-time process monitoring and control, and risk-based and integrated approaches have been introduced to the pharmaceutical community during the journey of implementing the cGMP initiative for the 21st century.

QbD CASE STUDIES FOR CAPSULE-FILLING PROCESS CONTROL AND PRODUCT QUALITY

In this section, case studies are created to illustrate the technical feasibility of applying innovative tools and methodologies to several critical formulation and process issues to achieve desired yet consistent quality attributes of the capsule products. The discussion will focus on how raw material properties (such as particle size, particle morphology, etc.), formulation compositions, and process variables (such as capsule fill machine settings, etc.) affect both intermediate product performance (e.g., segregation tendency [ST] of blends) and final capsule product quality attributes (e.g., capsule weight uniformity).

EFFECTS OF PARTICLE SIZE AND PARTICLE DENSITY ON ST

Background

For capsule filling, the raw materials properties and flow characteristics, such as particle size and particle morphology of each component and particle size differences between various powder components, have a great impact on the capsule-filling process and final capsule fill product quality. During the raw material feeding and capsule-filling process, powder segregation could take place as a result of factors such as particle size difference, which can eventually affect capsule-filling content uniformity. Segregation is a process through which a powder blend becomes nonuniform, with regions of varying composition. Any process that causes relative particle movement can introduce powder segregation if the components of the powder blend have different flow characteristics. Depending on powder flowability, segregation can occur owing to a number of reasons. For free-flowing powders, segregation can occur when set in motion by a mixer, during handling after mixing, during material transfer (e.g., discharge from a hopper), and during transport of stored blends. The primary particle properties that influence the segregation blends include particle size, density, shape, and surface texture.[14–16] Secondary factors include coefficient of friction, moisture, shape and surface of the container, and the difference in resilience of the particles. On the other hand, for cohesive powders, which do not flow well, segregation involves overcoming interparticulate bonding forces, for example, van der Waals, electrostatic, and hydrogen bonding. The primary mechanisms of segregation are percolation (sifting or void filling),[17–19] trajectory (rolling),[18,20–23] fluidization,[14,24] push-away effects,[25] angle of repose, and stratification.[26–28] Previously powder segregation and its effect had been examined quite intensively.[29–35]

Various quantitative studies on the ST of powder blends, including computer simulation, mathematical modeling, and experimental methods, have received increased attention as discussed in previous reviews.[36,37] Computer simulations were used to study the segregation of binary mixtures in a bladed mixer.[38] A simple mathematical tool was adapted for the study of the behaviors of continuous chemical reactors with classical fluid flows, to evaluate the tendency of a binary granular mixture to segregate.[39] The glass beads with different colors and sizes were used to visualize the state of segregation during gravity flow through vertical pipes.[40]

As a standard device, the ASTM D 6940 segregation tester has been used for testing the ST of a powder.[41] It uses powder flow to measure the ST of a powder blend. Bench-scale segregation tests were found to be a predictor of blend sampling bias.[42] However, very few QbD research studies[43] are available to discuss the effects of testing parameters and formulation variables on the ST of pharmaceutical powder measured by the ASTM D6940-04 segregation tester. As discussed below, a case study based on our published study[43] examines the effects of particle size and particle density on ST.

Materials and Methods

Aspirin (ASP) was received from AnMar International Ltd (Aspirin, Lot # 98626, Crystals, 20–60 mesh, USP, Metuchen, New Jersey). Coarse particles were collected from those retained on a 35-mesh (500-μm) screen and fine particles were obtained by twice milling with a Comil (Model: 197S, Quadro Engineering Inc., Waterloo, Ontario, Canada). The mill was operated at 80 rpm with a number 200 washer. The mesh used was 2A019R014/19. The temperature of the processing environment was 20°C ± 0.5°C, and the relative humidity was 40% ± 5%. The particles that could pass through a 200-mesh (75-μm) sieve were collected and considered fine ASP particles for this study.

MCC from FMC (Avicel PH200 Lot # M414C, and Avicel PH301, Lot # M445C, Mechanicsburg, Pennsylvania) was used as received. Magnesium stearate (MgS) was obtained from Spectrum (NF/USP, Lot # RH0744, New Brunswick, New Jersey).

Powder blends of 200 g were blended in the PK twin shell V-blender (4 quarts) (Patterson-Kelley Co., East Stroudsburg, Pennsylvania), and powder blends of 400 g were blended in the PK twin shell V-blender (8 quarts) (Patterson-Kelley Co.). The 200- and 400-g powder blends were mixed at a rotating speed 28 rpm for 30 min. If a lubricant was included, it was added after first mixing the drug and filler. MgS was blended for 30 min to achieve complete lubricant coverage. To minimize segregation before testing, the powder collected from the V-blender was carefully handled to minimize the free-fall distance, and the powder blends were transferred into the top hopper of the segregation tester in a manner that minimizes the power free-fall height.

Segregation Tester

The segregation tester shown in Figure 15.1 conforms to the ASTM D 6940-04 standard and was custom built for this study (Pride Machining, Upper Falls, Maryland). Minimal segregation should occur as the blend discharges the mass flow hopper. As the particles free fall into a heap in the lower hopper, various mechanisms can contribute to segregation based on the size, density, shape, and flow properties of the particles that make up the binary mixture components. Particles that are smaller, denser, and rougher in shape and have a larger angle of repose tend to stay in the center of the heap. Particles that are larger, less dense, and smoother in shape and have a smaller angle of repose tend to migrate to the base of the heap near the sides of the hopper. The blend is then discharged out of the lower hopper. Since the lower hopper is a funnel flow hopper, discharge occurs so that the mixture is separated based on the location in the lower hopper. The particles in the central core (from bottom to top) are discharged first followed by discharge (from top to bottom) of the particles located near the outer wall of the hopper. The difference between the first and the last samples, for example, the ratio of drug concentrations between the first and the last sample discharged from the tester (L/F), can be used as an indicator of segregation potential given by

$$L/F \text{ ratio} = \frac{\text{Drug concentration in the last sample}}{\text{Drug concentration in the first sample}} \quad (15.1)$$

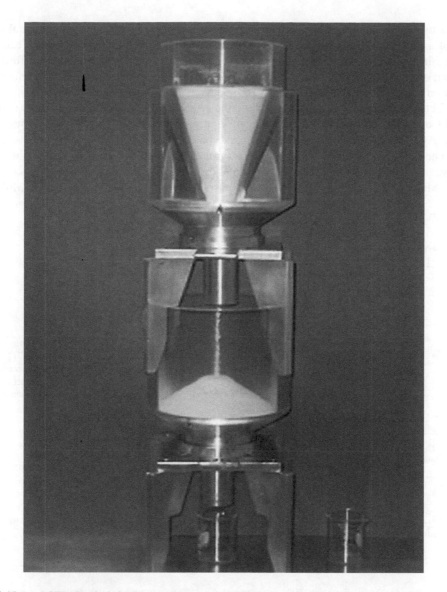

FIGURE 15.1 ASTM D 6940-04 Segregation tester (with the top slide gate open and the powder flow from the mass flow hopper down to the funnel flow hopper). Fifty-milliliter glass beakers were used as sample collector. (Reprinted from *Journal of Pharmaceutical Sciences*, 97(10), Xie L, Wu H, Shen M et al., Quality-by-Design (QbD): Effects of testing parameters and formulation variables on the segregation tendency of pharmaceutical powder measured by the ASTM D 6940-04 Segregation Test, 4485–97, Copyright 2008, with permission from Elsevier.)

The binary powder mixture can be classified into two categories: (1) minimal ST if an L/F ratio equal to or close to one is obtained, in which case the powder mixture is stable and more likely to maintain uniformity under free-flowing conditions; (2) strong ST if an L/F ratio deviates from 1 significantly, in which case the tested powder mixture is unstable and the blend is prone to segregate.

Objective, Study Design, and Testing Results

The objective of this study was to examine the effects of testing parameters and formulation variables on the ST of pharmaceutical powders measured by the ASTM D 6940-04 segregation tester using a DOE approach. To ensure our limited resources focused on the most critical areas and factors, a fishbone diagram[44,45] was created to highlight the variables that have potential to affect the ST of a binary powder system, as shown in Figure 15.2. Given that many factors can be well controlled in the laboratory setting and thus be held constant could be eliminated for further consideration; on the basis of this preliminary risk analysis result, only certain testing parameters and formulation variables were selected for the DOE study.

A 2^2 factorial design was used to determine the effects of measurement parameters (amount of material loaded [W, 200 and 400 g], number of segregation cycles [1 and 5]) with number of replicates 6. Analysis of variance (ANOVA) showed that W was a critical parameter for segregation testing. The L/F value deviated further from 1 (greater ST) with increasing W. A 2^3 full factorial design was used to assess the effects of formulation variables: grade of ASP (unmilled, milled), grade of MCC (PH200 and PH301), and amount of lubricant MgS (0% and 0.5%). Multi-linear

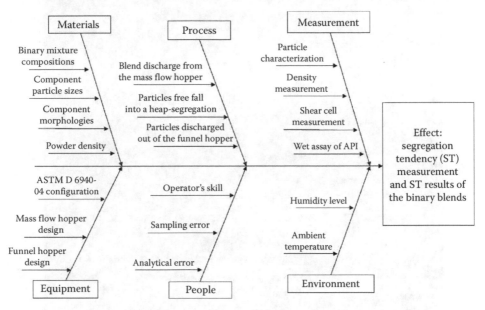

FIGURE 15.2 Fishbone diagram illustrating variables that could potentially affect the ST measurement and the ST results.

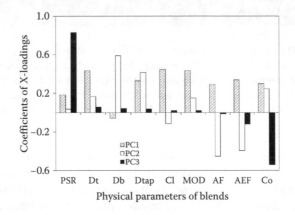

FIGURE 15.3 PCR model to link ST with physical properties for various formulations. PC1, PC2, and PC3 coefficients of X-loadings for model based on all nine physical properties. (Reprinted from *Journal of Pharmaceutical Sciences*, 97(10), Xie L, Wu H, Shen M et al., Quality-by-Design (QbD): Effects of testing parameters and formulation variables on the segregation tendency of pharmaceutical powder measured by the ASTM D 6940-04 Segregation Test, 4485–97, Copyright 2008, with permission from Elsevier.)

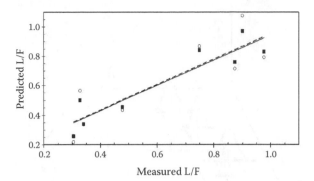

FIGURE 15.4 Predicted L/F versus measured L/F. PCR model is based on PSR and Co only. Solid line is the regression line for calibration model (■); dotted line is the regression line for leave-one-out cross-validation results (o). (Reprinted from *Journal of Pharmaceutical Sciences*, 97(10), Xie L, Wu H, Shen M et al., Quality-by-Design (QbD): Effects of testing parameters and formulation variables on the segregation tendency of pharmaceutical powder measured by the ASTM D 6940-04 Segregation Test, 4485–97, Copyright 2008, with permission from Elsevier.)

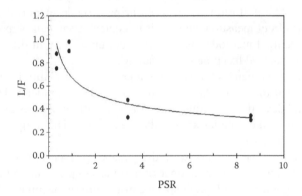

FIGURE 15.5 Dependency of ST on ASP/MCC PSR for the second DOE study. (a) L/F mean versus PSR; the curve represents the best fit using a power model. (Reprinted from *Journal of Pharmaceutical Sciences*, 97(10), Xie L, Wu H, Shen M et al., Quality-by-Design (QbD): Effects of testing parameters and formulation variables on the segregation tendency of pharmaceutical powder measured by the ASTM D 6940-04 Segregation Test, 4485–97, Copyright 2008, with permission from Elsevier.)

regression (MLR) and ANOVA showed that the grade of ASP was the main effect contributing to ST. Principal component regression (PCR) analysis established a correlation between L/F and the physical properties of the blend related to ASP and MCC, the ASP/MCC particle size ratio (PSR), and powder cohesion (Figures 15.3 and 15.4). The physical properties of the blend related to density and flow were not influenced by the grade of ASP and were not related to the ST of the blend. The direct relationship between L/F and PSR was determined by univariate analysis. ST increased as the ASP/MCC PSR increased (Figure 15.5). This study highlighted critical test parameters for segregation testing and identified critical physical properties of the blends that influence ST.

Effects of Formulation Compositions on Capsule Weight Variation

Background and Methodology of Capsule-Filling Process Characterization

Capsule weight variation is a CQA for capsule product. Typically, weight variation and content uniformity problems are caused by poor powder flow and drug segregation in the powder bed.[13,37,46]

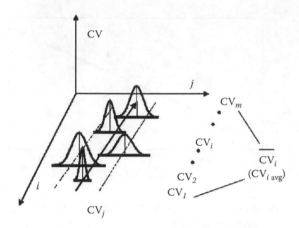

FIGURE 15.6 Scheme demonstration of the data collection and calculation profile for the different CVs.

For batch release, the United States Pharmacopeia (USP) <911> requires that the batches pass tests for weight and drug content uniformity. However, during early development stage when the supply of drug is limited, the direct measurements of drug content assay can be prohibitively expensive. In this regard, using indirect methods to assess product uniformity in the laboratory with a relatively small amount of material has practical advantage.

One of the most common metrics for assessing a product's variability is the coefficient of variation (CV), which is equal to the standard deviation divided by the mean. The CV is also termed as the relative standard deviation.[47] In this study, the CV will be used as an index to evaluate the dispersion or variability of the samples around the mean value. The sampling practice used in our study is illustrated in Figure 15.6.

As shown in Figure 15.6, the solid arrow on the ij plane represents the progression of the manufacturing process with time. A certain number of capsule samples can be taken from the process at various time points. For a relatively high-speed capsule-filling machine, 10 consecutive capsules can be taken in less than 1 min; thus, for an extended run, these samples are considered to be collected at a single specified sampling time point. The individual CV at each sampling time point, CV_i, is calculated by Equation 15.2. In addition, the mean of all the individual CV_i can be abbreviated as $CV_{i\ avg}$. To study how the capsule weight changes with the manufacturing time along the j axis in Figure 15.6, the average weight value (W_{avg}) and CV during the entire manufacturing process, CV_j, can be calculated by Equation 15.3. Furthermore, a total CV, which is the CV of all the capsules analyzed, CV_{ij}, can be calculated by Equation 15.4.

$$CV_i = \frac{(STD)_i}{(Mean)_i} = \frac{\sqrt{\dfrac{\sum_{i=1}^{n}(X_i - \bar{X}_n)^2}{n}}}{\bar{X}_n} \tag{15.2}$$

$$CV_j = \frac{(STD)_j}{(Mean)_j} = \frac{\sqrt{\dfrac{\sum_{j=1}^{m}(\bar{X}_j - \bar{X}_m)^2}{m}}}{\bar{X}_m} \tag{15.3}$$

$$CV_{ij} = \frac{(STD)_{ij}}{(Mean)_{ij}} = \frac{\sqrt{\dfrac{\displaystyle\sum_{j=1}^{m}\sum_{i=1}^{n}(\bar{X}_{ij} - \bar{X}_N)^2}{N}}}{\bar{X}_N} \tag{15.4}$$

where X is the quality parameter to be studied. $\bar{X}$ is the average of X, n is the number of capsules collected at each sampling time point at the i axis, and m is the number of sampling time points at the j axis. N is the total number of samples measured ($N = m \times n$). The j axis represents the time length of a process run. It is very important to understand the variation of the capsule product quality attributes and the contributing factors.

Previous Work on Capsule-Filling Formulation Study

The effects of various physical properties of formulation components (such as type and source of excipients, particle size and shape, lubrication, etc.) on capsule filling and solid dosage forms have been an active area for research and development. For microcrystalline cellulose (MCC),[48] it was found that a fine-grade MCC such as Avicel PH105 cannot be used in capsule filling because of unsatisfactory flow properties. Medium and coarse grades of MCC can be classified as a good capsule-filling excipient, but not all sources are suitable. The Lüdde–Kawakita constant a and Hausner's ratio are good indicators of the capsule-filling performance, in terms of interchangeability of different sources, possibility of filling above maximum bulk density, and flow problems producing large coefficients of fill weight variation. For the effect of particle shape on the mechanical properties of powders,[49] it was found that (i) for materials that consolidate by plastic deformation (e.g., Starch 1500 and NaCl), there is a large increase in compressibility, a large decrease in yield value, and a small decrease in elastic recovery in going from regular to irregular particles; and (ii) for materials that consolidate by fragmentation (e.g., lactose and Emcompress), the shape of the particles has practically no effect on the above properties. However, the irregular particles fracture to a greater extent than the regular ones as shown by the fragmentation propensity. For the effect of drug particle size on content uniformity of low-dose solid dosage form,[50] it was shown that the computer model was able to qualitatively simulate the observed potency profiles using only the particle size distribution of the drug and assuming ideal mixing. The effects of particle size and shape on the angle of internal friction and flow factor of unlubricated and lubricated powders were quite interesting.[51] For unlubricated powders, the angle of internal friction was found to depend on particle size and shape in a nonlinear manner, whereas the flow factor depended only on particle shape. For lubricated powders, both the angle of internal friction and the corresponding concentration of MgS depended only on the particle shape. A large aspect ratio as obtained for needle-shaped particles was accompanied by a particularly high angle of internal friction. In addition, the optimal MgS concentration was least for needle-shaped or round particles. While the flow factor depended only on particle shape, the corresponding optimal MgS was found to depend only on the particle size. It is important to note that the function of a lubricant in formulations for capsule filling is not limited to its effect on flowability. Lubricants (like MgS) relieve sticking of powders to tooling and other metal parts, facilitate ejection of plugs into capsules, can affect drug dissolution, and can affect plug mechanical strength. Too much MgS can adversely affect the ability to pick up and transfer plugs of uniform weight to capsules filled in dosator machines. In another independent study, the flowability of size fractions of five pharmaceutical excipients had been related to their capsule-filling performance.[52] Capsule fill weight and weight uniformity were monitored and the CV (X_{cv}) of the fill weight of 20 capsules was used as an indicator of capsule-filling performance. Flowability was dependent on the particle size, morphology, and bulk density of the powder. Significant correlation was found between the values of X_{cv} and the flow parameters of Carr's compressibility, Hausner's ratio, angle of repose, Kawakita's equation constant (a), and

Jenike's flow factor. X_{cv} was also related to the CV of the powder bed bulk density and the variation of the compression stress.

While all of the abovementioned studies helped to improve our understanding of how formulation variables affect capsule filling, unfortunately, only a univariate approach was used and is thus limited by its common drawback. A QbD approach that utilizes DOE and multivariate data analysis can offer certain advantages as described in the FDA's PAT Guidance and ICH Q8(R2). The objective of this second case study is to examine the relationships between the important powder formulation parameters and capsule weight and content uniformity via a DOE approach.

Materials and Manufacturing Process

The same materials (ASP, MCC, and MgS), API milling, and sieving process were used as described in "Materials and Methods" section. The coarse ASP particles were collected from those retained on a #35 mesh screen. The fine ASP particles were collected from those passed through a 75-µm (200-mesh) sieve. The particle size was measured by laser diffraction using a Malvern Mastersizer (Malvern Inc., Worcestershire, UK). The Malvern dry powder feeder was operated at an air pressure of 60 psi. A sample size of 1 to 1.5 g was used. The sample size reduction method was cone-and-quartering. The materials were stored at room temperature in sealed plastic bags. The powders were mixed in a twin shell V-blender (8 quarts) (Patterson-Kelley Co.) for 30 min. For lubricated formulations, lubricant was added at the end of the blending time of 30 min and blended for another 30 min.

The capsules were filled at a speed of 66 capsules per minute using either a Zanasi LZ-64 (Zanasi Nigris, Bologna, Italy) or a Harro-Hofliger KFM/3 capsule-filling machine (M.O. Industries Inc., East Hanover, New Jersey). The target capsule-filling weight was from 200 to 300 mg for size #1 and 300 to 400 mg for size #0. Powder bed height was set at 40 mm for both machines and was manually controlled through the entire filling process. The piston height for Zanasi LZ-64 was set at 15 mm and the plug height was 12 mm. The piston settings for the Harro-Hofliger KFM/3 machine were as follows: 20 mm for tapping pins set 1, 15 mm for set 2, and 12 mm for set 3; these settings were chosen to match the final plug height of the Zanasi machine plugs when PH200 was used. The piston height setting contributes to the capsule fill weight. It is expected that a different combination of piston heights will affect the final capsule plug fill weight; thus, the effect of formulation and processing variables can be studied when fixed machine settings are used for all the batches manufactured. For each sampling time point, 30 capsules were collected in 1 min. A capsule sample was collected at 5- or 10-min intervals through the entire filling process and were immediately transferred into plastic Ziploc bags and stored at ambient temperature (22°C ± 2°C, 40% ± 5% RH). The manufacturing time of one batch varied from 60 to 120 min depending on the bulk density of the formulation.

Capsule Product Weight and Content Analysis

From the 30 capsules collected at each sampling time point, 10 capsules were randomly selected and numbered 1 through 10, and weighed to the nearest milligram using analytical balance. The capsules numbered 1 to 6 were used to measure content variation; these six capsules were individually analyzed for the weight of the capsule plug (i.e., without the shell) and the amount of ASP. For the ASP assay, the capsule shells were carefully opened, avoiding any powder loss. The capsule plug was dissolved in 50 mL of 0.1 N NaOH at room temperature. To extract the drug from the suspension, the sample was degassed for 5 min and then sonicated for 30 min. The suspension was centrifuged for 15 min at 2000 rpm and was diluted with 0.1 N NaOH in a 25-mL volumetric flask. The UV absorbance of the supernatant was measured at 298 nm with 0.1 N NaOH as a blank (Spectronic Genesys 2, Thermo Electron Corporation, Rochester, New York).

The drug concentration of each capsule can be calculated using the formula below:

$$ASP\% = \frac{\text{Drug(ASP) content in a capsule (mg)} * 100}{\text{Fill weight of the capsule (mg)}} \%$$

(15.5)

Different from the drug amount per capsule, the drug concentration calculated here gives the drug amount per capsule normalized by capsule plug weight. This is needed when comparing the uniformity data of capsules with difference sizes.

Capsule-Filling Process Characterization and Effect of Formulation Composition on Capsule Fill Weight Variation via a DOE Approach

A previous study[43] indicated that the differences in a formulation's ST owing to PSR changes could be measured by the ASTM D 6940-04 segregation tester. In this work, powder systems with different segregation tendencies were selected to test the capsule-filling process. It has been reported[39,40] that powders with large PSRs and big differences in particle density and spherical particles with smooth surfaces such as glass beads produce the most segregation. For a better understanding of powder movement in the hopper during the capsule-filling process, the movement of dyed MCC particles in the powder bed was examined. First, the purple MCC was layered at the bottom of the powder bed and covered with MCC that was not dyed at the beginning of the manufacturing process. Then, a continuous capsule-filling process was started via a Zanasi-LZ 64 machine. The capsule plugs were collected from the continuous capsule-filling process and aligned per the sequence of their manufacturing order as shown in Figure 15.7, with number "1" representing the first capsule plug collected and number "262" representing the last capsule plug collected. The picture in Figure 15.7 shows clearly that the colored powder initially placed at the bottom of the powder bed quickly migrates throughout the powder bed along with the machine parts movement during the course of the capsule-filling process. It suggests that extensive mixing occurs in the hopper.

A DOE was created to measure the effects of capsule-filling formulation compositions on the capsule weight and drug content uniformity, as shown in Table 15.1. The experimental results are shown in Figures 15.8 through 15.11.

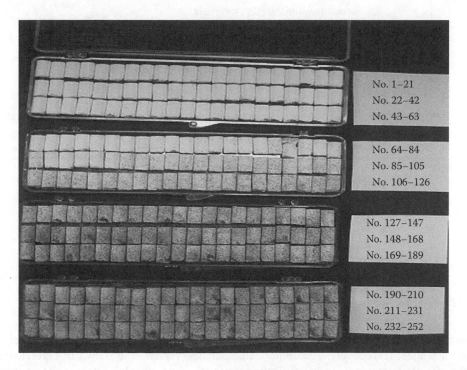

FIGURE 15.7 Capsule plugs collected and aligned according to their manufacture order (beginning from left to right and from top to bottom). Powder bed has purple MCC on the bottom and white MCC on the top. It is evident that two types of materials are mixed well at the end of the capsule-filling process.

TABLE 15.1
DOE Protocol of the Capsule-Filling Study, Filler Type: 1 = Avicel PH301, 2 = Avicel PH200, Machine Type: Zanasi LZ-64

Formulations Symbol	API Grade ASP% = 4% (D50)	Filler Grade FT(D50)	Lubricant Level LL (%)	Capsule Size CS
F1	Fine ASP (72 μm)	2 (208 μm)	0	1
F2	coarse ASP (608 μm)	2 (208 μm)	0	1
F3	Fine ASP (72 μm)	1 (72 μm)	0	1
F4	Coarse ASP (608 μm)	1 (72 μm)	0	1
F5	Fine ASP (72 μm)	2 (208 μm)	0.500	1
F6	Coarse ASP (608 μm)	2 (208 μm)	0.500	1
F7	Fine ASP (72 μm)	1 (72 μm)	0.500	1
F8	Coarse ASP (608 μm)	1 (72 μm)	0.500	1
F9	Fine ASP (72 μm)	2 (208 μm)	0	0
F10	Coarse ASP (608 μm)	2 (208 μm)	0	0
F11	Fine ASP (72 μm)	1 (72 μm)	0	0
F12	Coarse ASP (608 μm)	1 (72 μm)	0	0
F13	Fine ASP (72 μm)	2 (208 μm)	0.500	0
F14	Coarse ASP (608 μm)	2 (208 μm)	0.500	0
F15	Fine ASP (72 μm)	1 (72 μm)	0.500	0
F16	Coarse ASP (608 μm)	1 (72 μm)	0.500	0

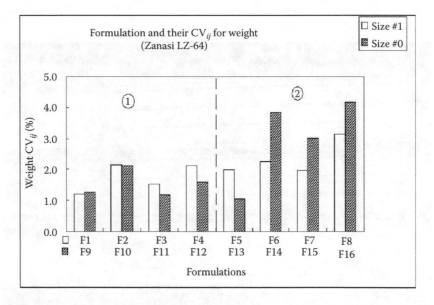

FIGURE 15.8 The plot of the weight CV_{ij} versus formulations (region 1: unlubricated batches, region 2, lubricated batches).

Figures 15.8 and 15.9 show the effects of capsule size and lubrication on capsule weight and content variations, respectively. For unlubricated batches (region 1 as shown in Figures 15.8 and 15.9), the effects of capsule size on capsule weight variation and capsule content variation seemingly follow similar trends: capsule size #0 exhibits either comparable or a slightly smaller capsule weight variation than capsule size #1; in addition, capsule size #0 always exhibits smaller capsule content

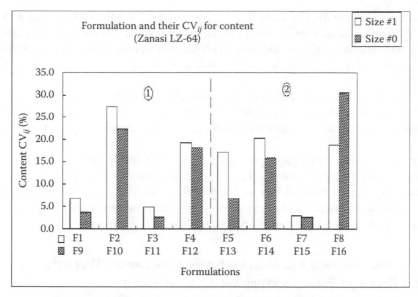

FIGURE 15.9 The plot of the content CV_{ij} versus formulations (region 1: unlubricated batches, region 2, lubricated batches).

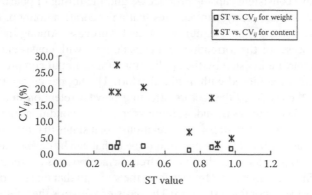

FIGURE 15.10 The plot of weight CV_{ij} and content CV_{ij} versus ST on a Zanasi LZ-64 machine.

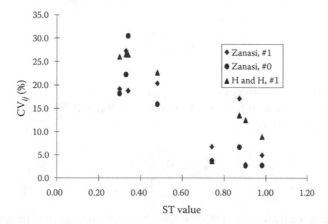

FIGURE 15.11 The relationship between the ST value and the content variation demonstrated on different equipment with size 1 or 0 capsules.

variation than capsule size #1. For lubricated batches (region 2 as shown in Figures 15.8 and 15.9), the effects of capsule size on capsule weight variation and capsule content variation seemingly follow opposite trends: capsule size #0 exhibits larger capsule weight variations in most cases; on the other hand, capsule size #0 exhibits smaller capsule content variations in most cases than capsule size #1.

Figures 15.10 and 15.11 show that (i) the ST parameter measured in this study has a strong correlation to the final product content variation. As expected, the content variation decreases as the ST decreases; (ii) there is no obvious correlation between the capsule weight variation and the ST parameter.

These experimental findings might be useful for evaluating the physical behavior of a blend during early formulation development. The ST value measured might help to predict the capsule content uniformity. On the basis of selecting appropriate material grade and checking the ST, the likelihood of producing batches that are prone to segregation can be reduced largely. Thus, it helps to move toward QbD from a formulation and materials science perspective.

EFFECTS OF PROCESS VARIABLES AND MACHINE SETTINGS ON CAPSULE WEIGHT VARIATION: A REVIEW OF PREVIOUS WORK AND CURRENT STATUS

How process variables and machine settings affect capsule weight variation has been a main area of research and development for the capsule-filling process. Taking the dosator nozzle system as one example, to achieve consistent capsule product weight, the filling of pharmaceutical hard gelatin capsules by the dosator nozzle system requires that an accurate amount of powder is picked up and retained within the cylinder nozzle, during a transfer process. Among those steps involved in the capsule-filling process for the formation of a capsule plug with consistent weight, retention is a critical step, which may be assisted by the application of a minimal compressive stress such that subsequent ejection can be achieved with minimal effort. The hopper design theories proposed by Walker[53] and Walters[54] considered the factors affecting powder retention in a tall cylinder (e.g., a capsule-filling nozzle). The theories include solutions for arching conditions in tall cylinders and are based on two main concepts: (i) the stress–span relationship; it states that the maximum span across which arching can occur is limited by the maximum shear that can be developed at the walls, to support the powder; and (ii) powder beds that have a free surface possess a strength that is the unconfined yield strength. Since an arch has a free surface, the strength that must be present in the powder for arching to occur is the unconfined strength. The basis of Walker's theory for arching conditions is the combination of the concepts of the stress–span relationship and the powder strength required at a free surface. The strength required in a powder bed for arching to occur was derived as

$$f_c = \frac{r\gamma g}{\sin 2\phi},\tag{15.6}$$

where f_c is the unconfined yield strength, r is the span radius, γ is the bulk density, g is gravity acceleration, and ϕ is the angle of wall friction. A critical flow factor (FF$_c$) above which arching would not occur could be calculated as

$$FF_c = \frac{\bar{\sigma}_z \sin 2\phi}{r\gamma g},\tag{15.7}$$

where $\bar{\sigma}_z$ is the mean vertical compressive stress. For arching to occur, the material must have a flow factor equal to or less than the critical flow factor, that is, a minimally stable arch has an FF equal to FF$_c$.

These theoretical foundations were applied to the powder retention by a dosator nozzle. It was concluded[55] that (i) the angle of wall friction is important in determining the stress distribution of a powder bed in the nozzle, especially in the vicinity of the wall; (ii) the angle of friction has an optimal value for which the compressive force required to cause stable arch formation is a minimum. Therefore, the efficiency of this type of capsule-filling system could be improved by considering the angle of wall friction, which depends on the properties of the nozzle wall surface and of the powder. The theory and equations proposed by Walker[53] and Jolliffe et al.[55] were applied[56] to predict the minimum stress requirement for arching and powder retention within a capsule dosator nozzle during the filling of different size fractions of five pharmaceutical excipients. It was found that (i) higher compressive stress requirement for arching, $\sigma_{z\,req}$ at the arching zone also required the application of a greater compressive stress, $\sigma_{z,\,o\,req}$ at the top of the powder bed; (ii) the magnitude of these stresses was particle size and material dependent; and (iii) these stresses are not the main controlling feature of capsule-filling performance, although the magnitude of f_c and $\sigma_{z\,req}$ may influence capsule fill weight uniformity to some extent.

In addition, the influence of the compression setting ratio on the capsule fill weight variability has been assessed for a series of particle size fractions of Avicel, calcium carbonate, lactose, maize starch, and Starch 1500, on a capsule-filling simulator.[57] It was found that for most of the systems tested, the most uniform weights were achieved when no compression was applied to the powder during the filling process. The finest particle size fractions of lactose and maize starch do however require some compression to aid powder retention. For the largest particle size fractions, providing high compression settings could induce the piston to jam in the nozzle, resulting in failure to fill a capsule at all. The degree of coating of the wall of the nozzle increased with decreasing particle size and increasing compression setting. Furthermore, the Tan and Netwon[58] found that the values of the observed plug density (γ_{po}) were particle size and material dependent. Deviations in the values of γ_{po} from the expected plug density (γ_{pe}) were attributed to differences between the observed and expected fill weights. Large deviations in the values of γ_{po} from γ_{pe} were generally observed with fine powders and higher compression settings. Although the findings[56–58] were based on experimental studies of limited powder systems and definitely needs further validation if applying for new powder systems, the findings could provide certain insights for optimization of both the compression settings and formulation system to achieve optimal capsule-filling performance.

For the investigation of various factors affecting encapsulation on the In-Cap automatic capsule-filling machine,[59] the fill weight and weight variation were found to depend on the flow property of the material. In addition, appropriate selection of pin settings and bed height can reduce the weight variability seen, especially with poorly flowing high-dose formulations. A recent work[60] nicely demonstrated a better understanding of how changes in powder flow of binary blends can lead to weight variability in pharmaceutical capsule filling. Percolation theory was considered to explain abrupt changes in the observed flow properties. Capsule weight variability displayed a threshold behavior as a function of the mixture fraction and correlated with the angle of internal friction as well as with the angle and energy of avalanches. The effect of the speed of capsule filling and the inherent machine vibrations on fill weight for a dosator nozzle machine was reported recently.[61] It revealed a correlation between powder densification under more intense vibrations and larger fill weights. Therefore, evaluating the effect of environmental vibrations on material attributes constitutes an important aspect for powder-based product QbD.

CURRENT CHALLENGES AND FUTURE OUTLOOK

Based on ICH Q8(R2), a QTPP for a hypothetical capsule drug product is provided in Table 15.2. The CQAs were established during the development, based on their potential impact to the performance and manufacturability of the drug product. The CQAs of the drug product include appearance, assay, degradation products, dissolution, content uniformity, microbiological limits, and stability. The CQAs of the API include impurities (organic and inorganic impurities, residual

TABLE 15.2
QTPP for a Hypothetical Capsule Drug Product

Critical Quality Attribute	Acceptance Criterion
Description	Size 1 capsule
Identification	Positive identity for the drug (e.g., by spectroscopic method)
Assay	95.0–105.0% of label claim
Degradation product	Total degradation products ≤2.0%
	Unspecified degradation product ≤0.2% at end of shelf life (meet ICH Q3B acceptance criteria)
Dissolution	Immediate release, $Q = 80\%$ in 45 min
	Meet acceptance criteria
Content uniformity	Meet compendial acceptance criteria for content uniformity
Microbiological limits	Meet compendial acceptance criteria
Stability	Stable throughout the proposed shelf life
	Meet acceptance criteria

solvents, water, and metals), polymorph, and particle size. Given the potential impact on the manufacturability or performance of the drug product, two key physicochemical characteristics of API including polymorph and particle size deserve special attention for monitoring and control: (i) if the drug substance involves polymorphism, typically the thermodynamically most stable polymorph is selected and controlled during the manufacturing process and is confirmed by identity testing at API release. In addition, the drug product primary stability and validation batches are monitored on stability for identity of polymorph; and (ii) particle size has the potential to affect drug product dissolution. However, API particle size distribution, bulk density, and surface area have the potential to affect drug product dissolution and each could be inter-correlated. Thus, it might be possible to predict and control the impact of API physical properties on drug product dissolution by controlling one of the three API physical properties.

It is important to recognize that some of the earlier work on intelligent hybrid systems for hard gelatin capsule formulation development[62–64] and dissolution performance analysis[65,66] of hard gelatin capsules of BCS II model drugs has laid the groundwork for some of the current QbD approaches to capsules. Although hard gelatin capsules were perceived to be a simple dosage form, the design of formulations for capsule can present significant challenges. A research group had created a prototype hybrid system[62,63] by linking a decision module (expert system) with a prediction module (artificial neural networks) capable of yielding formulations of a model BCS Class II drug (piroxicam) that meet specific drug dissolution criteria. This prototype expert network of a single drug was successfully expanded for use in the analysis of multiple BCS Class II drugs,[64] including carbamazepine, chlorpropamide, diazepam, ibuprofen, ketoprofen, naproxen, and piroxicam. The expanded hybrid network was generally able to predict the amount of drug dissolved within 5% of the model drugs. In addition, through validation, the system was proven to be capable of designing formulations that met specific drug performance criteria. Furthermore, by including parameters to address wettability and intrinsic dissolution characteristics of drugs, the hybrid system was shown to be suitable for analysis of multiple BCS class II drugs. As part of research that supports SUPAC-IR,[67] an FDA guidance that provided relaxed testing and filling requirements for scale-up and post-approval changes to immediate-release oral dosage forms, the impact of formulation and process changes on *in vitro* dissolution and the bioequivalence of piroxicam capsules was evaluated.[65] A 2^{5-1} + start point (resolution V) experimental design was used to investigate the effects of piroxicam particle size, excipient levels, and lubricant blending time on capsule dissolution. The in vitro study identified the main formulation factors and their interactions that influenced piroxicam dissolution. The in vivo study examined the effect of formulation changes on bioavailability via a randomized, single-dose, crossover design. It was concluded that the major changes incorporated into these formulations did not result in major differences in bioavailability. Additionally, the dissolution profiles that discriminated between the formulations in vitro did not accurately represent the in vitro bioavailability results. For evaluation of dissolution performance of BCS Class II model drugs,[66] it was found that the Box–Behnken experimental design was useful in assessing primary and secondary excipient effects on dissolution, The Bayesian network developed for the data set mirrored the key excipient effects on dissolution performance.

Novel technologies[68,69] are available for real-time monitoring and control of polymorph[70] and particle size[71] during the development, manufacturing, and storage of solid dosage form. From a scientific point of view, applying PAT tools to the manufacturing, storage, and even dissolution characterization of a pharmaceutical product may provide insights to what has been happening during those different processes.[72] It is anticipated that the application of the emerging technologies to the capsule fill process and capsule drug substance/drug product would provide tremendous opportunities to advance the control strategies of this type of dosage form manufacturing.[73–75]

After the development studies, a final quality risk assessment (QRA) is conducted as per ICH Q9 guideline. This objective of the QRA exercise was to identify the formulation component and unit operations that have the highest impact (greatest risk areas) on the quality attributes such that further studies, if necessary, may be conducted. For example, if the development studies concluded that API physical properties, particularly API particle size distribution, are critical to drug product quality (i.e., dissolution), then control of the API milling process variables and establishment of API particle size specification are used to mitigate its potential risk to the drug product quality.

In addition to the product and process engineering approach previously discussed, statistical sampling is another essential aspect to be addressed to ensure product quality consistency and capsule fill process robustness. Although a detailed discussion is out of the scope of this chapter, several critical aspects of statistical sampling are worthy to mention briefly, such as representativeness, randomness, and scale of scrutiny. For processes involving particulate matter where segregation is a concern, scale of scrutiny is especially important for developing PAT real-time process monitoring and control strategy. For traditional processes where end-product testing is heavily relied for QA, representativeness, randomness, and sample size are critical for developing QA strategy and release specifications.

Pharmaceutical drug product development focuses mainly on the therapeutic effect of new molecular entities by measuring the impact on the clinical parameter and biomarkers of a disease. The recent ICH Q8(R2) guideline[4] states that, "In all cases, the product should be designed to meet patients' needs and the intended product performance. The approach to, and extend of, development can also vary." Therefore, it is important to understand the different patient populations and patients' capabilities, perceptions, and behaviors within their diseases, as well as their therapeutic schedule. Over the past decade, many capsule manufacturing technologies have become available to meet the needs of various process scales across the pipeline, from preclinical, R&D, clinical, pilot-scale, to large-scale production. A recent list of suppliers of two-piece capsule fillers and softgel encapsulation equipment can be found elsewhere.[76]

Much work has been done to study encapsulation, including machine instrumentation, compression analysis, formulation requirements, powder densification predictions, and modeling. More knowledge is needed to further reduce empiricism in unit operation, formulation, and process development. Scarcity of the API especially at the early development stage limits encapsulation experiments. Encapsulation process modeling[77,78] provides a material-sparing approach to estimate encapsulation fill weights in accordance to the QbD principles. The encapsulation process model was evaluated experimentally. The results indicated that the model is a potentially useful in silico analysis tool that can be used for capsule dosage form development in accordance to the QbD principles. Given the various primary concerns at different levels (particle, powder, and dosage form), a recent paper[79] illustrated that understanding the properties and behaviors at each scale constitutes key elements in developing a multiscale process understanding of a pharmaceutical process. It pointed out that using informatics to manage data from advanced analytics across multiple scales is a key aspect in leveraging engineering and science to improve pharmaceutical quality while bringing down the cost of product development and manufacturing.

In summary, much experimental work on capsule-filling formulation and process development has been done, which laid out a good foundation and starting point for the QbD development. The capsule-filling formulation and process development and manufacturing presents unprecedented yet unique opportunities for QbD research, development, and implementation in the pharmaceutical community. To the best of our knowledge, to realize the full benefits of QbD, much collaborative efforts are needed in certain vital aspects, such as adapting system-based design concept,[62–64] developing process monitoring and control strategy,[6,7,68,72] and moving toward predictive manufacturing.[77–79]

ACKNOWLEDGMENT

This work was financially supported by the FDA Center for Drug Evaluation and Research (CDER) Regulatory Science and Review (RSR) Grant RSR-04-16. The statistical support from Dr. Meiyu Shen at DBVI/OB/OTS/CDER/FDA is acknowledged.

REFERENCES

1. Woodcock J, Woosley R, The FDA Critical Path Initiative and Its Influence on New Drug Development. *Annu. Rev. Med.* 2008; 59: 1–12.
2. FDA, 2004. *Pharmaceutical CGMPs for the 21st Century—A Risk-Based Approach. Final Report.* Available at: http://www.fda.gov/downloads/Drugs/DevelopmentApprovalProcess/Manufacturing/Questions andAnswersonCurrentGoodManufacturingPracticescGMPforDrugs/UCM176374.pdf (accessed on 08/30/2014).
3. FDA, 2004. *Guidance for Industry. PAT—A Framework for Innovative Pharmaceutical Development, Manufacturing, and Quality Assurance.* Available at: http://www.fda.gov/cder/guidance/6419fnl.pdf (accessed on 08/30/2014).
4. FDA/ICH, 2009. *Guidance for Industry, Q8(R2) Pharmaceutical Development.* Draft available at: http://www.fda.gov/downloads/Drugs/GuidanceComplianceRegulatoryInformation/Guidances/ucm073507.pdf (accessed on 08/30/2014).
5. FDA/ICH, 2006. *Guidance for Industry. Q9 Quality Risk Management.* Available at: http://www.fda.gov/cder/guidance/7153fnl.pdf (accessed on 08/30/2014).
6. FDA/ICH, 2009. *Guidance for Industry. Q10 Pharmaceutical Quality System.* Available at: http://www.fda.gov/downloads/Drugs/GuidanceComplianceRegulatoryInformation/Guidances/UCM073517.pdf (access on 09/06/2014).
7. Wu H, Hussain AS, and Khan MA, Process control perspective for process analytical technology: Integration of chemical engineering practice into semiconductor and pharmaceutical industries. *Chem. Eng. Commun.* 2007; 194: 760–779.
8. Yu LX, Pharmaceutical quality by design: Product and process development, understanding, and control. *Pharm. Res.* 2008; 25(4): 781–791.
9. Yu LX, Amidon G, Khan MA et al., Understanding pharmaceutical quality by design. *AAPS J.* 2014; 16(4): 771–783.
10. ICH, 2002. *The Common Technical Document for the Registration of Pharmaceuticals for Human Use: Quality-M4Q(R1). Quality Overall Summary of Module 2 Module 3: Quality.* Available at: http://www.ich.org/fileadmin/Public_Web_Site/ICH_Products/CTD/M4_R1_Quality/M4Q__R1_.pdf (accessed on 09/08/2014).
11. Montgomery DC, *Introduction to Statistical Quality Control* 4th ed. 2000; John Wiley & Sons, Hoboken, NJ.
12. Taguchi G, Chowdhury S, Taguchi S, *Robust Engineering* 2000; McGraw-Hill, New York.
13. Youngberg BJ, *Principles of Risk Management and Patient Safety.* 2011; Jones & Bartlett Learning, Sudbury, MA.
14. Chowan ZT, Segregation of particulate solids, part I. *Pharm. Technol.* 1995; 19(5): 56–70.

15. Williams JC, Continuous mixing of solids—A review. *Powder Technol.* 1976; 15: 237–243.
16. Lim HP, Hoag SW, Particle size and shape. In *Pharmaceutical Dosage Forms: Tablets* Volume I, 3rd ed., 2008. Stephen W. Hoag and Larry L. Augsburger, Editors; Informa Healthcare, New York.
17. Savage SB, Lun CKK, Particle size segregation in inclined chute flow of dry cohesionless granular solids. *J. Fluid Mech.* 1988; 189: 311–335.
18. Samadani A, Pradhan A, Kudrolli A, Size segregation of granular matter in silo discharges. *Phys. Rev.* 1999; E 60: 7203–7209.
19. Dolgunin VN, Kudy AN, Ukolov AA, Development of the model of segregation of particles undergoing granular flow down an inclined chute. *Powder Technol.* 1998; 96: 211–218.
20. Dolgunin VN, Ukolov AA, Segregation modeling of rapid powder gravity flow. *Powder Technol.* 1995; 83: 95–103.
21. Khahar DV, McCarthy JJ, Ottino JM, Mixing and segregation of granular materials in chute flows. *Chaos* 1999; 9: 594–610.
22. Drahun JA, Bridgwater J, The mechanisms of free surface segregation. *Powder Technol.* 1983; 36: 39–53.
23. Olivieri G, Marzocchella A, and Salatino P, Segregation of fluidized binary mixtures of granular solids. *AIChE J.* 2004; 50: 3095–3106.
24. Salter GF, Farnish RJ, Bradley MSA et al., Segregation of binary mixtures of particles during the filling of a two-dimensional representation of a hopper. *Proc. IMechE* 2000; Part E 214: 197–208.
25. Makse HA, Havlin S, King PR et al., Spontaneous stratification in granular mixtures. *Nature* 1997; 386: 379–382.
26. Cizeau P, Makse HA, Stanley HE, Mechanisms of granular spontaneous stratification and segregation in two-dimensional silos. *Phys. Rev.* 1999; E 59: 4408–4420.
27. Makse HA, Stratification instability in granular flows. *Phys. Rev.* 1997; E 56: 7008–7016.
28. Duffy SP, Puri VM, Primary segregation shear cell for size-segregation analysis of binary mixtures. *KONA* 2002; 20: 196–207.
29. Staniforth JN, Rees JE, Kayes JB, Relation between mixing time and segregation of ordered mixes. *J. Pharm. Pharmacol.* 1981; 33: 175–176.
30. Staniforth JN, Rees JE, Segregation of vibrated powder mixes containing different concentrations of fine potassium chloride and tablet excipients. *J. Pharm. Pharmacol.* 1983; 35: 549–554.
31. Carson JW, Royal TA, Goodwill DJ, Understanding and eliminating particle segregation problems. *Bulk Solids Handling* 1986; 6: 139–144.
32. Johanson JR, Predicting segregation of bimodal particle mixtures using the flow properties of bulk solids. *Pharm. Technol.* 1996; 20: 46–57.
33. Wong LW and Pilpel N, Effect of particle shape on the mixing of powders. *J. Pharm. Pharmacol.* 1990; 42: 1–6.
34. Alexander A, Roddy M, Brone D et al., A method to quantitatively describe powder segregation during discharge from vessels. *Powder Technol. YEARBOOK 2000*, 2000; 6–21.
35. Venables HJ, Wells JI, Powder mixing. *Drug Dev. Ind. Pharm.* 2001; 27: 599–612.
36. Swaminathan V, Kildsig DO, Polydisperse powder mixtures: Effect of particle size and shape on mixture stability. *Drug Dev. Ind. Pharm.* 2002; 28, 41–48.
37. Williams JC, The segregation of particulate materials. A review. *Powder Technol.* 1976; 15: 245–251.
38. Chowan ZT, Segregation of particulate solids, part II. *Pharm. Technol.* 1995; 19(6): 80–94.
39. Zhou Y, Yu A, Bridgwater J, Segregation of binary mixture of particles in a bladed mixer. *J. Chem. Technol. Biotechnol.* 2003; 78: 187–193.
40. Abatzoglou N, Simard JS, Prediction of segregation tendency occurrence in dry particulate pharmaceutical mixtures: Development of a mathematical tool adapted for granular systems application. *Pharm. Dev. Technol.* 2005; 10: 59–70.
41. Liss ED, Conway SL, Zega JA et al., Segregation of powders during gravity flow through vertical pipes. *Pharm. Technol.* 2004; 79–94.
42. ASTM International, *D6940-04 Standard Practice for Measuring Shifting Segregation Tendencies of Bulk Solids*. ASTM International, West Conshohocken, PA, 2004.
43. Prescott JK, Ramsey PJ, Bench scale segregation tests as a predictor of blend sampling bias. *AAPS Pharm. Sci.* 2000; 2(2), Abstract 235(2000). Available at: http://www.aapspharmaceutica.com/search /abstract_view.asp?id=2065&ct=00Abstracts.
44. Xie L, Wu H, Shen M et al., Quality-by-Design (QbD): Effects of testing parameters and formulation variables on the segregation tendency of pharmaceutical powder measured by the ASTM D 6940-04 Segregation Test. *J. Pharm. Sci.* 2008; 97(10): 4485–4497.

45. Wu H, White M, Khan M, Quality-by-Design (QbD): An integrated process analytical technology (PAT) approach for a dynamic pharmaceutical co-precipitation process characterization and process design space development. *Int. J. Pharm.* 2011; 405: 63–78.

46. Wu H, White M, Khan M, An integrated process analytical technology (PAT) approach for process dynamics-related measurement error evaluation and process design space development of a pharmaceutical powder blending bed. *Org. Process Res. Dev.* 2015; 19(1): 215–226.

47. Hoag SW, Augsburger LL, *Pharmaceutical Dosage Forms: Tablets.* 3rd ed., 2008; Informa Healthcare, New York.

48. Patel R, Podczeck F, Investigation of the effect of type and source of microcrystalline cellulose on capsule filling. *Int. J. Pharm.* 1996; 128: 123–127.

49. Wong LW, Pilpel N, The effect of particle shape on the mechanical properties of powders. *Int. J. Pharm.* 1990; 59: 145–154.

50. Zhang Y, Johnson KC, The effect of drug particle size on content uniformity of low-dose solid dosage form. *Int. J. Pharm.* 1997; 154: 179–183.

51. Podczeck F, Miah Y, The effect of particle size and shape on the angle of internal friction and flow factor of unlubricated and lubricated powders. *Int. J. Pharm.* 1996; 144: 187–194.

52. Tan SB, Newton JM, Powder flowability as an indication of capsule filling performance. *Int. J. Pharm.* 1990; 61: 145–155.

53. Walker DM, An approximate theory for pressures and arching in hoppers. *Chem. Eng. Sci.* 1966; 21: 975–997.

54. Walters JK, A theoretical analysis of stresses in axially-symmetric hoppers and bunkers. *Chem. Eng. Sci.* 1973; 28: 779–789.

55. Jolliffe IG, Newton JM, Theoretical considerations of the filling of pharmaceutical hard gelatin capsules. *Powder Technol.* 1980; 27: 189–195.

56. Tan SB, Newton JM, Minimum compression stress requirements for arching and powder retention within a dosator nozzle during capsule filling. *Int. J. Pharm.* 1990; 63: 275–280.

57. Tan SB, Newton JM, Influence of compression setting ratio on capsule fill weight and weight variability. *Int. J. Pharm.* 1990; 66: 273–282.

58. Tan SB, Newton JM, Observed and expected powder plug densities obtained by a capsule dosator nozzle system. *Int. J. Pharm.* 1990; 66: 283–288.

59. Nair R, Vemuri M, Agrawala P et al., Investigation of various factors affecting encapsulation on the In-Cap automatic capsule-filling machine. *AAPS PharmSciTech* 2004; 5(4): Article 57.

60. Nalluri VR, Puchkov M, Kuentz M, Toward better understanding of powder avalanching and shear cell parameters of drug–excipient blends to design minimal weight variability into pharmaceutical capsules. *Int. J. Pharm.* 2013; 442: 49–56.

61. Llusa M, Faulhammer E, Biserni S et al., The effect of capsule-filling machine vibrations on average fill weight. *Int. J. Pharm.* 2013; 454: 381–387.

62. Guo M, Kalra G, Augsburger LL et al., A prototype intelligent hybrid system for hard gelatin capsule formulation development. *Pharm. Technol.* 2002; 26(9): 44–60.

63. Kalra G, Peng Y, Guo M et al., *A Hybrid Intelligent System for Formulation of BCS Class II Drugs in Hard Gelatin Capsules.* Neural Information Processing, *ICONIP '02.* Singapore Proceedings of 9th International Conf. on Neural Information Processing 2002; 4: 1987–1991.

64. Wilson W I, Peng Y, Augsburger LL, Generalization of a prototype intelligent hybrid system for hard gelatin capsule formulation development. *AAPS PharmSciTech* 2005; 6(3): E449–E457.

65. Piscitelli DA, Bigora S, Propst C et al., The impact of formulation and process changes on in vitro dissolution and bioequivalence of piroxicam capsules. *Pharm. Dev. Tech.* 1998; 3(4): 443–452.

66. Wilson W, Peng Y, Augsburger LL, Comparison of statistical analysis and Bayesian networks in the evaluation of dissolution performance of BCS Class II model drugs. *J. Pharm. Sci.* 2005; 94: 2764–2776.

67. FDA, 1995. *Guidance for Industry. Immediate Release Solid Dosage Forms. Scale-up and Postapproval Changes: Chemistry, Manufacturing, and Controls, In Vitro Dissolution Testing, and In Vivo Bioequivalence Documentation.* Available at: http://www.fda.gov/downloads/Drugs/Guidances/UCM070636.pdf (accessed on 09/15/2014).

68. Wu H, Khan M, THz spectroscopy: An emerging technology for pharmaceutical development and pharmaceutical process analytical technology (PAT) applications. *J. Mol. Struct.* 2012; 1020: 112–120.

69. Wu H, White M, Khan M, Quality-by-Design (QbD): An integrated process analytical technology (PAT) approach for a dynamic pharmaceutical co-precipitation process characterization and process design space development. *Int. J. Pharm.* 2011; 405: 63–78.

70. Lee AY, Erdemir D, Myerson AS, Crystal polymorphism in chemical process development. *Annu. Rev. Chem. Biomol. Eng.* 2011; 2: 259–280.

71. Lionberger RA, Lee SL, Lee L et al., Quality by design: Concepts for ANDAs. *AAPS J.* 2008; 10(2): 268–276.

72. Wu H, Dong Z, Li H et al., An integrated process analytical technology (PAT) approach for pharmaceutical crystallization process understanding to ensure product quality and safety: FDA scientist's perspective. *Org. Process Res. Dev.* 2015; 19(1): 89–101.

73. FDA, 2011. *Advancing Regulatory Science at FDA: A Strategic Plan.* August 2011. Available at: http://www.fda.gov/downloads/ScienceResearch/SpecialTopics/RegulatoryScience/UCM268225.pdf (accessed on 07/15/2014).

74. FDA, 2011. *Guidance for Industry, Process Validation: General Principles and Practices.* Available at: http://www.fda.gov/downloads/Drugs/GuidanceComplianceRegulatoryInformation/Guidances/UCM070336.pdf (accessed on 07/15/2014).

75. FDA/ICH, 2012. *Guidance for Industry. Q11 Development and Manufacture of Drug Substances.* Available at: http://www.fda.gov/downloads/Drugs/GuidanceComplianceRegulatoryInformation/Guidances/UCM261078.pdf (accessed on 07/15/2014).

76. Suppliers of two-piece capsule fillers and softgel encapsulation equipment. *Tablets & Capsules. Supplement to Tablets & Capsules.* May 2014: 8–12.

77. Khawam A, Modeling powder encapsulation in dosator-based machines: I. Theory. *Int. J. Pharm.* 2011; 421: 203–209.

78. Khawam A, Schultz L, Modeling powder encapsulation in dosator-based machines: II. Experimental evaluation. *Int. J. Pharm.* 2011; 421: 210–219.

79. Hamad M, Bowman K, Smith N et al., Multi-scale pharmaceutical process understanding: From particle to powder to dosage form. *Chem. Eng. Sci.* 2010; 65: 5625–5638.

Index